Clinical Measurement of Speech and Voice

Clinical Measurement of Speech and Voice

R. J. Baken, Ph.D.

Professor of Speech Science
Teachers College
Columbia University
New York, New York

ALLYN AND BACON
Boston London Toronto Sydney Tokyo Singapore

Library of Congress Cataloging in Publication Data
Main entry under title:

Baken, R. J. (Ronald J.), 1943-
    Clinical measurement of speech and voice.
    Includes index.   1. Speech, Disorders of—Diagnosis. 2. Speech—
Measurement. 3. Voice—Measurement. I. Title.
[DNLM: 1. Speech Production Measurement. WV 501 B167c]
RC423.B28   1987   616.85'5075   86-9725

Dr. Joan Wald Baken
uxori meae hoc libellum
D.D.D.
a.d. iiii Kal Iul MCMLXXXVI

Centum sunt causae cur ego semper amem.

—*OVID*

Contents

Preface

Several years ago, a group of doctoral candidates in speech pathology urged Dr. Carol Wilder and me to organize and lead a seminar that would provide a formal framework for consideration of the state of the art of speech and voice diagnosis. As a group, we were strongly committed to clinical practice as well as to research in diagnostic and therapeutic methods. We also shared an interest in various facets of speech science. It seemed like an interesting and potentially useful undertaking, and so we met each week for a semester. We argued philosophies, debated view points, proposed paradigms. But mostly we dug into the literature to see whether it could be mined for nuggets of methodology—founded on viable theory and validated by adequate research—that could be refined and cast into a cohesive whole of diagnostic and therapeutic procedure, at least in some small corner of the vast realm of communicative disorders.

As so often happens in academe, we had hardly begun when the semester ended. But we had found a lot of very useful material. And we reached a consensus that, indeed, the resources were there to sharpen diagnoses and perhaps greatly improve therapy. Our discussions uncovered plausible reasons why so much of what was in the literature should have achieved so little application.

Rather than let the issues die, I volunteered to write a brief report of our findings and conclusions. I did, but the resulting document clearly was not good enough or long enough to do the subject any real justice. So I began drafting a more complete version, that grew and developed a life of its own and became this book. It is, in some very real ways, a belated report to my erstwhile students—now my colleagues—on our seminar.

Although this book deals with a considerable array of instrumentation, it is different from the few "speech instrumentation" texts that have appeared so far. One of my primary goals has been to cull, from the literature of speech pathology and related fields, assessment methods that can be said to be "objective" and valid. Another major goal was to summarize methods that offer relatively precise measurement of physiologic events during speech or of characteristics of the speech signal itself. The objective was to consider methods and techniques that are consistent with our present understanding of speech processes on the one hand and with acceptable engineering principles on the other. The prime emphasis has been on techniques that are applicable in the context of speech rehabilitation settings. Occasionally, more complex or more invasive methods have been included, either because they are common tools of researchers or because, in instances of real need, they may be done by physicians or other technical personnel available to the speech clinician.

Almost everything discussed in this book depends on instrumentation, so there is a very heavy emphasis on "machines." Where different instruments are available to achieve the same objective, they are considered and compared. Because I have always believed that valid use of instrumentation requires a clear understanding of operating principles, there are sometimes-lengthy explanations of what is inside the various "black boxes." For the same reason, there is a separate chapter on the elementary principles of electronics. Finally, there are occasional microtutorials on important, but sometimes overlooked, aspects of the physiology or acoustics of speech.

There is no point in informing the reader about tests that can be performed without also providing information about what the test results should look like. Therefore, tabulations of data that approximate "norms" for the various test methods have been provided wherever possible. They are intended to serve as guidelines to interpretation of test results.

There is only passing reference to microcomputers. This is not meant to denigrate them or to deny that they are in fact the wave of the future. And it is emphatically not because the author hates them (at least not most of the time). Rather, the decision to forego discussion of microcomputers was based on the observation that, at least for the present, they are doing no more in the domain of diagnosis and appraisal than what more traditional analog methods do. They can usually do it faster, often do it more conveniently, and—on occasion—can do it much better. But what they do is not *different*. And, the computer takes its input from the same analog instrumentation discussed in this book, so it seemed better to stick with what a clinician—or computer—must do to obtain data than to devote a great deal of space to consideration of computer function and mechanics. Fortunately, a great many other books are starting to appear on that subject.

The organization of this book posed genuine problems. Many test methods are useful for a wide range of disorders, so a division of the text by classes of pathology did not seem optimal. But there are exceptions to this rule, and so, for example, there are separate chapters on laryngeal and velophargeal dysfunction. A glance at the table of contents will show that no general principle was found to divide the material of the book into chapters. The organization may be inscrutable (in places, even to the author!), but it is hoped that reference to the index will allow a reader to find whatever is needed.

The text is very liberally sprinkled with references. Their function is not so much to assure that what is presented is "true," but rather to guide the reader to more complete explanations and to the original data. (Despite the size of the book, a great deal has been left out.) Sometimes references have been included for historical purposes; we have too often forgotten where we came from and to whom we owe what we have.

Although the title page recognizes just one author, in fact many people contributed to this undertaking in diverse but important ways. My wife, Joan, considered this book another of my esoteric hobbies and was good natured and understanding throughout its gestation. She and Dr. Jeannette Fleischner (whom some think is my alternative spouse) spent untold hours listening to my meanderings in the arcane lore of speech pathology and to my all-too-frequent groaning when the work was going badly. And, somehow, they usually managed to keep smiling.

A number of my colleagues read major segments of the first versions and offered helpful comments and insights. Among them are Drs. Elizabeth Allen, Steve Cavallo, Ray Daniloff, Kathy Harris, Honor O'Malley, Nick Schiavetti, Phil Schneider, and Carol Wilder. Bob Orlikoff gamely tried out segments of the book on the unsuspecting graduate students in his course on clinical laboratory techniques and broke the news of their responses to me as gently as possible. Dr. Ed Mysak, chairman of my department, was very encouraging and tolerant of the many quirks in my work style that developed as this book matured. Dr. Miriam Goldberg often applied those psychological insights for which she has gained a worldwide reputation, doing a wonderful portrayal of the gadfly to my reluctant role of Io. She managed to apply frequent motivating prods where she thought they would do the most good.

Finally, my doctoral students suggested revisions in the text, relishing the opportunity to do unto me as I often do unto them. They also volunteered—with somewhat less enthusiasm—to be subjects as I tested out various methods and procedures. I know how much happier they will all be now that I can, once again, devote all my creative energies to the task of making their lives more interesting.

CHAPTER 1

Introduction

This book addresses ways of measuring speech. It deals with the means available for determining what the various parts of the speech system are doing to produce a speech product and with the ways of specifying the characteristics of the acoustic output in a quantitative manner. It is intended for all medical and rehabilitative professionals who assess and treat disorders of voice and speech, but mostly it is aimed at speech pathologists, with whom the major responsibility for communicative rehabilitation ordinarily rests.

Ever since the inception of the field, speech pathologists have relied heavily, almost exclusively, on their highly trained ears for judgments of speech acceptability. When disorder was detected, the clinician typically relied upon his own auditory perception for insight into its origins. Based upon careful listening, clinicians often would make judgments such as "inadequate velopharyngeal closure," "vocal fold hyperfunction," or "inadequate breath support."

Nothing in this book is meant to deny the importance of the therapist's listening skills in assessing and treating speech disorders. The first step in diagnosis, after all, is determining whether or not a problem exists. There is no instrument, no technique, no computer that can begin to match the human auditory system for detecting subtle acoustic variations or for determining whether they represent varieties of normal or nonnormal speech. Still, it is clearly a major premise of this book that listening is not enough, that clinician perceptions cannot provide the sole and universal basis for mapping and guiding the course of therapy. To many practitioners, this axiom is already self apparent, but for others some explanation is in order.

A major problem with simple listening as a diagnostic method is that the auditory system is inherently configured for dealing with the speech signal as a whole entity and for detecting linguistically relevant features in it. It is this highly evolved aptitude that makes the auditory system so efficient in speech communication. Unfortunately, from the speech pathologist's point of view, auditory processing often does not leave the listener with a conscious awareness of the acoustic details that have combined to generate a given perception. Yet, for the speech pathologist, it is commonly the individual acoustic components, the ingredients of the speech product, that must be evaluated. It is the specific defective aspects of the speech signal that must be the target of therapy. The ear is too easily fooled. Pitch peculiarities can be due to the spectral composition of the vocal signal, rather than to its frequency. Perceived hypernasality may be the result of abnormal velar timing, rather than inadequate velopharyngeal closure.

Then there is the problem of *degrees of freedom*. Almost any speech sound, normal or otherwise, can be produced in a variety of ways. There is often no way, based on listening alone, to be sure of exactly what the vocal tract is doing to produce a given output. The problem here is analogous to fixing a stereo that has become distorted and noisy. The trouble might be in the stylus, the cartridge, the amplifier, or the speaker. Listening to the system can provide hints about where to look for the trouble. But only careful testing of the several components can really pinpoint the source of difficulty and indicate appropriate solutions.

Dealing with aberrant mechanisms, rather than simply modifying unacceptable products, often offers distinct advantages. It is entirely possible for better-sounding speech to result from worse function—severely increased muscle tension, more injurious vocal fold behavior, more bizarre or inefficient motor patterns. Adequate assessment of function is likely to help the clinician avoid the possibility of maladaptive, but good-sounding, speech production. Conversely, it is possible that specific parameters of speech behavior are indeed normalizing as a result therapy, although overall speech quality may not yet show much positive change. Well-chosen measurement methods may reveal therapeutic progress before the therapist hears much improvement.

It is a major tenet of this book that observation and measurement of speech and its physiologic correlates offers significant advantages over unaided perceptual judgment. Specifically, these advantages are:

1. Increased precision of diagnosis, with more valid specification of abnormal functions that require modification;
2. More positive identification and documentation of therapeutic efficacy, both for short term assessment (is a given approach modifying the abnormal function?) and long term monitoring (how much has speech behavior changed since the inception of therapy?);
3. Expansion of options for therapy modalities. Most measurement techniques offer a means of demonstrating to the patient exactly what is wrong, and they can usually provide feedback on the degree of his success in modifying the fault.

In one form or another, many speech measurement techniques have been around for a long time. It is reasonable to ask why, if they offer significant advantages, it has taken so long for them to gain currency in diagnosis and therapy.

Almost everyone is aware of the technological revolution of the last two or three decades. It has changed our homes, our ways of conducting business, our preferred recreations. It has revolutionized research laboratories and advanced medical practice in quantum leaps. The development of technology has also had its effect on our ability to observe speech behavior. Early clinicians and researchers commonly had to spend hours obtaining data about speech system function, and their primitive (by today's standards) instruments were often incapable of giving them a clear picture of the variable being evaluated. In many instances this is no longer the case. Instrumentation today tends to be more reliable, more valid, much easier to use, less esoteric, and more readily available. Measuring vocal fundamental frequency is a case in point. In the 1920s it took several hours of work to produce a record of the fundamental frequency characteristics of just a few seconds of speech. The process involved generating a record of the speech waveform on moving film, developing the film, projecting it and measuring the wavelengths by hand, tabulating the results, and deriving the summary means, wave-to-wave variations, and other measures of interest. Today, with several instruments available commercially, measuring fundamental frequency and obtaining a record of its changes during speech production can be done while the patient is speaking—in "real time," to use the current jargon.

While today's instruments are often much more complex, more accurate and more reliable than the devices of the past, they are nonetheless much easier to use. It has taken a while for the changes wrought by technological advance to be applied to clinical needs in speech pathology, and it has required a bit longer for an awareness of the improvements to spread. Thus, there has been a significant lag in their adoption in the speech clinic.

Instrumentation tends to be expensive. Equipment requires capital investment, and budgets are often tight (to say the least). Whether the investment is made depends on the importance attached to offering state-of-the-art service to patients. Much greater expenditures are needed to equip a physician's office, yet no physician would consider practicing without the tools of the art. Closer to home, perhaps, is the large investment needed to set up an audiologist. Tuning forks are orders-of-magnitude cheaper than audiometers. Impedance bridges are a very expensive way of documenting eardrum deflections. Brainstem evoked-response audiometry is a vastly more complex and infinitely more costly means of documenting auditory reception than watching for an eyeblink when a book is slammed against a table. Yet it would be a rare audiologist who felt that an acceptable and professional assessment could be done without many, if not all, of these instruments. Audiologists have concluded that the cost to benefit ratio warrants the investment in good tools.

If better measurement can improve therapeutic efficacy and efficiency (and it is the author's firm conviction that it can), then it is very likely to be cost effective. If it is cost effective, it warrants the investment.

The investment will be made when speech clinicians insist on it, as their colleagues in related areas have done.

Part of the reluctance to embrace advanced technology can be traced to the fact that many speech and language pathologists view their profession as part of the social and behavioral disciplines. The result is that speech pathologists often have little exposure to the "hard" sciences in their professional background. Acoustic and physiologic instrumentation are perceived as parts of an alien tradition. However valid the "behavioral" categorization of the field might have been, the fact is that biology and physics are having an increasing impact on it and are destined to become ever more important as knowledge of speech and language processes advances. Professional speech pathology has been evolving, and the discomfort associated with hardware is likely to continue to diminish.

A major share of the blame for the alienation of so many clinicans from the technological and scientific end of the profession must be assigned to the members of the research community. While there are notable exceptions, most speech scientists (and even many clinical investigators) have simply not taken the trouble to ensure that their methods and findings are accessible to clinical practitioners. To be sure, mathematics may be the best language for the expression of many complex concepts, but translations into more common prose are possible and obviously useful, even if some precision and subtlety is lost in the process. Technical jargon is used because it tends to be precise, unambiguous, and economical, but less esoteric explanations can be composed. (Let it be noted that the journals have not always encouraged "popularization." Their content, however, is largely governed by researchers.)

Finally, the adoption of technology has been impeded by the fact that relevant and important information is scattered throughout a large number of different sources, often highly specialized, published by many different professional groups. It is unreasonable to expect any working professional to winnow the haystack of literature looking for needles of methodologic utility.

A number of considerations have determined the structure of this text. It is intended to introduce clinicians to the techniques and instruments for observing and evaluating the activity of the speech system. All of the methods have been culled from the literature of speech pathology and related disciplines. None is hypothetical or untried (although some need further validation.) They have been collected from widely dispersed sources together with whatever normative or quasinormative data are available for them.

It is the author's unshakable conviction that a professional must understand his tools. Maybe a technician can use a device as a simple "black-box", unaware of what is inside and unconcerned with how it functions. A professional, however, is not let off so easily. If judgments are to be based on evidence, that evidence must be beyond reasonable reproach or, failing that, its limitations must be clearly understood and accounted for in drawing conclusions. In practical terms, this boils down to solid comprehension of where the data came from, and how they were obtained. Therefore, this text includes explanations of instrumentation functions as well as the rationales and assumptions underlying test procedures. Another reason for including (sometimes lengthy) explanations of equipment function is to provide enough information to allow clinicians to use or adapt laboratory equipment that, particularly in academic settings, is often available but perceived as off-limits to the clinician or inapplicable to clinical problems. And finally, advanced students and more sophisticated clinicians may find that a solid understanding of the equipment at hand allows them to modify or interconnect it in novel and creative ways to solve complex measurement problems.

Speech scientists may protest that important details of physics or biology have been omitted. That the text is oversimplified or that the methods presented are less precise than they could be. Some speech path-

ologists, on the other hand, may object that there is too much physics, too much discussion of engineering, too much complication of what has always been a more interpersonal, "humanist" activity. Within their different frames of reference, perhaps both sides have a point, which highlights an important issue. The speech pathologist has the right to insist that the needs of a clinic are different from those of a research laboratory. Very small differences between sets of data may be of great importance to the scientist trying to validate or refute a theoretical position. By and large, however, small differences are not likely to indicate anything that is clinically useful. (The statisticians remind us that significant differences are not necessarily meaningful.) While refinement of method and increased measurement precision are very important to the laboratory worker, there comes a point where increased precision and subtlety cease to improve the therapeutic process.

There is, admittedly, a case to be made for maximal understanding of every aspect of all that is a part of professional practice. Yet a balance must be struck—clinicians do not want to be research scientists or engineers. They want to be well-informed and solidly grounded specialists in an applied field. Clinicians have a right to get on with their own work, and scientists must recognize this.

On the other hand, those advocating a purely social or solely behavioral approach to speech pathology must be made aware of the increase in scientific understanding of speech production that has taken place. They must be made sensitive to the impact that that understanding and the technological advances that make its application to clinical work possible will have on the field. There can be little doubt that changes will continue to occur, probably at a greater rate than we have seen so far. The only question is whether the speech pathologist or members of other fields who are more comfortable with acoustic and motor theory, electronics and instrumentation, will be doing the applications in the future.

Some speech clinicians, more psychologically oriented in their approach, have protested that increasing technology "dehumanizes" therapy. There is no reason why this need be so. Humanism is a function of the therapist. It does not necessarily flourish in the absence of technology, nor does it automatically wither when instruments come on the scene.

This book is admittedly incomplete. It could not be otherwise. The topic is far too vast to be covered adequately in any single volume. To compensate, extensive references to the literature are provided. In a research paper, their purpose would be to validate the statements made in the text, but their function is different here. They are intended to tell the reader where to find more complete information, explanations to fill in the gaps of this book which is, after all, only an introduction to this aspect of speech pathology.

One final, perhaps all important, consideration. This volume is not a textbook of diagnostics. Nothing in it says "here are the things you should do in dealing with this or that kind of disorder." It is assumed that the reader has already had sufficient grounding in, and experience with, speech disorders to decide what needs to be known, what measures are likely to be useful in evaluating a given patient and in designing a therapeutic course. What is to be done with a patient is a matter for the clinician to decide anew on the basis of each individual case. No book could possibly lay down specific procedures to be applied according to disorder category, even if it were deemed advisable to do so. Only after a skilled clinician has formulated diagnostic hypotheses about the problem, can an evaluation procedure be implemented. The author has assumed that anyone approaching the area of speech measurement techniques already has an adequate background in speech pathology and a good understanding of the mechanisms of speech production. It is taken as a given that the reader can decide what, specifically, needs to be examined in a given case. None of the procedures described in this book, none of the instruments, can achieve a diagnosis. That can be arrived at only on the basis of all of the evidence—biological, physical, psychological, and social—as interpreted by a professional who is well versed in theory and who has wideranging knowledge of how speech is produced. Diagnosis rests, in the final analysis, on the abilities of a single super-instrument: a competent professional. ■

CHAPTER 2

Fundamentals of Electronics

Electronics is the medium through which measurements are made. Ingenious mechanical means of observing the action of the speech system were devised in the early days of the profession, but modern instrumentation is almost always electronic. This development is not the result of any perverse desire on the part of scientists to mystify or confuse their professional public. It simply reflects the fact that electronic circuits can perform measurement functions much faster and more accurately than mechanical systems can, while interfering far less with the process being evaluated. In fact, in most cases only electronic circuits are capable of doing the job at hand.

By no means does using an electronic instrument guarantee valid or reliable measurements. An instrument or circuit must be used in ways that are consistent with its characteristics, with its capabilities and, sometimes, with its quirks. Otherwise, the validity of the information obtained will be compromised, often to the point of seriously misleading the unsuspecting user. If they are to obtain maximally useful evaluations

of their clients' speech behaviors, clinicians will need to know at least a little bit about electronics. This does not mean that speech pathologists need to be biomedical engineers. Just a little understanding, creatively applied, goes a remarkably long way.

There seems to be a widespread tendency to panic or despair when approaching basic electronic theory. On the assumption that these reactions are provoked by the mathematical approaches commonly used, this chapter will try to develop an understanding of the most basic electrical phenomena by relying on more intuitive explanations. The objective is not to train the reader to design circuits but to help her or him understand enough electronics to use those that are available intelligently, productively, and creatively. It is the intent of this very cursory review to provide just enough background to understand the instrumentation and methods discussed in the following chapters. A list of basic textbooks is provided at the end of the chapter for those who are motivated (or driven by necessity) to delve more deeply into this area.

ELECTRICITY: CURRENT, VOLTAGE, AND RESISTANCE

In the simplest sense, electricity is the flow of electrons from a place where thay are abundant to a region where they are relatively scarce. The path that the electrons follow is called a *circuit*. Nothing moves without being pushed, so the electrons obviously must be driven by some force. Each electron has a negative charge. Since like charges repel each other, the electrons in any region tend to push away from each other. It is this mutual repulsion that provides the pushing force. The more crowded a space is with electrons, the greater the mutual repulsion will be. Therefore, if there is a path they can follow, electrons will flow from a zone of tight electron packing (with consequently great repulsive force) to an area where the packing is not so dense (and the outward pushing force is therefore less). The flow of electrons will continue until the electron concentration is equalized in the two areas. One can imagine an analogous situation involving two identical balloons, one fully inflated (having tight packing of air molecules) and the other blown up only slightly (and therefore having less crowding of the air molecules). If the two balloons are connected by a tube, air will flow out of the fully inflated one into the less inflated one. When both have the same density of air molecules the flow stops.

In the everyday world of practical electronics, the source of electrons is called a *power supply*. It may be a device that plugs into the wall outlet or a simple battery. Whatever its form, it has a region where electrons are abundant and a region where electrons are scarce. There is some way of connecting wires to each region. The electrons cannot flow from one zone to another inside the power supply. The only route for them to take to equalize the imbalance is via an external device that the user connects to the terminals. Hence, a power supply provides a flow of electrons for activitating electronic devices.

The flow of electrons is called *current*.

The symbol for current is "*I*." It is measured in *amperes* (A). One ampere (1 A) represents the flow of a given number of electrons every second. (The number happens to be 6.25×10^{18}. It is of importance to physicists and chemists, but doesn't really matter to the user of electronic instrumentation.) The *pressure* or force pushing the electrons is called the *voltage* or *potential* (symbol: *E*).* Voltage is measured in volts (V). *Voltage* is the difference in electrical pressure between two points. Current and voltage in an electrical circuit are the equivalent of flow and pressure in a plumbing system. Just as the flow through a pipe might be measured in gallons per minute, current is quantified in amps. The pressure of water in a pipe might be described in pounds per square inch, and in the same way the electrical "pressure" in a wire is described in volts.

All other things being equal, the greater the voltage (difference in pressure between two points) the greater the flow. One is directly proportional to the other:

$$I \propto E$$

Direct and Alternating Current

There is a fundamental distinction to be made between electron flows that are steady (or that change only *very* slowly) and those that vary from one instant to the next. Steady flow is called *direct current* (DC) while variable flow is known as *alternating current* (AC). The distinction is important because there are several electronic components whose characteristics are different depending on whether, and how fast, the current is changing. In fact, it is this property that makes such components useful. (More will be said about this later.)

It is easy to understand DC. It might be exemplified by current in a flashlight: After the switch is turned on electrons flow at a

---

*There is a difference between voltage and potential. In essence it is the distinction between the actual and the ideal. Any electronics text can provide further information about this distinction, but it will not concern us here.

constant rate—out of one pole of the battery, through the lamp, and back to the battery's other pole—until the switch is turned off again. Except for the instants when the switch is moved (and current flow suddenly begins or ends) the flashlight works on DC. But there are two common misconceptions about AC that may interfere with understanding basic electronic circuits. First, current in an AC circuit does not necessarily reverse direction from time to time. Reversal is the case in many systems, but it is not reversal that makes them AC devices. What characterizes AC is not changes in direction of current, but changes in the *amount* of current. Second, the changes in flow need not be periodic. That is, there is no requirement that there be a regular waveform. Any current change, according to any pattern or following no pattern at all, makes an AC signal.

Because information can only be conveyed by a change in some quantity, it is not surprising that most useful electronic devices are built around AC circuits. However, AC signal processing is much more complex than the handling of DC signals. To facilitate understanding of the most basic aspects of electrical circuits, the discussion to follow will consider only DC circuits. The more complex phenomena relating to AC will be deferred until later.

Conductors, insulators, and resistance

Because of differences in atomic structure, some materials allow electrons to pass more easily than others do. Substances through which electrons can move with relative ease are called *conductors*. Most metals are good conductors. This is why copper and aluminum, which are excellent but reasonably priced conductors, are used to make wire. On the other hand, it is very difficult to get current to flow through some other materials, including wood, air, glass, and many plastics. These substances are called *insulators*. Under normal conditions all materials, even the best conductors, present *some* impediment to the flow of electricity. The impediment is

referred to as *resistance* (R), and it is measured in "ohms" (symbol: Ω). A good conductor has very low resistance; an insulator has extremely high resistance. At a given voltage (driving force, pressure) more current will flow through a low resistance than through a high resistance. In other words, current is inversely proportional to resistance:

$$I \propto 1/R.$$

Ohm's Law

Taking the relationships between current and voltage and between current and resistance, a general rule of electrical flow can be formulated. **Current is proportional to voltage and inversely proportional to resistance.** This principle is known as Ohm's law. It is the foundation upon which most of the field of electronics rests. If the units used to measure resistance (R), current (I), and potential or voltage (E) are chosen properly (and they have been!) Ohm's law can be stated as an equation:

$$I = E/R.$$

Expressed in words, the equation says that flow (current in amperes) is equal to pressure (in volts) divided by impediment to flow (resistance, in ohms). This relationship can be manipulated algebraically to derive two alternate forms:

$$R = E/I$$

(resistance equals voltage divided by current) and

$$E = IR$$

(voltage equals current times resistance). This last form of Ohm's law has a very significant implication that may not be immediately apparent. It really says that a voltage (pressure difference) results from the flow of current through a resistance. That is, when a flow of electrons encounters an obstacle (the resistance) the electrical pressure will be higher on the "upstream" side of the resistance than on the "downstream" side. The voltage (or pressure) "drops" across the resistance. If there is no resistance there is no pressure difference between two points, which is to say that there is no voltage.

A couple of examples will demonstrate the usefulness of even these simple electronic principles.

1. According to the manufacturer's specification sheet, a transducer for sensing intraoral air pressure has a resistance of 300 ohms. It can tolerate a current through it of no more than 0.5 A. (Greater currents may destroy it.) Can the transducer be safely connected to the 20V power supply available in your clinic?

   The problem is to find out how much current will flow through the pressure transducer when 20 V is applied to it. We need to determine the current (I). Therefore

   $$I = E/R = 20 \text{ V}/300\Omega$$
   $$I = 0.067 \text{ A}.$$

   The 20 V supply on hand will not overpower the transducer and can safely be used.

2. The manufacturer of a flow sensor recommends that it be heated by a current of 0.1 A. The heater element has a resistance of 250 Ω. How much voltage is needed to provide the necessary heating? We are interested in determining the voltage (E) that produces a current (I) of 0.1 A through the heater's resistance (R)of 250 Ω. Therefore,

   $$E = IR = (0.1 \text{ A})(250 \text{ }\Omega)$$
   $$E = 25 \text{ V}.$$

Proper heating will require a 25 V supply.

Power

Another important concept can be derived from Ohm's Law. Both pressure and flow represent the energy that is available to do work in a system. In electrical terms the voltage drop and the current determine the power (P) being used or dissipated. *Power*, then, is

$$P = EI$$

(power equals voltage times current). Power is measured in *watts* (W).

Because voltage, current, and resistance are all related to each other there are a number of formulae by which power can be calculated, depending on which variables are known in a given situation. For instance, because $E = IR$, we can substitute IR for E in the power equation. That is,

$$P = EI,$$
but since $E = IR$,
$$P = (IR)I,$$
which can be simplified to
$$P = I^2R.$$
Similarly,
$$P = EI,$$
but since $I = E/R$,
$$P = E(E/R),$$
$$P = E^2/R.$$

Power may be dissipated as sound pressure, light, or motion, among other forms. Mostly, however, power is lost as heat. Sometimes generating heat is the goal (as in the case of the flow-system heater), but usually it is only a by-product. Many electronic systems are housed in ventilated cases so that the waste heat can be carried away easily.

Ohm's law, then, relates four electrical quantities: current, voltage, resistance, and power. By using algebraic substitutions again, a number of forms of Ohm's law can be derived to express any one of the quantities in terms of the others. All of the alternative forms are summarized in Table 2-1.

TABLE 2-1. Summary of Ohm's Law*

Current	Voltage
$I = E/R$	$E = IR$
$I = P/E$	$E = P/I$
$I = \sqrt{P/R}$	$E = \sqrt{PR}$

Resistance	Power
$R = E/I$	$P = EI$
$R = P/I^2$	$P = E^2/R$
$R = E^2/P$	$P = I^2R$

I = current in amperes; R = resistance in ohms; E = potential across R in volts; P = power in watts

Schematic diagrams

It is very much easier to describe an electronic circuit with a diagram than to use words to explain how its various elements are connected to each other. For this reason more-or-less standardized symbols are used according to a generally agreed upon set of rules to generate what are called "schematic diagrams." Some of the basic principles of reading them are considered here in order to facilitate further consideration of circuitry.

Figure 2-1 is a set of schematics for a very simple electrical circuit: two lamps

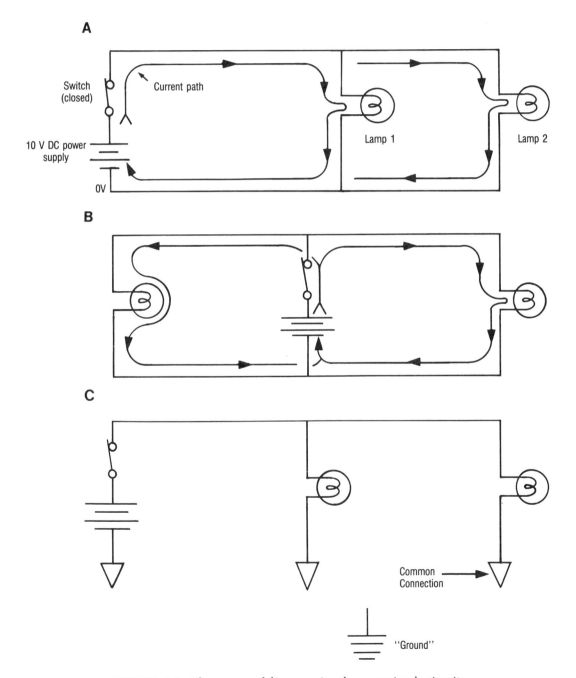

FIGURE 2-1. Three ways of diagramming the same simple circuit.

connected to a DC source. In Figure 2-1A the flow of current is from the + 10 V side of the source (which might be a battery) through a switch. After the switch the current pathway has two branches, one through each lamp. The circuit paths merge again to carry the current to the 0 V side of the DC source, completing the circuit. Note the symbols used for the DC supply, the lamps, and the switch. (A summary of standard electronic symbols will be found in Appendix H). Straight lines represent wires (or other conductors). The layout of the schematic diagram is intended to make the circuit easy to understand. It does not necessarily have any relationship to the actual physical placement of the wiring that would be used in building the circuit. The circuit diagrammed in Figure 2-1B is identical in every way to the one shown in Figure 2-1A although it looks different on the page: in each case the current flow is from the source, through a switch, through one of two branches that includes a lamp, and back via a final single path to the power source.

In complex circuits many elements may share a common current path back to the power source. In order to simplify their diagrams the convention shown in Figure 2-1C has been adopted. The triangular marker indicates a "common" connection, a single point or wire in the actual circuit to which the marked points are connected. In reading these diagrams all points marked with the triangle should be considered to be joined together.

Ground

The common return path for current in a circuit is often referred to as the circuit's *ground*, a term that goes back to the very early days of electronics. Often the ground is the metal chassis on which an instrument is built, and the metal parts of the instrument case are often attached to the ground for safety (see "Electrical Safety," this chap.). These days it is not uncommon for the ground of a circuit to be physically connected to the earth itself by a separate wire

(the third contact on a three-prong plug), but this is not the case for older devices, in which the ground is "floating" — unconnected to anything that is actually in contact with the earth. The symbol for ground is shown in Figure 2-1.

Series and parallel circuits

Figure 2-2 shows the two basic ways in which components can be arranged in any circuit. In Figure 2-2A the current path is through a set of elements (in this case, light bulbs) in sequence. Each electron traveling around the circuit must pass through every component. This is called a *series* circuit. The electrons are like cars traveling bumper-to-bumper along a single-lane road through a series of towns. Each car must go through each town in sequence and all the cars must travel at the same rate, which is the overall speed of traffic. In a series circuit, then, all the electrons (cars) move at the same speed everywhere in the circuit (road). In electronic terms, the current in a series circuit is everywhere the same.

In a *parallel* circuit, on the other hand, there are alternative paths that the electrons

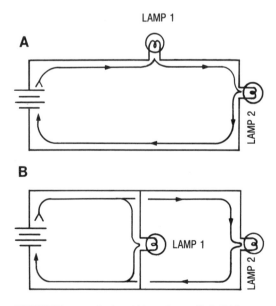

FIGURE 2-2. Series (A) and parallel (B) lamp circuits.

can travel. Some electrons in Figure 2-2B go through lamp 1, while others are routed through lamp 2. If the lamps have different resistances the current through the two branches of the circuit will be different. The total current flowing from the power source is the *sum* of the currents through lamps 1 and 2 in the parallel circuit. This contrasts with the series circuit, in which the current from the power source is the same as the current through either lamp 1 or lamp 2, since the current in a series circuit is everywhere the same.

Most real circuits are combinations of series and parallel arrangements. The circuit depicted in various ways in Figure 2-1 provided a good example of this, although it was not mentioned. The switch in that circuit is in *series* with the lamps, while the two lamps are themselves connected in *parallel*. Since all current flows through a series element, opening the switch in Figure 2-1 interrupts the current to both lamps, turning them off. On the other hand, if lamp 1 of Figure 2-1 should burn out, lamp 2 will be unaffected because it represents an alternative current path through which electrons can flow without going via lamp 1 first.

Resistance Networks

While some amount of resistance is inherent in any circuit component (even wires), circuit function usually depends on having exact amounts of resistance at specific places. This is arranged by using *resistors*, components which are characterized by specific amounts of resistance. Resistors can be made of many different materials— carbon powder, special metal wire, carbon films, and so forth—to optimize them to meet different requirements (such as stability in the face of temperature change, or minimization of aging effects). They are available with values ranging from a fraction of an ohm to several million ohms (megohms). (The value of a resistor is most commonly marked on it in the form of a series of colored bands.) Resistors dissipate

power (Ohm's law: $P = I^2R$) and they are available to handle different amounts of power without overheating. The conventional schematic symbols for resistance are shown in Figure 2-3.

Series and parallel resistance

Each resistor represents a certain impediment to the flow of current. When resistors are arranged in series, as in Figure 2-4A, the current flow must pass through all of them, and the total resistance encountered by the electrons will be the sum of all the resistances in the series. Therefore, given a set of resistors in series, $R_1, R_2, R_3, \ldots R_n$, the total resistance is

$$R_{series} = R_1 + R_2 + R_3 + \ldots + R_n.$$

The total resistance of a set of resistors connected in parallel may be somewhat less easy to grasp. Consider the very simple circuit of Figure 2-4B, which (except for the absence of a switch) is the same as the parallel lamp circuit of Figure 2-1. Here, however, resistors R_1 and R_2 have taken the place of the light bulbs. We will need to evaluate the current through each of them (I_1 and I_2) as well as the total current (I_T) flowing from the power supply. The circuit of Figure 2-4B is rearranged to the form of Figure 2-4C to facilitate the evaluation. It is clear from the rearrangement that R_1 and R_2 are both directly connected to the supply voltage, V. Therefore, according to Ohm's law, the current through R_1 must be $I_1 = V/R.$ Similarly, the current through R_2

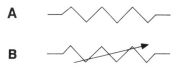

A

B

FIGURE 2-3. Resistors. (A) Fixed   (B) Variable.

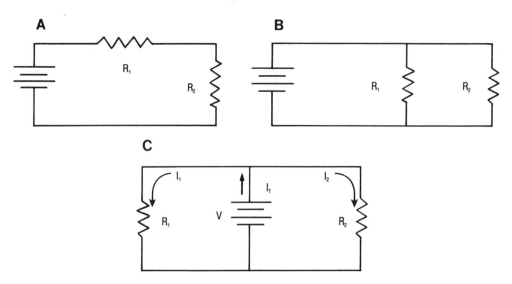

FIGURE 2-4. Total resistance of series and parallel circuits. (A) is series resistance, $R_T = R_1 + R_2$; (B) Parallel resistance. (C) shows Rearrangement of B.

must be $I_2 = V/R_2$. The total current (I_T) from the supply must be equal to the sum of these two currents, so that $I_T = I_1 + I_2 = (V/R_1) + (V/R_2)$. As the power supply "looks out" at the circuit it sees its voltage, V, causing a current flow of I_T amperes. Therefore, from the point of view of the supply, the resistance of the total circuit must be

$$R_T = V/I_T$$
$$= \frac{V}{\dfrac{V}{R_1} + \dfrac{V}{R_2}}$$

which can be reduced to

$$R_T = \frac{1}{\dfrac{1}{R_1} + \dfrac{1}{R_2}}$$

This relationship can be generalized to any number of resistors in parallel. The total resistance is equal to the reciprocal of the sum of the reciprocals of the resistances:

$$R_T = \frac{1}{\dfrac{1}{R_1} + \dfrac{1}{R_2} + \ldots + \dfrac{1}{R_N}}$$

In the case of only two resistors a little mathematical manipulation provides a more convenient formula:

$$R_{1+2} = (R_1 R_2) / (R_1 + R_2).$$

The need to evaluate the sum of resistances in series and parallel frequently arises, as a simple example can illustrate. Many audio amplifiers provide several different connections for loudspeakers or earphones. Very often there are three, labelled "4 ohms," "8 ohms," and "16 ohms." These designations refer to the resistance of the speaker (or earphones) to be hooked up to the amplifier. Most speakers have a resistance of 8 Ω. If only one is to be connected to the amplifier, it should obviously be wired to the 8-ohm connection. But suppose that two sets of earphones (one for the client, and one for the clinician) are to be used to listen to some audio material. Each earphone set, according to its label, has a resistance of 8 Ω. In order for both listeners to hear the same material, the two sets of earphones must be connected to the same output of the amplifier. This means that current coming from the amplifier can follow either of two alternate paths. That is, the earphones will be in parallel. To which connector on the amplifier should both earphones be connected? Four ohms, 8 Ω, or 16 Ω?

Since the earphones are to be connected in parallel, the total of their resistances must be $R_T = (R_1 R_2)/(R_1 + R_2)$. Therefore, $R_T = (8 \times 8)/(8 + 8) = 64/16 = 4\,\Omega$. Since the total resistance of the parallelled devices is 4 Ω, the audio output should be taken from the 4 Ω connection on the amplifier.

Voltage dividers and potentiometers

Figure 2-5A shows a simple circuit in which two resistors in series are connected to a power supply. Measurement points are provided at the positive side of the supply (point A), at the junction of the two resistors (point B), and at the negative side of the supply (point C) to allow the voltage differences between several points in the circuit to be determined. The total voltage of the circuit (V_T) is the 10V provided by the supply. This is the voltage difference between measurement points A and C. The total resistance of the circuit is R_T = $R_1 + R_2$, which is $100 + 400 = 500\,\Omega$. Current through the series resistances must therefore be $I = E/R_T = 10/500 = 0.02$ A.

Now, since this is a series circuit, the current must be everywhere the same. That means that the current through R_1 equals the current through R_2, equals 0.02 A. Ohm's law states that current interacts with resistance to produce a voltage difference across a resistor. The voltage difference or drop produced by the 100 Ω of R_1 must be $V_1 = IR_1 = 0.02\text{A} \times 100 = 2$ V. This is what a voltmeter connected to point A and point B would read. On the other hand, the voltage created by the 400 ohms of R_2 is $V_2 = IR_2 = 0.02 \times 400 = 8$ V. A voltmeter connected to points B and C would show this much voltage. Note that the two voltages, from A to B and from B to C, total 10V. This is as it should be, since the total voltage drop in the circuit (the voltage difference between the two poles of the power supply) must occur across the total of the elements in the circuit. What the resistive circuit has done is to split the total available voltage provided by the supply into

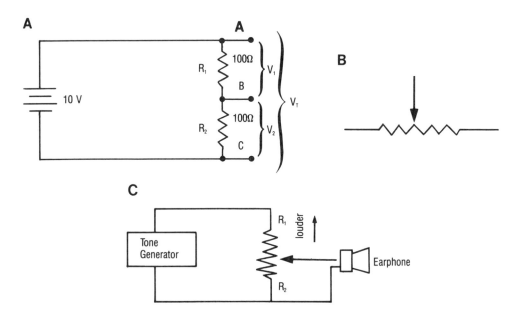

FIGURE 2-5. (A) Voltage divider circuit. (B) Potentiometer. (C) Potentiometer as a variable voltage divider in an intensity-control function. R_1 and R_2 are resistors. V_1 and V_2 are the voltages across R_1 and R_2. V_T is the total voltage. A and C are measurement points at the positive and ground side of the power supply, B is a measurement point at the junction of the two resistors.

two parts. For this reason this circuit arrangement is called a *voltage divider*. Any number of resistors can be included in series to allow the total available voltage to be split into as many smaller voltages as there are resistors in series. The analysis of voltage division by any number of resistors is the same as the evaluation for the circuit of Figure 2-5.

There is a simpler way of describing (or, for that matter, of computing) the voltage drops in a voltage divider. Note that, in Figure 2-5, R_1 is 1/5 of the total resistance and the voltage drop across it is 1/5 of the total applied voltage. Similarly, R_2, which accounts for 4/5 of the total resistance in the circuit, produces a voltage drop that is equal to 4/5 of the applied voltage. To generalize, in a voltage divider the voltage drop across a resistor is to the total applied voltage as the resistance in question is to the total resistance. That is, $V_x: R_1 = V_T : R_T$. Therefore, the voltage across a given resistor R_x is

$$V_x = (R_x/R_T) \times V_T.$$

Because any practical circuit is likely to need a great many different voltages, fixed voltage-divider networks are quite common. However, there is often a need for *variable* voltage division. For instance, a clinician might want to use a sine wave generator to produce a tone to be matched by the client's phonation. The voltage produced by the generator might produce too loud a tone when it is fed to a set of earphones. A voltage divider between the generator and earphones would reduce the voltage, and thereby the tone intensity, but perhaps by too much. In order to adjust the sound intensity to the client's preference an *adjustable* voltage divider network is needed.

Variability is easily provided by a device known as a *potentiometer*, shown in Figure 2-5B. Usually it is made of a resistive element (perhaps a strip of carbon film or a resistive wire winding) that is contacted by a "wiper." The two ends of the resistive element correspond to points A and C of the voltage divider, while the wiper is

point B. The wiper contact really separates the total resistance of the potentiometer into two resistances and, because the wiper can be moved along the resistive element, the two resistances can be adjusted to any proportionality. If the tone generator and speaker are connected via a potentiometer, as in Figure 2-5C, the client could control the sound intensity over a continuous range simply by adjusting a knob on the potentiometer shaft. This use of a potentiometer is familiar to anyone who has ever adjusted a radio's volume.

Wheatstone bridge

One of the most useful and widely employed circuits in electronic instrumentation is called the Wheatstone bridge. It lies at the heart of many measurement devices, including, for example, pressure gauges (Chap. 7) and motion transducers (Chap. 11). Given its importance in so many measurement applications, it seems worthwhile to examine it in some detail here.

As shown in Figure 2-6A, the Wheatstone bridge is a purely resistive network and so can be analyzed at this point in our discussion. To simplify slightly, the Wheatstone bridge produces a voltage that is proportional to the change in the resistance of R_x, which could be a pressure gauge, for instance.

In Figure 2-6B the circuit has been redrawn, and the resistors assigned values, to facilitate analysis. The two schematics show exactly the same circuit, except that a meter has been added in Figure 2-6B so that the circuit output can be measured. (We will assume that the meter does not allow any current to flow between points 1 and 2. In other words, the meter is considered to have infinite resistance. Any detector that *does* allow a significant current to flow across the bridge behaves like a resistor connecting the two sides, greatly altering circuit function. In real-life situations, of course, points 1 and 2 would more likely be connected to an amplifier or other electronic system. Anything connected across the bridge must meet the

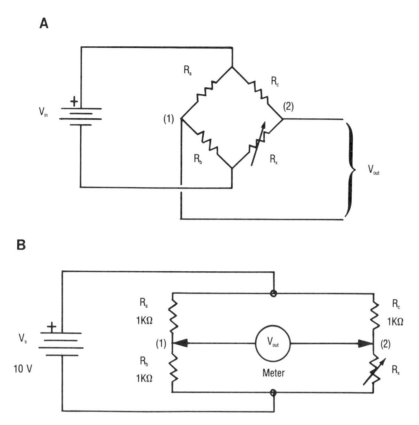

FIGURE 2-6. The Wheatstone bridge. (A) As commonly drawn in schematics. (B) Redrawn (with the addition of a meter) for analysis. R_a, R_b, R_c = constant resistors, R_x = variable resistor.

requirement of essentially infinite resistance if the bridge circuit is to function correctly.) It is worth noting at this point that, while the circuit we are considering has a DC "excitation" (supply) voltage, a Wheatstone bridge will work just as well with any sort of AC signal. Indeed, this is one of its major attractions.

The redrawn bridge circuit looks very much like two voltage dividers, connected in parallel to a voltage source. One of the resistors (R_x) is variable. (In the real world of measurement, that variable resistance would be a strain gauge or other sensing device whose resistance changes in response to some outside phenomenon to be evaluated.) For the moment, let us assume that the variable resistance has the same value as the other resistors. If this is the case, then the two voltage dividers are identical, and the voltage drops across each

one of their resistors must be the same. Therefore, the meter connected to points 1 and 2 sees no voltage difference, and registers 0 V. The bridge is said to be "balanced." But suppose that something happens to change the resistance of R_x. (Perhaps a pressure has been applied to the gauge that R_x represents.) Now the two voltage dividers are *not* the same (the bridge is "unbalanced") and the voltage at point 1 is no longer the same as the voltage at point 2. The meter now detects a voltage difference. The greater the difference between R_x and the other resistors in the bridge, the greater the voltage seen by the meter.

Table 2-2 summarizes the meter readings that result as R_x varies over a range of values. Note that the voltage across the bridge is directly and fairly linearly related to the value of R_x, at least over the narrow range of resistances in question.

TABLE 2-2. Bridge Voltages for Different Values of R_x in Figure 6*

R	V_1	Meter Reading
900	4.736	−0.263
920	4.791	−0.208
940	4.845	−0.155
960	4.898	−0.102
980	4.949	−0.051
1000	5.000	0.0
1020	5.050	+0.050
1040	5.098	+0.098
1060	5.146	+0.146
1080	5.192	+0.192
1100	5.238	+0.238

*$R_A = R_B = R_C = 1000$ ohms.

From an applied point of view the value of the Wheatstone bridge lies in the fact that many sensing devices have a detecting element whose resistance changes as a function of the variable of interest. By including the resistive detector in a Wheatstone bridge, the resistance change is converted to a voltage that can be used by analysis circuits or display devices, such as oscilloscopes, amplifiers, chart recorders, and the like. There are many variations of the basic Wheatstone bridge. For example, diagonally opposite resistors in the bridge are often made to vary by equal amounts, doubling the sensitivity of the bridge and providing temperature stability. Other resistors are often added to regulate current or provide a means of calibration. These modifications are discussed in most basic textbooks.

PRINCIPLES OF ALTERNATING CURRENT

In the real world, most signals are *time dependent*: something about them changes with time. Such signals constitute "alternating current" or AC.* It is worth repeat-

---

*Technically, of course, a signal that shows voltage, rather than current, change should be referred to as "alternating voltage." However, the rather sloppy application of the term "alternating current," even to voltage changes, is well established.

ing here that, despite the term "alternating," there is no requirement that the flow of current or the polarity of the voltage actually reverse. Any change with time makes a signal AC.

The simplest kind of time variation is the sine wave, the basic building block of all other periodic waves. And the simplest kind of sine wave is, in fact, one in which the current actually does reverse direction (which implies that the driving voltage reverses polarity). A simple sine wave of this type will be used to elucidate some of the basic properties of AC signals and the ways in which AC differs from DC.

AC Current and Voltage

Because an AC signal is continuously changing a simple measure of voltage or current is inadequate to describe it completely. Its frequency and phase, with which speech pathologists are already familiar, must also be specified. The fact that the amplitude of an AC signal is constantly changing creates problems in describing the voltage or current, since any single reading is valid for only one point in time. To cope with this, several standard measures have been adopted. They are illustrated in Figure 2-7.

Instantaneous current or voltage is the amplitude of the wave at a given point in time. To distinguish this value from a more global, overall measure it is generally symbolized by a lower-case letter. Hence, instantaneous voltage is "e", while instantaneous current is "i."

Peak-to-peak current or voltage of the wave is the difference between its most negative and most positive value. In other words, it is the height of the wave from the bottom of a trough to the top of a peak. In Figure 2-7 the peak-to-peak voltage is 2 V_p-p.

Peak voltage or current is defined as the amplitude of the wave above (or equivalently, below) the zero-voltage or zero-current line. In Figure 2-7 the peak voltage is 1 V_p.

Average current or voltage. It is often useful to have an overall average of all of the

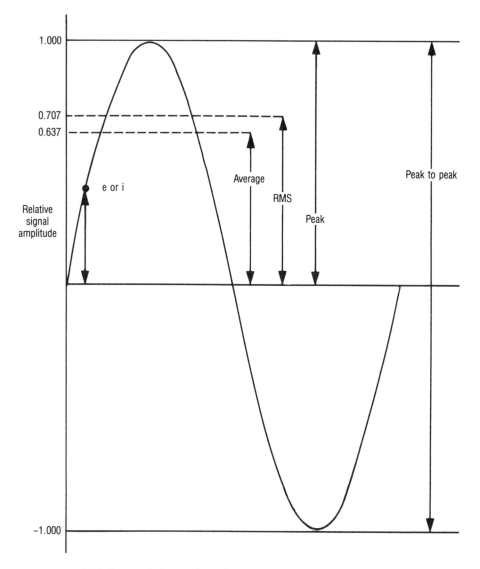

FIGURE 2-7. Relationship of AC measures of voltage or current.

instantaneous voltages or currents. A problem with taking the simple average of all the instantaneous values should be obvious: If the waveform is symmetrical about the zero point, the average of all the negative- and positive-signed points must equal zero. The way around this is, of course, to limit the averaging process to half of the cycle—that is, to either a positive or negative alternation. Then, when the averaging is performed (by a process known in the

calculus as integration), the average value (V_av or I_av) of a *sine wave* will be 0.637 times its peak amplitude. (It must be emphasized that this relationship of peak to average value is valid *only* for a sine wave!)

Root-mean-square (RMS) current or voltage. Perhaps the most common specification of an AC signal is its *equivalent* or *effective* amplitude. This is the amplitude that a DC voltage (or current) would need in order to deliver the same power as a given AC signal. Since power is proportional to the square of the voltage or current, deriving the equivalent amplitude involves (in theory) taking the square of the amplitude of the wave at every point in time, finding the average or mean of these squared values, and then finding the square root of the mean. Hence, this amplitude measure is referred to as the *root-mean-square* value, commonly denoted as "RMS." In practice, of course, there is no real need to do the mathematics (which are specified by the calculus of integration). For a sine wave (but *only* for a sine wave) the RMS voltage (or current) will be equal to the peak voltage (or current) times 0.7071. Thus, if the peak voltage of a particular sine wave is 1.00 V, its rms voltage is 0.7071 V_{RMS}. This means that the power delivered by a sine wave of 1 V peak amplitude is equal to the power that would be delivered by a DC flow at 0.7071 V in the same circuit.

It is important to reemphasize that the constant 0.7071 is valid only for the relationship between a *sine wave* and a DC signal. If the waveform being evaluated is not a sine wave, some other constant will apply. If the waveform is complex it may not be possible to determine exactly what the constant should be. This last point is of importance to the speech pathologist, who has frequent occasion to measure the amplitude of complex periodic waves, such as speech waveforms. A problem arises because most meters (whether digital or analog) actually determine average voltage (or current) and then apply a correction factor to derive RMS values. But the correction factor is valid only for sine waves, not for complex waveforms. The difference between the scale reading and the actual RMS value can be substantial. For complex waves a "true RMS" meter (that actually performs the required calculation) is needed. Table 2-3 provides the appropriate factors by which to multiply readings to convert voltage readings of one form to another. The conversions are fully valid only for sine waves, but can provide useful approximations in other cases.

TABLE 2-3. Relationship among AC Voltage and Current Values

TO DERIVE:	MULTIPLY*		
	Peak	Average	RMS
		by	
PEAK	—	1.57	1.41
AVERAGE	.637	—	0.9
RMS	.707	1.11	—

*Example. To derive *average* equivalent of a measured RMS voltage, multiply RMS voltage by 0.9.

DC Bias

Very often the voltage or current of an AC signal does not, in fact, reverse direction. An example of a sine wave for which this is the case is shown in Figure 2-8. What is happening here is that the waveform is alternating around some middle value that is not zero. (In Figure 2-8 a dashed line has been drawn at the level of that central value.) A moment's reflection reveals that the central value is equivalent to a DC signal. The AC wave, then, really represents the addition of a varying voltage (an AC signal) to a DC level. The AC wave is said to be associated with a "DC bias." To completely specify the wave of Figure 2-8 we need to state not only its amplitude (peak, RMS, and average) but also the DC bias associated with it.

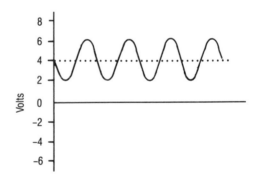

FIGURE 2-8. A sine-wave signal without reversal of current or voltage. The voltage varies by about 2 V above and below a nonzero "center" value indicated by the dashed line. This "DC bias" amounts to 4 V for this signal.

REACTANCE

A prime difference between DC and AC circuits is the fact that AC circuits are subject to the effect of *reactance*. This special property is a function of energy storage by components of the circuit. Mechanical systems store energy in analogous ways. A pendulum, for example, swings because the energy of the starting push is stored as momentum and is released in a controlled fashion. Energy can also be stored by stretching a rubber band. The elasticity of the rubber converts the stretch into a force that can be released later to do work. The electrical analogs of momentum and elasticity are called "inductance" and "capacitance." They affect the flow of alternating current by means of inductive and capacitative *reactance*.

Inductance

A magnetic field surrounds any wire through which current is flowing. The strength of the magnetic field is proportional to the current. As the current changes the magnetic field enlarges or contracts. Conversely, a conductor placed in a magnetic field will have a current generated in it (or a voltage produced across it) whenever the strength of the field changes. The induced voltage is referred to as an *electromotive force* or EMF. Considering the magnetism and electricity phenomena together, it should be clear that a conductor carrying a current not only produces a magnetic field, but it is itself caught in the very magnetic field it produces. Any time the current in the conductor changes, the resulting expansion or contraction of the magnetic field will induce a current in the conductor that is producing the field in the first place. Furthermore, Lenz's law states that the current induced by the change will be in the direction that *opposes* the generating current. Therefore, a conductor is caught in a sort of "Catch-22" situation: Any change in the current through it causes a change in its magnetic field that opposes the change in current. It is precisely this effect—self-opposition to change of current—that an inductor exploits. It does so by storing some of the energy of the electrical flow in the form of a magnetic field. If the current increases, energy is withdrawn from the current flow to enlarge the magnetic field, leaving less energy to push the electrons and thereby slowing down the rate of flow increase. If the flow diminishes, the magnetic field gets smaller, returning energy to the conductor and helping to push the electrons along, thus partially making up for the diminished driving force. In short, an inductor represents electrical momentum: It tends to keep electrons moving when the force pushing them lessens, and it opposes their rapid acceleration when the pushing force increases. The momentum effect in an electrical system is called *inductance*, which is symbolized as "L." Real inductors are generally made of a coil of wire wound on a form of paper or some magnetic material. (Coiling the wire concentrates the magnetic field produced.)

The key phrase in understanding inductance is "change in current." While any current produces a magnetic field, only a *changing* magnetic field can induce a current in a wire. Therefore, the inductor only interacts with a current when that current is changing. In other words, the inductor affects only AC. Furthermore, the faster the rate of change of the current the more strongly it is affected by the inductance. Since *rate of change* is another way of describing frequency, the degree to which a given inductance influences a signal depends on the signal's frequency.

The unit of inductance is the *henry* (symbol: H). (One henry is defined as the amount of inductance that will generate an EMF of 1 V when the current is changing at the rate of 1 ampere per second.) The faster the rate of change (the higher the frequency of the signal) the greater the opposition of the inductor to the change. The opposition effect is called the *inductive reactance* (symbol: X_L). Since it is an opposition to current, it is measured in ohms. The inductive reactance clearly depends jointly on the inductance (L) and on the rate of change, or frequency. The inductive reactance grows linearly with increasing frequency. Since the reactance is an impediment to current change it constitutes a kind of special resistance that increases with frequency.

PHASE SHIFT. The reactance is not really a resistance, for a very important reason. In a true resistance the current through the resistor and the voltage across it are in phase. When the current through the resistor is greatest, the voltage across it is greatest. This is not true in an inductor. Because of the storage phenomenon and the fact that the opposition comes from the interaction of the conductor with its own magnetic field, a peculiar time lag is generated between the current through and the voltage across the inductor. The two are out of phase by 90°. That is, the voltage and current waveforms have the same shape, but the voltage wave leads the current wave by 90°, as shown in Figure 2-9. It is this phase

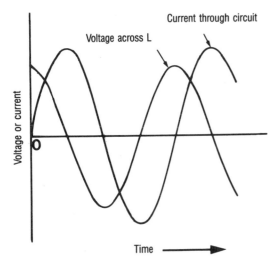

FIGURE 2-9. Relationship of voltage and current when an AC (sine wave) signal is applied to an inductive circuit. Note how voltage reaches its maximum 90° before current does.

shift and the complications that it introduces that makes a reactance different from a resistance.

At this point it is useful to look at a simple circuit that will illustrate another important property of reactive circuits and, at the same time, demonstrate at least one everyday use of inductance. The circuit, shown in Figure 2-10, looks very much like the voltage divider configuation discussed earlier, except that an inductor has been substituted for one of the resistors. It is known as an *RL circuit*. As in previous instances, values have been assigned to the circuit components in order to facilitate analysis.

IMPEDANCE. The circuit of Figure 2-10 contains a resistor and inductor in series. The inductor has a reactance, X_L, that is, in many ways, like a resistance. Therefore, the *total resistance* of the circuit is the series sum of the resistance and the reactance. The reactance of a 100 mH inductor (such as the one in the figure) at 1000 Hz happens to be about 628.3 ohms. Therefore, it might seem that the total resistance of the circuit should be $R + X_L = 1000 + 628.3 = 1628.3\ \Omega$. But there is a catch. According to Ohm's Law resistance equals voltage divided by current ($R = E/I$). The value of the resistor could be calculated from the voltage across it and the current through it. But this will not work for the inductor because the current through it is not in phase with the voltage across it. This means that, at least in the sense that Ohm's law requires, at any given instant the inductor's "E" does not correspond to its "I." The presence of the inductor's 90° phase shift makes the total resistance of the circuit very different from an ordinary resistance. To distinguish it from everyday resistance, it is called *impedance*. The phase shift implies that the impedance of the RL circuit must be found by vector addition, such as is studied in elementary algebra. So, for an RL series circuit, the impedance, Z, is

$$Z = \sqrt{R^2 + X_L{}^2}$$

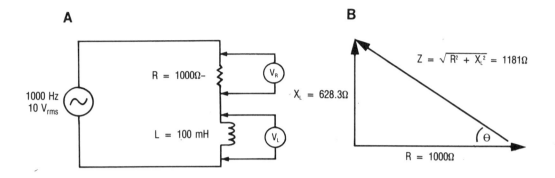

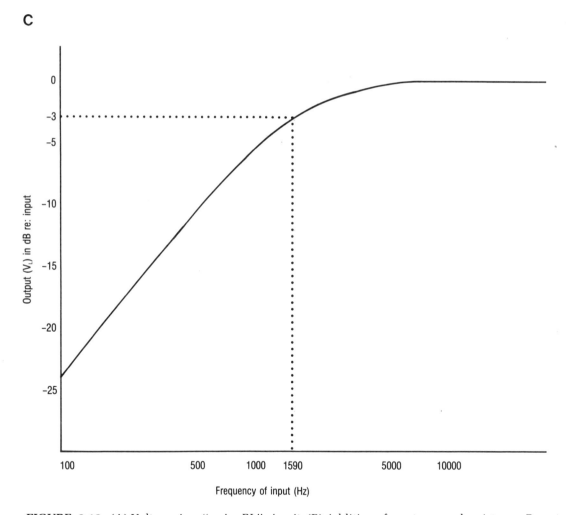

FIGURE 2-10. (A) Voltages in a "series RL" circuit. (B) Addition of reactance and resistance. Because of the 90° phase shift the R and X_L vectors are perpendicular, and the net sum of the two is the hypotenuse (Z) of a triangle. The net phase shift of the circuit is the angle θ. (C) Voltage (in dB) across the inductor in the RL circuit. Low frequency sine waves are attenuated. The cutoff frequency is defined as that frequency where the output amplitude is 3 dB below the input amplitude. The cutoff frequency in this example is about 1590 Hz.

decreased

23

For the specific example of Figure 2-10, the impedance is

$$Z = \sqrt{1000^2 + 628.3^2}$$
$$= 1181\Omega.$$

Although it is sometimes necessary, most clinicians will not have to calculate the impedances of circuits. What they will have to remember, however, is the important effect of frequency in determining the "equivalent resistance" of a circuit that contains a reactance, and the fact that there is a phase shift present.

FILTERING. The fact that the reactance of an inductor increases with the frequency of the applied signal makes the circuit of Figure 2-10 very useful. Analyzing the circuit as a voltage divider (but taking account of the phase shift by using vector addition), it turns out that, when the applied signal is 1000 Hz at 10 V, the amplitude of the sine wave as it appears across the inductor is about 5.3 V. If the frequency of the signal is increased to 1400 Hz, the reactance of the inductor increases. Therefore, the voltage divider is different, and the signal across the inductor increases to 6.6 V. With an input of 2500 Hz the signal across the inductor is 8.4 V, for 5000 Hz it is 9.5 V. If a graph (Table 2-4) is prepared to show the voltage across the inductor as a function of the input frequency, the curve will look like the one in Figure 2-10C. This curve describes the "transfer function" of the circuit. lt shows that, below a certain point, the circuit discriminates against low frequencies. That is, when taking the output across the inductor, the lower the frequency, the less the output. The circuit is a *high-pass filter* that attenuates all frequencies below a certain "cutoff" frequency (f_{co}). That *cutoff* is defined as the frequency at which the output is 3 dB less than the input. (Hence, the cutoff frequency is commonly known as the "3 dB-down" point.) If the output of the circuit were to be taken across the resistor, then the observed wave would grow smaller as the frequency increased. This configuration is called a *low pass filter.*

Filters, (of the inductive type just discussed or of the capacitive variety, yet to be considered) are extremely useful for removing unwanted components of complex signals. For example, a high-pass filter with a cutoff of, say, 90 Hz could be used to remove unwanted hum from a speech recording. A low-pass filter could be used to eliminate high-frequency noise in a data signal. Filter circuits are very common in all kinds of instrumentation.

A NOTE ON FILTERING. The fact that filtering circuits are almost ubiquitous presents a problem that may seem esoteric and unimportant, but can seriously affect the validity of data signals. The trouble derives from the fact that the phase shift created by a filter changes quite a bit with frequency. Recalling that all complex periodic signals (such as speech) are composed of sine waves of different frequencies, it should be apparent how a speech signal might be seriously distorted by the presence of reactance in a circuit (such as a tape recorder amplifier) that processes the signal. Figure 2-11, for example, shows the vowel /a/ as transduced by a microphone lower trace), and as it appears across the resistor of a RL circuit such as the one we have been discussing. The cutoff frequency of the filter circuit was about 400 Hz. The distortion of the /a/ waveform is due to the progressive attenuation of frequencies above the cutoff and to the different phase shifts of the different frequency components.

Mutual inductance and transformers

The changing magnetic field that surrounds an inductor can induce a current in any conductor that lies within it. If a second inductive coil is placed near one that is carrying an alternating current, a current will be induced in it. The current induced in the second coil, however, produces its own magnetic field, and this affects the first coil. Thus, the coils influence each other. This situation is referred

TABLE 2-4. Parameters for the Circuit of Figure 2-10 as a Function of Frequency

f	X_L	Z	V_R		V_L		PHASE ANGLE
Hz	ohms	ohms	volts	dB	volts	dB	degrees
100	62.83	1001.97	9.98	−0.02	0.63	−24.01	3.59
200	125.66	1007.86	9.92	−0.07	1.25	−18.06	7.16
300	188.50	1017.61	9.83	−0.15	1.85	−14.66	10.67
500	314.16	1048.19	9.54	−0.41	3.00	−10.46	17.44
700	439.82	1092.45	9.15	−0.77	4.03	−7.98	23.74
1000	628.32	1181.01	8.47	−1.44	5.32	−5.48	32.14
1200	753.98	1252.39	7.98	−1.96	6.02	−4.41	37.02
1300	816.81	1291.19	7.74	−2.23	6.33	−3.97	39.24
1400	879.65	1331.83	7.51	−2.49	6.60	−3.61	41.33
1500	942.48	1374.14	7.28	−2.76	6.86	−3.27	43.30
1590	999.00	1413.52	7.07	−3.01	7.07	−3.01	44.97
1600	1005.31	1417.97	7.05	−3.04	7.09	−2.99	45.14
1650	1036.73	1440.42	6.94	−3.17	7.20	−2.85	46.03
1700	1068.14	1463.19	6.83	−3.31	7.30	−2.73	46.88
1800	1130.97	1509.67	6.62	−3.58	7.49	−2.51	48.52
2000	1256.64	1605.97	6.23	−4.11	7.82	−2.14	51.49
2100	1319.47	1655.60	6.04	−4.38	7.97	−1.97	52.84
2500	1570.80	1862.10	5.37	−5.40	8.44	−1.47	57.52
3000	1884.96	2133.79	4.69	−6.58	8.83	−1.08	62.05
4000	2513.27	2704.91	3.70	−8.64	9.29	−0.64	68.30
5000	3141.59	3296.91	3.03	−10.37	9.53	−0.42	72.34
7000	4398.23	4510.48	2.22	−13.07	9.75	−0.22	77.20
10000	6283.18	6362.26	1.57	−16.08	9.88	−0.10	80.96

X_L = $2\pi fL$ (inductive reactance).
Z = $\sqrt{R^2 + X_L^2}$ (impedance).
V_R = Voltage across resistor.
V_L = Voltage across inductor.
dB = voltage level re: $10V_{RMS}$ (source voltage).

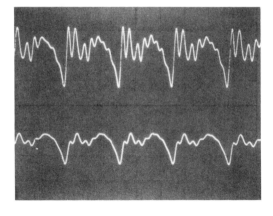

FIGURE 2-11. Waveform of sustained /a/ as actually produced (upper trace) and after passage through a 400 Hz low-pass filter.

to as *mutual inductance*. Mutual inductance can be used to transfer electrical power from one circuit to another in a device called a *transformer*, illustrated in Figure 2-12. The two inductor coils are wound on a single form. The one carrying the input signal is called the primary coil, while the one in which a current is induced is designated the secondary coil. All other things being equal, the relationship between the applied and induced voltages is a function of the ratio of the number of turns in the two coils. If, for example, the primary coil has 10 turns of wire and the secondary has 20 turns, the voltage induced across the secondary coil will be twice the voltage applied to the primary. In other words, the

A

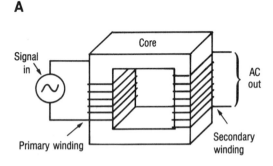

B

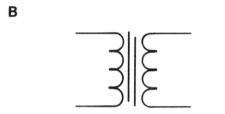

FIGURE 2-12. (A) A transformer and (B) its schematic symbol.

voltage output can be determined from the "turns ratio": $N_{secondary}/N_{primary}$, where N is the number of turns in the coil. The voltage across the secondary coil ($V_{secondary}$) is simply

$$V_{secondary} = V_{primary} (N_{secondary}/N_{primary}).$$

If the secondary coil has more turns that the primary ($N_{secondary}/N_{primary} > 1$) the output voltage is greater than the input and the transformer is of the "step up" type. Fewer turns in the secondary than in the primary coil ($N_{secondary}/N_{primary} < 1$) results in a "step down" transformer whose output voltage is less than the input voltage. When both coils have the same number of turns the output and input voltages are the same.

Transformers serve many functions. Obviously they are useful for converting AC voltages to the levels needed for circuit operation. For example, most modern instruments are designed to operate on 5 to 20 V DC. Yet the standard wall outlet in the United States provides about 120 V AC. The voltage mismatch is almost always resolved by a transformer in the power supply that is built into a given

instrument. (How the AC is converted to DC is discussed later.) It is not uncommon for a single device to require several different operating voltages. An oscilloscope, for instance, needs low voltages for its amplifier circuits but several hundred volts for its display tube. Different voltages can be obtained from a transformer with several secondary coils, each having an appropriate number of turns.

Only the *changes* in primary coil current can induce a current in the secondary coil. If an AC signal having a DC bias is applied to the primary, only the changing (AC) portion of the signal will be effective in producing a voltage in the secondary coil. The output of the transformer in such a situation will be the primary coil input without the DC bias. Hence, transformers also see service as "DC blockers."

Finally, because there is no direct electrical connection between the primary and secondary coils, transformers are often used to isolate devices from the main power supply, particularly in cases where instrumentation makes physical contact with a patient. In electrolaryngography, for instance, a very weak current must be passed through the neck (see Chap. 6). The presence of transformers at appropriate points in the electrolaryngograph circuit ensures that the neck-current supply is in no way connected to the wall outlet. If the very worst happened, and something went catastrophically wrong with the instrument, the patient would be protected from the large current capability of the wall outlet by the isolation provided by the transformers.

CAPACITANCE

A *capacitor* stores electrons. It is constructed of two metalic plates that face each other but are separated by a very thin layer of insulating material (called the *dielectric*) as shown in Figure 2-13. When the plates are connected to a DC voltage, electrons flow until their packing into the dielectric under one plate becomes dense

A

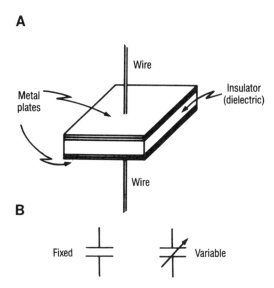

B

Fixed ⊣⊢   ⊣⊬ Variable

FIGURE 2-13 The capacitor. A. Construction B. Schematic symbol

enough to produce a voltage that equals that of the driving voltage. The accumulation of electrons near one plate causes electrons near the opposing plate to be driven away (since like charges repel) They are pushed to the other pole of the DC source. During the period when electrons are being packed into one region and driven away from the facing region of the dielectric, there is an electron flow (current) in both of the wires connecting the capacitor to the DC source. (Note, however, that the electrons do not cross the insulating barrier in the capacitor.) Shortly after the capacitor has been connected to the source, the applied DC voltage will have caused as many electrons to be packed into the dielectric as it can hold. If the capacitor is then disconnected from the voltage supply, the electrons remain in the dielectric, leaving the plates charged to the same voltage as the original driving source.

The unit of capacitance (C) is the *farad* (F). It describes how many electrons can be stored under the plate per volt of packing pressure. That is, *capacitance* is a measure of the storage ability of the capacitor. Capacitance increases with the area of the metal plates. (Obviously, increasing the size of the plates increases the electron storage area, allowing more electrons to be packed in.) Capacitance can also be increased by making the insulating layer between the metal plates thinner. This allows the electrons on one side of the dielectric to repel more effectively electrons from the other side. In practice, the "plates" take many forms—foil or metallic coatings, for example—while the dielectric can be paper, ceramic, mica, air, or a layer of metal oxide. The three layers are usually rolled up or molded to occupy the smallest possible volume.

The fact that storage occurs implies that a capacitor will have reactance. While that reactance is similar to the reactance of an inductor, the different storage mechanism implies different reactance characteristics. In a capacitor the reactance *decreases* as the frequency increases. That is, as the rate of change of the voltage applied to the capacitor increases, the capacitor has an easier time passing it through. A steady state (DC) voltage, however, is totally blocked. To a DC signal the capacitor seems to be an insulator. The energy storage that occurs in the capacitor introduces a phase-shift of 90° between the voltage across the capacitor and the current flowing into it. In the capacitor, however, the current leads the voltage; whereas in the inductor, the voltage leads the current. In many ways, a capacitor can be viewed as an inverse inductor.

The capacitor's frequency-dependent reactance allows the construction of simple filter circuits, analogous to those using inductors, as shown in Figure 2-14. Again, values have been assigned to R (1000 Ω) and

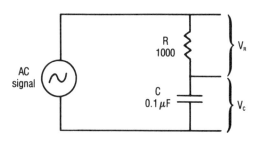

FIGURE 2-14. A simple RC filter circuit.

C (0.1 microfarad) for the sake of this example. As was the case for the inductive filter, this circuit can be analyzed as a kind of frequency-dependent voltage divider. As the frequency of the input increases, the reactance (equivalent resistance) of the capacitor falls, while the resistance of the resistor remains fixed. Therefore, as the frequency rises, the ratio of R to X_C rises, and less and less voltage appears across the capacitor. Therefore, the higher the frequency of the input, the less signal appears at the output. The circuit discriminates against high frequency, and so it is a low-pass filter. The cutoff point of the filter is defined just as it was for the inductive filter seen earlier: It is the frequency at which the amplitude of the output is 3 dB less than the amplitude of the input. Also like the inductive filter, if the output is taken across

the resistor then the circuit behaves as a high-pass filter.

Band-Pass and Band-Reject Filters

What happens if the output of a high-pass filter is used as the input to a low-pass filter, as shown in Figure 2-15A? The components in the two filters have been chosen so that the cutoff frequency of the high-pass circuit is about 2000 Hz while that of the low-pass section is about 8000 Hz. The transfer function of this circuit is shown in Figure 2-15B. The high-pass section discriminates against any frequency below its 2 kHz cutoff and the low-pass section attenuates signals above 8 kHz. The only signals that will escape attenuation are those that lie in the "pass-band" between the two cutoff frequencies.

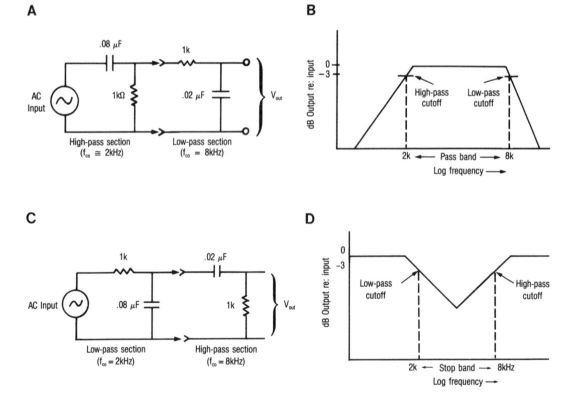

FIGURE 2-15. Band-pass and band-reject filters. (A) High-pass and low-pass RC sections (B) Tansfer function of the filter in A. C. "Reversed" version of the circuit in A. D. Transfer function of the "reversed" circuit.

Hence this circuit (and any other that behaves like it) is called a *band-pass filter*.* (Such a circuit might be useful for transmitting the fricative noise of /v/ or /z/ while suppressing the voicing component.)

What if the cutoff frequencies had been reversed? That is, what would be the result if f_{co} for the *high-pass* section were 8 kHz while f_{co} for the low-pass portion were set at 2 kHz? This is easily arranged by inverting the circuit, as in Figure 2-15C. The low-pass section now attenuates frequencies above 2 kHz and the high-pass portion rejects those below 8 kHz. Therefore any signal between the two cutoffs is rejected. This type of circuit is called a *band-stop* or *band-reject* filter. It is often used to eliminate unwanted components (such as 60 Hz hum from power-line interference) from signals.

Resonant Circuits

Suppose that R, L, and C are all combined in a series circuit, like the one shown in Figure 2-16. What is the transfer function like? Because capacitive reactance (X_C) decreases with frequency, while inductive reactance (X_L) increases with frequency, there will be one frequency at which $X_C = X_L$. When the reactances are equal the phase shifts produced by L and C are equal in magnitude. However, the shifts are of opposite sign, since current leads voltage for the capacitor but lags behind voltage in the inductor. Therefore, when the reactances of L and C are equal they exactly cancel each other and the net reactance of the circuit is zero. The only remaining obstruction to current (that is, the only component of the impedance of the circuit) is the series resistance, R. Therefore, when $X_L = X_C$ circuit impedance is minimized, current is greatest, and the voltage across either of the reactive elements,

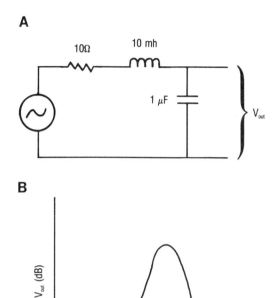

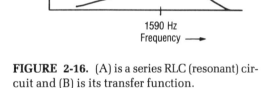

FIGURE 2-16. (A) is a series RLC (resonant) circuit and (B) is its transfer function.

C or L, is maximal. The circuit is said to be *resonant* at the frequency for which $X_C = X_L$. The output of the circuit is illustrated in Figure 2-16B. It happens that the resonant frequency of the circuit of Figure 2-16 is 1590 Hz. At this frequency $X_L = X_C \doteq 100 \, \Omega$.

When L and C are connected in parallel, as in Figure 2-17A, a similar situation prevails. At one single frequency X_L equals X_C. Since, at that frequency, the phase shifts are equal but opposite, L is always storing energy when C is losing it and vice versa. The two components trade electrical energy back and forth in perfect synchrony. At the resonant frequency the impedance of the circuit is maximal, and thus the output voltage of the circuit is maximized (Figure 2-17B). The circuit is a resonant band-pass filter. (If the output were taken across the resistor a band-stop filter would result.)

---

*Obviously such a filter could also be built with inductors. But capacitive circuits are much more common because capacitors are easier to work with.

A

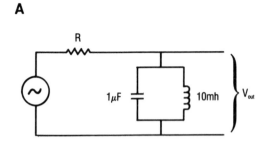

B

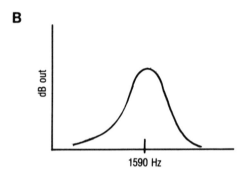

C

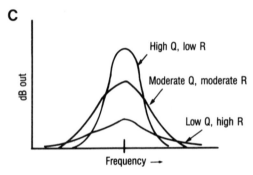

FIGURE 2-17. Parallel LC circuit (A) and its transfer function (B). C. shows the effect of increasing the value of R, resulting in lower Q.

BANDWIDTH AND Q. The sharpness of the peak in the transfer function of a resonant circuit is measured by Q. It is defined as the ratio of the reactance at resonance to the series resistance in the circuit:

$$Q = X/R.$$

The greater the value of Q the narrower the resonant peak, as illustrated in Figure 2-17C. The bandwidth of a resonant circuit (its pass-band) is defined as the difference between the two points on the transfer-function curve at which the output amplitude is 3 dB less than maximal. As Q

increases the bandwidth is reduced and the resonant circuit is said to be more sharply tuned. Filter sharpness and its consequences are important in many ways, not the least of which is in deciding on the proper filter setup for sound spectrography (see Chap. 9).

Loading and Impedance Matching

In all of the circuits considered so far it has been tacitly assumed that connecting a measuring device (such as a voltmeter or oscilloscope) to the circuit output has no effect on circuit function. This is not really the case. Some current flows out of the circuit to any device that is connected to it. Therefore, anything connected to the circuit output behaves like an impedance in parallel with it. This has important implications in instrumentation.

Consider, for example, a situation that is extremely common in speech pathology. The clinician wants to observe a client's vocal waveform and so connects a microphone to an amplifier and then connects an oscilloscope to the amplifier output, as diagrammed in Figure 2-18. But at its output the amplifier has a series capacitor whose function is to block any DC bias that the amplifier might create from being transferred to the next instrument.

Now, the signal from the amplifier is not merely applied to the oscilloscope. A certain amount of signal current actually flows into it. That is, the amplifier "sees" the oscilloscope's input connection as a parallel resistor. Therefore, we can show the oscilloscope as a "load resistor" (R_L) connected to the amplifier. Notice that, viewed in this way, the capacitor in the amplifier and the load resistor of the oscilloscope form a capacitative high-pass filter. Recalling that the cutoff frequency of a filter is the one at which the capacitive reactance (X_C) is the same as the resistance (R_L) and remembering too that X_C rises as frequency decreases, it is clear that the cutoff frequency of the transmission filter must be high if the oscilloscope allows a lot of current to flow

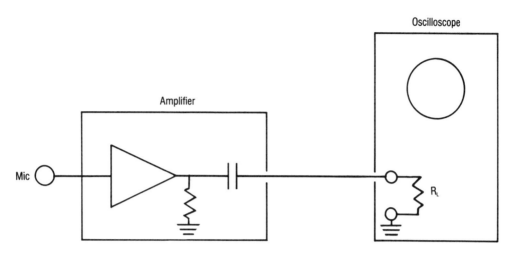

FIGURE 2-18. Effect of load resistance. Note that the capacitance at the output of the amplifier and the internal "load" resistance (R_L) of the oscilloscope form a high-pass filter. As R_L decreases the cutoff frequency of this filter increases, causing greater distortion of the signals.

from the amplifier (i.e., if R_L is small). As the input impedance of the oscilloscope gets less, more low-frequency components in the complex signal coming from the amplifier are attenuated and lost to the oscilloscope, which will therefore show an increasingly distorted version of the speech signal. Clearly, in situations such as this one, the higher the input impedance of the oscilloscope the better. Loading can also have very serious consequences for the fidelity of microphones, a problem that is discussed in Chap. 3.

Distortion of the signal is perhaps the most serious consequence of connecting an inappropriate impedance to a circuit's output, but it is certainly not the only deleterious consequence. Consider the situation diagrammed in Figure 2-19. A voltage divider has been designed to deliver 5 V from a 10 V source, as shown. To verify that the circuit is correctly designed and connected, it is tested by connecting a voltmeter across R_2. Now, the voltmeter draws current, which is to say that it has an internal resistance (R_m). When it is connected across R_2 the voltage-divider circuit is changed because it now consists of R_1 and the parallel sum of R_2 and R_m. If the voltmeter is a good one R_m will be very large,

say 250 k Ω. A bit of calculation shows that the parallel combination of $R_2 = 5k\ \Omega$ and $R_m = 250k\ \Omega$ is 4902 Ω. So connection of the voltmeter in this case changes the voltage divider to the equivalent of 5 k Ω and 4902 Ω in series. The voltage across the modified R_2 will be 4.95 V, which is what the meter will read. While less than the voltage divider's theoretical output of 5.00 V, this is not a bad estimate. However, if a cheap voltmeter were used, one with a very low R_m of, say, 10 k Ω, the $R_2 + R_m$ combination becomes only 3333 Ω, and the meter will read only 4.00 V. In short, the "loading" by the meter has reduced the output of the voltage divider by 20%. In this situation one might be tempted to believe that there was something wrong with the voltage divider, when the problem actually lies with the inadequate resistance of the voltmeter.

The lesson in all of this is that the input impedance of one circuit must be suitable in terms of the output impedance of the device to which it will be connected. (Any standard textbook of electronics will provide guidance about determining "suitability.") The input and output impedances of the instruments that the clinician will use are usually clearly indicated on the

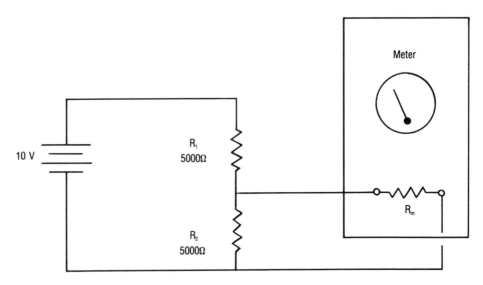

FIGURE 2-19. Loading of a voltage divider by a meter. The meter's internal resistance (R_M) is connected in parallel with R_2 of the voltage divider, changing its net value. If R_M is very large the change is negligible, but a small value of R_M will seriously alter the voltage divider's characteristics.

devices themselves or in their operating manuals. This information should be used when setting up equipment arrays.

SEMICONDUCTOR DEVICES

There are some substances whose inherent properties make them fall somewhere near the middle of the insulator-conductor continuum. Such materials, called *semiconductors*, are the foundation of the miniaturization revolution in electronics. Silicon (Si) and germanium (Ge) are the most common semiconductors. After small amounts of "dopant" substances (such as gallium or arsenic) are added, the electrical properties of crystals of these elements can be changed in a known way by varying the voltage applied to them. This is the basis of the transistor and all the devices related to it. The physics of semiconductors, which rests on quantum theory, is far too complex for consideration here, although adequate discussions can be found in most basic electronics textbooks. For the present purposes it will be sufficient to accept on faith that these devices perform as described.

Diodes

Diodes (Figure 2-20) behave as good conductors when current flows in one direction (when they are said to be *forward biased*), but they act as insulators when the current reverses (and they are *reverse biased*). That is, they are electrical one-way valves. This is an extremely useful property and finds widespread use for "rectification." Consider the circuit shown in Figure 2-20B, in which a diode is wired in series with a resistor to a sine-wave generator. During one alternation of the sine wave the current will flow in the direction indicated by the solid line. The diode is a good conductor of current in this direction, and hence presents very little resistance — certainly less than the 10 k Ωof the resistor. Consequently, most of the voltage drop in the resistor-diode "voltage divider" occurs across the resistor. By monitoring the output across the resistor, as shown, the postive alternation of the sine wave will be detected. During the sine wave's negative alternation the current goes the other way, in the direction indicated by the dashed line. The diode is a very poor conductor in this direction and behaves as a

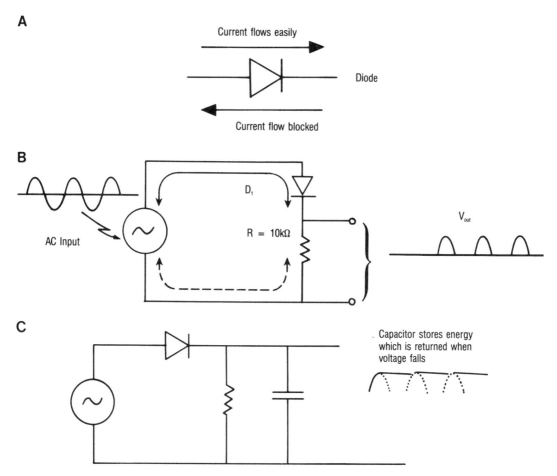

FIGURE 2-20. The diode. (A) Symbol and current characteristics. (B) Half-wave rectifier. The diode functions much like a resistance whose value depends on the direction of the current. (C) Using a "filter capacitor" to store charge and reduce ripple at the rectifier's output.

very large resistance—much greater than 10 k Ω. Therefore, most of the voltage drop during the negative alternation will occur across the diode itself, with very little observable across the resistor. Monitoring the output across the resistor indicates almost no voltage during a negative alternation. When the current again reverses, the voltage will appear mostly across the resistor. The diode-resistor circuit, known as a *half-wave rectifier*, has converted the bidirectional AC into a unidirectional flow of half sine-waves, sometimes called *pulsating DC*.

Usually a half wave rectifier, like the one in Figure 2-20B, is terminated with a capacitor, as shown in Figure 2-20C. The capacitor creates a low-pass filter. It stores energy during the voltage peaks and returns it when the voltage falls. The DC pulses are averaged out, or smoothed. Except for some residual ripple, the original AC signal has been converted to DC.* This is obviously useful in deriving the DC needed to power instruments from the AC supplied at the wall outlet. Rectification is also the basis of deriving information from an amplitude-modulated wave and so is an important function of carrier amplifiers (see Chap. 3).

---

*There are many more sophisticated circuits that perform rectification more efficiently or with less residual ripple. Consult any electronics text for details.

Transistors

Since its invention in the 1940s the transistor has almost completely replaced the vacuum tube as an amplifying element. A host of related semiconductor devices has since evolved to meet special needs. Among them are FETs, MOSFETs, thyristors, SCRs, VMOS, and many others, with new ones constantly appearing on the market. It is patently impossible to consider all of these here. The description that follows will be limited to the "bipolar" transistor, which is the classic type, the one originally developed at Bell Telephone Laboratories that ushered in the transistor era. Even for this single type, our discussion will have to be a very superficial one.

Transistors are made of semiconductor elements, usually silicon or germanium. By the addition of impurities to crystals of these metals they can be made into conductors of either electrons (N-type semiconductor) or positive charges (P-type semiconductor). A transistor is constructed by making a sandwich of these two types of "doped" semiconductor, as shown in Figure 2-21. Depending on what kind of material is in the center of the sandwich, a transistor is of either the NPN or PNP type. A connecting wire is connected to each layer in the sandwich. The layers are designated the emitter (e), the base (b), and the collector (c).

A junction of P and N material forms a diode. The bipolar transistor has two such junctions and, therefore, can be represented (Figure 2-21C) as two diodes connected back-to-back. The device can be wired to voltage sources, as shown for the diode model of an NPN transistor in Figure 2-21D, to provide amplification. (The very same wiring would work for a PNP transistor if the polarity of the batteries were reversed.) When connected, as shown, to the power supply, the collector diode is reverse biased so that it behaves as a very poor conductor. Hence, very little current flows through it from the power supply. The emitter diode is forward biased and creates a path for current from the base if, and only if, there is enough voltage there to push the current through a slight inherent electronic barrier. A small "bias" voltage is applied to the base to insure that current can always flow through the base-emitter pathway. The signal to be amplified (V_{in}) is also applied to the base, so that the current injected into the base of the transistor is the combined bias current and signal current. Now it turns out that a current flow into the base alters the conduction properties of the collector-base junction. That is, the diode representing the collector is no longer as reverse-biased as it was in the absence of a base current. (This is one of the phenomena that must be taken on faith in this discussion.) Therefore, within certain limits, the greater the current injected into the base, the more conductive the collector-emitter pathway becomes for current coming from the power supply. The greater the current in the collector, the greater the voltage drop produced by the resistor (R_c) in the collector line. This voltage can be tapped as shown. The current in the collector-emitter path is much greater than the current flowing into the base. The voltage drop across the collector resistor is, therefore, a much larger version of the base voltage. In short, amplification is achieved.

In the circuit shown there are two current paths: signal(+ bias) current flows through the base-emitter loop, while output current travels via the collector and emitter. The emitter is shared by both currents, which is why this configuration is known as a *common emitter* circuit. Other arrangements (common base and common collector) are possible and see service in special situations. Somewhat more detailed consideration of amplifiers (and a few of the problems that must be addressed in designing practical circuits) is provided in Chap. 3.

Integrated circuits

By adding appropriate impurities to it, the silicon that makes transistors can also be used to create resistors, diodes, and even

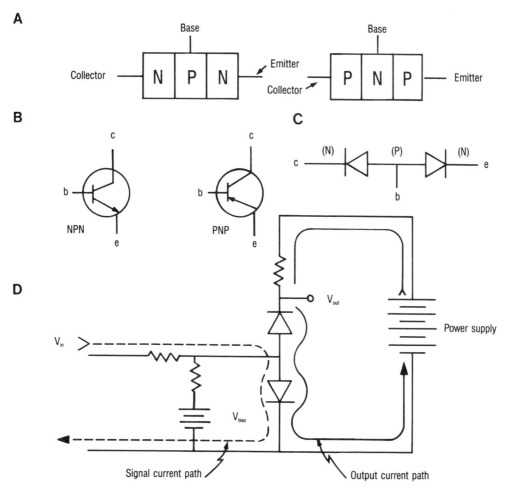

FIGURE 2-21. Transistors. (A) Three layer, two junction structure. (B) Standard schematic symbols. (C) An NPN transistor considered as back-to-back diodes. (D) Diode model of a very simple transistor circuit.

capacitors. Hence it is possible, by carefully controlling where different impurities are deposited, to create transistors and all the other elements of a fully functional circuit on a single piece of silicon crystal. Such a circuit then is monolithic (literally, made of a single stone) and integrated. Modern techniques of photoreproduction have made it possible to make such integrated circuits (ICs) very small indeed, packing thousands of transistors and other necessary support components into an area of a few tenths of a square inch. The IC "chip" is housed in a case (Figure 2-22) to facilitate handling, and the result is a complete plug-in circuit. There are literally thousands of different ICs

available: memories, microcomputer processors, audio amplifiers, complete instrumentation amplifiers, and so on. Because they are produced by automated processes in very large quantities their cost is almost always very low. The variety is staggering, and more appear each week. The importance of this lies in the fact that complete instrumentation systems can now be constructed with very little need for highly developed engineering skills. Even the neophyte, once he or she has chosen the appropriate ICs, can assemble complex electronic systems that are not only better than much of what was available in the "old days" of discrete components,

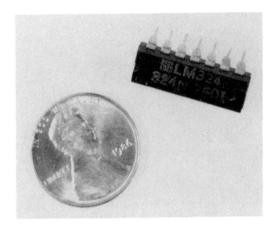

FIGURE 2-22. An integrated circuit, in its package. This particular integrated circuit has four complete operational amplifiers in it.

but are very much cheaper as well. Speech pathologists should make an effort to familiarize themselves with the range of ICs available and to experiment with using them as building blocks in circuits they need.

DIGITAL CIRCUITS

Analog and Digital Electronics

All electronic circuits fall into two broad categories: analog and digital. In *analog* circuits some electrical characteristic (often the voltage or the current) represents the information being processed. For example, the voltage produced by a pressure gauge is *analogous* to the air pressure that the gauge is sensing. Devices, such as the amplifier that follows the pressure gauge or the pen recorder that produces a written record of the pressure, operate on this voltage analog. The flow of information through the system is in the form of an "analogy" which implicitly says (at least in this case) "let this amount of voltage represent the air pressure that the gauge is sensing at this instant in time." Even the final output, the curve traced by a recording pen on a sheet of paper, is an analog of the pressure. It says

"the height of this tracing above the zero line is analogous to the amount of pressure that the gauge sensed."

Digital instruments have recently become much more common. They handle information as discrete numbers, coded in a way that fairly simple circuits can deal with. Usually the format is binary: numbers are expressed to the base 2. The only binary digits (usually called *bits*) are 0 and 1. They can be represented by the presence of an electrical voltage ($=1$) or its absence ($=0$). In other words, "on" $=1$, "off" $=0$. Without exception, any number can be represented to the base 2 by a series of 1s and 0s. Thirty five, for example, is binary 100011, while 255 is binary 11111111. The output of a pressure gauge (to continue with the earlier example) could be sampled at very brief intervals, and its output over time expressed as a series of binary numbers. (This process is called *analog-to-digital conversion.*) The binary numbers could then be arithmetically manipulated to produce, let us say, a series of numbers representing the rate of change of the pressure. The data could be displayed on a digital meter or fed to a computer (which is a digital arithmetic processor).

The proliferation of digital clocks in the past few years has made the differences between analog and digital systems obvious to everyone. On the standard (old fashioned) wall clock the position of the hands is an analog of the time. Each hand moves continuously around the circumference of the clock face and, therefore, it is possible to read *any* time. For example, if the second hand is between two markings at a given instant, a fairly good estimate can be made of the fraction of a second represented. In digital systems continuity is not the case. A digital time display that reads 12:05:42 is very difinite about what time it is—up to a point. The fraction of a second is not shown and there is no way of estimating what it might be. Digital systems provide a very unambiguous display of information with no need for the user to estimate intermediate values. Analog systems are less definite and somewhat harder to read, but they often present more information.

Despite the growing popularity of digital systems, most of the instrumentation that the speech pathologist will encounter will be analog. Even in those systems that use digital methods an analog stage will be required to sense the variable of interest (pressure, flow, acoustic wave) and generate a signal that can be converted to digital form. Still, some knowledge of the basic concepts of digital circuitry is increasingly important.

In digital circuits voltages represent discrete numerical values rather than analogs of an input signal. Most commonly there are only two digits in the number system, 0 and 1. Such a system is said to be *binary*. The two digits correspond to "on" and "off", or, in a transistor, conducting maximally (*saturation*) or not at all (*cutoff*). In digital applications the transistors really serve as electronically operated switches, and we can represent them that way in order to see how digital logic operates.

Figure 2-23A shows two switches (representing transistors) wired in series with a power supply and a light bulb. When both switches are open (=off) the light obviously must be off. If switch A is closed (=on) but switch B remains off, then the light bulb still remains off. Likewise, if switch B is on, but A remains off, the light stays off. For the light to go on switch A

and switch B must be closed. In the terminology of digital electronics, the series switches form an *AND gate*, because "light on" requires that A *and* B be on.

In Figure 2-23B the circuit is redrawn with transistors replacing the switches. The transistor-switches, of course, can be "closed" (turned on) by voltages applied to their bases. If we let the digit 1 represent a voltage, while 0 is taken to mean no voltage, then we can set up a formal tabular description of how this AND gate works. Known as a *truth table*, such a description for an AND gate looks like this:

Truth Table for an AND gate

Input A	Input B	Output (Lamp)
0	0	0
1	0	0
0	1	0
1	1	1

Other logical arrangements of switches (transistors) are possible. Let us consider one more, the switching circuit of Figure 2-24A (switch version) and 2-24B (transistor version). In this case when switch A is closed (transistor A conducting) the light will go on. Similarly, closing switch B (activating transistor B) also allows the light to turn on and so does closing both switches. In this circuit activating A or B completes

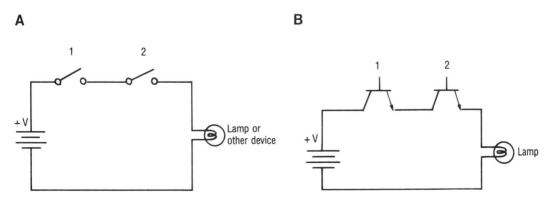

FIGURE 2-23. AND gate implemented with switches (A) and transistors (B).

A

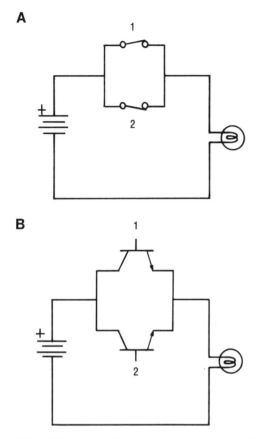

B

FIGURE 2-24. OR gate implemented with switches (A) and transistors (B).

the circuit. Hence, this is an OR *gate"* The truth table for this OR gate is

Input A	Input B	Output (Lamp)
0	0	0
1	0	1
0	1	1
1	1	1

(In this particular logic circuit an output is obtained when either A or B, or A and B are activated. There are other OR gates, designated *exclusive* OR (XOR) that produce an output when A or B but not both are activated. It is easier to produce such a

gate with transistors than to show it with switches.)

Before proceeding to other types of logical gates, it seems useful to pause and ask "So what?" The fact is, the gates can be said to be making decisions. The AND gate decides that if "A" and "B" are both happening, then a light will be turned on. A very simple example shows how even so easy a decision could be used clinically. Imagine that a client (perhaps hearing impaired) has trouble with voiced fricatives. A microphone and amplifier system could be used to monitor the client's speech. Two filters (see section entitled "Band-Pass and Band-Reject Filters) could be put at the amplifier output: a low-pass filter to pass only the vocal fundamental frequency, and a band-pass filter to transmit only those high-frequency components that indicate fricative production (see Chap. 9, Sound Spectrography). Now when both filters generate an output, a voiced fricative is being produced. If the filter outputs (after some simple electrical modification) are applied to an AND gate the light will go on whenever a voiced fricative is produced, providing client feedback. The system could be used with suitably constructed therapy materials for unsupervised client practice.

Many other logic gates are in everyday use. They are available as integrated circuits that have been standardized so that they need only be connected to each other to form arrays that can handle very complex logical processes. A few of the simpler digital logic circuits are summarized in Figure 2-25.

Although the specific circuits that are involved cannot be explored here, it is possible to arrange logic gates to perform addition and subtraction of numbers represented by binary digits (bits), that is, of numbers expressed to the base 2. Logic gates and transistor memory circuits are the components of digital computers. In the next few years they promise to revolutionize clinical speech pathology in much the same way as they have already dramatically changed so many other fields.

FIGURE 2-25. Digital logic gates.

Schematic Symbol	Truth Table

Buffer

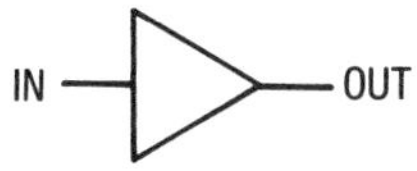

In	Out
1	1
0	0

Not or Invert

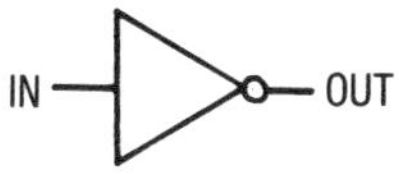

In	Out
1	0
0	1

Or

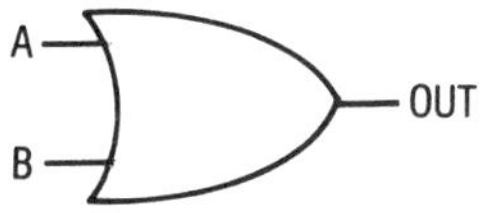

A	B	Out
0	0	0
0	1	1
1	0	1
1	1	1

Nor

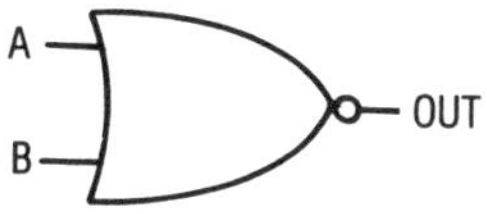

A	B	Out
0	0	1
0	1	0
1	0	0
1	1	0

3-input Or

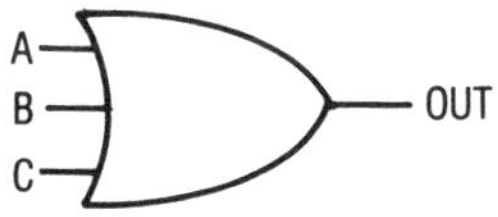

A	B	C	Out
0	0	0	0
	all other combinations		1

Exclusive Or (XOR)

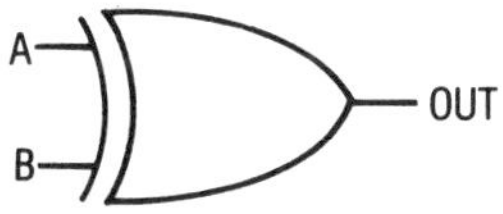

A	B	Out
0	0	0
1	0	1
0	1	1
1	1	0

And

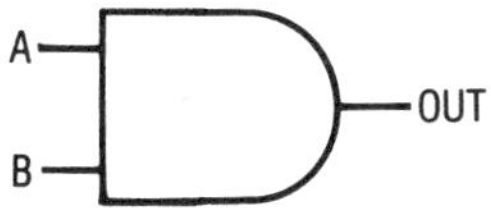

A	B	Out
0	0	0
0	1	0
1	0	0
1	1	1

Nand

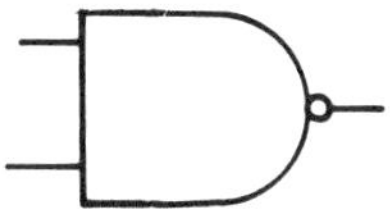

A	B	Out
0	0	1
0	1	1
1	0	1
1	1	0

ELECTRICAL SAFETY

At some time or other, everyone has suffered an electric shock. We all know from experience that electricity can be unpleasant. And reports of people who were accidentally electrocuted occassionally appear in newspapers. We are aware that carelessness with current can be lethal. It goes without saying that the instrumentation used by the speech professional should not expose a client to risk. Electrical safety must be a serious professional concern.

To understand where danger lurks and how to eliminate risk it is necessary to understand how the power company delivers its product to us via the electrical "mains" and how we tap into it in our clinics and labs.

The first thing to consider is that the zero reference against which mains voltages are measured is the potential of the earth itself. This is because we, and everything around us, are all connected with the earth and, under normal conditions, we are all at just about the same potential—at least in theory. Also, the earth is an enormous conductor, so big, in fact, that we assume that any amount of current could be injected into it without significantly altering its voltage.

Power is sent out from the utility's generator along three wires, each of which carries current at very high voltage (Figure 2-26). The wires are said to be "hot." A fourth cable at the power plant is attached to a very large metal plate sunk deep in the earth. This true ground connection, the "cold" side of the current-delivery system, will be part of the pathway by which current returns to the generator.

Somewhere between the electric company's cables (under the streets or on poles) and the outlets in our walls is a transformer system. It combines the current on the three cables and reduces their voltage to produce two "hot" lines that feed the building's electrical distribution system. The voltage difference between these two wires is 220 V. A "neutral" wire, connected to the power company ground wire and to another ground just outside the building, travels with the hot wires. Each of the hot wires in our buildings has a voltage of 110 V with respect to the neutral wire. One of the contacts in each outlet in our walls is connected to one of the 110 V wires; the other is connected to the neutral wire.

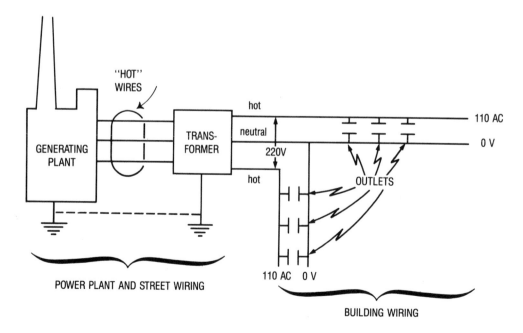

FIGURE 2-26. Electrical power distribution.

It is important to recognize that the "neutral" contact in the outlet is NOT ground. The wire that connects it to true ground can be quite long, and it has a real resistance. Now, electricity flows from the hot side of outlets, through any electrical device that is turned on, and back to ground through the neutral wire. So the neutral line is carrying all of the current being used by all of the active devices (appliances, lightbulbs, whatever) along it. Obviously, this can be quite a bit of current. And Ohm's law states that the current interacts with the neutral wire's resistance to generate a voltage. Therefore, the so-called "neutral" wire can have a voltage significantly above zero.

Now consider a client using a tape recorder in a therapy room. Wires connected to the wall outlet bring power to the recorder. So, inside the instrument there is a hot wire (at 110 V) and a neutral wire, ostensibly at 0 V. The metal framework inside the tape recorder serves as the internal "ground" for the instrument; through it current is returned to the neutral wire which carries the "spent" current back to ground and thence to the power plant.

Something goes wrong inside the tape recorder: the insulation on a wire cracks and suddenly the metal frame is in contact with 110 V. So are the control knobs on top of the tape recorder and maybe even the metal case on the microphone. When the client touches a metal part on the tape recorder current flows through him as it seeks a path to the 0 V of ground. The resistance of the human body is only moderate, but the resistance of furniture, floors, concrete building supports and the like is fairly high. So not much current is likely to flow through the client. He might feel a slight tingle. Bad enough, but if the client happens to be in contact with a relatively low-resistance path to ground (another piece of equipment), then a relatively large current will pass through the client, who may experience quite a jolt. The situation is getting worse. If the pathway to ground is really quite conductive (a radiator pipe), a truly large current flow might result, with terrible consequences! The scenario is not a likely one, but it is certainly possible. How do we guard against it?

The most important way is by connecting a very low-resistance pathway to ground to the exposed parts of all electrical devices. This is why three-prong plugs and outlets are now the rule. The third (round) contact is to a wire that is separately grounded. It does not ordinarily carry any current to speak of, so its voltage really is zero. The exposed parts of electrical devices are connected to this ground lead so that, if anything goes wrong, current finds it very easy to travel to ground through it, sparing people the experience of being unwilling conductors.

If your clinic has the old two-prong electrical outlets, have them changed by an electrician. Never use the three-prong "adapters" if there is any way to avoid them. If you must use them, be very certain that the green (ground) wire on the adapter is in excellent contact with a good ground. And, if you have to use adapters, use the equipment connected through them with extreme caution.

Most equipment is provided with fuses. When too much current is drawn the wire in the fuse melts, opening the circuit and cutting off power to the device. The prime purpose of the fuses is to protect the equipment, but they might also limit the amount of current that can pass through a person accidentally connected to the power line. **Do not substitute larger fuses for the ones specified by the manufacturer.** If the fuse blows, there is likely to be something wrong with the equipment. Have it repaired.

See to it that patients are not in contact with an external low-resistance path to ground. Do not use metal tables, or seat patients near pipes, or have ungrounded outlet boxes within reach.

While it may seem a bit paranoid, the best advice is to trust no one about electrical supplies. Electrical supply stores sell cheap testers that can be plugged into outlets and that indicate if the ground connection is faulty or if the hot and neutral wires have been reversed. Every outlet should be tested and any faults immediately corrected. ∎

SELECT BIBLIOGRAPHY

Brown, P. B., Maxfield, B. W., and Morall, H. *Electronics for Neurobiologists.* Cambridge, MA: MIT Press, 1973.

Buchsbaum, W. H. *Complete Handbook of Practical Electronic Reference Data.* Englewood Cliffs, N.J.: Prentice-Hall, 1973.

Carr, J. J. *CMOS/TTL—A User's Guide with Projects.* Blue Ridge Summit, PA: TAB Books, Inc., 1984.

Diefenderfer, A. J. *Principles of Electronic Instrumentation.* Philadelphia: Saunders, 1972.

Geddes, L. A. and Baker, L. E. *Principles of Applied Biomedical Instrumentation* (Second edition). New York: Wiley, 1975.

Hawkins, H. M. *Concepts of Digital Electronics.* Blue Ridge Summit, PA: TAB Books, Inc., 1983.

Hoenig, S. A. and Payne, F. L. *How to Build and Use Electronic Devices without Frustration, Panic, Mountains of Money, or an Engineering Degree.* Boston: Little, Brown, 1973.

Horn, D. T. *How to Design Op Amp Circuits with Projects and Experiments.* Blue Ridge Summit, PA: TAB Books, Inc. 1984.

Jackson, H. W. *Introduction to Electric Circuits* (4th ed.). Englewood Cliffs, N.J.: Prentice-Hall, 1976.

Kaufman, M. and Seidman, A. H. Eds. *Handbook of Electronics Calculations.* New York: McGraw-Hill, 1979.

Stout, D. F. and Kaufman, M. *Handbook of Operational Amplifier Circuit Design.* New York: McGraw-Hill, 1976.

. . . . and many, many others, available at any academic bookstore.

CHAPTER 3

General-Purpose Tools

There are certain devices that are the workhorses of measurement systems. They tend to be highly versatile and form the core of most instrumentation arrays. Several are essential to many of the measurement procedures a speech pathologist is called upon to do. They are to the speech clinician what hammers and screwdrivers are to a carpenter: indispensible general-purpose tools of the trade. The purpose of this chapter is to consider several such devices in order that clinicians can select intelligently among the varieties available and use them appropriately.

ORGANIZATION OF INSTRUMENT ARRAYS

Before moving to a discussion of instrumentation components, it is useful to consider the way in which any instrumentation system is organized. In a general sense, any measurement system must do at least three things.

1. First, there must be some means of detecting the phenomenon of interest (motion, pressure, airflow, sound pressure) and converting it into a *signal* that is acceptable for electronic processing. Sound waves, for example, will need to be converted to electrical waves before they can be recorded on a tape deck.

2. Then the system must be equipped to manipulate or modify the signal in a controlled and reliable way and to process it, if required, to derive useful information. It is almost always necessary to amplify a signal (make it stronger), but other processing may be needed as well. For instance, it might be necessary to filter the signal to get rid of unwanted components, such as noise.

3. Finally, the electronic signal must be reconverted to a form that can be displayed in a convenient way for evaluation by the user. The signal might be written by a pen writer, or shown on an oscilloscope screen, or converted to a numeric value on a digital indicator.

Almost any instrumentation system will therefore have at least three "stages" of operation. They are diagrammed in Figure 3-1.

A *transducer* converts one form of energy into another. Usually this means translating some phenomenon into an electrical signal. A microphone, for example, converts sound pressure waves into a variable voltage. Hence, a microphone is an "electroacoustic" transducer. Sometimes the transduction is accomplished in more than one stage. In fact, the microphone is really an example of a two-stage process. First the sound pressure is converted to movement of an energy-collecting surface (acoustic-to-mechanical transduction), and then the motion of the energy-collector is converted into an electric signal (mechanical-to-electrical transduction). A microphone thus has a primary transducer (sound-to-motion) and a secondary transducer (motion to voltage). The process by which an instrument interfaces with the physical world is known as *input transduction*.

Modification of the signal from the input transducer is called *signal conditioning*, a general term that conceals a vast number of processing possibilities. Sometimes the signal needs only to be made larger (amplified), but it may be necessary to derive its fundmental frequency, to eliminate some of its parts, to find the average of its peak amplitudes, to compress it, expand it, code it, and so on. All of these processes (and many others) fall under the heading of "signal conditioning."

The results of the instrument's processing are made available via *output transduction*, the process of converting the information from an electrical signal into some form that people can perceive and deal with. Output

transduction is the process by which an instrument communicates its "findings" to us, the users.

AMPLIFIERS

The output of most transducers is very small: Strain gauges produce signals in the microvolt range, microphones only a few millivolts. On the other hand, most display devices require significant voltages or currents. The cathode-ray oscilloscope's display tube needs several volts of input; speaker systems can require currents well in excess of an ampere. In short, most transducers cannot, of themselves, deliver enough power to show us directly what they observe. The discrepancy between what transducers can produce and what display systems demand is resolved by introducing amplification into instrumentation systems. The need is so universal that amplifiers are virtually ubiquitous. It is hard to imagine an electronic device that does not include at least one, and a sophisticated instrument may well have dozens. Aside from those already incorporated into clinical devices, the speech clinician will frequently have occasion to use separate, special-purpose amplifiers for handling audio or physiological signals.

The invention of the transistor, its reduction to nearly microscopic size, and its incorporation into integrated circuits has led to the marketing of hundreds of prefabricated amplifier "building blocks." These blocks permit individuals with only a minimal background in electronics to construct all sorts of special amplifiers to serve their particular needs. Even if one never plans

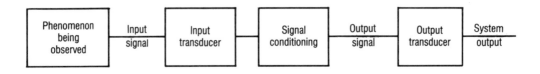

FIGURE 3-1. Components of an instrumentation system.

to actually design and build an amplifier, however, it is vitally important to understand them in order to use them successfully. What amplification is, how it is achieved, and what characterizes the variety of amplifiers among which the professional user must choose are discussed in this section. While not every clinician, and perhaps not even most, will need to master all the details, at least a broad familiarity with what follows is important. The success of most measurement procedures rests, at least in part, on the competent use of amplifying devices.

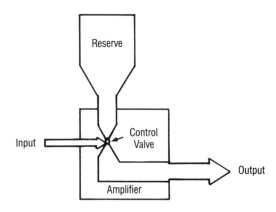

FIGURE 3-2. Conceptual diagram of an amplifier.

Basic Principles of Amplification

Amplification is the process whereby the magnitude of an electrical signal is increased. The increase may be in voltage, current, or both (that is, in power) according to the amplifier design. In fact, it is common to categorize devices as *voltage amplifiers, current amplifiers,* or *power amplifiers* depending on which parameter is augmented. Figure 3-2 provides a conceptual schema of what is involved in achieving this.

The diagram underscores the fact that the signal to be amplified is not, itself, magically enlarged. Rather, the input regulates the flow of power from a reservoir by acting on some sort of control valve. For example, we may assume that the reserve in Figure 3-2 represents a source of large quantities of current. Changes of the input signal, which might be a current of only a milliamp or so, cause the control valve to open or close. As the input signal current increases, the valve is opened wider; as it decreases, the valve closes more and more. Depending on how wide open it is, the valve can permit large amounts of current to flow to the output, and the valve is operated by the small current of the input signal.

In many ways an automobile is a mechanical analog of an amplifier. The power reserve is the gasoline in the tank, while the control valve is the accelerator pedal and the throttle system attached to it. The input signal is the force of the driver's foot on the pedal. As the driver's foot pushes down, more gasoline is fed to the engine from the reservoir, and the engine's power output increases. A very small amount of force (foot pressure) is used to control a large force (engine output power) by drawing energy from a reservoir (the gas tank). In some sense, then, the automobile is really an amplifier of foot power.

It is important to remember that the power that moves the car forward does not come from the driver's foot; it comes from the gas tank in which the necessary energy has been stored. The foot power *controls* reservoir output. In an analogous way, the output of an amplifier does not come from the input signal, which serves only as a control function, but from an energy reservoir, called the power supply. The control element in an electronic circuit is now almost always a transistor, although older instruments and some very specalized devices use vacuum tubes.

An electronic diagram of Figure 3-2 might look like the circuit shown in Figure 3-3. The control valve is now a transistor. A small input signal is applied between ground and one of the transistor elements (the "base") which causes a very small current to flow along the path shown by the solid line. This small input controls the amount of current the transistor will al-

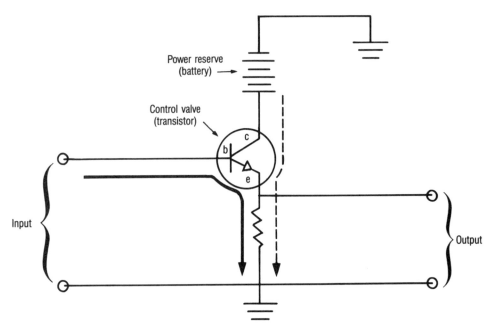

FIGURE 3-3. A simple amplifier. Input current flows along the path indicated by the solid line, while output current follows the dashed line. The transistor leads are b = base, c = collector, e = emitter.

low to flow from the reservoir (a battery) through the transistor's "collector" and "emitter" and along the dashed-line current path. The resistor in this part of the circuit develops a voltage proportional to the current through it (Ohm's Law: E = IR, voltage = current times resistance), and this larger voltage is "tapped" to serve as the output.

Real transistors are complex devices, and their use demands that special voltage requirements be met. For this reason practical transistor amplifiers must be more elaborate than the one shown in Figure 3-3 would indicate. Nonetheless, even if the circuit shown is actually impractical, it points up several critical variables in amplifier design or implementation. These, in turn, lie behind the specifications that manufacturers provide for their units.

Gain

The term *gain* describes the degree of amplification achieved by a circuit. It is most conveniently defined as the output to

input ratio. If, for example, an amplifier produces an output of 15 V when the input signal is 0.1 V it is said to have a *voltage gain* of 15/0.1 = 150. Similarly, if a unit produces a current of 250 mA at its output when the input is 2 mA, it has a *current gain* of 250/2 = 125. If the output is smaller than the input, the gain figure will be fractional. In such a case, of course, the circuit is functioning as an attenuator.

Gain is also frequently expressed according to the decibel (dB) scale, already quite familiar to speech and hearing specialists. Thus, an amplifier with an output to input voltage ratio of 150 has a gain of 20 log (150) = 43.5 dB, while a current gain of 125 represents current amplification of about 42 dB.

The current and voltage gains of a single amplifier are usually quite different, and units are generally designed to optimize one or the other. The selection of an amplifier will, in the first place, be governed by which parameter—current or voltage—is important, as well as by the amount of gain required. These specifications will depend on the use to which the amplifier will be put. Amplifying the output of a microphone for display on an oscilloscope, for instance, will require only a voltage amplifier. Since an oscilloscope is a voltage-sensitive device that draws very little current, adequate voltage gain is vital, but current gain is unnecessary. On the other hand, if the microphone output is to be fed to earphones (e.g., to achieve enhanced auditory feedback) current gain will be very important, because earphones are quite likely to require a great deal of current.

Amplitude linearity

An amplifier is said to show amplitude linearity if its gain is constant for all input magnitudes. That is, for a voltage amplifier, the gain should be the same whether the input is 0.01V, 0.1V, or 1.0V. If the output to input ratio is different for different input levels severe distortion of the signal will result. Some special amplifiers, however, are designed to be nonlinear. The most common of these is the logarithmic amplifier, in which the output voltage is proportional to the logarithm of the input. This is a useful way of compressing a signal with very large voltage variations.

The power supply imposes an inherent upper limit on an amplifier's linear range. Consider the case of an amplifier that has a gain of 10 and works on a power supply that provides 15 V. If a 0.5 V signal is applied to the input, an output of 5.0 V will result. Similarly, a 1 V input produces a 10 V output. But what happens if 2 V are applied to the input? The output (under *ideal* circumstances) will be only 15 V, not the expected 20 V. The amplifier's gain drops from 10 to 7.5 when the input is 2.0 V. The reason for this is not hard to understand. Recalling that the output is derived from an "energy reservoir" (the power supply), it is clear that the voltage output cannot exceed the reservoir's capacity. If the amplifier has a 15 V supply, it cannot provide an output of more than 15 V, no matter what the gain is supposed to be. The device cannot give what it has not got. As

the input magnitude increases, there will come a point at which the maximum output is reached. Beyond this point, increasing the input does not increase the output. Hence the gain (output to input ratio) falls. The amplifier is said to be overloaded or, more precisely, *saturated*.

Figure 3-4 shows the results of amplifier saturation. The sine wave shown at the top of Figure 3-4A has a peak voltage of 2 V. It has been applied to an amplifier that is set for a gain of 10, but the amplifier has only a 15 V power supply. The lower trace of Figure 3-4A shows that the amplifier out-

A

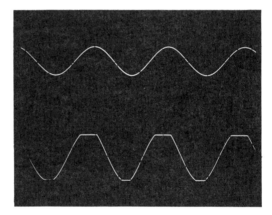

B

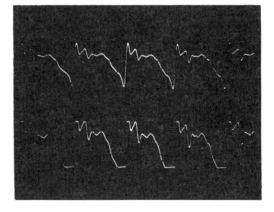

FIGURE 3-4. Peak-clipping due to amplifier saturation. The upper trace in each oscillogram is the input signal, the lower one is the amplifier's output. (A) Sine wave. (B) The vowel /a/.

put "follows" the signal as long as the power supply voltage is not exceeded. When it is, the output remains at maximum until the input voltage falls, when the output again follows the input. The result is severe distortion of a type known (for obvious reasons) as *peak clipping*. This sort of gross distortion of the signal is very obvious in a sine wave, but it may be less so when speech or other complex waves are at issue. Note how, in Figure 3-4B, only the very tops of the peaks of the speech waves are lost. These are very rapid events, and the distortion does not seem too severe. In fact, however, the distorted speech waveform may be utterly unsuitable if, for example, procedures such as spectrographic analysis are planned.

Permitting amplfier saturation and its consequent peak clipping is one of the most common errors made by the novice. Many amplifiers have a meter that shows if they are operating in their linear range. The gain must be set so as to avoid saturation at the greatest expected input amplitude. Figure 3-4B shows that the overload may be fleeting, and thus it may be too rapid to produce a noticeable deflection of the relatively sluggish meter pointer. To avoid clipping occasional peaks of very brief duration, then, amplifiers are usually operated at a gain that is significantly lower than that which produces observable saturation.

Frequency response and bandwidth

Just as the gain of an amplifier should be the same for all input magnitudes, so it also should be constant for any input frequency. That is, a sine wave of 100 Hz should be amplified exactly as much as one of 5 Hz or 25,000 Hz or, for that matter, of 0 Hz. Unfortunately, for reasons that are beyond the scope of the present discussion, this ideal situation cannot be achieved in practice. (In any case, it is sometimes undesirable to have and amplifier handle all frequencies equally—a concept that will be discussed later.)

It is common to describe an amplifier's response to different frequencies by a graph of amplification (in dB) over input frequency. This kind of plot is familiar to anyone who has worked with hearing aids or similar electroacoustic devices. Figure 3-5A shows an ideal frequency-response curve. Very low-and very high-frequencies are amplified less than those in the middle range, which are amplified with absolute equality. The frequency response of the ideal amplifier, whose characteristics are plotted in Figure 3-5A would be described as absolutely "flat" over this middle range, with "roll off" at the high and low ends, indicating that beyond certain lower and upper limits the amplifier is less effective. By convention, these limits are taken to be the frequencies at which the gain has fallen by 3 dB. One refers to these as the "cutoff frequencies" or, somewhat more descriptively, as the "3-dB down points." The *bandwidth* of the amplifier is then defined as the range between the cutoff frequencies. In Figure 3-5A the cutoff frequencies are 20 Hz and 10000 Hz, and the bandwidth is therefore 9980 Hz.

The frequency response curve of an actual amplifier is shown in Figure 3-5B. The cutoff frequencies are approximately 40 Hz and 13,000 Hz, and, as is typical of real electronic devices, the flatness of the response between those limits is not perfect. For this reason, manufacturers generally specify a tolerance for the gain characteristic. Thus, the amplifier characterized in Figure 3-5B may be said to have a frequency response that is flat ± 2 dB over its bandwidth. Modern components have made it easier to implement electronic designs that achieve excellent frequency response characteristics, and these specifications should be examined before acquiring a unit. It is wise to avoid purchasing any amplification system whose response is not specified.

Input and output impedance

The input impedance of an amplifier describes how great a load it imposes on the device providing the input signal. Consider the following example. Suppose one wishes to observe the electromyographic

A

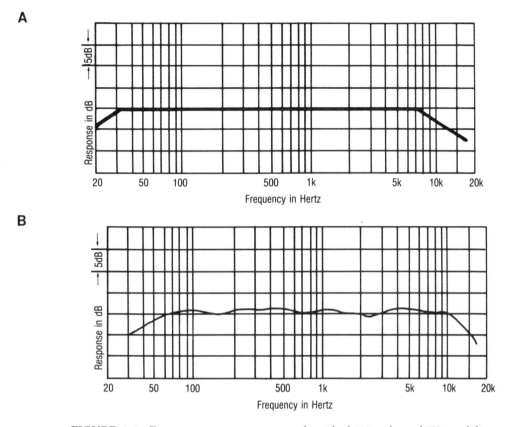

B

FIGURE 3-5. Frequency response curves of an ideal (A) and a real (B) amplifier.

response of the superior orbicularis oris muscle. Appropriate electrodes are glued onto the lip over the muscle to sense the voltages accompanying contraction. Since these voltages are very small (very much less than a millivolt) considerable amplification will be required to increase their magnitudes to levels suitable for display. Now, it turns out that, while the muscle is a fairly good voltage generator, it is not capable of producing large currents. Therefore, the amplifier that is connected to the electrodes must be capable of using a very small current for operating the "control valve" at its input. If the amplifier should draw anything but a miniscule control current it will overtax the generating capacity of the muscle. While this will not damage the muscle, it will probably lower its output voltage quite significantly. This, of course, means that drawing too much current may well eliminate the electromyo-

graphic voltage that is to be observed. A roughly analogous situation constantly arises in everyday life: Voltage drops, and so lights dim, when too much current is drawn from a household electrical outlet. In the same way, it is possible to overload a signal-source by connecting it to an amplifier that draws too much current.

The input impedance of an amplifier is a way of stating how much input current the amplifier will draw, since Ohm's law states that current equals voltage divided by the impedance. If, for example, a transducer whose output is 0.01 V is connected to an amplifier with an input impedance of 1 M Ω, a current of 0.01 V/1,000,000 = 0.00000001A (1 x 10^{-8} A or 0.01 μ A) will flow into the amplifier. This is unlikely to overload the current-producing capability of most transducers and so would be considered an adequate input impedance for most transducer amplifiers. Ideally, a voltage amplifier would have an infinite input impedance; that is, it would draw no current at all. The laws of physics tell us that this is an unattainable goal—some current must always flow into the amplifier. But extremely high input impedances are attainable with modern semiconductors, especially with a device known as a field-effect transistor (FET). If needed, for instance, amplifiers can be obtained with an input impedance of about 10^{11} (one hundred billion) ohms.

The inference should not be drawn that a higher input impedance is necessarily better than a lower one. It all depends on the device providing the input signal. Some transducers (certain types of microphones, for instance) have current, rather than voltage, outputs. Amplifiers to be used with them should have relatively low-input impedances that will permit these currents to flow freely. It is best that the input impedance of an amplifier be matched to the output impedance of the signal source. In a gross sense, this means that the tendency of an amplifier to "absorb" current should match the transducer's capacity to produce it.

The need for an appropriate input impedance (either high or low) must be borne in mind when selecting an amplifier for a given job. Transducer manufacturers usually indicate the requirements of their units in this regard, and amplifier suppliers always state the characteristics of their systems. Many audio or general-purpose amplifiers have both high- and low-impedance input connections to accomodate different devices.

At the other end of the amplification process one must consider the amplifier's ability to supply current. This is primarily of importance if the input of the next item in a series of devices requires large current inputs. Suppose, for instance, that a speech signal is to be amplified and then displayed on an oscilloscope for evaluation. Typically, an oscilloscope has an input impedance on the order to 1 M Ω. This implies that it will not draw significant amounts of current from the amplifier, and thus the latter

could have a moderately high output impedance without compromising the quality of the oscilloscope display. If, on the other hand, the amplified speech signal is to be fed to a loudspeaker the situation is very different. Typically, speaker systems have impedances of about 8 Ω, and so they draw large amounts of current. If the amplifier has an output impedance of, say, 1000 Ω it can provide no more than 0.002 A when its output is 2 V. At the same voltage, the speaker would draw 0.25 A, more than 100 times what the amplifier can deliver. With this kind of mismatch the amplifier's output voltage will drop enormously and the output waveform will be terribly distorted.

Amplifier Classification

It is common to describe different kinds of amplifiers by functional category, that is, according to the uses for which they are intended. Audio amplifiers, for example, are optimized for acoustic signals, while electromyography amplifiers are designed to handle certain bioelectric events. It might seem, therefore, that there is a very large number of different types of amplifiers. In fact, this is not really the case. Despite the myriad specializations for particular purposes that these functional categories represent, almost all amplifiers fall into a few relatively distinct electronic categories. It is important that these electronic distinctions be understood if the actual differences that separate the functional categories are to be appreciated.

Electronic classifications

Two sets of characteristics can be used to categorize almost any amplifier: response to a DC input and the nature of the reference (zero voltage point) against which the input is measured.

AC AND DC AMPLIFIERS. A single-transistor amplifier, such as the one in Figure 3-3, usually does not provide sufficient gain for most purposes. Consequently the output of one transistor is usually used as the input to another, which then further amplifies the signal. A typical circuit of this type, in which the transistor *stages* are *cascaded* is shown in Figure 3-6 in somewhat simplified form. The two stages are identical, and each is of the basic type illustrated in Figure 3-3, although some of the components required for the operation of a real circuit have been added. In spite of the possibly forbidding look of the schematic, it warrants careful consideration.

In this circuit, as in the simpler version of Figure 3-3, the input signal is applied to the base of the transistor, which serves as the control device that regulates the flow of the power supply's current through the R3-collector-emitter-R4 path. This current flow results in a voltage at the R3 = collector junction that is larger than, but proportional to, the voltage of the input signal. In short, amplification is achieved. Unfortunately a transistor, by its very nature, is unlikely to be able to handle the input signal in its unaltered form. For instance, the input must exceed a certain minimal voltage before the transistor can use it as a control signal, and (at least in the circuit shown) the actual voltage at the base must never reverse its polarity. It is for these (and other) reasons that R1 and R2 have been added. They serve to keep the base at a giv-

en voltage (referred to as the *bias*) to meet the transistor's requirements for linear operation. In reality, the input voltage is *added to* the bias voltage at the base, and the transistor amplifies them both. Therefore the output of the first stage is the amplified version of the sum of the input and bias voltages. The bias voltage is generally much larger than the input voltage, and if their amplified combination were to be directly applied to the base of the second transistor for further amplification, it would be very likely to saturate it. The final output would thus be a grossly distorted representation of the original input.

This situation is avoided by connecting the output of the first stage to the input of the second stage through a capacitor, C1. Since a capacitor blocks a steady (DC) current while passing a changing (AC) current, the amplified form of the steady bias at the input is blocked from passage to the next stage while the changing voltage of the input is passed for further amplification. Another capacitor, C2, at the final output of the amplifier performs a similar function and prevents the bias created for the second stage by R5 and R6 from appearing in the final output.

Capacitive coupling of the amplifier stages neatly solves the problem of cascad-

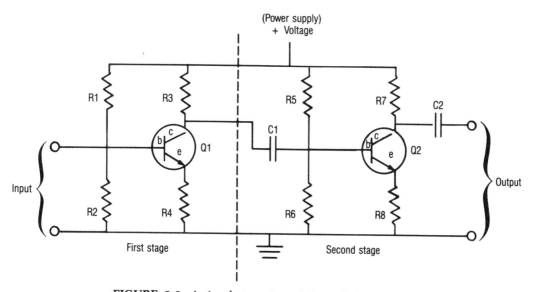

FIGURE 3-6. A simple two-stage, AC coupled amplifier.

ing transistors without overload due to bias voltages. The solution is achieved at a price, however. The amplifier will only work for AC inputs. Any steady-state (or even slowly changing) voltage at the amplifier input will be blocked by the coupling capacitors.* This is clearly shown in Figure 3-7. The top trace is the square-wave signal applied to the input of an AC coupled amplifier; the lower trace is the amplifier output. The flat portions of the square wave represent (temporarily) steady voltages. The output trace shows that the amplifier has, in essence, failed to handle them, while the transitions (changes in voltage) between the steady-state portions are amplified quite well.

There are techniques for cancelling out the bias, rather than blocking it. Semiconductor technology has produced transistors that have identical characteristics except that they are, in a sense, mirror images of each other. This reversal applies to their biasing requirements: When these *complementary* transistors are used in successive amplifier stages, the bias of one stage is cancelled out by the opposite biasing of the next stage. The final output thus represents simply the amplfied input, without the bias voltage. With the elimination of the DC-blocking elements, the circuit is capable of amplifying a DC input.

Amplification of DC inputs is crucial to many physiological measurements. It is not uncommon for the magnitude of a physiological variable (for instance intraoral air pressure) to change very slowly (by electronic standards). In some cases (such as the measurement of subglottal pressure) the steady-state period can be quite long. In these instances the measurement transducer will produce an output that is essentially a DC voltage. Clearly the amplifier must be capable of handling this situation.

AC amplifiers, then, can deal with AC inputs only, whereas DC amplifiers can

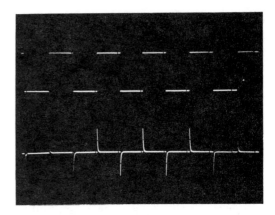

FIGURE 3-7. Blocking of steady-state (DC) voltages by an AC-coupled amplifier. The unchanging (flat) portions of the square-wave input (top trace) are blocked, and thus only the transitions appear at the output (lower trace).

handle both AC and DC signals. The logical question is: Why bother with the functionally-restricted AC amplifiers at all? Why not use DC amplifiers for all purposes? The answer is twofold. DC amplifiers are more difficult to design and build. They must, for instance, include compensation for inherent temperature instability. But their problems, with today's technology, are not overly difficult to manage, although the resultant circuits are somewhat more expensive. More important is the fact that many transducers and instrumentation systems produce outputs that have their own useless bias voltages associated with the AC signal of interest. Certain types of microphones, for example, require DC working voltages, and their outputs are composed of a DC voltage plus the changes produced by audio transduction. Since it is only the varying (AC) portion of the microphone output that is of interest, use of an AC amplifier that will ignore the DC bias is obligatory.

Single-ended and differential amplifiers

The amplification techniques discussed thus far have shared an important characteristic that has not been mentioned. Reference to Figures 3-3 and 3-6 shows that,

---

*The stages of the amplifier may also be coupled through transformers, which also serve to block transmission of the DC bias from one stage to another. The effect on overall amplifier function is essentially the same.

in each case, the input current and output current loops have part of their paths in common. They both feed their current to ground, which serves as a common connection point for both input and output. (The concept of circuit ground is considered more fully in Chapter 2.) The result of this arrangement is that the amplifier really senses the voltage difference between a single input line and ground, and produces an output voltage that is proportionally "distant" from ground. All of this is a rather elaborate way of saying that the point common to the two portions of the circuit—the input and output loops—serves as a zero reference, with all voltages being measured from that common zero level. An amplifier whose output shares such a common ground reference with its input source is known as a *single-ended amplifier*, because it senses the voltage on a single "active" input wire.

Unfortunately, a single-ended amplifier is inadequate in those situations (and there are many) in which the input source cannot share a common ground with the amplifier. Consider the following example. Certain apsects of labial control are to be evaluated in a dysarthric client. Electromyography will be done on two opposing muscles, orbicularis oris and depressor labii inferior, in order to study their coordination. If only single-ended amplifiers are available the electrode and amplifier arrangement would have to be as shown in Figure 3-8.

The single active input of each amplifier is connected to an electrode that picks up the electrical activity of the muscle on which it is positioned. The other input connection of each amplifier is, of course, connected to a common, neutral reference point, ground. In order for the client's muscles to serve as an input to the amplifiers he must be connected to the same ground. This is accomplished by connecting a grounded electrode to some site near both of the muscles being examined. A number of problems instantly arise. First, each amplifier is "looking" at the voltage difference between the "ground" electrode and the electrode connected to its active input. From a physiological point of view, there is a vast distance between these two points, a distance within which all sorts of bioelectric events may be going on. Most

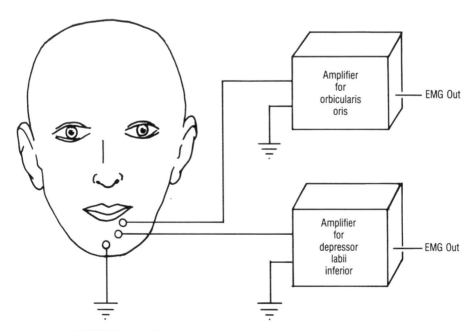

FIGURE 3-8. Electromyography using single-ended amplifiers.

of these events have nothing to do with the activity of the specific muscle being monitored. Because these events are all between the active and common electrode, they all contribute (in unpredictable ways) to the voltage seen by the amplifier. If the contributions are unpredictable, the final output is uninterpretable. The problem could, of course, be solved by moving the common electrode much closer to one of the active electrodes, thus improving the quality of the signal from one muscle. But that means moving it further from the other electrode, exacerbating the problems of recording from it. If both muscles are to be examined at the same time, as they must be if their coordination is to be evaluated, the difficulties arising from the need to use a common reference point are insoluble. This is one reason why single-ended amplifiers won't do in this situation.

There is, however, another reason, somewhat more subtle but just as important. The environment in which we live is filled with electromagnetic waves: radio signals, electrical interference from motors and lamp dimmers, and—most important—60 Hz radiation from the power lines all around us. The body and the electrode wires serve quite effectively as antennas for all of these. Thus, the electrodes on the muscles also pick up voltages induced by atmospheric electromagnetic radiation. Since the single-ended amplifiers "see" any voltage difference between the electrode and the common ground, which is not affected by stray radiation, they amplify these interfering signals, confounding them with the muscle potentials being examined. Muscular electrical activity is very weak, generally of far lower amplitude than the interfering induced voltages. The electromyographic signals are quite likely to be completely lost in all the electrical noise.

While there are still other problems, the foregoing clearly emphasizes the need for an alternative amplification technique. It happens that a solution to all of the problems described above can be achieved by using what is known as a *differential* amplifier. This type of circuit, in fact, was originally developed by electrophysiologists confronted with the kind of problem just described.

Put briefly, the differential amplifier is designed to amplify the voltage difference between two active input lines, neither of which (in contrast to the single-ended amplifier) is grounded. If, for instance, a differential amplifier with a gain of 100 has an input of 1.00 V at one input connection and 1.01 V at the other, its output will be 1 V, which is the difference between the two inputs (1.01 - 1.00 = 0.01) times the gain (100). The way in which this is achieved, although complex in actual implementation, is not difficult to conceptualize and is illustrated in Figure 3-9.

Careful examination shows that this circuit is really very similar to the amplifier shown in Figure 3-6. The key to seeing this is the recognition that there are really two identical amplifiers that have been drawn as mirror images of each other: The bottom amplifier is "upside down" compared to

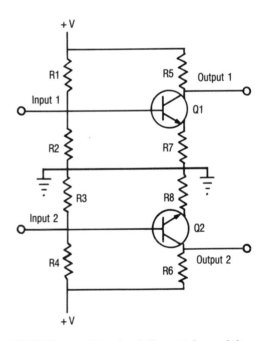

FIGURE 3-9. Simple differential amplifier. Note that there are actually *two* amplifiers, drawn upside-down with respect to each other. Both are connected to a single ground, but neither input line is grounded.

the top one. (This refers only to the way in which the circuits are drawn; it has nothing to do with their function.) Note, for example, the power supply connections, which represent a single power supply connected to two different points, and the location of ground, the common point to which the amplifiers are connected.

What this arrangement provides is a separate amplifier for each input line, thus permitting both lines to be active. Each of the inputs is amplified separately and appears at an output. The resistor networks serve the same function as their counterparts in Figure 3-6. A critical feature of this circuit resides in the fact that both output lines are active, an arrangement that confers important advantages.

Recall that voltage is the difference in electrical pressure between two points. In a single-ended amplifier the two points are an active line and ground, but in the circuit shown in Figure 3-9 the two points are both active, meaning that they carry real voltages. Taking the output as the difference in voltage between two amplifier outputs (which is what is involved here) yields a major benefit that is best explained by an example.

Consider the situation diagrammed in Figure 3-10. A differential amplifier has been connected to a pressure gauge that transduces a short period of high intraoral pressure to a positive voltage pulse on one of its output lines. The two wires from the transducer, however, serve as antennas and

pick up significant 60 Hz voltage from the electromagnetic radiation in the environment. The result is that both of the inputs to the differential amplifier carry 60 Hz signals of about equal amplitude and phase, since the two wires from the transducer are equally effective as antennas, but one input wire also carries the positive voltage pulse representing the pressure event. Both inputs are amplified and appear at the outputs. But the final output of the circuit is the voltage difference between the two output lines, and thus the difference between the lines will always be zero for the 60 Hz component. On the other hand, the voltage pulse representing the pressure event appears on only one line, and so for it, and it alone, the difference between the two output lines is real and large. By taking the output as the difference between the output lines, the 60 Hz noise signal, because it is the same at both outputs, is cancelled out and eliminated from the final result.

By the same process a differential amplifier will cancel out a DC voltage that is present at both inputs. So, for example, if a measurement device has both of its output terminals at, let us say, 2 V DC in its baseline state, the differential amplifier to which it is connected will turn out 0 V. If *one* of the transducer outputs goes to 3V when transducing an event, the differential amplifier will amplify only the 1 V difference that represents the meaningful signal.

An identical voltage at both amplifier

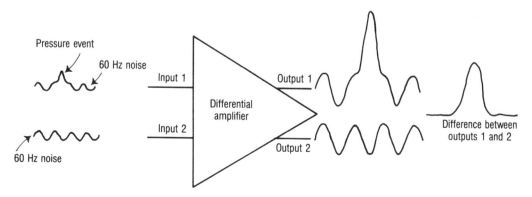

FIGURE 3-10. Cancellation of a common-mode signal by a differential amplifier.

inputs is called a *common mode* voltage. The ability to eliminate such a signal from the final output is a very important feature of differential amplifiers. It is often the prime reason for using them. This capability is quantified by the *common mode rejection ratio* or CMRR. In essence, the CMRR is the gain of a common mode signal. That is, it is the ratio of the voltage output to voltage input (V_{out}/V_{in}) for a signal applied to both inputs, usually expressed in dB. Common mode rejection ratios of -85 dB or greater are common in commercially available circuits.

It is important to understand the significance and value of the CMRR and, once again, a concrete example may help in clarifying the matter. Consider a differential amplifier with a differential gain of 100 and a CMRR of 90 dB. Suppose that it is operating in an electrically noisy environment with the result that there is a 60 Hz common mode noise signal of 0.1 V at both inputs. At the same time there is a meaningful 0.1 V signal at one input only. The meaningful signal will be amplified by a factor of 100, and so this component appears as 0.1 V x 100 gain = 10 V at the output. The common mode signal, however, faces a CMRR of 90 dB, meaning an output to input (gain) ratio of about 0.00003. The output for the 60 Hz noise signal is therefore 0.1 V x 0.00003, or 3 *micro* V. The signal-to-noise ratio is clearly vastly improved, from a 1-to-1 ratio to greater than 3 million to 1 (>110 dB).

The ability to amplify the voltage difference between two points, neither of which is ground, and to selectively amplify a signal in the presence of relatively high levels of common-mode background noise makes the differential amplifier very important. It will be encountered often in measurement systems.

Functional classification

Although all amplifiers can be categorized as AC or DC, single-ended or differential, specific circuits are designed for optimal performance with certain kinds of input signals. Therefore, it is common to refer to amplifiers according to their intended function. In some cases the functional description of an amplifier makes its characteristics obvious. For example, one would guess that audio amplifiers, intended to amplify music or speech, are AC, single-ended devices with a flat frequency response from about 50 to over 15,000 Hz. The first several stages of such a device would probably be voltage amplifiers, but, if speakers are to be connected, the last stages will no doubt be a power amplifier. Other functional descriptions, however, might not be as immmediately comprehensible to the nonspecialist. Some of these are briefly described below.

PREAMPLIFIERS. Any amplifier designed to accept a low-level input signal (generally directly from a transducer) and provide enough gain to make the signal suitable for further electronic processing is called a preamplifier. The term itself is not rigidly defined, and the circuit referred to can be AC or DC coupled, differential or single-ended. The essential characteristic is that the circuit serve as a first stage "signal conditioner" at the input of a more elaborate array of circuits. For example, the voltage amplifier that boosts a small voltage from a microphone is an audio preamplifier for the power system that drives the loudspeakers.

BRIDGE AMPLIFIERS. These meet the special requirements for amplifying the outputs of bridge-type transducers (see Chap. 2), especially those using DC excitation. These circuits are differential DC amplifiers with high gain, great stability, and high CMRR. Their very large input impedance draws very little current, thus preventing the amplifier from acting as a shunt across the bridge to which it is connected. Bridge amplifiers commonly also provide the required excitation voltage for the transducer.

CARRIER PREAMPLIFIERS. These are really composed of at least three different circuits housed together for convenience. They incorporate a highly stable oscillator (excitation source), a high-gain differential AC amplifier, and a demodulator circuit that extracts the transducer analog voltage from the modulated carrier signal. Together with the transducer, carrier preamplifiers provide for a complete amplitude modulation and demodulation system for generating a voltage analog of an external phenomenon. Carrier preamplifiers are commonly used with bridge transducers.

INSTRUMENTATION AMPLIFIERS. Although this term is only loosely defined, in general it is used to describe a precision DC differential amplifier with very high input impedance, high gain, and very low noise. This type of circuit is used when a very weak signal must be greatly amplified without loading the signal source.

OPERATIONAL AMPLIFIERS. A special type of high-gain, DC, differential amplifier whose characteristics are determined by feedback networks is called an *operational amplifier* (or "op amp" for short). While the definition might not immediately suggest it, op amps may well be the most useful circuits ever devised for processing analog signals. There is scarcely any kind of signal modification, from simple amplification to complex mathematical transformation, that these circuits cannot do. (The term *operational amplifier*, in fact, derives from their early use in analog computers, in which they performed the actual mathematical operations.) It is important to remember that op amp circuits do far more than amplify. Addition of a few components to an op amp produces an electronic filter, or an oscillator, or rectifier, voltage summer, integrator, differentiator, comparator, and so on, almost without end.

High-quality operational amplifiers are available as ultraminiature integrated circuits at exceptionally low cost. In many cases it is possible to buy four of them in a single miniature package for well under $2.00. Given their extreme versatility, precision, convenience, and exceptionally low cost, it is not surprising that they have become absolutely ubiquitous. Using them, many laboratories now routinely construct special circuits as needed, overcoming instrumentation problems in a few hours that would have entailed enormous effort, much time, and great expense just a few years ago.

It is not possible, in this text, to present a discussion of sufficient depth to make the reader competent at operational amplifier circuit design. Many volumes have been written with that objective in mind: Several are listed at the end of the chapter (Hoenig and Payne [1973] is one of the best for the beginner). Integrated circuit manufacturers have also produced extensive applications literature. While it takes some effort and time, but very little money, to develop creative skill in the use of op amps, most clinicians will find that the relatively small investment pays off quite handsomely. It takes only a little competence with these devices to permit construction of *usable* precision circuits that can greatly enlarge one's measurement capability. In fact, much of the electronic circuitry described throughout this text can be designed (if necessary) and built quite easily with op amps—even by relative novices. Therefore, the reader is strongly urged to consult the appropriate references and start learning.

MICROPHONES

Microphones produce an electrical analog of acoustic waves. They are, by far, the most common input transducer used by the speech pathologist. Perhaps it is because they are so common that most users give them little thought, with the result that their mechanisms and characteristics are often poorly understood. This is unfortunate for two reasons. First, there is a truly vast array of microphones available, and a wise choice among them must be based on knowledge rather than advertising hyperbole. Second, audio reproduction can be no better than the worst of the components through which the audio signal passes. The microphone is the first component, the link between the acoustic world and the audio electronics. If it is not matched to the audio task on the one hand and to the electronic system on the other, if it is used in ways that are not in keeping with its inherent characteristics, sound reproduction will suffer, perhaps drastically. While casual users might find a poor or noisy audio signal acceptable, the speech pathologist cannot afford to be so tolerant. Every client recording must be as good as reasonable effort can make it; every transduced speech signal to be analyzed must be as perfect as possible. Therefore, it is apparent why the speech clinician will want to pay particular attention to the choice of the microphone. The following material is intended to provide basic information in this regard. Further discussions of specific engineering details and application techniques can be found in the references at the end of the chapter.

Microphone Specifications

There are four different specifications that are most important to the microphone user: sensitivity, impedance, frequency response, and directionality.

Sensitivity

A microphone's sensitivity rating quantifies its effectiveness in converting acoustic to electrical energy. The microphone can be considered to be an electrical generator, and *sensitivity* is stated as the amount of electrical power produced for a standard sound pressure input. The rating most commonly used is the electrical output in dB re: 1 mW when the sound pressure input is 10 dynes/cm.^{2} For audio microphones this value is commonly measured at a frequency of 1000 Hz. Most microphones have sensitivities in the range of -50 to -60 dB, which indicates power outputs of 0.00001 to 0.000001 mW when the microphone is driven by a sound pressure of 10 d/cm.^{2} This is obviously very little power, but audio amplifiers are designed to accept this low

level, and so a sensitivity of -50 dB is perfectly acceptable for ordinary uses. If the microphone is to be connected directly to other kinds of devices, such as an oscilloscope, for display of the acoustic waveform, some type of preamplifier will be necessary. If *precisely* known, the microphone's sensitivity rating may be used to determine the sound pressure of an audio signal.

Impedance

The impedance of a microphone specifies its ability to deliver current to the amplifier or other circuit to which it is connected. Unless one intends to design a special amplifier, the actual current output levels are not overly important. What does matter, however, is the degree to which the impedance of the microphone matches that of the amplifier's input stage. A gross mismatch of the two will significantly reduce microphone sensitivity and increase the noise level. Worse, the mismatch may compromise the microphone's frequency response, with the result that the audio input to the amplifier becomes unacceptably distorted.

Achieving an adequate microphone-to-amplifier impedance match is fortunately not a major problem, thanks to the fact that the audio industry has, by and large, achieved some degree of standardization in this regard. Most microphones have an impedance of about 200 Ω and audio amplifiers have been designed around this value. There are exceptions, however, and the impedance rating of a microphone should be checked to be sure that it is suitable for its intended use. Instances of serious mismatch can often be corrected by insertion of a special miniature matching transformer or a resistive "pad" (available from microphone manufacturers) into the amplifier input line. But it is better to have a matched system.

Frequency response

Like the human ear, no microphone is equally sensitive to all audio frequencies. The microphone frequency response is depicted in the equivalent of an audiogram: A given microphone's sensitivity in dB is plotted over frequency. An example is shown in Figure 3-11. This kind of specification should be easily intelligible to any speech pathologist.

An ideal microphone would be equally sensitive to all frequences over (at least) the range of human hearing, from about 20 Hz to approximately 20,000 Hz. While this degree of perfection is not readily achieved, a good quality microphone comes reasonably close. Thanks to the large popular interest in audio reproduction that recreates the original acoustic event as precisely as possible (high fidelity) there are many acceptable models among which to choose.

Directionality: The polar response

The design of a microphone will strongly affect the variability of its sensitivity to sounds arriving from different directions. The directional sensitivity characteristics are typically detailed in a "polar response" graph of the type shown in Figure 3-12. The radii on the graph represent the angles from which the test sound arrives. The concentric circles are spaced 5 dB apart. The pattern of the response plot shows the direction(s) from which sound is best picked up. The microphone whose polar response is plotted in Figure 3-12, is most sensitive to sounds coming from the front, within 60° of the microphone's axis. As the sound source moves further to the side, sensitivity falls off. The microphone is least sensitive to sounds coming from directly behind: The response in this direction is 20 dB below that of head-on incidence.

Microphones are often categorized according to their directionality characteristics, and several standard patterns are available. The pattern shown in Figure 3-12 is described as *cardioid* (heart shaped) and typifies most undirectional microphones. Clearly this kind records best those sounds coming from the direction in which it is pointed. Its great advantage is that sound coming from other sources tends to be attenuated. A microphone with a unidirectional sensitivity pattern, then, would be chosen when the ambient noise levels are higher than one would like and when the speaker remains in front of the microphone. A unidirectional microphone would normally be used, for example, to obtain a recording of a speech sample from a seated client.

Figure 3-13 shows the two other common polar response types. The *omnidirectional* microphone (Figure 3-13A) is almost equally sensitive in all directions. It is, therefore, the unit of choice in those circumstances in which a single microphone must be used to pick up sounds coming from all around it. For recording a child moving around a playroom, for example, this response pattern may be ideal. On the other hand, extraneous noises coming from any point in the

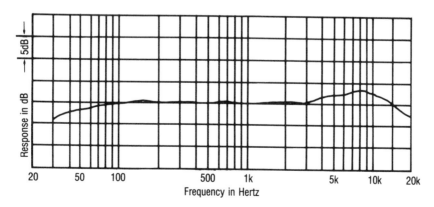

FIGURE 3-11. Typical frequency-response curve for a high-quality microphone. The response is acceptably flat over the range of human hearing.

recording area will be picked up just as clearly as the child's utterances.

Finally, Figure 3-13B shows a *bidirectional* response pattern. The microphone picks up sounds from either side (or from front and back) equally well, but it is very much less sensitive to sounds arriving from other directions. This type may be useful in those situations where two speakers (perhaps therapist and client) are facing each other with a microphone between them.

Microphone Mechanisms

There are innumerable methods available whereby audio energy may be converted to an electrical signal. Almost all have been tried in microphones. Some techniques have been found suitable for highly specialized purposes, and a few have proven to be so versatile and easy to implement that they have become the workhorses of audio transduction. It is with these that we are concerned.

Almost all microphones have some sort of diaphragm that is exposed to the incoming sound wave. The sound pressure acts on the diaphragm and causes it to move. The diaphragm, then, serves as a collector of acoustic energy; its movement affects an active element that does the actual transduction.

Carbon button microphone

Ordinary carbon, say in the form of graphite, is a fairly good conductor of electricity. The resistance of a pile of *powdered*

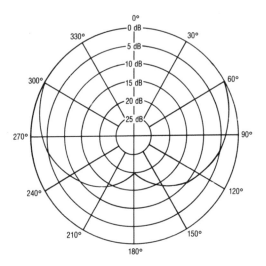

FIGURE 3-12. Polar-response or directionality plot for a typical microphone. The microphone is assumed to lie in the center of the graph, pointed at the 0° mark. (A microphone having this particular response pattern is said to be "unidirectional.")

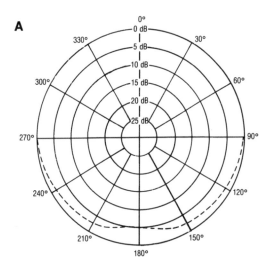

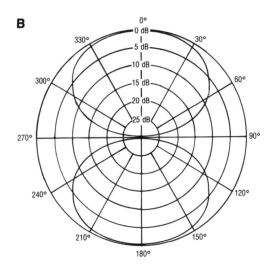

FIGURE 3-13. Polar response plots of (A) an omnidirectional and (B) a bidirectional microphone.

carbon, however, will depend heavily on how tightly the fine particles are packed together: the tighter the packing, the lower the resistance. Carbon button microphones take advantage of this fact. A small chamber is filled with finely ground carbon through which an electrical current flows. The front wall of the chamber moves with the diaphragm, which collects the sound energy. As the wall moves it compresses and decompresses the carbon granules, and the electrical resistance of the carbon powder changes accordingly. The resultant variations in the flow of current through the carbon-filled chamber are analogs of the original sound waves.

The carbon button microphone is one of the oldest types still in general use. (It is the microphone found in a typical telephone handset.) While it is reliable and very inexpensive, it has quite serious limitations: Its frequency response is poor and irregular, and it has an exceptionally low impedance that tends to change over time. These disadvantages effectively eliminate the carbon microphone as a viable alternative for work in speech pathology.

Crystal (piezoelectric microphones)

Crystals of certain substances generate electrical voltages when they are mechanically deformed. The voltage is proportional to the rate of deformation. The phenomenon, known as the *piezoelectric effect*, is used in piezoelectric, or crystal, microphones, in which the movement of the diaphragm is used to deform the crystal. These microphones are very inexpensive, but that is their chief virtue. They do not do a very good job with respect to fidelity, having poor low-frequency response and suffering seriously from frequency nonlinearity. Although they are sometimes provided with recording equipment, they are not well suited to the needs of the speech clinician.

Dynamic microphones

Dynamic microphones take advantage of the fact that a voltage is produced across a conductor when it moves through a magnetic field. When, as in a microphone, the conductor is moved by acoustic pressure, the voltage produced will be an analog of the audio input. There are two common types of dynamic microphones, diagrammed in Figure 3-14. In the moving-coil type, a single-layer coil of very fine wire is attached to the sound-collecting dia-

A

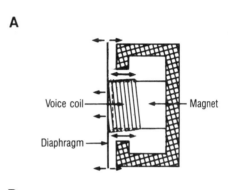

B

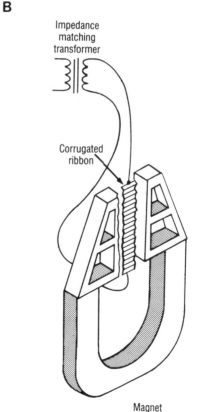

FIGURE 3-14. Dynamic microphones. (A) moving coil. (B) ribbon.

phragm. This coil is positioned around a cylindrical permanent magnet. Displacement of the diaphragm by a sound wave moves the coil within the magnetic field, and an electric flow through the coil is produced. In a very real sense, this type of microphone is an electrical generator, working on much the same principle as the enormously larger generators that produce power for utility companies. The *ribbon* microphone uses a very thin sheet of metal suspended between the poles of a magnet. The ribbon is acted on directly by the impingent sound wave; a separate energy-collecting diaphragm is not needed. Movement of the metal ribbon produces a voltage in it. (Ribbon microphones are less common than coil-type dynamic microphones.)

Because the impedance of the actual microphone element is very low, dynamic microphones usually include a transformer within the microphone housing to meet the requirements of the amplifier input. On the whole, dynamic microphones are rugged, can be made with excellent frequency-response characteristics, and are moderately sensitive. These features, together with their moderate cost, make them the best all-around choice for routine audio work.

Condenser microphones

The charge on the plates of a capacitor (see Chap. 2) varies as a function of several variables, one of which is the distance separating them. This fact forms the basis of yet another method of acoustic transduction, exploited in the condenser microphone. (Condenser is the obsolete term for capacitor.)

The mechanism of a condenser microphone is illustrated (in greatly simplified form) in Figure 3-15. A very thin metallic diaphragm acts as the energy collector and at the same time serves as one plate of a capacitor. The other plate is held rigidly fixed behind, but extremely close to, the diaphragm. A power supply maintains a fairly large voltage difference between the two plates. Since they are a pair of conductors separated by an insulator (air), the microphone elements form a capacitor that stores a charge imposed by the power supply. When the diaphragm moves in or out under the pressure of sound waves the distance between the plates changes by a microscopic amount. This is sufficient, however, to significantly alter the capacitance of the system, which means that the charge-storage capability changes, causing

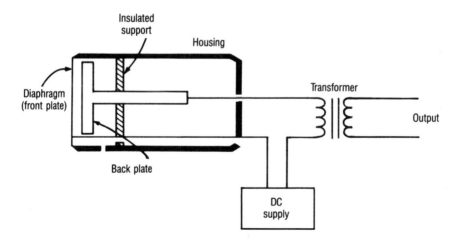

FIGURE 3-15. Simplified construction of a condenser microphone. The diaphragm and back plate form a capacitor. Movement of the diaphragm changes the capacitance, causing current to flow to or from the power supply through the transformer.

electrons to flow to and from the plates. The current is made to flow through a transformer that is part of the power-supply circuit. The transformer's primary coil generates a voltage proportional to the magnitude of the current flow, which is transferred to the microphone amplifier by the transformer's secondary coil.

The condenser microphone has a flat frequency response over a wide range, excellent stability, fairly high sensitivity, and very little self-generated internal noise. For these reasons it is the transducer of choice for precision measurement of sound pressure and for similarly demanding transduction tasks. It is, for example, the type of microphone used by audiologists for calibration of audiometric equipment.

The condenser microphone usually costs more that other types, and it also has certain drawbacks. First, it will not tolerate abuse. Physical shock can easily damage the capacitor elements or their positioning, as can exposure to high-pressure bursts, such as powerful puffs of air directed at the diaphragm. Second, there is the extra complication of a separate power supply which, in practice, means that a special preamplifier must be used. These factors usually rule out the use of condenser microphones for everyday purposes. On the other hand, the fidelity of their audio transduction more than compensates for their problems where precision is of prime concern.

Some of the problems are solved by a special type of microphone that uses an *electret* as one of the capacitor elements. An *electret* is a device that retains an electric charge indefinitely. Although the principle has been known for over 150 years, it is only in the past couple of decades that electret materials suitable for microphone use have been available. Present electret microphones use a thin, metal-plated plastic membrane that permanently holds a charge which is applied to it in the manufacturing process. The permanence of the charge eliminates the need for a special power supply in the microphone. In essence, the power supply is built-in. There is, however, a small problem: The resultant electret capacitor can function only when connected to an amplifier with an *extremely* high input impedance. The most effective way to deal with this requirement is to make a special preamplifier part of the microphone itself. Modern transistor devices make this easy to achieve, but it means that the electret microphone will still need an external power supply—not for the capacitor, which is permanently charged, but for the transistor in the preamplifier. Despite this, the electret condenser microphone's advantage is a significant one, because a transistor requires only very low voltages, meaning that a miniature battery is all the power supply that is needed. Furthermore, these microphones can be made very small, making them very useful as probe microphones (Harford, 1980, 1981; Villchur and Killion, 1975).

Contact microphones (accelerometers)

There are instances in which one is interested in only a specific aspect of the speech signal, such as the fundamental frequency of phonation. Occasionally one might need simply an indication of the presence or absence of speech, as in reaction-time determination. In these cases the use of a contact microphone, or accelerometer, should be considered. These devices are specially designed to pick up acoustic signals, or vibrations, from the body surface. They are almost totally insensitive to airborne sounds. They are held in intimate contact with the skin by an adhesive or strap mounting.

The speech signal is badly degraded by transmission through the tissues of the body (Figure 3-16), but vocal fundamental frequency is unaltered. Koike (1973) found that the improvement of signal-to-noise ratio afforded by a contact microphone in the pretracheal region made it preferable to a standard microphone for analysis of fundamental frequency perturbation. While neck placement is usual, more esoteric locations (forehead, ear canal, mastoid, nose) have been evaluated by Snidecor, Rehman, and Washburn (1959).

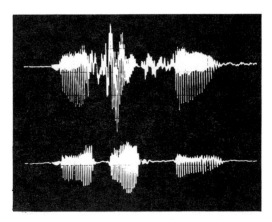

FIGURE 3-16. Airborne (top) and neck-surface (bottom) pickup of audio signals. (The spoken phrase is "I think so.")

TAPE RECORDERS

The tape recorder may be the one item of technical electronics with which absolutely every speech pathologist is familiar. It has become an indispensible tool in therapy and an invaluable aid in the maintenance of adequate client records. Yet the way in which the ordinary tape recorder works is a mystery to many, which prevents them from gaining maximal advantage from it.

Actually, tape-recording devices are usually classed into two categories. Tape *decks* provide a system for recording, playing back, and erasing the tape but do not amplify the output. Typically, then, they must be used with external power amplifiers that can drive a speaker system. Tape *recorders*, however, have their own power amplifiers and, usually, a built-in set of speakers. Each is a complete, portable, sound system. By and large, better recording quality is obtained in tape decks, which, freed from the necessity of providing power amplification, can be optimized for the best possible record and reproduce functioning. Furthermore, the amplifiers that are built in to tape recorders are very unlikely to offer the quality obtainable in free-standing amplifiers, and high-fidelity speakers cannot be built into a tape recorder. While speech pathologists may wish to take advantage of the convenience of tape recorders for routine recording tasks, it is obvious that they will also need a tape deck-amplifier-speaker system for their more serious recording needs.

When asked what a tape recorder does, most users are likely to answer that it stores speech or music on a magnetic tape and allows it to be played back to reproduce the original material with high fidelity. For the general public, this is a perfectly adequate view, but for the speech professional such a formulation is far too narrow. What a tape recorder *really* does is store *information* on a magnetic tape. That information might be (and most commonly is) speech or music, but it could just as easily be voltages representing intraoral pressure, jaw position, nasalization ratio, or any of the many measurements that a speech pathologist might make on a client. Almost any kind of information can be stored on magnetic tape with just a little ingenuity and a bit of knowledge about the recording process. This section provides a basic introduction to the tape recorder. More complete information is available in several of the references listed at the end of the chapter. For the neophyte, Johnson and Walker (1977) is particularly recommended.

Basic Principles

Magnetic tape recording depends on the fact that an electric current causes a magnetic field to be produced around the conducting element. Conversely, movement of a magnetic field near a conductor causes an electric current to flow in it. Magnetic fields can be "frozen" and stored by allowing them to magnetize a susceptible material. A tape deck does all this with (1) a record system that generates magnetic fields; (2) a transport system that moves magnetically sensitive material (the tape) into those magnetic fields in order to "capture" them; and (3) a playback system that detects the currents generated when the magnetic fields that have been captured on the tape are moved past a transducer (see Figure 3-17).

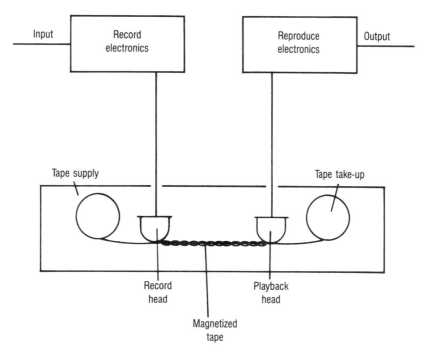

FIGURE 3-17. Functional components of a tape recorder.

Tape-Recorder Components

Record transducers (heads)

The flow of current through a wire generates a magnetic filed around the wire; the strength of that field is proportional to the magnitude of the current (Chap. 2, Inductance). The magnetic field can be concentrated by winding the wire into a coil. Given these facts, it is easy to see how transduction of a tape-deck's input to a magnetic field is accomplished. The signal (a varying voltage that represents sound, or pressure, or air flow, or whatever) is fed to an amplifier whose variable-current output is connected to a recording head, which is constructed as shown in Figure 3-18. The wire coils in the head generate a magnetic field that is further concentrated and directed by the metal core on which the coils are wound and by a set of "pole pieces." The net result is that a magnetic field whose strength is proportional to the current appears in the gap at the top of the head. (The gap itself is very narrow, on the order of 0.00025 inches.) The entire head is really

nothing more than a specially shaped electromagnet. One side of the gap is the magnet's north pole, the other side the south pole. Not only does the magnetic strength change with the magnitude of the current, but magnetic polarity reverses when current flow changes direction, as it periodically does in most AC signals.

The storage medium: Recording tape

Recording tape consists of a very thin plastic-film backing on which is deposited an even thinner layer of microscopic crystals of easily magnetized material (Figure 3-19) embedded in a binder. Each particle of magnetic material can be individually magnetized. In the recording process the gap of the record head is brought into intimate contact with the surface of the tape. As they travel past the record head each of the particles is magnetized to a degree proportional to the strength of the head's magnetic field and with a polarity that matches it. Each particle therefore serves as a permanent record of the record-head's magnetic status at the time it passed by. From one end to the other, the tape preserves a record of the magnetic field of the record head over time, which in turn represents the input signal over time.

The original magnetic material for tape recording was ferric oxide (Fe_2O_3), and it remains the workhorse of recording. Special low-noise and high-output oxides have been developed in recent years. They have smaller, more densely packed magnetic par-

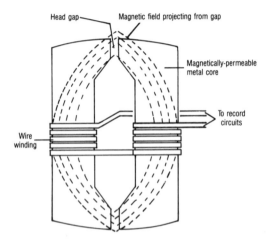

FIGURE 3-18. Tape-recorder head. A wire coil is wound on a core of magnetically-permeable material. When current flows through the coil a magnetic field is generated in the core and projects into space at the head gap. Tape passing near the gap is magnetized.

ticles and can provide an output up to 8 dB greater than older formulations. The increased output capability allows faithful reproduction of a wider range of signal intensities—a factor that is important to the speech pathologist because of the wide dynamic range of speech. Another development that has increased recording quality is the use of magnetic materials other than ferric oxide as the recording medium. Chromium dioxide (CrO_2) provides very high output levels, low signal distortion, and excellent frequency response. Tapes that use metal particles rather than an oxide are also available. They offer extremely high output levels and have a particularly good response at high frequencies, an important characteristic that can help overcome a major limitation of cassette tape decks. Furthermore, they tend to be less prone to saturation at high signal levels, thus offering greater protection from distortion. While the performance of metal tape is significantly better than that of ferric oxide tape, it is considerably more expensive. Metal tape also needs stronger biasing than is provided for on most cassette tape units. More important than the specific material, however, may be the specific formulation and manufacturing technique used to produce a given tape: The binders and finish used to produce it significantly affect its performance. Fortunately, the quality of the major

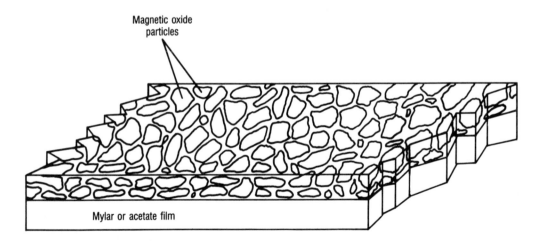

FIGURE 3-19. Recording tape.

brands of tape (Memorex, BASF, TDK, Scotch, and the like) is uniformly quite high. Differences in their ability to reproduce sound are likely to be small. More important, for most clinics, is the quality of the tape deck itself.

Tape can be made with any number of backing materials, but acetate and polyester (Mylar®) have generally proven most useful. Acetate is less expensive and can be made to closer thickness tolerances than polyester. But it turns brittle with age and is less dimensionally stable in the face of temperature and humidity changes. These factors are important in situations where long-term storage is planned. Polyester tapes are much stronger than acetate and are better able to withstand the forces of tape starts and stops without parting, which usually makes them superior for routine clinical work. However, while polyester will not tear, it may stretch very badly when subjected to excessive tensile force. In contrast, acetate tends to snap fairly cleanly when it separates. A badly-stretched segment of a tape represents a significant length of recording forever destroyed. A clean break, on the other hand, can often be spliced, keeping the loss to a small fraction of a second. Under some circumstances, then, a recording is better protected when done on acetate tape.

The thickness of the backing material also varies, from a minimum of 0.5 mil (thousandths of an inch) to over 2 mils. (The thinner the backing the greater the length of tape that can be wound on the reel.) Very thin tape should be avoided for two reasons. First, it is weaker and, therefore, is more likely to tear or deform. Second, as the backing is made thinner the magnetized coatings on the tape surface lie much closer to each other when the tape is wound on the reel. In storage, the magnetic fields in one layer can magnetize the coating in the next layer. On playback, one hears the original recording and an echo of material on the next tape layer. Such "print-through" can be distracting and disturbing to a listener and can interfere with analysis of the stored information. Print-through

is minimized by using thicker tape (1 1/2 mil is adequate) and by avoiding tight winding of the tape. (Because fast forward and rewind cause tight packing, recorded tapes are often stored on the take-up reel and rewound only before replaying.)

Reproduce transducers (heads)

Recall that moving a magnetic field near a wire causes a current to flow in it. Therefore, to reconvert the information stored in the tape's magnetic domains back to electrical signals, the tape need only be moved past the very same sort of coil-on-a-metal-core assembly that produced magnetic fields originally. As the magnetic domains on the tape pass the head, they induce currents that are sensed by the output amplifiers, and the original signal is recreated.

It turns out that the current induced by the magnetic domains is proportional to their strength and *to the rate of change* of magnetization as the magnetic domains move along. This implies that signals of similar amplitudes but different frequencies (that is, signals whose rates of change are different) will induce very different currents in the reproduce head. In fact, the amplitude of the output of an ideal reproduce head increases with frequency at the rate of 6 dB per octave. Tape decks have "equalization" circuits (discussed in the section labelled "Equalization") that compensate for this distortion of AC signals. It should be clear that when the rate of change (i.e., the frequency) of the stored signal drops to very low levels, the current induced in the playback head will ultimately become less than the random noise inherent in the system, and hence the signal will be irrecoverable.

Recording and Playback

Multichannel recording and tracking

It is possible to build a composite head that contains two or more record- or reproduce-transducers "stacked" above each other, as in Figure 3-20. If each head in a stack is associated with its own circuitry, then different signals can be simultaneously recorded as magnetized stripes, or *tracks* on the tape, with each track separated from its neighbors by a *guard band* of unrecorded tape.

Instrumentation (data) tape decks may be able to record up to 14 channels on a single (1-inch wide) tape. Clinicians are most likely to encounter 2-channel tape decks, however. These are usually called *stereophonic*, but this term tends to obscure their real value to the speech pathologist: One channel can be used to store the speech signal while the other records simultaneous physiological data (for instance, nasal air flow, or intraoral pressure).

Multichannel recording requires decisions about *tracking*—where on the tape the

A

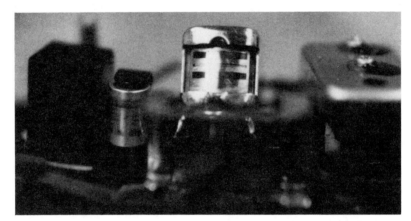

B

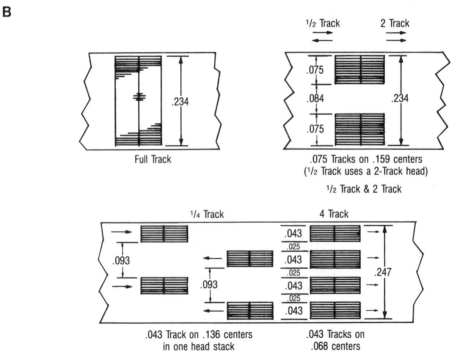

FIGURE 3-20. (A) Example of a two-head stack, such as is found in a "stereophonic" tape recorder. (B) Standard track patterns for various recording formats on 1/4 inch tape.

recording is to be located. Even a single channel of information need not occupy the entire width of the tape. Most 1-channel tape decks have record and playback heads that are somewhat narrower than half the tape width. They lay down a recorded track only on the upper half of the tape. This makes it possible to turn over the filled take-up reel and feed the tape through again to do another recording on the other half of the tape's width, doubling the effective length of the tape. A tape deck that uses this scheme is said to be single-channel, half-track. Two-channel (stereo) recorders use less than 1/4 of the tape width for each channel, and lay down a *two-channel, quarter-track* pattern, as shown in Figure 3-20. Multitrack usage of the tape means that the recorded material can only be played back on a machine that uses the same tracking pattern as the original recording unit. Note also that using the "other side" of the tape does not really mean using the other tape surface, but rather using the other half of the tape's width.

Biasing

There is a problem in the storage (tape magnetizing) process that has been ignored up to this point: The degree of magnetization achieved by the tape particles is by no means a linear function of the strength of the magnetic field produced by the record head. Typically, the strength of the magnetic field left on the tape (called the *remanent magnetic flux*) changes as shown in Figure 3-21A as the magnetizing force produced by the head increases. This "bent" transfer function has dire consequences for

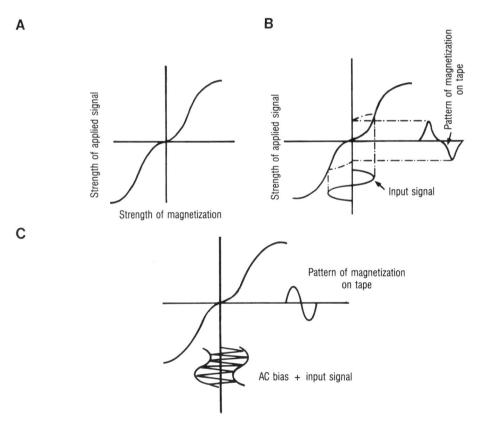

FIGURE 3-21. Recording-head AC bias. (A) demonstrates that magnetization of the tape is not a linear function of the magnetizing field. Hence, as shown in (B), a recorded signal will be severely distorted. Linearization is achieved by adding a high-frequency wave to the signal to be recorded (C), causing it to be stored in an undistorted form. The high-frequency signal is called an "AC bias."

the accuracy of representation of the stored signal, as shown in Figure 3-21B. Clearly, unless some corrective steps are taken, the magnetic analog representation on the tape will bear little resemblance to the original input signal, and the reproduced output will be an unrecognizably distorted version of what the record head laid down. A corrective measure has been developed empirically. It is called *AC bias*, and, as shown in Figure 3-21C, it involves adding a high-frequency complex waveform to the signal sent to the record head. When affected by the nonlinear transfer function, the composite signal produces a magnetic representation that is a *much* closer approximation of the original wave. The optimal frequency and amplitude of the bias signal depend on the range of frequencies to be recorded and on the characteristics of the record head and the magnetic material of the tape. Generally, a bias signal of around 100 kHz is used for audio recording, but the variety of tape materials (ferric oxide, chromium compounds, metallic particles) require different bias-current amplitudes. Therefore, producers of tape decks provide a way of changing the bias levels of their machines to suit the kind of tape being used. (It is unwise to buy a tape deck that does not have this feature.) Older machines that have a single, fixed bias, are generally optimized for standard ferric oxide tape. For best results, this is the only kind of tape that should be used with them.

Three-head tape recorders

Optimizing record, reproduce, and erase functions requires that the head be slightly different for each. While it is perfectly possible to get acceptable recordings from a head that serves both record and reproduce function, audio quality is significantly improved if separate, specially designed heads are used for the two functions. Accordingly, better-quality tape decks are usually "three head" machines. This feature should be considered essential when selecting a tape deck for purchase. There

are two reasons. The first, of course, is the increased audio fidelity that it affords. The second relates to the way in which the recording is monitored for quality. A combined record and reproduce head can only perform one function at a time. When it is recording, it cannot at the same time reproduce what is on the tape. Therefore, when listening to the tape to check for quality during actual recording, what the listener is hearing is not the recording itself (the single head is operating in record mode and so is not available to transduce what has been put onto the tape), but rather what is coming in to the recorder's amplifier. If there is any problem in the way in which the signal is laid down on the tape (incorrect bias, tape damage, and so on) it will not become apparent until later, when the tape is played back. On the other hand, a separate reproduce head can function while the recording is being made by the record head, so it is possible to monitor what has actually been laid down on the tape. (In fact, three-head tape decks allow the user to choose between listening to the input amplifier or the tape itself.)

Erasure

One of the advantages of magnetic tape storage of information is the ease with which the magnetic domains on the tape can be eliminated and the recorded information expunged. To erase the tape it must be exposed to a slowly diminishing cyclic magnetic field. This is accomplished very easily by passing it across a record head producing strong and rapidly alternating magnetic fields. As a given point on the tape moves further from the head, the effect of the head's magnetic field weakens, satisfying the "slowly diminishing" requirement. After this treatment, the magnetic domains on the tape are left very weakly magnetized (*degaussed*). Tape decks have a separate degaussing or erase head built into them. It is energized in the record mode and erases the tape just before it reaches the record head. Separate *bulk eras-*

ers are also available that can erase an entire reel of tape to a level at least 60 dB below that of a recorded signal.

Equalization

Mention was made earlier of the fact that the playback head inherently boosts the amplitude of signals of different frequencies at a rate of about 6 dB per octave.

There are also non-linearities in the frequency versus output amplitude curve due to inevitable losses produced by a number of physical phenomena. When these effects are taken together, the record-to-reproduce signal relationship is likely to resemble the one shown in Figure 3-22. Without correction, a reproduced signal will be very different from the signal originally applied to the record circuits.

The correction for these effects is called

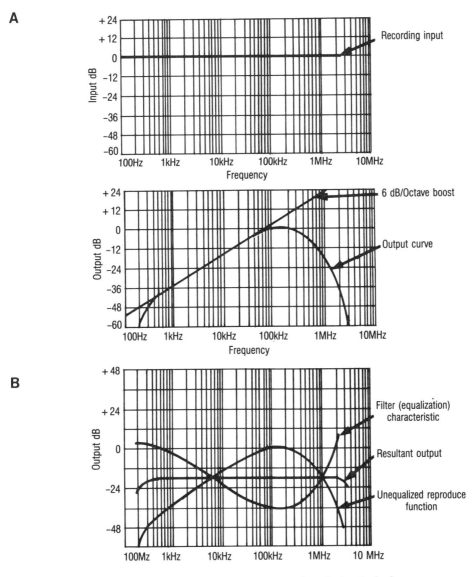

FIGURE 3-22. Equalization. (A) Because of electrical and physical phenomena, equal amplitude recordings at different frequencies will be reproduced with different amplitudes. Applying a special filtering function (B) results in a linearized signal.

equalization. Basically, it simply involves tailoring both the record and reproduce amplifiers' frequency responses to compensate for the inherent distortions of the tape-recording process. Tape decks designed to handle instrumentation signals exclusively (rather than audio signals) achieve equalization by making the frequency response curve of the recorder's electronics the inverse of the record and reproduce curves, as in Figure 3-22B. The result, on playback, is a faithful reproduction of the original input.

Audio signals, however, present greater complications, because the perceived loudness of equal-amplitude signals varies with frequency (Chap.4). The equalization characteristics of audio tape decks compensate for these effects as well, and therefore are more complex Figure 3-23). Furthermore, the different magnetic properties of the various kinds of tape now available call for different equalization curves. Fortunately, industry-wide standardization of equalization characteristics ensures that audio recordings made on one tape deck can be played back with equal fidelity on another. The U.S. standard equalization curve for

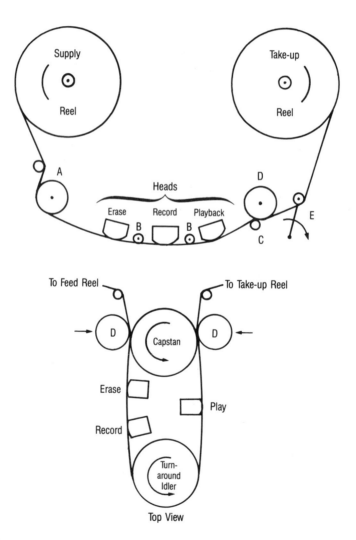

FIGURE 3-23. Tape transports. Top: Open loop; bottom: closed loop. A = inertia idler system; B = tape guides; C = capstan idler (pinch roller); D, E = loss-of-tension switch.

consumer audio recorders is called the National Association of Broadcasters (NAB) curve.

Noise reduction

Recording tapes have inherent random magnetic fluctuations that reproduce as tape hiss, and the tape deck electronics also contribute unwanted background noise. Optimalizing the signal-to-noise ratio of recorded material is important, therefore. One way to do this is to record at high signal levels to produce strong magnetic fields. Sometimes, particularly with the thinner and narrower tape used in cassettes, this is of limited effectiveness, especially if it increases print-through. Ways have been sought to improve the signal-to-noise ratio by electronic manipulations of the signal.

The most widely used noise reduction method is the Dolby system. The *Dolby-B* process (designed for incorporation in consumer devices) provides a prerecording emphasis of low-level input signals in the mid- and high-frequency ranges, where tape noise is most objectionable. On the tape, then, the amplitude of the higher frequencies is exaggerated. On playback, however, a matching deemphasis is applied, so that the signal is restored to its original spectral characteristics. The playback deemphasis restores the recorded material to original levels, but it also reduces unwanted hiss and noise in the frequency range of the de-emphasis. Since the noise signals were not boosted originally (because they were not part of the input, but rather came from the tape itself) they are attenuated in the final output. Recorded signals are reproduced at their real amplitudes. The net effect is that noise is reduced, and the signal-to-noise ratio improved by 5 to 10 dB. It is this noise reduction as much as any other factor that makes a cassette recorder capable of high-fidelity recording.

Transports: Moving the Tape

Moving the tape past the record and reproduce heads is the function of the tape transport system. Ideally, it would pull the tape at an absolutely constant rate, with no long-term or short-term speed variations. It would ensure that tape motion is always precisely perpendicular to the gaps in the heads and that the tape maintains a constant position vertically with respect to the heads, even when the tape is improperly or unevenly wound on the supply reel, so that tracking errors do not occur. The transport would not wear or damage the tape, and it would be compact, easy to maintain, and cheap to build.

Needless to say, no transport system fully meets these requirements. Improvement in one area often means compromise in another. And every performance increase is likely to be reflected in increased cost. A good transport, however, is likely to be worth its added expense.

From the speech clinician's point of view, the two most important transport specifications are those relating to *wow* and *flutter*. In audio work, wow generally refers to moderately slow tape speed variations, having a rate of less than 10 Hz. Wow is caused by small irregularities in movement of the mechanical components of the transport system, such as the capstan, drive belts, rollers, and the like. Flutter, on the other hand, describes tape speed changes of higher frequency. It is usually caused by vibrations of unsupported lengths of tape that result from friction with elements in the tape path, such as tape guides and the heads themselves. Well-designed tape transports can reduce both wow and flutter to a small fraction of one percent.

Two basic kinds of tape transport are used in audio tape decks. They differ in their effectiveness in keeping the tape properly aligned with respect to the record and reproduce heads and in their minimization of wow and flutter.

Open-loop drives

Figure 3-23A diagrams an open loop drive system, which is the simplest, most popular, and least expensive type in general use. Tape is drawn from a supply reel mounted on a spindle at the left and is ultimately wound on a take-up reel on the right. Tape movement is *not* due to rotation of the take-up reel. If it were, the speed of the tape past the heads would increase as the diameter of the tape pack on the take-up reel increased. Instead, the tape is pulled past the heads by a rotating *capstan*, against which the tape is held by a *pinch roller* or *capstan idler*. The capstan is turned by a special motor that maintains a steady speed.

If the tape were otherwise unsupported along its relatively long route between reels, it would be likely to flutter and drift up and down. Therefore, a number of guides are provided to position the tape correctly with respect to the heads. A relatively massive *inertia idler* serves to isolate the tape near the heads from the influence of irregularities in the supply reel or variations in the packing of the tape on it. On most recorders there is also some system that switches the transport off if the tape breaks or runs out.

Closed-loop drives

More expensive tape decks may use a closed-loop drive system like the one shown in Figure 3-23B. The main elements are the same as in the open-loop drive, but the tape path is "folded" around a turnaround idler, and two pinch rollers hold the tape on opposite sides of the capstan. This arrangement limits the distances over which the tape is unsupported, thereby providing much greater stability of tape travel.

Direct and FM Recording

The kind of recording process discussed thus far, in which instantaneous amplitude of the recorded signal is related to intensity of the stored magnetic field, is called *direct* or *amplitude modulated* recording. It was mentioned earlier that the voltage produced by the reproduce head of a tape deck is proportional to the rate of change of the magnetic field that it senses. As the frequency of a recorded signal falls, the rate of change of the magnetic strength

of the domains on the tape is reduced. Therefore, as frequency falls, the amplitude of a reproduced signal gets smaller. An attempt to record DC by direct recording is doomed to total failure. Since the rate of change of a DC signal is zero, the reproduce head will be unaffected by it. Many physiological signals (air flow and air pressure, for instance) characteristically have very low rates of change, and some come very close to being DC. The direct recording techniques discussed thus far will not work for them. What is needed is some way of coding them into a form that can be successfully recorded and decoded during reproduction. There are many ways of doing this, but the most widely used method is *frequency modulation* (FM).

In frequency modulation a waveform (called the *carrier*) is made to vary in frequency in proportion to the amplitude of some other signal. An example is shown in Figure 3-24. A sine wave carrier (lower trace) changes frequency as the voltage of a *modulating signal* (upper trace) rises and falls. The frequency of the carrier when the modulating voltage is zero (extreme left) is, in this case, 100 Hz. This is the *center frequency* of the carrier. When the modulating signal has a voltage of +5 V, the carrier's frequency is 167.5 Hz; when it is -5 V the carrier is at 32.5 Hz. The amount of variation of the carrier frequency for a given change in the modulating voltage is an important parameter of frequency modulation. In this case, a change of the modulating voltage from 0 V to +5 V produced a frequency change of 67.5 Hz in the carrier. The "frequency deviation" of the carrier is therefore 13.5 Hz/V.

In frequency modulation, then, the *frequency* of a carrier waveform (usually a square wave) represents the amplitude of some other signal. Since the carrier is an AC wave, it can be tape recorded, allowing a coded representation of a DC signal to be stored on tape. The only restrictions (from the tape recorder's point of view) is that the highest and lowest frequencies that the carrier might assume must lie in the range of the tape deck. Information theory

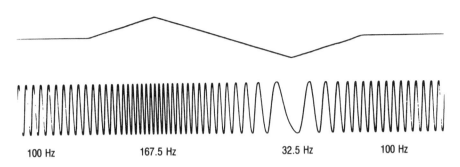

100 Hz   167.5 Hz   32.5 Hz   100 Hz

FIGURE 3-24. Frequency modulation (FM). The lower trace shows the frequency modulated form of the wave at the top. Note how the voltage of the top wave is represented by the frequency of the lower signal.

also indicates that the carrier frequency limits the frequency of the data that can be coded. It is not possible, for instance, to obtain an accurate frequency coding of a 100 Hz sine wave with a 150 Hz carrier frequency. In fact, for accurate data storage, the carrier frequency should be much higher than the highest frequency component in the modulating signal. For example, the instrumentation standards currently in effect call for a center frequency of 54 kHz to encode signals from DC to 10 kHz. It also turns out that the maximal deviation (produced by the maximal voltage change from 0 volts) must not be too great, or nonlinearities will occur. Industry standardization of FM tape decks permits a maximal deviation of $\pm 40\%$ about the center frequency. For a DC-10 kHz system, then, the center frequency of 54 kHz would vary from a minimum of 32.4 kHz to a maximum of 75.6 kHz.

FM tape decks contain all the necessary electronics for encoding an input into a frequency-modulated signal, storing it on the tape, and decoding it on playback. Usually these machines are multi-channel, to provide for simultaneous recording of different data, and there is often at least one direct-recording channel for recording voice or other audio information. These tape decks are moderately expensive, but are well worth their cost in situations in which a great deal of physiological recording must be done.

Most clinics, however, are unlikely to be enthusiastic about investing in a tape deck that is of very limited value for audio work. Fortunately, there is a relatively low-cost alternative to buying an FM tape system. The frequency modulation and demodulation system can be an external attachment to an ordinary tape deck, such as is found in every clinical setting. Such an *FM recording adapter* allows any direct-record machine to function as an FM unit whenever that is desirable. The most popular adapter units are produced by A. R. Vetter Co., one of whose instruments is shown in Figure 3-25. The DC or low frequency data signal to be recorded is input to the adapter unit, not to the tape deck. The adapter produces a frequency-modulated carrier, which is recorded on tape. On playback, the tape output is fed back through the FM adapter, which demodulates it to reproduce the original data signal. These adapters are designed to use center frequencies within the range of the audio tape deck. Their data frequency range is accordingly somewhat restricted, but is more than adequate for most physiological signals, which tend to be of low frequency. Adapters are available in dual-channel models, providing one adapter for each channel of a stereo tape system. Furthermore, Vetter offers three- and four-channel *multiplexed* adapters, which accept three or four inputs. Each input is modulated around a different center frequency. The results are then added together into a single composite signal

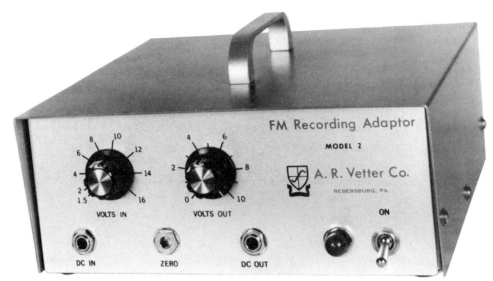

FIGURE 3-25. A Vetter Model 2 FM recording adapter. It converts a DC input into an FM signal suitable for tape recording. On playback it converts the FM signal back into the original waveform. (Courtesy A. R. Vetter Co., Rebersberg, PA.)

which requires only one tape-deck channel. Thus, for a very modest expenditure, any clinic can have a multichannel FM recording system.

Cassette Systems

In the last several years the popularity of the cassette tape format has grown enormously. This has resulted from improvements in tape materials and manufacturing techniques, from advances in tape-deck design, and from the introduction of noise reduction systems simple enough for use in consumer electronic products. Originally, cassette recording (which is always done at a speed of 1.875 ips) was not capable of sufficient fidelity for most uses in speech pathology, but that is no longer the case. Cassette tape decks can function quite adequately for client record-keeping or therapeutic feedback.

Cassette units offer convenience. But, all things being equal, they do not achieve the same recording quality as reel-to-reel tape decks. Furthermore, it is very difficult to splice or similarly edit cassette tapes. While clinicians may wish to make cassette tape

recorders the basic units in their recording instrument inventory, every clinical facility should have at least one high-quality reel-to-reel recorder, to be used when the best possible fidelity is needed, or when data recording demands recorder flexibility, such as high tape speeds that cassette units cannot deliver.

Recording Technique

Ideally, a microphone would produce a perfectly accurate electrical analog of a single acoustic signal (e.g., a client's speech) while disregarding all irrelevant sounds in the immediate environment. Ideally, that electrical analog would be precisely stored on the tape and would later be reproduced without any distortion. In a perfect world, an exact acoustic duplicate of the original sound waves would be generated by a loudspeaker system, recreating the original acoustic event. Perfection is not achieved in the real world, but with a little care it can be approached. What is required is a high-quality microphone, an excellent tape deck, and a well-designed speaker system. Clearly, every speech pathologist should be equipped with the best audio system possible. Much of the clinical work of the speech professional is founded on very careful listening. It is probably foolish to focus the finely honed auditory skills of a first-rate therapist on a noisy, distorted, second-rate recording. First, then, clinicians will want to purchase the best possible recording instrument. The specifications of Table 3-1 can be used to guide in selecting an adequate unit.

Just as important as the quality of the equipment is adherence to a few basic, common sense recording principles.

1. Choose quiet surroundings. Unlike the human auditory system, a microphone cannot be selectively attentive. It cannot "focus in" on a single sound source and suppress all others. Except for directionality effects, a microphone transduces all sounds that reach it: The client's speech, the clanking of a radiator, the rumble of passing trucks, and loud speech in the next room. It follows that the environment must be as quiet as possible. Excessively "live" or reverberant spaces should also be avoided: the

acoustic reflections may produce significant distortion of the audio signal. The sound isolation rooms used for audiometric work serve quite well for recording and should be used whenever possible. It is worth the scheduling problems that may have to be worked out.

2. Isolate the microphone from vibration. A microphone must be supported on (or from) something. The choice of support is far from trivial, since vibration of the microphone support will be transduced along with the sound input. A number of relatively simple steps can, and should, be taken to minimize this problem. The microphone should never be placed on the same surface with a tape recorder: the vibration of the recorder's motors will produce significant background noise in the recording. Whenever possible, mount the microphone on a boom, rather than on a desktop microphone stand. This keeps it isolated from the vibratory noise produced by client or therapist when, for example, they drop something on the table, kick its leg, and so on. The boom

TABLE 3-1. Minimal Specifications for Tape Decks

Specification	Reel-to-Reel	Cassette
Frequency response		
@7.5 ips	30–20,000 Hz ± 3dB	(speed not used)
@3.75 ips	40–14,000 Hz ± 3dB	(speed not used)
@1.875 ips		30–15,000 Hz ± 3dB
Signal/noise ratio		
Without Dolby	55 dB or higher	55 dB or higher
With Dolby	60 dB or higher	60 dB or higher
Wow and flutter		
unweighted	0.15% or less	0.15% or less
weighted*	0.10% or less	0.10% or less
Stereo, Separation		
(signal leakage from left	50 dB or higher	40 dB or higher
to right channel or vice-versa)		
Cross-talk		
(signal leakage from between	60 dB or higher	60 dB or higher
adjacent tape tracks)		

*Different frequency components in the signal are given different prominence in the mathematical computation. Caution: there are a number of different weighting systems in use, and they produce slightly different values for the same quality of performance.

allows the microphone stand to be positioned to the side of the speaker (out of the way of inadvertent kicks and knocks) while allowing great flexibility of placement of the microphone itself.

Manufacturers can usually provide shock mounts for their microphones, which cushion them and provide isolation from floor and building vibration. They are worth their moderate cost.

3. Place the microphone correctly in relation to the speaker. "Correct" is determined by the directionality characteristics of the microphone being used. In general the microphone should be pointed toward the speaker, slightly below and about a foot away from the mouth. Closer placement may be useful, but it tends to subject the microphone to the puffs of air accompanying plosives and strong fricatives; this produces loud noise bursts. This problem can be alleviated by the use of a windscreen, a plastic foam hood that fits over the microphone head (Figure 3-26).

Microphone use is much more of an art than a science. Clinicians should experiment with different locations, microphone placements, and mounting techniques to optimize results in their own settings. A great many suggestions can be garnered from the sources at the end of the chapter.

OSCILLOSCOPES

The oscilloscope (Figure 3-27) makes electrical waveforms and voltage conditions visible on a screen. It allows us to "see" speech waveforms and physiological variables, such as air flow rate, movement patterns, or pressure. It can also show stimulus characteristics and provide information on the calibration status of other instruments. Although it is almost a symbol of the research laboratory, the oscilloscope should also be considered an absolutely indispensable item of equipment for any clinician who routinely performs any kind of objective measurement. It will be used for check-

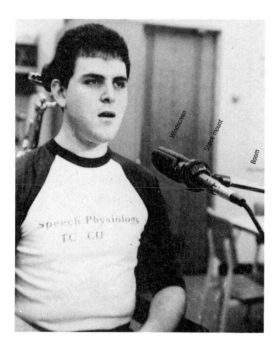

FIGURE 3-26. Microphone fitted with a shock-absorber and windscreen mounted on a boom for patient recording.

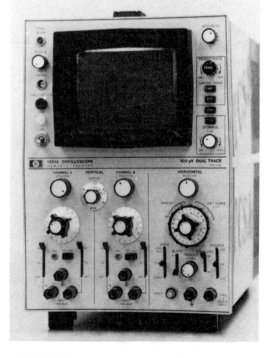

FIGURE 3-27. A typical oscilloscope.

ing the performance of almost every other electronic device, for obtaining basic measurements, and even for visual feedback to a client during the course of therapy.

Basic Principles and Design

Cathode Ray Tubes

The heart of any oscilloscope is the *cathode ray tube* (CRT, Figure 3-28), which looks very much like a TV picture tube, of which it is, in fact, the forerunner. The visual display appears on the front surface; the long neck contains most of the electronic elements. The tube is evacuated to a very high vacuum.

It has been known since the nineteenth century that electrons can be made to travel in straight lines in a vacuum if they are subjected to an accelerating force. The CRT elements that accomplish this are in the electron gun (Figure 3-28B). Here, electrons are "boiled off" a metal surface that is kept very hot by a filament heater. A cloud of electrons forms near the heated plate. Now, electrons are negatively charged, implying that they will be repelled by other negatively-charge bodies and attracted to positively-charged ones. The electron gun uses this fact. The metal plate from which the electrons are emitted is connected to the negative terminal of a voltage source, while the positive terminal is connected to a metal cylinder just in front of the emitting surface. The electrons are attracted out of the electron cloud toward and into the positively charged tube. The negative, or electron-producing, pole of the system is called a *cathode*; the positive pole is the *anode*. The stream of electrons drawn out of the electron cloud at the negative pole is called, therefore, a *cathode* ray.

The speed at which the electrons move toward the anode is proportional to the voltage difference between the cathode and anode. In the CRT very large voltages (perhaps 3000 V or more) are used.* The speed attained by the electrons will be so great that most of them will fly right on through

the accelerating anode tube, to encounter and be stopped by a plate that closes its far end. The plate, however, does have a small hole in its center, and the path of some of the electrons will carry them right through the hole and out of the electron gun. What has been created is a very thin beam (called a "pencil") of electrons travelling along the central axis of the CRT toward its face. Generally, the thin beam is made to pass through another anode at even higher voltage, to speed up the electrons still more. Along the path there will also be a special anode designed to compress the beam and focus it. (Other control elements may be included with the gun assembly, but they need not concern us here.) The high-speed electrons now race the length of the tube until, if they are properly focussed, they all crash into a single point on the inner surface of the face of the tube.

Unfortunately, the human eye is not sensitive to electron radiation: We cannot see the electron beam. However, there are a number of substances that give off visible light when they are excited by electrons. The inside of the screen is painted with a coating of such *phosphors*, and the coating gives off light wherever the beam strikes it. The electron beam's impact is thereby made visible.[†] Brightness of the phosphor glow depends on the number of electrons striking it. A front-panel control on the oscilloscope allows the birghtness level to be varied. Other controls adjust beam focus and astigmatism (directional inequality of focussing). A grid pattern, or graticule, etched on a plastic sheet covering the face

---

*The oscilloscope is one of the few instruments in clinical use that uses genuinely high voltages. The implication is that, unless very certain of what they are doing, untrained personnel should not attempt internal adjustments of these devices. Servicing is best left to a qualified technician.

---

†The phosphor coating cannot tolerate heavy electron bombardment for very long. Light is not the only result of electron radiation: significant heat is also produced. If the beam is focussed on a single spot for a long time, enough heat may be generated to burn away the phosphor, permanently damaging the CRT.

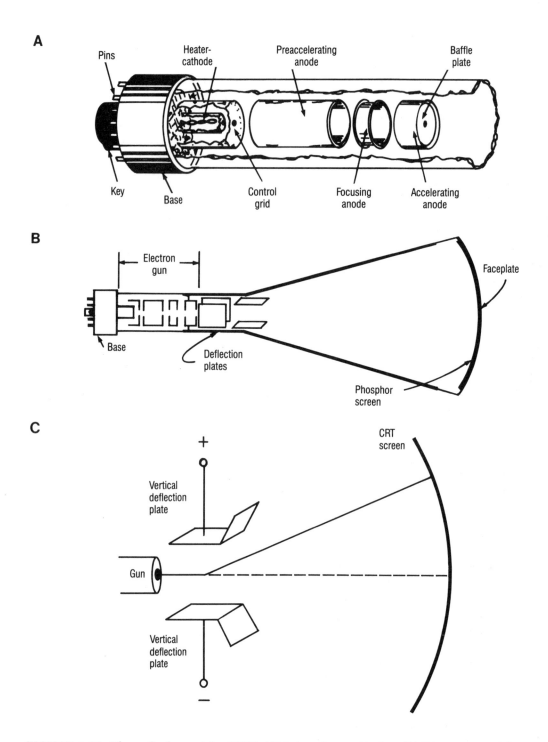

FIGURE 3-28. The cathode-ray tube (CRT). (A) Internal organization. (B) Generation and focusing of the electron beam. (C) Deflection of the electron beam (dotted line) by the plates. Equal charge on opposing plates allows the beam to pass undeflected; positive charge on the upper plate deflects the beam upward. (From Sessions, K. W. and Fischer, W. A. *Understanding Oscilloscopes and Display Waveforms.* New York: John Wiley and Sons, Inc. Figures 1-1, 1-2, and 1-3, pp. 3, 5, and 7. © 1978 by John Wiley and Sons, Inc. Reprinted by permission.)

of the screen or into the glass itself divides the usable screen area into squares on the order of 1 cm. on a side for easy measurement of spot position.

The method by which the beam, and hence the spot of phosphorescent light, is moved around in conformity with an input signal also depends on the attraction of electrons to (relatively) positively-charged bodies. Figure 3-28C shows how deflection of beam is achieved in most oscilloscopes. The speeding electrons pass between a pair of metal plates. If the two are at the same voltage the beam is unaffected. But if one of the plates is more positively charged than the other, the electrons are attracted toward it. Therefore, as the electrons whiz by, they are diverted somewhat from their straight-line path and the beam as a whole is deflected a bit. The result is that the spot of light moves toward the edge of the phosphor screen that corresponds with the position of the positively charged plate. The more positive that plate is, the more strongly the electrons are attracted to it and the greater the deflection of the beam. If the charge on the plate is controlled by the input signal to the oscilloscope, the location of the spot of light on the screen will represent the signal voltage. Oscilloscopes have two pairs of *defelction plates*. The *vertical* plates are oriented horizontally and deflect the beam vertically; the *horizontal* plates, oriented vertically, control side-to-side positioning of the spot. Neither set of plates is connected directly to the oscilloscope inputs, of course. Instead, they are controlled by amplifiers and other circuitry.

Oscilloscope electronics

Oscilloscopes are available with a very wide range of features that are designed to facilitate different kinds of displays or signal analyses. Certain functions, however, are fundamental and are included in all oscilloscopes. Some oscilloscopes are "dedicated" instruments: They are designed to perform one task and are permanently adjusted to optimize their function for that task alone. (A television set is an extreme example of just such a specialized oscilloscope.) In these units there is relatively little the user need do beyond turning the instrument on. But most oscilloscopes are designed to be as versatile as possible, which means that adjustment and "tuning" of the instrument must be done by the user for each task. Doing this is not difficult if the oscilloscope's functional components are well understood. Therefore, this section will provide an introduction to the oscilloscope's functional blocks, those that are common to all oscilloscopes and several that are optional but likely to be of special value to the speech clinician. Details of the specific electron circuits that perform the various functions will not be considered, but more information along these lines is available in Sessions and Fischer (1978), as well as in a host of books at all levels of sophistication available at most electronics shops.

Basic Functional Units

Figure 3-29 shows the organization of a minimal, "barebones" oscilloscope. Controlling the CRT defection plates are vertical and horizontal amplifiers, a sweep generator, and a trigger circuit.

Vertical and horizontal amplifiers

The basic function of the vertical and horizontal amplifiers is obvious: They modify the voltage of the input signal to a level that is adequate for the deflection plates (perhaps 25 V or so). In keeping with the objective of maximal versatility, the gain of these amplifiers can be varied by front-panel controls to accomodate inputs from just a few millivolts to over 100 V. (For very large signals the amplifier has fractional gain, and therefore acts as an attenuator.) Calibration of the amplifier is not in terms of gain, but rather is expressed as *sensitivity*—the input voltage required to deflect the beam 1 grid division on the screen's graticule. One gain setting of the amplifi-

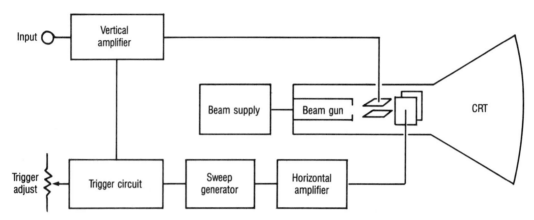

FIGURE 3-29. Organization of an oscilloscope.

er, for example, might read "5 mV/division," indicating that the gain is set to cause the deflection plates to move the beam exactly 1 screen division for each 5 mV of signal strength. (If the screen is 10 divisions high—or wide—then a change in input up to 50 mV could be seen.) Another setting might be labelled "1 V/div," another "5 V/div," and so on. Expressing the amplifier gain in this way makes the oscilloscope an easily read voltmeter.

The input amplifiers are almost always of the DC-coupled type (see section labelled "AC and DC Amplifiers), meaning that they will amplify unchanging or extremely low-frequency inputs. This is generally advantageous, since physiological signals, for instance, are very often quasi-DC. However, as mentioned previously, it is often desirable to eliminate a DC "bias" signal in order to be able to maximally boost a small AC component of interest riding on it. For example, in some types of dysphonia there is an uninterrupted flow of air during phonation, with only a small periodic fluctuation that represents the vocal signal. If a flow signal is being monitored on the oscilloscope, most of the beam deflection will be produced by the constant flow (DC signal) with the phonation showing as small ripples (AC signal) in the displayed trace. Amplification will enlarge the small AC ripple, but it will increase the DC level by an equal amount, perhaps driving

the entire display off the screen. Here is a case in which elimination of the DC signal would make it easier to see the AC ripple that might be of interest. To meet this need, the amplifier has a front-panel switch that allows the user to block DC and convert the circuit to an AC amplifier.

Usually the AC/DC amplifier switch has a third setting marked "ground." When the switch is in this position, the amplifier input is disconnected from the front-panel connections and is instead connected to ground. The amplifier then has a 0 V input, and the position of the beam on the screen represents the zero baseline, from which voltages are measured. The baseline itself can be changed by moving the beam by means of a control marked "position" or "center" on the front panel. It changes the no-signal voltage relationship of the deflection plates.

Sweep circuits (time base)

Although all oscilloscopes have vertical and horizontal amplifiers, most of the controls just described are provided only for the vertical one. It is always possible to connect an external signal to the horizontal amplifier, but it is really designed to handle internally generated voltages that will make the electron beam sweep from left to right across the screen at a known speed, establishing a *time base* for the display. If the beam is moving horizontally at a constant speed, then the horizontal axis of the screen is a *time* axis. Successive vertical deflections will occur further and further to the right in the display. The distance between any two points is a measure of the amount of time that separates them. An oscilloscope whose vertical deflection is produced by an input signal and whose horizontal deflection represents a time base generates a graph of the input over time — a very useful form of data display.

The timebase is established by a circuit called (for obvious reasons) a *sweep generator*. It is an oscillator that produces a "sawtooth wave" like the one in Figure 3-30. The voltage of this wave rises steadily from negative to positive, and then rapidly returns to the original negative level. If this voltage pattern is applied to one of the CRT's horizontal plates the beam will be deflected from its normally midline course in a pattern that matches the waveform.

At the start of the cycle, the beam is forced maximally away from the plate, which has a negative charge. As the charge becomes progressively less negative and then increasingly positive, the beam is deflected less and less away from one plate and then more and more toward the other one. The beam, then, is made to sweep across the screen at a constant rate during the period of time, $-t_s$, that the waveform's voltage is rising. At the end of this interval the voltage drops rapidly to its original negative level. Obviously during this *retrace* period, t_r, the beam is quickly returned to the starting point. As the cycle repeats, the beam moves relatively slowly from left to right (the voltages are applied to the plates to assure that directionality), and then it very quickly retraces its path back to the left and sweeps across again. Most oscilloscopes have a *blanking* circuit that dims the beam during the retrace portion of the cycle, so that the return stroke does not appear in the display. While the beam is being deflected across the screen, the vertical input signal is also producing vertical deflection. Thus, the input voltage produces a graph of its magnitude over time.

In Figure 3-30 the rising portion of the wave takes 100 msec, so this is the time required for the beam to cross the screen. If the graticule has ten divisions horizontally, the beam traverses each division in 10 msec. The sweep time can be varied by changing the repetition rate of the sawtooth wave. The higher its frequency, the less time required for a complete sweep. The time base control on the oscilloscope front panel is calibrated in sweep time per screen division. Commonly the settings range from 1 μsec/div to 5 sec/div. The higher sweep speeds spread out vertical deflections so that closely spaced (or high frequency) events can be seen clearly (Fig. 3-30). Very high sweep rates are of little use to the speech clinician, who is not often concerned with signals exceeding a few thousand hertz.

Triggering

Although a usable oscilloscope could be built with only the functional elements discussed so far, the addition of one more component will overcome one remaining inconvenience that results from the independence of the input and sweep signals. To appreciate the problem, consider the situation depicted in Figure 3-31. The sine-wave input (Figure 3-31A) has a period just slightly longer than the time base sweep-retrace cycle (Figure 3-31B). Therefore, each sweep of the beam across the screen begins a bit earlier in the input wave's cycle than the previous sweep, with successive representations of the waveform as shown in Figure 3-31C. Because the sweep repetition rate is very high, the display takes on the characteristics of a motion picture, and the waveform seems to drift across the display. Of course, this problem could be overcome by adjusting the sweep repetition rate to precisely match the frequency of the input signal, but such a solution has a number of inadequacies. Most signals that the speech clinician will want to see are not perfectly

A

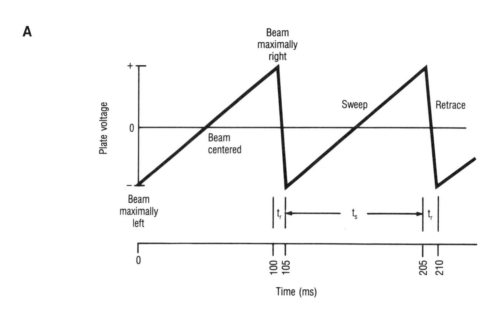

B

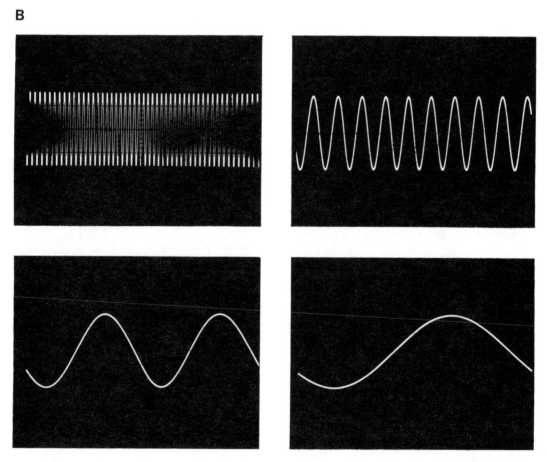

FIGURE 3-30. (A) The time-base generator's sweep signal. (B) Effect of increasing the sweep speed. A 1000 Hz sine wave is shown in each case. Slowest sweep speed is at upper left, highest speed at lower right.

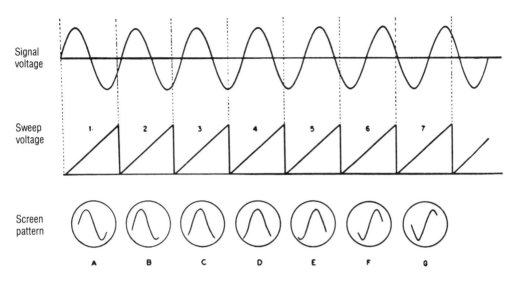

Signal voltage

Sweep voltage

Screen pattern

A   B   C   D   E   F   G

FIGURE 3-31. When the input signal and sweep signal are not synchronized each sweep starts at a different point in the input wave. The result is a display that seems to drift across the screen. (From Session, K. W. and Fischer, W. A. *Understanding Oscilloscopes and Display Waveforms.* New York: John Wiley and Sons, 1978. Figure 2-14, p. 36. © 1978 by John Wiley and Sons, Inc. Reprinted by permission.)

periodic—their repetion rate varies slightly from cycle to cycle. In order to get a stable display the sweep rate would have to be continually adjusted. Not only is this a practical impossibility, but, even if it could be achieved it would mean that the time axis of the display would be constantly changing, frustrating any attempt to derive time-based data, such as fundamental frequency. Even if these limitations were not objectionable, there would remain the problem of how nonrepetitive signals appear on the screen. If the sweep circuit is *free-running*, an isolated event could appear at any point in the sweep. Thus, it might show up anywhere from left to right on the screen, and it might even run off the right edge. Still worse, it could end up being continued into the next sweep cycle, which means that it would "wrap around" to continue on the left edge of the screen.

The solution to all these problems is called a *trigger* circuit. A trigger is a pulse that initiates the function of another circuit. In the case of triggered oscilloscopes, the trigger generator turns out a pulse that lets the sweep generator turn out a single sweep

wave. The trigger circuit itself can be controlled by an external signal that the user supplies (via a front panel connection) so that the beam will be swept across the screen once every time an external pulse is delivered to the scope. This is useful for synchronizing the display to some external event. For instance, a pressure probe in the mouth can cause the oscilloscope to trigger a sweep every time there is a pressure release for /p/, perhaps showing the acoustic waveform (transduced by a microphone) applied to the vertical input. The voice onset time for /p/ would then be easily determinable. But there is an even more helpful, and more common, use to which the trigger circuit is put. In almost all oscilloscopes the trigger circuit can be set to monitor the input signal itself and turn out a trigger pulse only when the amplitude and polarity of the input have certain minimal values. In short, this means that the oscilloscope sweep can be started at the same point in each of a series of repetitive input waves, as shown in Figure 3-32. This holds the display stable on the screen. Note that the sweep rate (the speed of the beam's

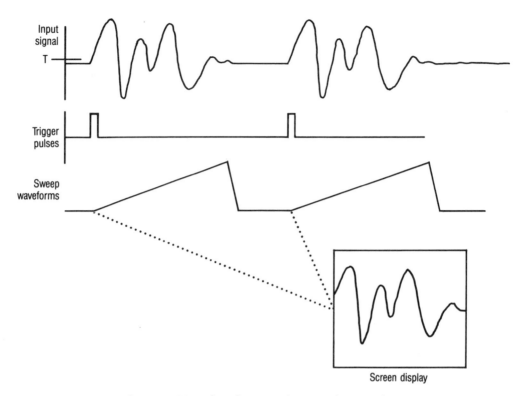

FIGURE 3-32. Triggered sweep. Note that the second sweep does not begin until a trigger pulse occurs.

travel across the screen) is not altered by the trigger: Each trigger pulse allows one sweep at whatever speed has been preselected. The time base calibration remains valid. But each sweep starts at the same point in the waveform (which point depends on the front-panel, trigger-control setting) and, when sweeps are retriggered in rapid sequence, a steady display is perceived.

Special Oscilloscope Features

The uitility of the oscilloscope can be greatly enhanced by a number of optional features that are offerred by almost all manufacturers. Those that are most helpful to the speech clinician are considered below.

Dual trace

Oscilloscopes are available that will allow two different input signals (e.g., the speech signal and oral airflow) to be shown on the screen at the same time. These *dual trace* or *dual channel* instruments use a single electron gun and one set of deflection plates that are shared by two separate vertical amplifiers. A switching circuit (called a *chopper*) alternately connects channel 1 and channel 2 to the deflection plates, so that the single beam is deflected for both of them. If each is associated with a different DC voltage (supplied by the oscilloscope circuitry) the segments representing channel 1 will appear at one level on the screen, and those representing channel 2 will appear at a different level.

Since a single deflection system is serving both signals, it is clear that both cannot be shown on the screen at exactly the same instant. Most dual-channel oscilloscopes offer a choice of methods for displaying the input signals alternately. They are illustrated in Figure 3-33. In the *alternate* mode, the chopper first connects chan-

A

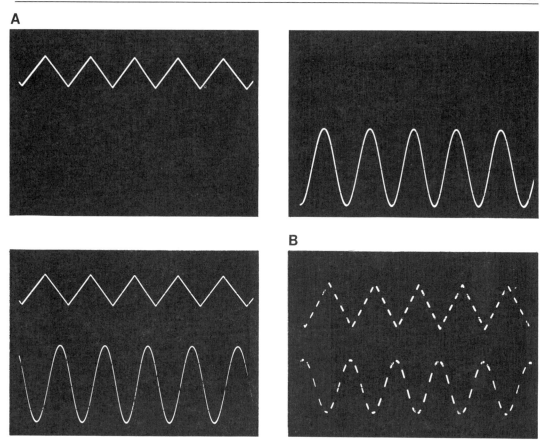

FIGURE 3-33. (A) "Alternate" display mode. The beam first traces the channel-1 signals, then does the channel-2 signals. When the traces alternate rapidly they appear to be on the screen at the same time. (B) "Chopped" display mode. The beam alternately traces short segments of each input. (Here the chopping has been greatly slowed for demonstration purposes. Under normal conditions each trace would appear to be continuous.)

nel 1 to the deflection plates for an entire sweep, and then connects channel 2 for the next sweep. The first-one-then-the-other pattern continues. When the sweep time is long, the user sees first the upper trace and then the lower one. But for fast sweeps, persistence of phosphorescence and of vision combine to produce the *illusion* that both traces are on the screen at the same time. Therein lies a problem that grows more serious as the sweep time grows longer. It is possible that something of interest might happen on one channel while the other is being displayed. If the event is short enough, it might be over by the time its channel is shown.

To counter this possibility a different form of alternation is provided. In the "chopped" mode the signals from the two channels are applied to the deflection plates for very brief periods in rapid succession during each sweep of the beam (Fig. 3-33B). The result is that a very short segment of the channel 1 signal is shown, then a very short segment of the channel 2 signal, and so on. Each trace is really a dashed line, with the dashes of one alternating with the dashes of the other. (Unless the sweep rate is exceptionally high the individual dashes cannot be seen, and each line looks solid.) The two lines are, of course, separated on the screen by the different DC level applied to each for just that purpose. In this mode not all of each trace is really present in the display, but the pieces that are missing are very short, and it is unlikely that any meaningful event will be missed—especially at the frequencies characteristic of speech events.

Display storage

The trace on the oscilloscope screen is very temporary, lasting only as long as the phosphor continues to glow after it has been excited. In the case of the most popular phosphor (P31), the glow persists for only 30 ms. If the waveform being observed is repetitive or continuous (e.g., a sustained speech sound), there is no problem. By the time one sweep's trace has disappeared, another, identical one, is written. Imagine, for example, that the therapist wants his client to see the noise component in her dysphonic voice. For this purpose the sweep rate of the oscilloscope can be quite fast, and there will always be a waveform to observe. Suppose, however, that the therapist's object is to provide feedback of intraoral air pressure to a client with velopharyngeal inadequacy. In this case, the beam will have to move slowly across the screen, because speech events are relatively slow and the client has to observe the pattern of air pressure change during an entire utterance. There is no problem in getting the beam to sweep slowly, but since the phosphor only glows for a small fraction of a second no trace is produced. All that appears on the screen is a dot, moving up and down according to the air pressure, leaving no trail to show what the pattern of change has been. Transient events, such as a plosive, present a similar problem. Their trace is gone from the screen far too fast for the clinician to clearly perceive, much less evaluate, them.

Storage oscilloscopes have modifications of the CRT which "freeze" a trace on the screen for a long period of time—typically up to an hour. The effect is achieved by a special second screen inside the tube made of a material such as magnesium oxide that serves as a charge-storage surface. The screen is placed in the beam's path, and

acquires a charge wherever the beam strikes it. The CRT also contains a second electron gun, which does not produce a narrow beam but rather floods the inside of the tube with electrons. These are accelerated toward the screen, but they are deflected back except from those areas that have been charged by the beam. Therefore, they pass through these areas and strike the phosphor coating, causing it to glow. A single sweep of the beam creates an electron "gate" through which the phosphor is excited. The storage screen can hold its acquired charge for a considerable period of time and, therefore, the pattern can be seen long after the sweep is over. Special electrical pulses delivered to the storage screen system erase it and ready it for the next display.

A modification of the storage principle allows for "variable persistence" displays, in which the path that the beam has taken across the screen can be kept glowing for a variable amount of time, adjusted by the user. Slowly changing phenomena, such as breathing movements, can be displayed with slow sweeps, and the trace persistence adjusted so that the trace remains visible for the duration of the entire sweep before fading away. The advantage of variable persistence over simple storage is that the display can be slow and continuous; with storage oscilloscopes a single "screenful" is stored, meaning that intermittent samples of an ongoing signal are acquired.

Oscilloscope cameras

A permanent record of the oscilloscope trace requires that the display be photographed. Special cameras (Figure 3-34) make this fairly easy to do. Typically, such a camera has a hood that attaches to a mounting in front of the screen. The hood excludes ambient light and keeps the lens a fixed distance from the screen surface. (The camera lens is permanently focussed for this distance.) The back of the camera holds standard Polaroid film providing instant copies of the trace at reasonable cost. (More elaborate, and expensive, cameras are available that have interchangeable

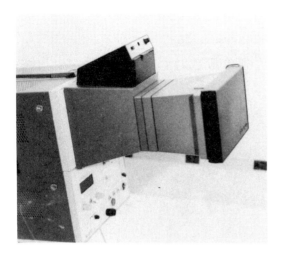

FIGURE 3-34. An oscilloscope camera.

backs to accept a variety of film types.) These cameras are available for almost any type of oscilloscope at very moderate cost.

CHART RECORDERS

Only a few seconds worth of data can be accommodated on the oscilloscope screen, and the data traces are quite small. Therefore, if events occurring over a relatively long time are to be permanently recorded, or if careful measurement of the data needs to be done, a single photograph of the oscilloscope screen is obviously inadequate. Imagine, for instance, having to evaluate the fundamental frequency pattern of a reading passage on the basis of an oscillograph trace. It is possible to arrange for a continuous strip of film to be drawn past the vertically moving spot on the screen and thereby produce a very long photographic negative of the oscilloscope's display over time and, in fact, this was a much-used method in the early years of research. One could also take motion pictures of the oscilloscope screen. Both of these procedures, however, are tedious, time-consuming (since the film needs to be developed) and, perhaps worst of all,

expensive. What is needed, really, is a chart recorder, a device that writes one or more oscilloscope-type traces on a continuous strip of paper. Chart recorders fall into at least three main categories: pen recorders, light-beam oscillographs, and cathode-ray oscillographs (Figure 3-35). They differ in how the trace is written onto the paper, but they also have many features in common.

Basic Organization

The basic organization of a typical chart recorder is schematized in Figure 3-35B. The elements are, by and large, analogous to the functional units of an oscilloscope. The input preamplifier generally corresponds to the oscilloscope's vertical amplifier. (It may be followed by a power amplifier to meet the high current demand of a pen motor.) The writing element (to be described later) is equivalent to the oscilloscope's cathode-ray beam: It produces the trace, in this case on paper. The osilloscope's time base is replaced by the chart recorder's paper transport system, a mechanical assembly that moves the paper at a steady rate (selected by the user, and generally ranging from from less than 1 cm/s to more than 1 m/s). This creates a time base in a way that is the reverse of the oscilloscope's method: The writing device stays still, but the display surface (paper) moves.

In most chart recorders the preamplifiers are plug-in modules. Manufacturers usually offer many different interchangeable modules for their units: Each is specialized for a given function. For example, one preamplifier may be designed for bridge transducers—it provides an excitation voltage for the bridge and any demodulation that may be needed. Another may provide the very high gain and other characteristics needed for bioelectric signals, such as electromyograms. Still other preamplifiers may have differential inputs, be DC or AC coupled, or perform mathematical functions, such as integration or rate computation, on the input. The ability to select the amplifier best suited to the job at hand accounts

A

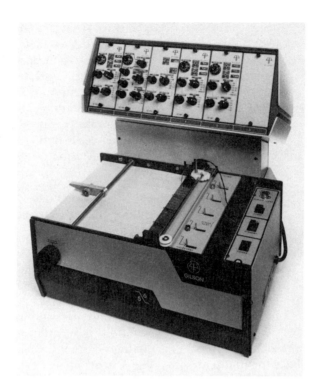

B

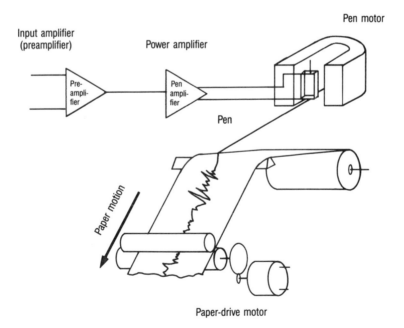

FIGURE 3-35. (A) A multichannel chart recorder. (Courtesy of Gilson Medical Electronics, Middleton, WI). (B) Basic organization of a pen recorder.

for a great deal of the utility of the chart recorder.

The most important feature of any chart recorder, and the one that most determines its capabilities, is the writing element. It is here that the major differences between various chart recorders lie.

Pen Recorders

In a pen recorder the input signal drives an electromechanical system that moves a pen across the surface of the paper, tracing out a graph of the input voltage. The pen (or *stylus*) is moved by a pen motor (Figure 3-36) which is actually a special galvanometer. After amplification the signal is applied to a wire coil located within the field of a very strong permanent magnet inside the pen motor. The magnetic field generated by the signal current flowing through the coil interacts with the magnetic field of the permanent magnet, causing the coil to rotate to an extent proportional to the strength of the interaction (which is

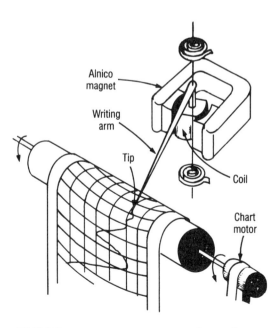

FIGURE 3-36. Pen motor (recording galvanometer).

determined by the strength of the coil's magnetic field and, hence, by the magnitude of the signal current). Attached to the pivot on which the coil is mounted is a rod that carries the writing stylus.* Rotation of the coil is therefore translated into displacement of the stylus tip, which marks the paper.

A moment's thought indicates a (relatively minor) problem inherent in the fact that the stylus tip rotates about a central pivoting point: Displacements of the pen trace arcs, rather than straight lines, on the paper. The result, called a *curvilinear* trace, is shown in Figure 3-37A. It does not take long to become accustomed to reading curvilinear records, especially when special chart paper, with the vertical divisions ruled as arcs to match the displacement of the pens, is used. In fact, this format is standard in many areas of biomedical work. The real problem with them is seen when the temporal location of a point needs to be evaluated. Figure 3-37A shows that it may be difficult to estimate exactly where on the time scale a peak is. Largely because of this problem, special pen linkages have been devised to convert the rotary movement of the pen arm to a linear motion and thereby produce a trace that lies on rectangular coordinates Figure 3-37B). The added mechanical components needed to achieve this may reduce somewhat the frequency response of the writing system. Despite this drawback rectilinear pen systems are likely to be more useful to speech pathologists, who are very often interested in intertrace time relationships.

The moving pen motor components and the stylus attached to them constitute a relatively massive structure. The fairly large mass and the inertia it represents greatly limits the speed with which the pen can be accelerated. What this means, of course, is that the frequency response of the writing system is poor. High-frequency com-

*The stylus may be an inking device, or a heated tip that exposes an underlying colored surface on special, wax-covered paper. The latter system tends to produce sharper traces.

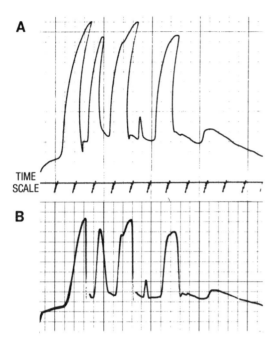

FIGURE 3-37. A record of intraoral pressuring during speech as produced by (A) curvilinear and (B) rectilinear pen recorders. The distortion of the curvilinear trace makes it difficult to judge where the pressure peaks actually occur on the time scale. In this record some of the peaks in the curvilinear trace are actually further to the right than the end of the pressure event.

ponents in the input signal will not be reproduced well, if at all. (In many pen-writer systems the cutoff frequency of the pens—the frequency at which the pen excursion is reduced by 3 dB compared to full excursion—is on the order of only 20 Hz). This may be a minor problem in the case of some physiological data (for instance subglottal pressure, which might not change very rapidly), but it means there will be significant distortion of many signals. And writing out the speech wave itself is utterly out of the question. Sometimes the problem can be circumvented by lowering all the frequency components in the data signal. This can be accomplished by playing back a tape recording of the data at a speed very much less than the recording speed. But often this is either not possible, because a sufficient speed reduction

cannot be achieved, or else it introduces unacceptable distortions. It is clear that, despite their relatively low cost, pen-writers are not ideally suited to the needs of speech clinicians.

Light-Beam Oscillographs

In the nineteenth century, before amplifiers were available, scientists confronted with the need for very sensitive voltage detectors often resorted to the "taut-wire galvanometer." This instrument was essentially a standard galvanometer movement, but the pointer system was replaced by a taut wire that was twisted by the galvanometer movement. Cemented to the wire was a small mirror, onto which a beam of light was projected. As the wire twisted the mirror rotated, and the reflection of the beam of light swept across space. The moving light spot could be observed on a graduated screen, or, if it was focused on a sheet of photosensitive paper, it could be recorded permanently.

The light-beam oscillograph operates in very much the same way, except that the galvanometers are miniaturized, enclosed in glass envelopes, and greatly improved. Several of them are lined up in the instrument, one for each data channel to be recorded. Their internal mirrors reflect an ultraviolet light beam onto photosensitive paper that requires no chemical developing.

The moving elements of the reflecting galvanometers constitute a very small mass, and the frequency response of the system is accordingly quite good. Upper frequency (3 dB down) limits are generally on the order of 1000 Hz. This is more than adequate for recording almost any physiological signal. It is even possible to get a relatively good record of the speech signal itself. Generally, light-beam oscillographs also contain lighting systems that cause rectangular grid lines to be printed on the paper at the time of recording. Grid spacing is automatically adjusted to the paper speed (usually in the range of a fraction of a centimeter to 2 m/s) that the user has chosen. Optical event-markers and other features are also available.

The largest single disadvantage of oscillographs lies in the recording paper: It is extremely expensive. If high-frequency signals are being recorded, paper speed must be high in order to separate the vertical deflections that would otherwise be too closely spaced to be individually resolved. Therefore, a great deal of paper may be used for the recording of a single event, again increasing cost significantly. Furthermore, the paper record is not truly permanent. The light sensitivity of the medium remains after the data are written on it, and further exposure to light slowly darkens the background against which the traces appear. In time, unless shielded from light or chemically treated, the entire chart becomes gray, and the traces can no longer be seen.

Because of these limitations, most laboratories use a pen recorder for low-frequency data, and they reserve the oscillograph for those cases in which it is really needed.

Cathode-Ray Oscillograph

If really high-frequency signals must be evaluated, there is a variation of the optical writing system that can be of use. Instead of light-beam galvanometers, the writing beam can be a spot of light on a long, thin cathode ray tube associated with an oscilloscope. No horizontal sweep is provided; the beam simply moves back and forth along the cathode-ray tube, driven by the "vertical" amplifier. The photosensitive paper is pulled at a constant rate and is pressed into intimate contact with the cathode- ray tube, whose spot of light exposes it. Because the beam is not associated with any moving structure, except for the electrons in it, it can be moved *very* quickly and, therefore, the system can record signals of much higher frequency than is otherwise possible. This system has the same disadvantages with respect to cost that are associated with the light-beam oscillograph and, because it also represents more frequency response than is generally needed by speech clinicians, it is not often used in speech work. It is available, however, for those special situations where its special capabilities are needed. ∎

SOURCES OF INFORMATION

Cobbold, R. S. C. *Transducers for Biomedical Measurements*. New York: John Wiley, 1974.

Cooper, W. D. *Electronic Instrumentation and Measurement Techniques* (2nd ed). Englewood Cliffs, NJ: Prentice-Hall, 1978. Pp. 500.

Eargle, J. *Sound recording* 2nd edition). New York: Van Nostrand Reinhold, 1980. Pp. 355.

Eargle, J. *The Microphone Handbook*. Plainview, NY: Elar Publishing, undated.

Geddes, L. A. and Baker, L. E. *Principles of Applied Biomedical Instrumentation* (2nd edition). New York: John Wiley, 1975.

Harford, E. R. The use of a miniature microphone in the ear canal for the verification of hearing aid performance. *Ear and hearing*, 1 (1980) 329–337.

Harford, E. R. A new clinical technique for verification of hearing aid response. *Archives of Otolaryncology* 107 (1981) 461–468.

Hoenig, S. A. and Payne, F. L. *How to Build and Use Electronic Devices without Frustration, Panic, Mountains of Money, or an Engineering Degree*. Boston: Little, Brown, 1973.

Johnson, K. W. and Walker, W. C. *The Science of Hi-Fidelity*. Dubuque, IA: Kendall/Hunt Publishing Co., 1977.

Johnson, K. W., Walker, W. C., and Cutnell, J. D. *Laboratory Manual: Science of Hi-Fidelity*. Dubuque, IA: Kendall/Hunt Publishing Co., 1978.

Koike, Y. Application of some acoustic measures for the evaluation of laryngeal dysfunction. *Studia Phonologica*, 7 (1973) 17–23.

Lowman, Charles E. *Magnetic Recording*. New York: McGraw-Hill, 1972. Pp. 285

Sessions, K. W. and Fischer, W. A. *Understanding Oscilloscopes and Display Waveforms*. New York: Wiley, 1978.

Sheingold, D. H. (Ed.) *Nonlinear Circuits handbook: Designing with Analog Function Modules and IC's*. Norwood, MA: Analog Devices, Inc., 1976.

Sheingold, D. H. (Ed.) *Transducer Interfacing Handbook: A Guide to Analog Signal Conditioning*. Norwood, MA: Analog Devices, Inc., 1980.

Snidecor, J. C., Rehman, I. and Washburn, D. D. Speech pickup by contact microphone at head and neck positions. *JSHR*, 2 (1959) 277–281.

Stout, D. F. and Kaufman, M. *Handbook of Operational Amplifier Circuit Design*. New York: McGraw-Hill, 1976.

Villchur, E. *Reproduction of Sound*. New York: Dover, 1965.

Villchur, E. and Killion, M. C. Probe-tube microphone assembly. *Journal of the Acoustical Society of America*, 57 (1975) 238–240.

Woram, John M. *The Recording Studio handbook*. Plainview, NY: Sagamore, 1977. Pp. 496.

CHAPTER 4

Intensity

BACKGROUND

Sound is the perception of changes in air pressure. The changes to which the human ear is sensitive are very rapid and exceptionally small, but they are conceptually no different from the slow fluctuations in air pressures measured by a weather barometer. Loudness is the perceptual attribute that corresponds to the magnitude of the pressure changes. The psychological scaling of loudness is very complex and is strongly influenced by the fundamental frequency and spectral properties of the stimulus. Figure 4-1, which is taken from Fletcher (1934) shows this quite clearly. There is no simple instrumental method for scaling loudness, but the physical correlates, intensity and sound pressure, are easily measured.

Intensity Level

The intensity (I) of an acoustic signal is its *power* per unit area in watts (W).* It

---

*The theory of sound intensity and its measurement is concisely summarized in Gade (1982a,b).

turns out, however, that using a simple power designation is inconvenient in a number of ways. First, the human auditory system is sensitive to a vast range of powers, from a just barely audible $1 \times 10^{-16}\,\mathrm{Wcm^2}$ (0.0000000000000001 W/cm²) to a very painful $1 \times 10^{-3}\,\mathrm{W/cm^2}$ (0.001 W/cm²). This is a range of about 1 to 10 trillion. Describing sound intensities by power values would require the use of very cumbersome numbers. Second, the relationship between intensity and loudness is by no means a linear one (any more than the frequency/pitch relationship is linear). It was discovered long ago that all sensory perception tends to be exponentially related to stimulus magnitude. Loudness grows irregularly with intensity and is strongly influenced by frequency (Fletcher and Munson, 1933) but the underlying exponential relationship is well documented. Finally, we are usually interested in one sound only in terms of its relationship to another. For instance, in assessing hearing we are generally more concerned with how much greater than the minimum required for perception a sound is than what its absolute power may be. On

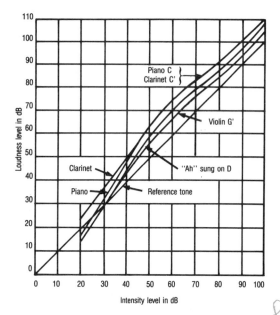

FIGURE 4-1. Relationship of loudness to intensity and timbre. (Fletcher, H. Loudness, pitch, and the timbre of musical tones and their relation to the intensity, the frequency, and the overtone structure. *Journal of the Acoustical Society of America* 6 (1934) 59–69. Reprinted by permission.)

the productive side, we are often concerned with a speaker's intensity range, that is, with how great the spread is from minimal to maximal sound intensity.

The need for intensity comparison provides a useful starting point for exploring the standard scaling system that has been universally adopted. Suppose a given speaker can phonate /a/ at a minimal intensity of 3.5×10^{-9} W/cm² and at a maximum intensity of 1×10^{-7} W/cm². His vocal intensity range obviously is $(3.5 \times 10^{-9}) - (1 \times 10^{-7}) = 9.65 \times 10^{-8}$ W/cm² (0.0000000965 W/cm²). But this number is not only less than useful; it is downright confusing. A better approach might be to generate a ratio of the speaker's two intensities. For the speaker in question, relative maximal intensity might more conveniently be expressed as $(1 \times 10^{-7})/(3.5 \times 10^{-9}) = 28.57$ times his minimal intensity. This is a more useful and comprehensible number, but the problems of the extent over which such ratios

might range and the nonlinearity of loudness perception have not been dealt with.

To express the total possible range of intensities and, at the same time, to scale intensity in keeping with the underlying principle of nonlinear loudness growth, relative intensity is quantified as the *logarithm* of the ratio of one sound power (W_1) to a reference power (W_r). When this procedure is applied, the resultant measure is called "intensity *level*"—designated *IL*. (The word "level" is an indicator of this sort of *relative* measure.) The unit of IL is the Bel (B). In standard notation,

(1) $IL = \log_{10}(W_1/W_r)$ Bel.

For the example under consideration,

Decibels

$$IL = \log_{10}(1 \times 10^{-7}/3.5 \times 10^{-9})$$
$$= \log_{10} 28.57$$
$$= 1.46 \text{ Bel.}$$

In practice, it turns out that the Bel is a little too coarse. (The one to ten-trillion range of normal hearing is covered by only 13 Bels, for example.) Therefore, intensity level is more commonly expressed in tenths of a Bel, or *decibels* (dB). The decibel value is derived by multiplying Bels by ten. Therefore, intensity level in dB equals

$$IL_{dB} = 10 \log_{10}(W_1/W_r). \quad (2)$$

A few examples will serve to demonstrate some important characteristics of the decibel scale. Given that the threshold of hearing at 1k Hz is 1×10^{-16} W/cm², what is the intensity level re: threshold of a stimulus having a power of 2×10^{-16} W/cm²? We are comparing the power of a stimulus (W_1) to a threshold power of 1×10^{-16} as the reference. Therefore,

$$IL = 10 \log_{10}(W_1/W_r)$$
$$= 10 \log_{10}(2 \times 10^{-16}/1 \times 10^{-16})$$
$$= 10 \log_{10}(2/1)$$
$$= 10 (.3010)$$
$$= 3.01 \text{ dB.}$$

Consider another case. A researcher measures the acoustic power of various phonemes, and determines that the average intensity of /m/ is 15 μW while /l/ has an average intensity of 7.5 μW. What is the intensity level of /m/ with respect to /l/? Clearly,

$$IL = 10 \log_{10}(\text{power } /m/ \div \text{power } /l/) \text{ watts}$$
$$= 10 \log_{10} (15 \, \mu W/7.5 \, \mu W)$$
$$= 10 \log_{10} 2$$
$$= 10 \, (.3010)$$
$$= 3.01 \text{ dB}.$$

Note that whenever the power doubles, there is a 3 dB increase in intensity level. It does not matter if one doubles 1×10^{-16} to 2×10^{-16} watts or 7.5 μW to 15 μW. The intensity level increase will always be 3 dB. Conversely, halving the sound power results in a change of -3 dB.

It is important to understand that the addition (or loss) of 3 dB for a doubling (or halving) of the sound power works anywhere on the dB scale. The following example may help clarify this point. Suppose that a patient with a serious problem initially produces /m/ at an intensity of 3×10^{-6} W/cm^2. This power is taken as a reference against which any therpeutic progress will be judged. After a couple of weeks of therapy the patient produces /m/ at 9×10^{-6} W/cm^2. The intensity level of this new /m/ with respect to his original /m/ is

$$IL_{\text{new } /m/} = 10 \log_{10} (W_{\text{new } /m/}/W_{\text{first } /m/})$$
$$= 10 \log_{10} (9 \times 10^{-6}/3 \times 10^{-6})$$
$$= 10 \log_{10} 3.0$$
$$= 4.77 \text{ dB}.$$

After more therapy, the patient manages to produce a maximally loud /m/ at 18×10^{-6} W/cm^2. What is the intensity of this better /m/ compared to his original /m/? By the same calculation,

$$IL = 10 \log_{10} (W_{\text{better } /m/}/W_{\text{first } /m/})$$
$$= 10 \log_{10} (18 \times 10^{-6}/3 \times 10^{-6})$$
$$= 10 \log_{10} 6$$
$$= 7.78 \text{ dB}.$$

The doubling of sound power (from 9 to 18 μW) has moved the intensity level up 3 dB—from about 4.8 to 7.8 dB.

SUMMARY: If a power of x watts represents intensity level y dB, then a power of $2x$ watts represents an intensity level of $y + 3$ dB, and a power of $x/2$ watts is equal to an intensity level of $y - 3$ dB.

By a similar process we could show that a tenfold increase (or decrease) in power raises (or lowers) the intensity by 10 dB, since

$$IL = 10 \log_{10}(10/1) = 10(1) = 10$$

Therefore:

If a power of x watts represents intensity level y dB, then a power of $10x$ watts represents $y + 10$ dB. A power of $x/10$ watts represents an intensity of $y - 10$ dB.

Intensity level, then, is a ratio of acoustic powers expressed on a logarithmic scale. By convention, the reference level is assumed to be 1×10^{-16} W/cm^2 (the threshold of normal hearing) unless stated otherwise.

Sound Pressure Level (SPL)

In actual practice, sound intensities are usually measured in terms of sound pressures as transduced by a very precise microphone. These pressures are converted to electrical voltages that are conditioned by the measurement circuitry and output as dB. Now, it happens that sound intensity (I),

$$I = P^2/Z_{\text{air}} \quad (3)$$

where P is pressure and Z_{air} represents the impedance of air as a transmission medium. Under ordinary circumstances, the air's transmissive characteristics are constant. Therefore

$$I \propto P^2.$$

That is, intensity is directly proportional to the *square* of the sound pressure. If we let P^2 substitute for power, we can express intensity level in dB as follows:

$$dB = 10 \log_{10}(W_1/W_r) \quad (4)$$
$$= 10 \log_{10} (P_1^2/P_r^2). \quad (5)$$

Recalling that

$$P_1^2/P_r^2 = (P_1/P_r)^2,$$

and that

$$10 \log_{10}(P_1/P_r)^2 = 2 \times 10 \log_{10}(P_1/P_r),$$

we have derived an expression for dB based on sound pressure:

$$dB_{\text{SPL}} = 20 \log_{10}(P_1/P_r).$$

The sound pressure *level* (SPL) is the logarithmic transform of the ratio of two sound pressures.

Because the logarithm of the pressure ratio is multiplied by 20, rather than by 10 as was the case for sound power, doubling a pressure raises the SPL by 6 dB, rather than by 3 dB. Similarly, increasing pressure by a factor of 10 increases SPL by 20 dB.

SUMMARY: Doubling sound pressure raises SPL by 6 dB; halving sound pressure lowers SPL by 6 dB. Increasing pressure tenfold raises SPL by 20 dB; dividing pressure by 10 lowers SPL by 20 dB.

By convention, the reference pressure for SPL is taken as 0.0002 dynes per square centimeter (d/cm^2), which is just at the threshold of normal hearing. (This, incidentally, is equivalent to a pressure of $0.000000204 cmH_2O$, which is a striking demonstration of the sensitivity of the human auditory system.) Since 1 d/cm^2 is also termed 1 microbar, this value is often expressed as 0.0002 microbar. In the standard version of the metric system this pressure is expressed as 20 micropascals (μPa). One Pascal is 1 newton (Nt) per square meter.

IL and SPL

The fact that doubling sound *power* increases both IL and SPL by 3 dB while doubling sound *pressure* raises both SPL and IL by 6 dB often leads to significant, but needless, confusion. Many seem to feel that there are different dB scales for quantifying different sounds. This is simply not the case.* Any acoustic signal can be measured in terms of either IL or SPL, and the resultant dB values will be the same, assuming that equivalent reference power and pressure have been used.

The confusion seems to stem from a failure to recall that power is proportional to the *square* of the pressure. Therefore, if pressure is doubled (i.e., multiplied by 2), the power is increased by 2^2, that is, by 4.

---

*See Kallstrom (1976), Kramer (1977), Feth (1977), and Ward (1977).

So $2P = 4W$ in our equations. Therefore,

$$dB_{SPL} = 20 \log_{10}(2P/P) = 20 \log_{10} 2$$
$$= 20(.3010)$$
$$= 6.02 \text{ dB,}$$

and, equivalently,

$$dB_{IL} = 10 \log_{10}(4W/W) = 10 \log_{10} 4$$
$$= 10(.6020)$$
$$= 6.02 \text{ dB.}$$

Conversely, pressure increases as the square root of the increase in power. So if the power of a signal doubles, the pressure has been multiplied by $\sqrt{2} = 1.414$. Therefore,

$$dB_{IL} = 10 \log_{10}(2W/W) = 3.01 \text{ dB}$$

while

$$dB_{SPL} = 20 \log_{10}(\sqrt{2P/P})$$
$$= 20 \log_{10} 1.414$$
$$= 20(.1505)$$
$$= 3.01 \text{ dB.}$$

It is clear that, if a signal is increased or diminished in strength, its magnitude changes by the same number of dB on either the IL or SPL scales.

INSTRUMENTATION

Determination of sound pressure level is, at least in principle, a relatively easy and straightforward procedure. It is only necessary to obtain a voltage proportional to sound pressure and then to electronically implement the equations presented earlier. While this might seem a formidable task, in practice it is not difficult. The block diagram of Figure 4-2 conceptualizes the requisite instrumentation.

The acoustic pressure is transduced to a voltage by a microphone. It should be obvious that the validity of the final SPL value depends very heavily on the accuracy of the initial pressure-to-voltage conversion, and therefore on the linearity of the input transducer. For this reason SPL measurements are almost always done with a condenser microphone (see Chap. 3), since this type has the best linearity and stability. A precision low-noise amplifier brings the

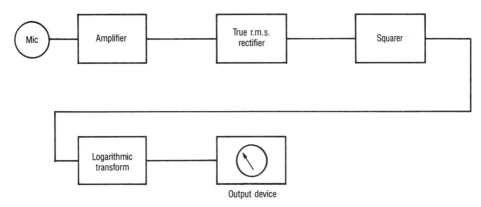

FIGURE 4-2. General scheme for measuring sound pressure level.

microphone's low output up to a usable level. The output of the amplifier is a voltage analog of the acoustic pressure.

Since it is not the voltage peak of each cycle that we are interested in, but rather the overall power of each wave, the next step is to derive the root-mean-square (rms) voltage of the waveform. This is accomplished by a special circuit whose output is proportional to the integral of the voltage. For the present purposes this can be considered to be a special "average" of the wave's amplitude. Because power is proportional to the square of the pressure (or, as in this case, the equivalent voltage) the next circuit element multiplies the rms voltage by itself. A final set of circuit components derives the equivalent of the logarithm of the squared rms voltage, which represents $\log P_{rms}^2$.

The process of comparing to a reference pressure (in order to obtain sound pressure *level*) is neatly achieved by adjusting all of the circuitry to produce an output reading of 0 whenever the reference signal is applied to the input. Once the instrument is adjusted in this manner, the output will always be so many dB above or below that reference. In fact, it is not even necessary to derive the logarithm of the pressure-squared signal. It is just as valid—and a lot easier—to have the output indicator (perhaps a meter) marked with a logarithmic, rather than a linear, scale. In a pen-recording system the calibration ruling on the paper can be logarithmically spaced. Com-

mercially available sound level devices use just these conversion strategies.

Fortunately, there is no need to construct one's own speech intensity system, since accurate and reliable measurement instruments have been readily available for a long time. While these are designed mainly for the engineer and the audiologist, they are very versatile and are likely to serve the needs of the speech pathologist quite well.

Sound Level Meter

The sound level meter (Figure 4-3A) is a portable, self-contained precision instrument system for determination of the SPL. It consists of several specially-matched and sequentially arranged elements that transduce the acoustic signal and perform the necessary mathematical operations on the resultant voltages. The output is shown on a meter; no permanent record is produced. The instrument described below (for which a simplified block diagram is shown in Figure 4-3B) is the B & K model 2203, which is something of a standard.* Other manufacturer's devices are similar.

Input to the system is from a high-precision condenser microphone. An input amplifier boosts the microphone signal (which is only a few millivolts). The output of this amplifier is fed to a variable

---

*The model 2203 is no longer made, having been replaced by the model 2230. A great many of them are still in active service, however.

A

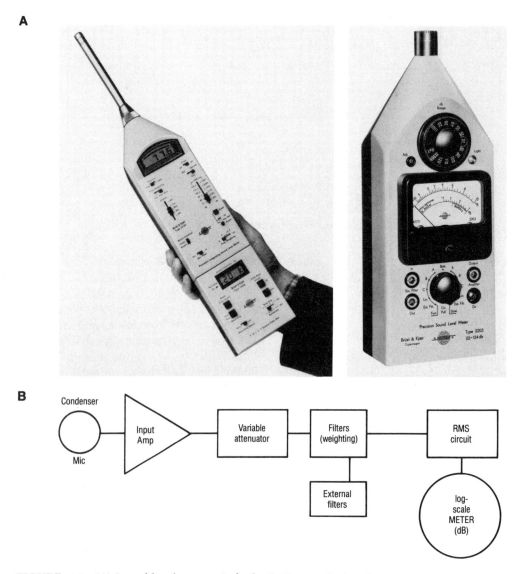

B

FIGURE 4-3. (A) Sound level meters. Left: the B&K 2230. Right: the B&K 2203. (Courtesy of Bruel and Kjaer Instruments, Inc., Marlborough, MA.) (B) Simplified block diagram of the B&K model 2203.

attenuator that is adjusted by the user. The attenuator divides the voltage by an adjustable amount to ensure that the rest of the circuitry is not overwhelmed by too strong a signal. In so doing, it subtracts a certain number of decibels from the signal, and the attenuator setting, therefore, is calibrated in dB.

Following the attenuator is a set of user-selected filter networks. These adjust the relative amplitudes of frequency components in the acoustic signal so as to *weight*

them according to their approximate contributions to the perception of loudness. Provision is also made for connecting external filters to the meter to allow the intensity evaluation of selected frequency bands, for example, to include only a speaker's fundamental frequency. Finally, a special rectifying circuit produces an output proportional to the rms voltage of the filtered signal. This voltage drives a meter whose logarithmic scale runs from -10 to $+10$ dB.

For use, the sound level meter is first

adjusted so that the meter reads 0 dB for a standard signal. This reference can be anything the user chooses, a 1 kHz sine wave at 0.0002 d/cm^2 or a patient's phonation of /a/, for example, but until it is readjusted the meter will indicate dB re: this reference. The microphone is pointed at the sound source and the variable attenuator is adjusted so that the meter pointer is somewhere on the scale. The SPL of the signal is then equal to the attenuator setting plus the meter reading.

Recently, digital processing has been used to make sound level meters more convenient and more versatile. In the newest models (such as the B&K 2230) the microphone signal is digitized (converted to a series of binary numbers) and then evaluated by a microprocessor. No attenuator settings are needed. Instead of a meter reading the intensity is shown (to the nearest 0.1 dB) on a numeric display. (Voltage outputs are also provided for chart recording.) Thanks to the microprocessor and its associated memory the display can also show the maximum, minimum, and average SPL of a sample.

The sound level meter has the advantages of simplicity, ease of operation, and portability. But in the absence of a graphic record of the data there is no way in which even relatively slow changes of SPL can be tracked. Therefore, the sound level meter is best suited to measurement of steady-state sounds, such as prolonged vowels. Somewhat more flexible sound meters, designed with the needs of the speech pathologist in mind, are now appearing on the market. The F-J Electronics model IM360, for instance, gives not only a *meter* reading of SPL in dB, but also it provides two analog voltage outputs—one that is linearly scaled representing dynes/cm^2 and the other, which is logarithmically scaled representing SPL—that may be plotted by an external chart recorder. The instrument also has two channels that can be used simultaneously. Thanks to the different and selectable filter characteristics associated with them, it is possible to compare the intensities of two portions of a speaker's frequency spectrum. In fact, one of the voltage outputs represents log (channel 1) − log (channel 2), which is mathematically equivalent to the *ratio* of the two input sound pressures.

Level Recorder

The sound level recorder (first described by Wente, Bedell, and Swartzel, 1935) produces a strip-chart record of SPL. It is an extremely versatile instrument whose characteristics can be adjusted to meet almost any intensity-measurement need. It is not, however, a complete system for sound measurement, nor is it self-contained or portable. It requires considerably more expertise and planning on the part of the user, but it can track fairly rapid changes in intensity level. All things considered, it is probably the best intensity-measurement device for the clinician.

The function of the level recorder (Fig. 4-4A) is very different from the level meter. It contains what is technically known as an automatic null balancing bridge. Because this application of cybernetic theory is an excellent example of important instrumentation principles and because the validity of the data generated by the instrument depends quite heavily on the user's intelligent application of a basic understanding of how the instrument works, the operative principles of this device are worth exploring.

The block diagram of Figure 4-4B shows the basic functional units of the (B & K 2307) level recorder. After initial attenuation (determined by the user), the input signal is further diminished by a potentiometer that serves as a second variable attenuator. Following this, it is amplified and rectified and fed to a comparator, which is really the heart of the instrument. Here, the amplitude of the input is compared to a stable reference voltage. The comparator produces a voltage that is proportional to the *discrepancy* between the reference and the (attenuated) input. It is known, therefore, as an *error voltage*, and it is used to power a magnetic drive mechanism that moves a mechanical linkage to both the recording

A

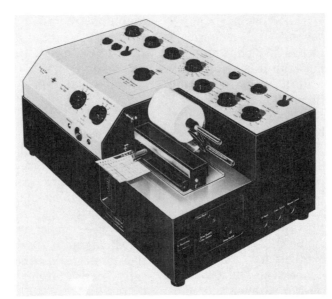

B

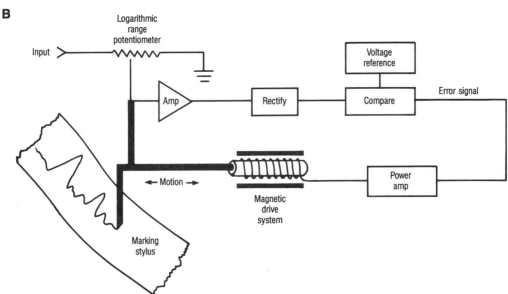

FIGURE 4-4. The B&K model 2307 sound level recorder. (Courtesy of Bruel and Kjaer Instruments, Inc., Marlborough, MA.) (B) A simplified block diagram of its organization.

pen and the attenuator control. The error voltage thereby adjusts the potentiometer and continues to do so until the (rectified) input to the comparator equals the reference voltage. When it does, of course, the error voltage disappears. If the input amplitude changes, the comparator again sees a difference between the reference and the input, and the new error voltage that it pro-

duces causes the mechanical drive to readjust the potentiometer so that the input is again attenuated just enough to exactly match the internal reference voltage of the instrument. In short, the entire system functions automatically to maintain a *null balance* condition in which the error voltage is zero.

The position of the potentiometer control is always proportional to the discrepancy between the input and the internal reference seen by the comparator. Since the pen is attached to the same mechanical linkage that controls the potentiometer, the record it produces on the strip-chart is an accurate record of this discrepancy over time. A permanent record of changes in sound intensity is produced, therefore. Logarithmic scaling, to create an output calibrated in dB, is assured by the fact that the potentiometer is itself designed with a logarithmic characteristic. That is, the position of the potentiometer's control rod and the degree of attenuation that position produces are logarithmically related. Because of the pen and potentiometer linkage, this means that the pen's position on the paper is logarithmically related to the amplitude of the input signal. Hence, the written record has a dB scale, with linearly spaced intervals. The setting of the (user-controlled) input potentiometer determines the baseline level to which the dB values of the strip-chart record are added.

The level recorder includes provisions for selecting any one of three different signal rectification methods—average, rms, or peak. In addition, there is provision for measuring DC levels. Although an acoustic signal cannot, of course, be DC, this capability does mean that the level recorder can write out data from other instruments if there should be a need to do so.

There is one other feature of the level recorder that must be understood if valid use of the instrument is to be made. This is the variable averaging time of the system, which is controlled primarily by the writing speed, a term which indicates the maximum speed at which the recording pen can move.* It is not hard to visualize the effect of writing speed on averaging time. Imagine an input signal, such as running speech, with very rapid changes in amplitude. An oscillogram of such a signal is shown in Figure 4-5A. Now suppose that the SPL of the

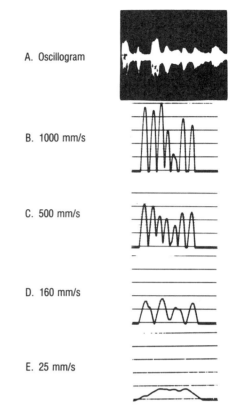

FIGURE 4-5. A speech utterance ("Joe took father's shoe bench out") and level recorder analyses (A through E) of it at successively slower writing speeds.

signal is analyzed with the level recorder set for a very high writing speed, perhaps 1000 mm/s, as in Figure 4-5B. The pen moves quickly enough to follow the peaks associated with the different syllables quite accurately, and so this read-out has a strong resemblance to the oscillogram. Now suppose that the writing speed is reduced significantly, say to 500 mm/s. Because of this reduction, the pen cannot move quite fast enough to keep up with the rapid changes in the signal. Before it can get to the "target" position on the paper that actually represents the SPL of a peak, the event to which it is responding is over and the pen is being influenced by the level of the signal at the next point in time. Figure 4-5C shows that the peaks in the record are lowered and the troughs raised because the pen

---

*The exact relationship between writing speed and averaging time has been investigated by Broch and Wahrman (1961).

is always responding to events over a moderately broad time interval. In fact, the write-out no longer represents the actual acoustic events, but rather a moving average of the them over an averaging time of about 0.02 s. When the writing speed is lowered to an even slower 160 mm/s (Fig. 4-5D) the pen is quite sluggish. Before it can fully respond to any major change in SPL several other changes have occurred. At this writing speed its position at any one time represents an average of what has been going on in the past 0.075 s. At an *extremely* slow writing speed of 25 mm/s or so, all rapid fluctuations are lost in the printout record (Figure 4-5E). With an averaging time of about 0.5 s what has been produced is an indication of the overall average SPL of the entire utterance.

The user must decide what averaging time best meets the measurement needs of the moment. If, for example, the intensity level of a given phoneme as it occurs in context is needed, then averaging time will have to be sufficiently short (that is, writing time must be adequately fast) to capture a transient event. But if the average SPL of, let's say, sustained /a/ is wanted, a long averaging time that will smooth out minor intensity fluctuations is probably more useful. Then again, if the degree of *instability* of a patient's intensity is to be quantified, a fast writing speed that will show all the sudden variations in the intensity of the sustained /a/ is in order. There are no general rules.

VU Meters

In theory, almost any meter or chart recorder can be used to measure IL or SPL. If a standardized measure, comparable to data gathered by others, is needed the acoustic signal must be conditioned as shown in the flow-chart of Figure 4-2 before being fed to the output device. But if an "in-house" comparison of the intensity of two comparable samples is all that is required, then much simpler means are suitable. A therapist might, for instance, want to establish that a given intervention im-

mediately results in increased intensity. For this, a simple pre-post comparison of phonatory intensity is adequate. Similarly, elaborate signal processing is not important in the provision of visual feedback of loudness.* In short, in everyday clinical practice situations often arise in which an informal measure of intensity suffices quite well. In these situations equipment found in most clinics can be pressed into service, provided their limitations are clearly understood.

Almost all good quality recording devices have a level indicator called a *VU meter* that is marked in decibels. "VU" stands for "volume unit," whose zero reference is a steady-state power of 1 mW in a circuit of 600Ω impedance. The meter itself has certain specified dynamic characteristics. The VU meter was developed to provide a useful measure of the average power of music and speech signals that typically have very rapid and large sound pressure fluctuations.

The complexity of the relationship between dB VU and dB SPL makes conversion from one to the other impractical. The readings of VU meters are, however, comparable to each other if test conditions are the same and if the same trained observer reads the meter. Special procedures have been proposed to meet the need for high reliability (Levitt and Bricker, 1970; Brady, 1971). Therefore, while not the method of choice, VU meters can be used quite successfully in clinical practice. VU measures can be recorded on paper by modifying the tape recorder slightly, and in this form they have been of some use in formal research studies of infant cry (Fisichelli, Karelitz, Eichbauer, and Rosenfeld, 1961).

Other Instruments

Many of the F_o-display devices being marketed include the capacity to show amplitude versus time, often along with the fundamental frequency data. Examples of

---

*A simple device that provides an acoustic cue of excessive loudness has been described by Holbrook, Rolnick, and Bailey (1974).

such instruments include Kay Elemetrics' Visi-Pitch, Voice Identification's PM100 intonation trainer, and Madsen Electronics' Vocal-2. These instruments display information on a CRT screen, but some include outputs that permit pen-recording of the data.

INTENSITY MEASUREMENTS

General Procedure

No matter how intensity is to be evaluated, there are certain general procedural rules that must be observed. The choice of a microphone is very important, since much depends on the accuracy of the sound pressure-to-voltage conversion that it performs. To the extent that the microphone response is not linear or deviates from acceptable flatness (see Chap. 3) the final measures will be less than valid. For this reason a condenser microphone should be used if possible. In its absence, the best quality microphone available should be selected. Microphone unidirectionality will help eliminate background noise.

Another factor that is often overlooked is the microphone amplifier, which might be part of a recording system if the speech sample is being saved for later evaluation. It is obvious that it must be a high-quality unit—a requirement easily met at very reasonable expense by equipment available commercially. Perhaps less apparent is the importance of matching the amplifier input characteristics to the microphone in order to preserve the fidelity and noise-free characteristics of the microphone signal. Some tape recorders have automatic level control circuits that adjust the unit's gain to compensate for changes in signal level. Such a circuit directly alters the intensity variable that is being evaluated, and so it must be turned off. Finally, it is very important that the amplifier never be overloaded by the signal. This means that some metering device should be available to check that the amplifier is functioning in its linear region over the entire range of sound intensities to be measured.

It is best to provide a standard signal of known intensity that can be used to calibrate the measurement. There are two basic means of achieving this. The easier way is to zero the sound measuring instrument using a sine-wave voltage of known amplitude produced by a precision generator. This calibration signal need not be played through a speaker; it can be directly coupled to the sound level meter or recorder. All sound level measurements done after this zeroing will be in dB re: the calibrating signal. They will be comparable across speech tasks and from one measurement session to any other that has used the same standard signal to represent 0 dB. Alternatively, the microphone-amplifier-metering system can be calibrated to a known sound pressure produced in an anechoic chamber by an audiometer or other precision source. Any clinical setting that has an audiologic unit should have the equipment to do this kind of calibration. Obviously, once calibrated, no part of the measurement system should be readjusted.

Special precautions must be taken to assure that the distance between the speaker's mouth and the microphone remains constant. The intensity of sound diminishes in proportion to the square of the distance from the source ($I \propto 1/d^2$). A relatively small change in position of the microphone can have, therefore, a significant effect on the intensity level. (Zaveri [1971] presents a good summary of how to measure sound in a free field.) There are a number of common techniques that help assure mic-to-mouth constancy. A rod may be fixed to the microphone, its free end placed in contact with some stable area (perhaps the forehead) of the speaker's face. Alternatively, the speaker's head can be held against a stable support and the microphone set on a stand at a convenient distance in front of him. If the microphone is sufficiently small it may be mounted on a short boom that is attached to a headband fitted on the patient. This works particularly well with children, who often cannot be induced to sit still. Finally, there are now extremely small but very accurate microphones (Villchur and

Killion, 1975) that can be simply taped to the upper lip. These provide an excellent solution to the distance-variation problem. Although contact microphones might seem an obvious choice for intensity measurements, there is some uncertainty about how transmission through soft tissue influences sound amplitude (Horii, 1982), especially as F_o changes.

Sustained Phonation

Maximum and minimum vocal intensity

Vocal intensity is dependent on an interaction of subglottal pressure and the adjustment status and aerodynamics at the level of the vocal folds, as well as vocal tract status (Isshiki, 1964, 1965, 1969; Bernthal and Beukelman, 1977; Rubin, LeCover, and Vennard, 1967). The range of intensities at which voice can be produced is a measure of the limits of adjustment of the phonatory system, and, therefore, has been proposed as a potentially important measure in the assessment of vocal disorder (Michel and Wendahl, 1971).

Given the interaction of pressure and laryngeal status, it is not surprising that maximum and minimum vocal intensity change with fundamental frequency. Several studies have confirmed the tendency of both to increase as F_o rises (Wolf and Sette, 1935; Wolf, Stanley, and Sette, 1935; Stout, 1938; Colton, 1973; and Coleman, Mabis, and Hinson, 1977). Stone and Krause (1980) have confirmed the effect on minimum SPL and have shown that the increase with F_o is roughly linear at a rate of from 7.5 to about 12 dB/octave. It has also long been recognized (Black, 1961) that speakers raise their F_o when asked to speak with greater effort. (A simple instrumentation array to display vocal intensity as a function of vocal F_o on an oscilloscope screen has been designed by Komiyama, Watanabe, Nishinow, and Yamai, 1977).

MEASUREMENT METHOD. Unless vocal intensity is to be measured at preselected frequencies, the first step in the assessment is to determine the patient's maximum phonational frequency range in the combined modal and loft registers. To provide the most useful data in the most efficient way, it is customary to test intensity capabilities at selected points in this range. One way of doing this is to sample intensities at 10% intervals of the frequency range; another is to use third-octave increments. Whatever the sample points decided on, their frequencies are computed.

For the test itself the patient is presented with stimulus tones (usually sawtooth or square wave) at the several sample frequencies and is required to sustain a vowel at a matching vocal pitch. Minimal sustainable intensity is elicited by instructing the patient to say the vowel as softly as possible without whispering; maximal intensity is generated by having him shout it as loudly as possible without screaming or squealing. A microphone, placed at a fixed distance from the lips, is connected to the intensity measurement system or, if analysis is to be done later, to a tape recorder. Several trials of each minimum and maximum are done. The extreme values for each condition are the data.

Quite recently, there have been attempts to standardize the testing methodology and plotting of F_o-SPL profiles to determine the vocal "space" (Komiyama, Watanabe, and Ryu, 1984). Schutte and Seidner (1983) recommend that the mouth-microphone distance be universally fixed at 30 cm and that the plots of the *phonetograms* be done on a standard form (reproduced in Figure 4-6C). Different vowels should be color coded: blue for /a/, green for /u/, and red for /i/.

Expected Values of Modal and Loft Registers. Coleman, Mabis, and Hinson (1977) tested young men and women at 10% intervals of their maximum phonational frequency range. SPL re: 0.0002 d/cm² was measured at 6 inches from the lips by a sound level meter set for a "fast" response. The data are summarized in Table 4-1. What the summary of values obscures, however, is the very real difference in performance at different F_o levels. Plots of the experimental

TABLE 4-1. Maximum, Minimum, and Range of Vocal SPL (in dB re: 0.0002 d/cm²)*

Measurement	Men	Women
Mean maximum SPL	117	113
Mean minimum SPL	58	55
Mean SPL range (at a single F_o)	54.8	51
Lowest single SPL	51	48
Greatest single SPL	126	122

From Coleman, R. F., Mabis, J. H., and Hinson, J. K. Fundamental frequency—Sound pressure level profiles of adult male and female voices. *Journal of Speech and Hearing Research*, 20 (1977) 197–204. © American Speech-Language-Hearing Assn., Rockville, MD.

*Method: 10 men, age 21–34 yrs; 12 women, age 20–39 yrs. Vowel sustained for at least 2 seconds; 10% intervals of pitch range; 6″ mouth-mic distance; means of 2 trials, > 48 hrs apart.

data (Figure 4-6) show that both minimum and maximum SPL do indeed tend to increase as F_o rises. Notice also that the SPL range is narrowed at the extreme frequency levels. At the upper end of the range this may be due, at least in part, to the use of the loft register, in which the intensity range is smaller than in the modal register (Colton, 1973).

Age seems to have a real, but not dramatic, effect on the maximum SPL of adults. Ptacek, Sander, Maloney, and Jackson (1966) had young and old adults shout /a/ as loudly as possible for at least 1 s at a self-selected pitch. SPL was measured 12 inches from the lips. The data, summarized in Table 4-2, show that maximum SPL falls off on the order of 6 dB (i.e., sound pressure drops by half) between young adulthood and old age. (Given the doubling of mouth-to-mic distance from one study to the other, the young adult data are consistent with the data of Table 4-1.)

Stone and his coworkers have evaluated the reliability of measures of minimum SPL. The mean data for young and middle-aged adults (Stone, Bell, and Clack, 1978) are very similar (after adjustment for different microphone placements) to the values given in Tables 4-1 and 4-2. They have also shown (Stone and Krause, 1980; Stone

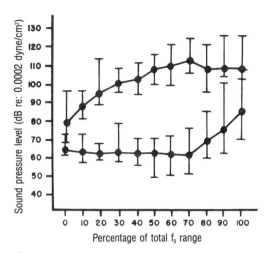

A

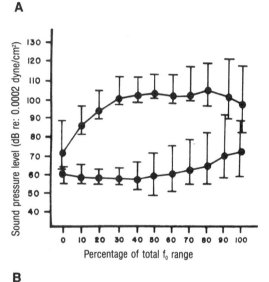

B

FIGURE 4-6. Range of sound pressure level as a function of fundamental frequency level for (A) men and (B) women. (Coleman, R. F., Mabis, J. H., and Hinson, J. K. Fundamental frequency—Sound pressure level profiles of adults male and female voices. *Journal of Speech and Hearing Research*, 20 (1977) 97–204. © American Speech-Language-Hearing Assn., Rockville, MD. Reprinted by permission.)

TABLE 4-2. Maximum Vocal Intensity: Age Effect*

No./Sex of Subjects	Age Range (yrs)	Maximum SPL (dB re: 0.0002 d/cm^2)		
		Mean	S.D.	Range
31 M	18–39	105.8	5.1	92–116
27 M	68–89	100.5	5.9	88–110
30 F	18–38	106.2	3.0	99–112
34 F	66–93	98.6	4.5	90–104

From Ptacek, P. H., Sander, E. K., Maloney, W. H. and Jackson, C. C. R. Phonatory and related changes with advanced age. *Journal of Speech and Hearing Research*, 9 (1966) 353–360. © American Speech-Language-Hearing Assn., Rockville, MD.

*Method: /a/ sustained > 1 sec, self-selected pitch, 12″ mouth-mic distance, three trials each.

and Ferch, 1982) that subjects tended to come within 3 dB of their original mean measurements when retested after 1 day and after 13 days. The perceptual insignificance of such a small difference is underscored by the fact that a perceived doubling of loudness requires an intensity increase on the order of 10 dB (Steinberg and Gardner, 1937). They have concluded that testing of minimum vocal intensity constitutes a generally reliable procedure.

Pulse Register. The limits of the vocal intensity range in pulse register have not been adequately explored. A study by Murry and Brown (1971a), however, provides some basis for initial and tentative conclusions. Five young adult men and five women were asked to sustain pulse register phonation for at least 4 s at the 25, 50, and 75 percent levels of their pulse frequency range. The mean (self-selected) SPL used by the subjects was a bit more than 50 dB at the lowest frequency, rising to close to 60 dB at the highest frequency. When corrected for differences in microphone placement, these data are close to the mean *minimum* SPL for the modal and loft registers reported by Coleman, Mabis, and Hinson (1977). The conclusion, confirmed by everyday perceptual experience, that pulse register phonation is produced at lower intensity seems reasonable.

Even more interesting is the fact that Murry and Brown's subjects not only changed intensity with F_o, but, when asked to change intensity by specific amounts, they did so by altering F_o. In the case of both F_o matching and intensity matching, the correlation coefficient of F_o with intensity level was about 0.85. F_o and intensity level seem very much more interdependent in pulse register than in other phonatory modes.

Vocal rise time

Acoustically, different types of vocal attack are discriminable by the vocal rise time, among other things. This is the duration of the interval between the onset of voice and the point at which amplitude reaches a stable value. Since vocal therapy may have modification of vocal onset characteristics as a goal, information concerning acoustic rise time is likely to be of clinical value. It is generally recognized that, perceptually, there are three broad categories of vocal attack: soft, breathy (or aspirate) and hard (or glottal). Oscilloscopic representations of the vowel /a/ initiated with each of the attack types are shown in Figure 4-7. Note that the rise time is different in each case.

Koike, Hirano, and von Leden (1967) and Koike (1967b) have studied vocal rise time together with F_o and aerodynamic variables in normal subjects. They derived the data of Table 4-3 from measurement of oscillograms.

Koike (1967b) has also measured the rise time associated with the softest vocal initiation that could be produced by patients with several different types of laryngeal pathology. These data are summarized in Table 4-4.

Speech

The intensity level of connected speech shows very large fluctuations over short time intervals. This is because speech contains periods of silence, because intensity is varied for syllable and word stress, (Lie-

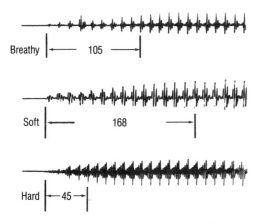

Breathy |←——— 105 ———→|

Soft |←——— 168 ———→|

Hard |←—45—→|

FIGURE 4-7. Oscillograms of three different vocal initiations. Vocal rise time (in ms) is measured from the onset of voice to the point at which the waves achieve the mean amplitude of the steady portion of the vowel. Top: breathy onset; Center: soft onset; Bottom: hard onset.

berman, 1960; Fry, 1955) and because different phonemes are characterized by very different acoustic powers. The comparability of intensity levels of different samples of connected speech therefore depends very heavily on the type of averaging used (e.g., peak, rms), the averaging time of the measurement system, and the utterances being spoken. Speech intensity also changes according to the communicative ambiance: One presumably speaks more loudly to an audience of 50 people than to a single interlocutor across a table. (Interestingly, while interspeaker distance does affect speech intensity, the magnitude of the change is not nearly as large as might be imagined (Markel, Prebor, and Brandt, 1972; Johnson, Pick, Siegel, Cicciarelli, and Garber, 1981). These considerations must be kept in mind when evaluating a speech sample.

TABLE 4-3.   Vocal Rise Time for Different Vocal Attacks*

Attack Type	Rise Time (ms)**		
	Mean	S.D.	Range
Hard (glottal)	29	9.5	18– 50
Soft	261	54.2	163–325
Breathy (aspirate)	148	66.6	65–243

From: Koike Y. Experimental studies on vocal attack. *Practica Otologica Kyoto*, 60 (1967) 663-688. Reprinted by permission.
*Method: 10 normal males (Japanese speakers). Voluntary production of each type of attack. "Optimal pitch." Loudness and pitch constant.
**"The time duration from the onset of sound to the point at which the envelope of acoustic waves reached the mean amplitude of the steady portion of the phonation" (Koike, 1967, p. 664).

Acoustic power of phonemes

As part of his broad investigations of the acoustics of speech, Fletcher (1953) reported the absolute and relative acoustic power of the phonemes of English. In presenting data derived by Sacia and Beck (1926), Fletcher warns that "although sixteen people were used in obtaining these data [on] sounds made in various combinations, they are still insufficient to give average values which can be said to be typical" (p. 83). Nonetheless, the findings presented in Table 4-5 do provide a firm idea of general orders of magnitude of the radiated power of the components of the speech signal.

TABLE 4-4.   Vocal Rise Time: Laryngeal Disorders*

Diagnosis	No./Sex of subjects	Mean Age	Rise Time (msec)**		
			Mean	S.D.	Range
Cancer, glottic	5 M	60	50.8	48.9	25–138
Unilateral paralysis	2 M	41.5	130.5	26.2	112–149
	2 F	35.5	120.5	19.1	107–134
Acute laryngitis	2 F	34.5	62.0	19.8	48– 76

From Koike, Y. Experimental studies on vocal attack. *Practica Otologica Kyoto*, 60 (1967) 663–688. Reprinted by permission.
*Condition: softest initiation possible.
**Calculated from author's data.

TABLE 4-5. Acoustic Power of Phonemes, Measured at the Mouth

| Phone | Peak Power (μW) | |
	Average	Maximum
/u/	235	700
/ʊ/	470	890
/o/	435	1300
/ɔ/	615	1500
/ʌ/	450	1700
/a/	700	1600
/æ/	650	1800
/ɛ/	500	1700
/e/	525	1700
/ɪ/	350	1300
/i/	310	1500
/m/	110	200
/n/	47	70
/ŋ/	97	170
/l/	130	230
/r, ɝ/	200	600
/v/	25	30
/f/	3	4
/z/	30	40
/s/	30	55
/θ/	1	1
/ð/	9	10
/ʒ/	40	55
/ʃ/	110	130
/b/	7	7
/p/	6	7
/d/	4	7
/t/	16	19
/dʒ/	24	36
/tʃ/	52	60
/g/	8	9
/k/	6	9

From Fletcher, H. *Speech and Hearing in Communication.* New York: van Nostrand, 1953. Reprinted by permission.

Fletcher (1953) has also done an analysis of the *phonetic power* of phonemes. This measure was based on two psychophysical determinations of power. *Threshold scores* represent the amount of attenuation required to render a sound inaudible to the listener. *Articulation scores*, on the other hand, give the average degree of attenuation required to reduce the sound to a level at which it is misunderstood some arbitrary percentage of the number of presentations. A combination of these measures has been

derived to represent the *phonetic power*. These data, indexed to the weakest phone (θ = 1) are given in Table 4-6.

Tables 4-5 and 4-6 both show that the vowels are the most intense phonemes, but they are not equally powerful. The differences among them have been explored by Fairbanks, House, and Stevens (1950) by Black (1949) and by Lehiste and Peterson (1959b). While the specific intensity rank orders of the vowels differ somewhat among these studies, all found that the intensities did differ significantly. The important lesson for the clinician is that comparative measures must be based on the same utterance each time, even if the utterance is a monosyllable.

Within syllables the intensity of a phoneme is influenced by the context in which it is found. This effect has been studied primarily for the syllables' vowel nuclei. Lehiste and Peterson (1959b) have determined that vowels are most strongly affected

TABLE 4-6. Relative Power of the Phonemes*

Phone	Relative Power	Phone	Relative Power
/ɔ/	680	/tʃ/	42
/a/	600	/n/	36
/ʌ/	510	/dʒ/	23
/æ/	490	/ʒ/	20
/o/	470	/z/	16
/ʊ/	460	/s/	16
/e/	370	/t/	15
/ɛ/	350	/g/	15
/u/	310	/k/	13
/ɪ/	260	/v/	12
/i/	220	/ð/	11
/r, ɝ/	210	/b/	7
/l/	100	/d/	7
/ʃ/	80	/p/	6
/ŋ/	73	/f/	5
/m/	52	/θ/	REFERENCE = 1

From Fletcher, H. *Speech and Hearing in Communication.* New York: van Nostrand, 1953. Reprinted with permission.

*Based on combination of "threshold" and "articulation" scores. (See text.) Ratio of power of a given phoneme to that of the least powerful (= θ). "As produced by an average speaker."

by neighboring semivowels and voiced plosives, next by glides, nasals, and voiced fricatives, and least strongly by voiceless fricatives and plosives. These findings generally support those of House and Fairbanks (1953). Blood (1981) has studied the average SPL of 20 English vowels and diphthongs in the same CVC contexts used by Lehiste and Peterson (1959a). The average intensity of the (pooled) vowel nuclei is shown for different categories of surrounding consonants in Table 4-7. Very similar results were obtained by House and Fairbanks (1953).

Correlates of phonemic intensity

The intensity (or, perceptually, the loudness) of a phone is correlated to a number of other variables. One of the clearest relationships is to intraoral air pressure (Pio), as has been documented by Malécot (1969), Brown and McGlone (1974), and Ringel, House, and Montgomery (1967). Hixon, Minifie, and Tait (1967) have found that, for /s/ and //, as produced by two speakers, SPL Pio$^{1.2}$–$^{1.4}$. Intraoral air pressure is itself correlated to speech effort (Hixon, 1966) or "force of articulation" (Malécot, 1966a, 1969) and, therefore, it is not surprising that effort level is correlated to SPL. Leeper and Noll (1972) found that SPL for /t/ and /d/ increased logarithmically (power function = 0.56) with effort level on a magnitude production task. It is possible, in fact, that the speaker's vocal effort plays a role in a listener's perception of loudness (Brandt, Ruder, and Shipp, 1969; Lehiste and Peterson, 1959b).

Connected speech

Reduced speech intensity is a symptom of some speech disorders, especially those involving CNS or ventilatory pathology. And, of course, achieving adequate loudness is a goal of therapy for the laryngectomee.

The intensity levels of connected speech are quite different from those of sustained phonations or isolated monosyllables. A

TABLE 4-7. Average SPL of English Vowels in CVC Monosyllables*

Consonant Category**	Average SPL (dB)
Voicing:	
Voiced (13)	82.5
Voiceless (10)	78.8
Mode of Production:	
Plosive (6)	80.3
Fricative (8)	80.4
Affricate (2)	80.9
Glide (5)	81.5
Nasal (2)	82.7
Place of production:	
Bilabial (5)	80.9
Labiodental (2)	81.8
Linguadental (2)	80.1
Alveolar (7)	81.6
Palatal (4)	80.3
Velar (2)	79.9
Glottal (1)	78.7

From Blood, G. The interactions of amplitude and phonetic quality in esophageal speech. *Journal of Speech and Hearing Research*, 24 (1981) 308–312. © American Speech-Language-Hearing Assn., Rockville, MD. Reprinted by permission.

*Three adult male speakers. 30 cm. mic-mouth distance. Utterance: "Say _____ again."

**Parentheses indicate number of consonants in each category.

major cause of the discrepancy resides in the significantly long pauses that are either physiologically or linguistically required in a complex utterance. To some extent, they are bound to reduce the overall average intensity. Therefore, intensity measures of connected speech are probably best obtained together with an estimate of the proportion of the sample occupied by pauses.

Elimination of pauses

Pauses may be removed from the computation of intensity level by ignoring any segment of a graphic sound level recorder output during which the SPL is zero. However, unless the writing time is very fast (that is, the averaging time is short) a silence will still significantly influence the height of the peak that follows it. Unfortunately, a fast writing speed means that averaging is not done by the instrument and, therefore, must be accomplished by the user if an overall intensity estimate is to be generated. The complexity of this task can be enormous to the point of impracticality unless a computer is available.

In the premicrocomputer era Bricker (1965) described a simple electronic system for performing "speech spurt averaging" in order to derive a measure called $\overline{V}$. This has been defined as "the ratio of the integrated, rectified, gated signal voltage to the integrated gating time, where the gate is operated . . . by the speech signal being measured" (p. 361).

This concept was very cleverly implemented and is not nearly as difficult to do as to describe. What is required is shown in Figure 4-8. The input signal (from a microphone and preamplifier or from a tape recorder) is fed to an attenuator, which the user adjusts to keep the signal within the range of the instrument. After rectification the signal causes a voltage-to-frequency converter to produce pulses at a rate that is always proportional to the signal amplitude. Each pulse out of the converter represents one *amplitude unit*. The number of pulses (or *amplitude units*) since the system was last reset is tallied by a pulse

counter. The input signal is also applied to a comparator that turns out a voltage only when the signal exceeds some threshold voltage. The comparator thus indicates when speech is present, and its output controls an electronic switch that connects the pulses to the counter only when there is a speech signal. So amplitude units accumulate only for speech—pauses are not tallied. When the electronic switch closes to allow counting of amplitude units it also connects 100 Hz pulses to a separate counter, which thereby keeps track of the total amount of time (in hundredths of a second) that a speech signal was present.

At the end of an utterance there is a record of the cumulative amplitude and of the time period of accumulation. The average speech intensity is the total amplitude divided by the time. Thanks to the electronic switch this average is for speech only, with silent periods ignored.

While this instrument may look very complex, it can be constructed very easily, and at little cost, from integrated circuits that are widely available. The comparator, electronic switch, amplifiers, voltage-to-frequency converter, and pulse generators all can be bought at any electronics store. Other parts needed are available as mod-

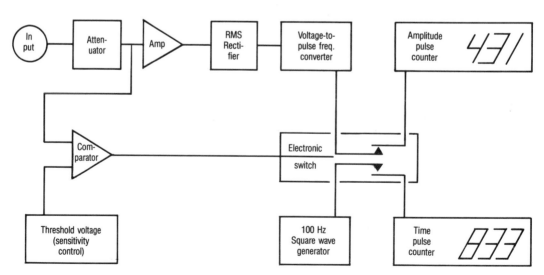

FIGURE 4-8. Block diagram of a "speech spurt averaging" system that eliminates silent periods from the average intensity measure. (After Bricker, 1965)

ules, and any technician should be able to assemble them into a small, highly portable package that can be calibrated in the same way as an intensity meter.

Expected values

By and large, the data of Table 4-8 indicate that the SPL of connected speech lies in the general range of 70 dB. Recall, however, that the communicative setting affects loudness and its physical correlate, intensity. One expects more power from a speaker addressing an audience; less from a speaker in a one-to-one conversation. In the studies cited speakers were asked to speak more or less naturally, as if to just a few people close by.

EFFECT OF DELAYED AUDITORY FEEDBACK. It was recognized quite early that delayed auditory feedback (DAF) has a clear effect on speech intensity (Lee, 1950). Clinicians who use DAF as a diagnostic or treatment modality may find the data of Table 4-9 useful as a guide to the assessment of the normality of a patient's response to this alteration of sidetone.

ALARYNGEAL PSEUDOPHONATION. The attainment of adequate pseudovocal intensity is one of the specific objectives of the rehabilitation of the alaryneal speaker. The intensity that can be produced will depend on many highly variable factors, including several, such as the type and extent of surgery performed, that are beyond the control of the therapist. In general, esophageal speakers will have noticeably lower SPLs (Blood, 1981), probably because of the limited power supply (esophageal reservoir) driving the pseudoglottis (Diedrich, 1968; van den Berg and Moolenaar-Bijl, 1959; Snidecor and Isshiki, 1965). Table 4-10, which includes some findings for the Singer and Blom (1980) and Staffieri and Serafini (1976) modifications, can be used as a yardstick by which expectations may be scaled.

One note of caution is in order. Tracheostomized patients often produce significant "stoma noise." The microphone used for measurement of their vocal intensity, therefore, should be placed so as to maximize pickup of the oral signal and minimize the transduced level of the ventilatory turbulence. Furthermore, it should be remembered that the signal-to-noise ratio is a very important factor in alaryngeal speech (Horii and Weinberg, 1975).

Amplitude Perturbation (Shimmer)

Measures of *amplitude perturbation*—generally called *shimmer*—are analogous to those of fundamental frequency perturbation discussed in Chapter 5. (That discussion should be read first by those unfamiliar with the concepts and terms related to perturbation.) Like frequency-perturbation scores, measurements of shimmer serve to quantify short-term instability of the vocal signal. In fact, there is reason to believe that shimmer is at least as important

TABLE 4-8. SPL of Connected Speech: Normal Speakers—Reading

No./Sex	Mean Age	Material	Misc. Distance	dB Peak	dB Average	Source
1 F 7 M	23.2	Song lyrics	12" (lavalier)	73.5 (0.31)	70.4 (0.29)	Colcord and Adams (1979)
15	Adult	Rainbow (2nd sent.)	6"		69.3 (2.94)	Robbins et al. (1981)
17 M	35-75 (56.7*)	Rainbow (1st para)	8"	78.5*		Carter (1963)
7 M 1 F	40-65	Grandfather	6"	79.		Hyman (1955)

*Median.

TABLE 4-9. Speech Intensity Increase Produced by Delayed Auditory Feedback*

Delay (s)	Mean SPL Increase (dB re: Simultaneous Feedback)			
	Adult		8 yr olds[a]	5 yr olds[a]
	Note a	Note b		
0.0 (simultaneous)	0.0		0.0	0.0
0.03	2.4			
0.06	3.0			
0.09	5.2			
0.12	5.6			
0.15	5.7			
0.18	5.6			
0.21	5.7			
0.25		5.4	7.71	6.1
0.24	6.4			
0.27	6.9			
0.30	6.4			
0.375		4.7	6.0	5.6
0.500		4.0	8.0	3.9
0.625		4.1	5.8	4.5

Note a. Adapted from Black (1951). 22 adult males, reading 5-syllable phrases

Note b. Adapted from Siegel, Fehst, Garber, and Pick (1980) 10 college undergraduates, 10 children age 7.1–8.8 yr, 7 children age 4.5–5.8 yr. Reading 30 simple sentences used by MacKay (1968). (Differences from simultaneous feedback have been computed from tabled data.) Age differences are not significant.

*22 adult males, reading of 5-syllable phrases.

as jitter in its contribution to the perception of hoarseness (Wendahl, 1966a,b), and possibly even more important (Takahashi and Koike, 1975).

Unfortunately, shimmer has not been as carefully studied as jitter. The effect on amplitude perturbation of neither fundamental frequency nor mean amplitude has been explored, for instance. Possible differences due to age or sex remain unclear. None the less, shimmer holds promise as a diagnostic tool and, for the same reasons that were invoked for examining jitter, will be reviewed in this section.

Measurement methods

The collection of a sample for shimmer analysis is simply a matter of eliciting sustained phonation of the type that requires evaluation. As is the case with any intensity measure, stability of mouth-to-microphone distance is very important. Whereas for frequency measurements a "clean"

signal can be obtained by using an accelerometer (contact microphone), this is not advisable for amplitude studies. Horii (1982) has found that shimmer values of accelerometer signals may be lower than those from an air microphone for the same utterances. (Presumably this is due to the fact that vocal tract phase-shifts affect the airborne wave but do not influence the neckwall vibrations.) Until the situation is clarified it is best to use a high-quality air microphone.

Amplitude perturbation is a measure based on the *peak* amplitude of each phonatory cycle. This is a very different value from the rms or average amplitude that is typically used as the basis of SPL, and the two must not be confused. The average peak amplitude that is derived for some of the shimmer measures is not the average that results from integration of the wave—which is what rms really represents. Without a very elaborate (and completely impractical) mathematical evaluation of the complex

TABLE 4-10. Speech SPL: Alaryngeal Speakers

N	Mean Age	Material	Mic. Distance	SPL (dB)	Source
		Esophageal			
15	48–80	Rainbow, 2nd sent.	15 cm.	59.3	*a, e*
8	40–65	Grandfather, 1st sent.	6″	73.	*b*
22	36–81	Rainbow, 1st para.	12″	62.4	*d*
10	61–67	Rainbow, 2nd sent.	30 cm.	70	*f*
		Singer-Blom			
15	53–65	Rainbow, 2nd sent.	15 cm.	79.4	*a, e*
10	52–68	Rainbow, 2nd sent.	30 cm.	82	*f*
		Staffieri			
2	55–69	Rainbow, 1st para.	12″	63.5	*c*

Adapted from
  [a] Robbins, Fisher, Logeman, Hillenbrand, and Blom (1981)
  [b] Hyman (1955)
  [c] Robbin, Fisher, and Logemann (1982)
  [d] Hoops and Noll (1969)
  [e] Robbins, Fisher, Blom, and Singer (1984)
  [f] Blood, 1984

vowel waveform, there is no way to convert average peak amplitude to another intensity measure.

A number of newer digital instruments that analyze speech intensity also provide measures of intensity variability. Users of these systems must be certain they understand the exact method by which such automatic shimmer data are derived before any comparisons are made to published data.

Measurement of a wave-by-wave graphic readout remains the most common way of deriving shimmer indices. Although somewhat tedious, the method is perfectly valid *provided* that the writing system has a frequency response good enough to assure accurate representation of the waveform peaks. This is not a problem with optical devices, such as oscillographs, but pen writers are almost always too slow to follow rapid waveform changes. This problem can be mitigated by recording the sample at the greatest possible tape speed and playing it back through the pen writer at the lowest tape speed available. If the speed reduction is great enough, the frequency components of the signal will be lowered into the range the pen writer can handle. It is best to use an FM tape system (see

Chap. 3) for any recording to be subjected to shimmer analysis, since direct recorders are very prone to momentary amplitude reductions (*drop-outs*).

Given an adequate record, the measurements for evaluation of shimmer are done in very much the same way as frequency measurements for jitter analysis. The data to be obtained, however, are the maximal peak-to-trough amplitudes of the individual waves, in whatever units (millivolts, millimeters, etc.) are convenient and compatible with the shimmer measure being applied. If necessary or useful, a calibrating signal of known amplitude should be recorded to provide a reference to standard intensity values.

Directional perturbation factor

Originated by Hecker and Kreul (1971) as a measure of period perturbation, the directional perturbation factor (DPF) can also be applied to amplitude variation. The measure tallies the number of times that the amplitude change between two successive waves shifts direction. Computation of the DPF sounds complex, but it is not really difficult in practice. The technique for calculating the DPF for fundamental periods is described (together with a computational example) in Chap. 5. If "amplitude" is substituted for "period" that discussion is fully applicable to the amplitude DPF.

Sorensen and Horii (1984) have studied the amplitude DPF in normal men and women. Their data (Table 4-11) may be taken as tentative norms for this measure.

Amplitude variability index

The amplitude variability index (AVI) of Deal and Emanuel (1978) resembles their period variability index. It is not an average of the cycle-to-cycle amplitude variation, but rather it represents the average degree of variation from the mean peak amplitude of the sample. It is unique among perturbation measures in this respect, and it is clearly not equivalent to the other amplitude variability indices that have been proposed.

The AVI is based on a *coefficient of variation* (CV) that can be applied to either periods or amplitudes. This is defined as

$$CV = \left[\frac{1}{n} \sum_{i=1}^{n} (x_i - \bar{x})^2 \right] / \bar{x}^2$$

where n = number of peaks measured, x_i = individual amplitude values, and $\bar{x}$ = mean peak amplitude. The CV, then, is the average of the deviations from the mean peak amplitude squared ($[x_i - x]^2$) divided by the square of the mean amplitude. The AVI is then calculated as

$$AVI = \log_{10} (CV \times 1000).$$

Deal and Emanuel (1978) evaluated their index with samples (originally collected by Sansone and Emanuel, 1970 and by Hanson, 1969) of sustained vowels produced by normal adult males and by clinically hoarse men with confirmed laryngeal pathologies. AVI values for both groups are summarized in Table 4-12. A peculiarity of the analysis method, however, requires the use of caution in interpreting these data. Before oscillographic write out, all signals

TABLE 4-11. Directional Perturbation Factor (% Sign Change) for Amplitude: Normal Men and Women*

	Vowel		
	/a/	/u/	/i/
Men			
Mean	59.47	58.91	61.13
Range	52.0-68.3	43.5-67.0	52.8-66.7
SD	3.89	5.40	3.91
Women			
Mean	63.13	59.76	61.71
Range	52.3-69.4	51.3-70.9	57.5-72.6
SD	4.27	4.66	3.56

From Sorensen, D. and Horii, Y. Frequency and amplitude perturbation in the voice of female speakers. *Journal of Communication Disorders* 16 (1983) 57–61. © 1983 by Elsevier Publishing Co., Inc. Reprinted by permission.

No correlation between DPF and actual shimmer magnitude values. Period perturbation (jitter) studied in same group (see Chap. 5).

*20 men, 20 women (all nonsmokers); age 25–49 yr (means: males 38.1 yr; females 36.4 yr); sustained vowels, 70–80 dB SPL for ~5 s.

were conditioned by an extremely narrow (10 Hz) bandpass filter with its center frequency at the first harmonic of the voice signal. Such a filter smooths out irregularities in the signal, but the exact extent to which it did so in the samples analyzed cannot be determined.

Shimmer in dB

Given that the decibel scale is based on a ratio of amplitudes, it is an easy matter to use this scale for quantifying shimmer. The ratio need only be that of two contiguous cycles (A_i and A_{i+1}) for which the amplitude difference in dB is

$$dB_{shimmer} = 20 \log_{10}(A_i/A_{i+1}).$$

The average shimmer for a sample of N cycles is then

$$dB_{shimmer} = \frac{\sum_{i=1}^{n-1} \left| 20 \log (A_i/A_{i+1}) \right|}{n-1}$$

TABLE 4-12. Amplitude Variability Index: Normal and Hoarse*

Vowel	Normal Mean	S.D.	Hoarse Mean	S.D.
/u/	− 0.1287	0.2241	0.4142†	0.6497
/i/	− 0.1330	0.4087	0.5706†	0.8831
/ʌ/	− 0.0389	0.2432	0.5977†	0.8486
/a/	− 0.0619	0.4036	0.2163	0.6389
/æ/	− 0.0216	0.2557	0.1550	0.5876
Overall	− 0.0768		0.3908†	

From Deal, R. E., and Emanuel, F. W. Some waveform and spectral features of vowel roughness. *Journal of Speech and Hearing Research*, 21 (1978) 250–264. © American Speech-Language-Hearing Assn., Rockville, MD. Reprinted by permission.

*Method: 20 normal males; 20 hoarse males with diagnosed laryngeal pathology. Analysis of 1-sec portion of 7-sec productions; vocal intensity 75 dB SPL; signal narrow-band filtered.

†All significantly different, p < .05.

TABLE 4-13. Shimmer in dB: Normal Adults*

Vowel	Men:** Mean (SD)	Women:† Mean (SD)
/a/	0.47 (0.34)	0.33 (0.22)
/i/	0.37 (0.28)	0.23 (0.08)
/u/	0.33 (0.31)	0.19 (0.04)
Overall‡	0.39 (0.31)	0.25 (0.11)

Data for men from Horii, Y. Vocal shimmer in sustained phonation. *Journal of Speech and Hearing Research*, 23 (1980) 202-209. American Speech-anguage-Hearing Assn., Rockville, MD.

Data for women from Sorensen, D. and Horii, Y. Frequency and amplitude perturbation in the voice of female speakers. *Journal of Communication Disorders* 16 (1983) 56-61. Elsevier Publishing Co., Inc.

*Method: 20 women, aged 25–49 (mean 36.8 yr); 31 men, aged 18–38 (mean 26.6 yr); sustained vowels, 5 s; 70–80 dB SPL; F_o controlled ± 10 Hz; 3 sec segment of the least variable 3 trials analyzed.

**Significant difference p = .05): /a/ > /i/ and /u/. 95% critical region: > 0.98 dB.

†Significant difference (p = .05): /a/ > /i/ and /u.

‡Male/female shimmer values are significantly different (p = .05) for /i/ and /u/ but not for /a/. The overall mean shimmer values for men and women are not significantly different.

This approach to the quantification of shimmer has the distinct advantage of freeing the measurement from the absolute amplitude. In this it is analogous to the F_o compensation used for several jitter measures. It is the method used by Horii (1980b) to generate the data of Table 4-13.

Compensation for long-term changes: APQ

Long-term changes in vocal intensity are not the issue in evaluation of shimmer, but they are bound to increase its measured magnitude. Eliminating the effects of amplitude "drift" in order to get a truer index of the underlying shimmer itself has been attempted by the same kind of trend-line smoothing used for jitter analysis. Kitajima and Gould (1976) proposed using deviation from a least-squares trend line, but their method is cumbersome without a computer.

Takahashi and Koike (1975) and Koike, Takahashi, and Calcaterra (1977) have suggested a measure they call the *amplitude perturbation quotient* (APQ), which is analogous to the relative average perturbation originally devised by Koike (1973). The function uses an 11-point average for smoothing and is defined as

$$APQ = \frac{\dfrac{1}{n-10} \displaystyle\sum_{i=6}^{n-5} \left| \dfrac{A_{i-5}+A_{i-4}+\ldots+A_i+\ldots+A_{i+5}}{11} - A_i \right|}{\dfrac{1}{n}\displaystyle\sum_{i=1}^{n} A_i}$$

where A_i = peak amplitude of each wave and n = number of waves measured.

Davis (1976, 1979, 1981) has evaluated the effect of window size (that is, the number of waves in the running average) and has found that the APQ function is optimalized at 5. He prefers, however, to evaluate the peaks of the residue signal after inverse filtering, which eliminates the effects of the acoustic characteristics of the vocal tract. Davis' data are not, therefore, directly comparable with those of Takahashi and Koike, but because they are reflective of the information derived by a commercially distributed system (ILS) the use of which is becoming more common, they are included in Table 4-14. Note also that Takahashi and Koike's samples were collected using a pretracheal contact microphone. Data for various pathologies are included in the table. Although not normative, they do provide an indication of the shimmer increases that might be expected.

Serial correlation function

The serial correlation function will be described more completely in connection with F_o perturbation (Chap. 5). It has been found (von Leden and Koike, 1970) that the same technique applied to amplitude measures can be a very sensitive indicator of the presence of laryngeal pathology. Von Leden and Koike emphasize that, because cyclicity of perturbation tends to be a relatively short-term phenomenon, it is only necessary to use lags of 1 to 15 for analysis. They have categorized amplitude-perturbation correlograms into four basic types, schematized in Figure 4-9.

The type 1 correlogram is typical of a normal speaker. The very high correlation at lag = 1 is indicative of the similarity of successive waveforms. The correlation decreases smoothly as the comparison is made across a greater lag, and the negative peak between lag = 10 and lag = 15 tends to show a longer-term periodicity of amplitude variation, perhaps like vibrato. The type 1 pattern is also seen in mild, transient laryngeal involvements.

TABLE 4-14. Amplitude Perturbation Quotients: Normal and Pathologic*

No./Sex	Mean Age	Mean F_o	APQ Mean	APQ SD	Note
			NORMAL		
Acoustic signal:					
7 M	27.7	108.1	40.3×10^{-4}	13.6×10^{-4}	a
2 F	29.5	206.0	32.9×10^{-4}	20.9×10^{-4}	a
Inverse-filtered residue signal:					
8 M	28.4	120.0	5.97%	3.10%	b
2 F	29.5	206.0	6.81%	3.15%	b
			PATHOLOGIC		
Chronic laryngitis:					
2 F	46.0	193.5	16.7×10^{-4}	8.3×10^{-4}	b
Unilateral paralysis:					
2 M	49.5	193.0	111.3×10^{-4}	0.64×10^{-4}	b
Nodules:					
2 M	54.5	118.5	41.0×10^{-4}	31.8×10^{-4}	b
1 M	11	271.	28.5×10^{-4}		b
1 F	33	205.	38.3×10^{-4}		b
Tumors:					
1 M	50	155	120.1×10^{-4}		b
1 F	61	149	137.3×10^{-4}		b
Partial laryngectomy:					
2 M	66	100.0	93.1×10^{-4}	4.1×10^{-4}	b

Adapted from:
   [a]Takahashi and Koike (1975). Eleven point smoothing. Pretracheal contact microphone.
   [b]Davis (1979). Five-point smoothing. Data based on samples collected by Koike and Markel (1975).
   *Sustained /a/, comfortable pitch, loudness, analysis of steadiest 1.5 s.

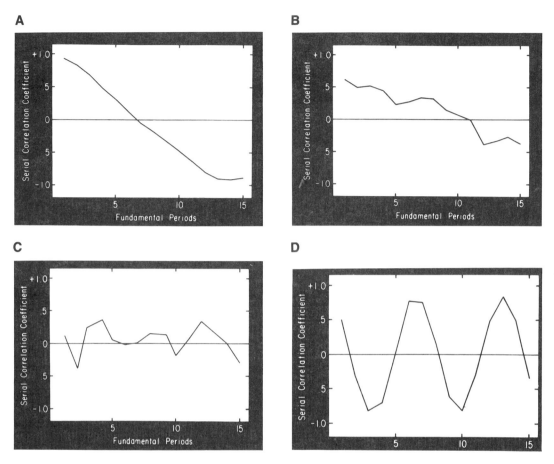

FIGURE 4-9. Amplitude perturbation correlogram categories. (A) Type 1—normal. (B) Type 2—inflammation, small nodules. (C) Type 3—incomplete closure, paralysis. (D) Type 4—malignancy, papillomatosis. (From von Leden, H. and Koike, Y. Detection of laryngeal disease by computer technique. *Archives of Otolaryngology* 91 (1970) 3-10. Reprinted by permission.)

The type 2 correlogram is similar to type 1, but the irregularity of the correlation decrease points to erratic, short-term amplitude perturbation. This pattern is commonly associated with benign changes of the vocal folds, such as fibrosis, inflammatory tumors, or severe inflammation. An absence of correlational periodicity is characteristic of the type 3 correlogram. It is a common concommittant of disorders that result in incomplete glottal closure, such as unilateral paralysis and benign neoplasms. Type 4 patterns are associated with serious laryngeal pathology, including malignant tumors of the vocal folds (Koike, 1969; Izdebski and Murry, 1980), and multiple papillomatosis. The clearly marked posi-

tive and negative correlational peaks indicate fairly rapid and strongly periodic amplitude modulation.

The research concerning serial correlation functions is not sufficiently rigorous or extensive to permit firm diagnostic conclusions, but the promise of great utility is clearly present. Further work may put this diagnostic technique on a firmer footing. ■

SELECT BIBLIOGRAPHY

Bernthal, J. E. and Beukelman, D. R. The effect of changes in velopharyngeal orifice area on vowel intensity. *Cleft Palate Journal*, 14 (1977) 63-77.

Black, J. W. Natural frequency, duration, and intensity of vowels in reading. *Journal of Speech and Hearing Disorders*, 14 (1949) 216-221.

Black, J. W. The effect of delayed side-tone upon vocal rate and intensity. *Journal of Speech and Hearing Disorders*, 16 (1951) 56-60.

Black, J. W. Relationships among fundamental frequency, vocal sound pressure, and rate of speaking. *Language and Speech*, 4 (1961) 196-199.

Blood, G. The interactions of amplitude and phonetic quality in esophageal speech. *Journal of Speech and Hearing Research*, 24 (1981) 308-312.

Blood, G. Fundamental frequency and intensity measurements in laryngeal and alaryngeal speakers. *Journal of Communication Disorders*, 17 (1984) 319-324.

Brady, P. T. Need for standardization in the measurement of speech level. *Journal of the Acoustical Society of America*, 50 (1971) 712-714.

Brandt, J. F., Ruder, K. F., and Shipp, T., Jr. Vocal loudness and effort in continuous speech. *Journal of the Acoustical Society of America*, 46 (1969) 1543-1548.

Bricker, P. D. Technique for objective measurement of speech levels. *Journal of the Acoustical Society of America*, 38 (1965) 361-362.

Broch, J. T. and Wahrman, C. G. Effective averaging time of the level recorder type 2305. *B & K Technical Review* 1-1961, 3-23.

Brown, W. J., Jr. and McGlone, R. E. Aerodynamic and acoustic study of stress in sentence productions. *Journal of the Acoustical Society of America*, 56 (1974) 971-974.

Canter, G. J. Speech characteristics of patients with Parkinson's disease. I. Intensity, pitch, and duration. *Journal of Speech and Hearing Disorders*, 28 (1963) 221-229.

Colcord, R. D. and Adams, M. R. Voicing duration and vocal SPL changes associated with stuttering reduction during singing. *Journal of Speech and Hearing Research*, 22 (1979) 468-479.

Coleman, R. F., Mabis, J. H., and Hinson, J. K. Fundamental frequency-sound pressure level profiles of adult male and female voices. *Journal of Speech and Hearing Research*, 20 (1977) 197-204.

Colton, R. H. Vocal intensity in the modal and falsetto registers. *Folia Phoniatrica*, 25 (1973) 62-70.

Davis, S. B. *Computer evaluation of laryngeal pathology based on inverse filtering of speech.* (SCRL Monograph No.13) Santa Barbara, CA: Speech Communications Research Lab, Inc., 1976.

Davis, S. B. Acoustic characteristics of normal and pathological voices. In Lass, N. J. (Ed.). *Speech and Language: Basic Advances in Research and Practice*, vol. 1. New York: Academic Press, 1979. Pp. 271-335.
Reprinted in:
Ludlow, C. L. and Hart, M. 0. (Eds.). Proceedings of the Conference on the Assessment of Vocal Pathology. *ASHA Reports* No.11 (1981), 97-115.

Deal, R. E. and Emanuel, F. W. Some waveform and spectral features of vowel roughness. *Journal of Speech and Hearing Research*, 21 (1978) 250-264.

Diedrich, W. M. The mechanism of esophageal speech. In Bouhuys, A. (Ed.) *Sound Production in Man.* (Annals of the New York Academy of Sciences, 155 (1968) 303-317.

Fairbanks, G., House, A. S., and Stevens, E. L. An experimental study of vowel intensities. *Journal of the Acoustical Society of America*, 22 (1950) 457-459.

Feth, L. L. Letter to the editor. *Asha*, 19 (1977) 225-226.

Fisichelli, V. R., Karelitz, S., Eichbauer, J., and Rosenfeld, L. S. Volume-unit graphs: their production and applicability in studies of infants' cries. *Journal of Psychology*, 52 (1961) 423-427.

Fletcher, H. Loudness, pitch and the timbre of musical tones and their relation to the intensity, the frequency, and the overtone structure. *Journal of the Acoustical Society of America*, 6 (1934) 59-69.

Fletcher, H. *Speech and Hearing in Communication.* New York: van Nostrand, 1953.

Fletcher, H. and Munson, W. A. Loudness, its definition, measurement, and calculation. *Journal of the Acoustical Society of America*, 5 (1933) 82-108.

Fry, D. B. Duration and intensity as physical correlates of linguistic stress. *Journal of the Acoustical Society of America*, 27 (1955) 765-768.

Gade, S. Sound intensity (Part I: Theory). *B & K Technical Review* 3-1982a, 3-39.

Gade, S. Sound intensity (Part II: Instrumentation and applications). *B & K Technical Review*, 4-1982, 3-32.

Hanson, W. Vowel spectral noise levels and roughness severity ratings for vowels and sentences produced by adult males presenting abnormally rough voice. Unpublished doctoral dissertation, University of Oklahoma, 1969.

Harris, J. D. Loudness discrimination. *Journal of Speech and Hearing Disorders*, monograph suppl. 11, 1963.

Hecker, M. H. L. and Kreul, E. J. Descriptions of the speech of patients with cancer of the vocal folds. Part I: Measures of fundamental frequency. *Journal of the Acoustical Society of America*, 49 (1971) 1275-1282.

Hixon, T. Turbulent noise sources for speech. *Folia Phoniatrica*, 18 (1966) 168-182.

Hixon, T. J., Minifie, F. D., and Tait, C. A. Correlates of turbulent noise production for speech. *Journal of Speech and Hearing Research*, 10 (1967) 133-140.

Holbrook, A., Rolnick, M. I., and Bailey, C. W. Treatment of vocal abuse disorders using a vocal intensity controller. *Journal of Speech and Hearing Disorders*, 39 (1974) 298-303.

Hoops, H. R. and Noll, J. D. Relationship of selected acoustic variables to judgments of esophageal speech. *Journal of Communication Disorders*, 2 (1969) 1-13.

Horii, Y. Vocal shimmer in sustained phonation. *Journal of Speech and Hearing Research*, 23 (1980) 202-209.

Horii, Y. Jitter and shimmer differences among sustained vowel phonations. *Journal of Speech and Hearing Research*, 25 (1982) 12-14.

Horii, Y. Jitter and shimmer in sustained vocal fry phonation. *Folia Phoniatrica*, 37 (1985) 81-86.

Horii, Y. and Weinberg, B. Intelligibility characteristics of superior esophageal speech presented under various levels of masking noise. *Journal of Speech and Hearing Research*, 18 (1975) 413-419.

House, A. S. and Fairbanks, G. The influence of consonant environment upon the secondary acoustical characteristics of vowels. *Journal of the Acoustical Society of America*, 25 (1953) 105-113.

Hyman, M. An experimental study of artificial larynx and esophageal speech. *Journal of Speech and Hearing Disorders*, 20 (1955) 291-299.

Isshiki, N. Regulatory mechanism of voice intensity variation. *Journal of Speech and Hearing Research*, 7 (1964) 17-29.

Isshiki, N. Vocal intensity and air flow rate. *Folia Phoniatrica*, 17 (1965) 92-104.

Isshiki, N. Remarks on mechanism for vocal intensity variation. *Journal of Speech and Hearing Research*, 12 (1969) 665-672.

Izdebski, K. and Murry, T. Glottal waveform variability: a preliminary inquiry. In Lawrence, V. and Weinberg, B. (Eds.), *Transcripts of the Ninth Symposium on Care of the Professional Voice*. New York: The Voice Foundation, 1980, vol. I pp. 39-43.

Johnson, C. J., Pick, H. L., Jr., Siegel, G. M., Cicciarelli, A. W., and Garber, S. R. Effects of interpersonal distance on children's vocal intensity. *Child Development*, 52 (1981) 721-723.

Kallstrom, L. A. A small portion falls short. (Letter to the Editor). *Asha*, 18 (1976) 879-880.

Kitajima, K. and Gould, W. J. Vocal shimmer in sustained phonation of normal and pathologic voice. *Annals of Otolaryngology*, 85 (1976) 377-381.

Koike, Y. Experimental studies on vocal attack. *Practica Otologica Kyoto*, 60 (1967) 663-688.

Koike, Y. Vowel amplitude modulations in patients with laryngeal diseases. *Journal of the Acoustical Society of America*, 45 (1969) 839-844.

Koike, Y. Application of some acoustic measures for the evaluation of laryngeal dysfunction. *Studia Phonologica*, 7 (1973) 17-23.

Koike, Y., Hirano, M., and von Leden, H. Vocal initiation: acoustic and aerodynamic investigations of normal subjects. *Folia Phoniatrica*, 19 (1967) 173-182.

Koike, Y. and Markel, J. Application of inverse filtering for detecting laryngeal pathology. *Annals of Otology, Rhinology, and Laryngology*, 84 (1975) 117-124.

Koike, Y., Takahashi, H., and Calcaterra, T. C. Acoustic measures for detecting laryngeal pathology. *Acta Oto-laryngologica*, 84 (1977) 105-117.

Komiyama, S., Watanabe, H., Nishinow, S., and Yamai, 0. A new phonometer. *Otologia* (Fukuoka), 23 (1977) 105-110.

Komiyama, S., Watanabe, H. and Ryu, S. Phonographic relationship between pitch and intensity of the human voice. *Folia Phoniatrica*, 36 (1984) 1-7.

Kramer, M. B. Kallstrom creates concern from a doctoral candidate. (Letter to the Editor) *Asha*, 19 (1977) 225.

Lee, B. S. Some effects of side-tone delay. *Journal of the Acoustical Society of America*, 22 (1950) 639-640.

Leeper, H. A. and Noll, J. D. Pressure measurements of articulatory behavior during alterations of vocal effort. *Journal of the Acoustical Society of America*, 51 (1972) 1291-1295.

Lehiste, I. and Peterson, G. E. Linguistic considerations in the study of speech intelligibility. *Journal of the Acoustical Society of America*, 31 (1959a) 280-286.

Lehiste, I. and Peterson, G. Vowel amplitude and phonemic stress in American English. *Journal of the Acoustical Society of America*, 31 (1959b) 428-435.

Levitt, H. and Bricker, P. D. Reduction of observer bias in reading speech levels with a VU meter. *Journal of the Acoustical Society of America*, 47 (1970) 1583-1587.

Lieberman, P. Some acoustic correlates of word stress in American English. *Journal of the Acoustical Society of America*, 32 (1960) 451-454.

Malécot, A. The effectiveness of intra-oral air-pressure-pulse parameters in distinguishing between stop cognates. *Phonetica*, 14 (1966a) 65-81.

Malécot, A. The effect of syllabic rate and loudness on the force of articulation of American stops and fricatives. *Phonetica*, 19 (1969) 205-216.

Markel, N. N., Prebor, L. D., and Brandt, J. F. Biosocial factors in dyadic communication: sex and speaking intensity. *Journal of Personality and Social Psychology*, 23 (1972) 11-13.

Michel, J. F. and Wendahl, R. Correlates of voice production. In Travis, L. E. (Ed.), *Handbook of Speech Pathology and Audiology*. Englewood Cliffs, N. J.: Prentice-Hall, 1971. Chap. 18, pp. 465-480.

Murry, T. and Brown, W. S., Jr. Regulation of vocal intensity during vocal fry phonation. *Journal of the Acoustical Society of America*, 49 (1971a) 1905-1907.

Ptacek, P. H., Sander, E. K., Maloney, W. H., and Jackson, C. C. R. Phonatory and related changes with advanced age. *Journal of Speech and Hearing Research*, 9 (1966) 353-360.

Ringel, R. L., House, A. S., and Montgomery, A. H. Scaling articulatory behavior: intraoral air pressure. *Journal of the Acoustical Society of America*, 42 (1967) 1209A.

Robbins, J., Fisher, H. B., and Logemann, J. A. Acoustic characteristics of voice production after Staffieri's surgical reconstructive procedure. *Journal of Speech and Hearing Disorders*, 47 (1982) 77-84.

Robbins, J., Fisher, H. B., Logemann, J., Hillenbrand, J., and Blom, E. A comparative acoustic analysis of laryngeal speech, esophageal speech, and speech production after tracheoesophageal puncture. Paper presented at the 1981 Convention of the ASHA.

Robbins, J., Fisher, H., Blom, E., and Singer, M. I. A comparative acoustic study of normal, esophageal, and tracheoesophageal speech production. *Journal of Speech and Hearing Disorders*, 49 (1984) 202-210.

Rubin, H. J., LeCover, M., and Vennard, W. Vocal intensity, subglottic pressure, and air flow relationships in singers. *Folia Phoniatrica*, 19 (1967) 393-413.

Sacia, C. F. and Beck, C. J. The power of fundamental speech sounds. *Bell System Technology Journal*, 5 (1926) 393-403.

Sansone, F. E., Jr., and Emanuel, F. Spectral noise levels and roughness severity ratings for normal and simulated rough vowels produced by adult males. *Journal of Speech and Hearing Research*, 13 (1970) 489-502.

Schutte, H. K. and Seidner, W. Recommendation by the Union of European Phoniatricians (UEP): Standardizing voice area measurement/phonetography. *Folia Phoniatrica*, 35 (1983) 286-288.

Siegel, G. M., Fehst, C. A., Garber, S. R., and

Pick, H. L., Jr. Delayed auditory feedback with children. *Journal of Speech and Hearing Research*, 23 (1980) 802-813.

Singer, M. and Blom, E. An endoscopic technique for restoration of voice after laryngectomy. *Annals of Otology, Rhinology, and Laryngology*, 89 (1980) 529-533.

Snidecor, J. C. and Isshiki, N. Air volume and air flow relationships of six male esophageal speakers. *Journal of Speech and Hearing Disorders*, 30 (1965) 205-216.

Sorensen, D. and Horii, Y. Frequency and amplitude perturbation in the voice of female speakers. *Journal of Communication Disorders*, 16 (1983) 57-61.

Sorensen, D. and Horii, Y. Directional perturbation factors for jitter and for shimmer. *Journal of Communication Disorders*, 17 (1984) 143-151.

Staffieri, M. and Serafini, I. La riabilitazione chirurgica della voce e della respirazione dopo laryngectomia totale. *Atti del 29 Congresso Nazionale, Bologna*, 1976.

Steinberg, J. C. and Gardner, M. B. The dependence of hearing impairment on sound intensity. *Journal of the Acoustical Society of America*, 9 (1937), 11-23.

Stone, R. E., Jr., Bell, C. J. and Clack, T. D. Minimum intensity of voice at selected levels within pitch range. *Folia Phoniatrica*, 30 (1978) 113-118.

Stone, R. E., Jr. and Ferch, P. A. K. Intra-subject variability in F_o-SPL_{min} voice profiles. *Journal of Speech and Hearing Disorders*, 47 (1982) 134-137.

Stone, R. E., Jr. and Krause, P. Intra-subject variability in minimum SPL of voice at selected fundamental frequencies. Paper presented at the 1980 Convention of the ASHA.

Stout, B. The harmonic structure of vowels in singing in relation to pitch and intensity. *Journal of the Acoustical Society of America*, 10 (1938) 137-146.

Takahashi, H. and Koike, Y. Some perceptual dimensions and acoustical correlates of pathologic voices. *Acta Oto-Laryngologica*, suppl. 338 (1975) 1-24.

van den Berg, J. and Moolenaar-Bijl, A. J. Cricopharyngeal sphincter, pitch, intensity, and fluency in oesophageal speech. *Practica Oto-Rhino-Laryngologica*, 21 (1959) 298-315.

Villchur, E. and Killion, M. C. Probe-tube microphone assembly. *Journal of the Acoustical Society of America*, 57 (1975) 238-240.

von Leden, H. and Koike, Y. Detection of laryngeal disease by computer technique. *Archives of Otolaryngology*, 91 (1970) 3-10.

Ward, W. D. . . . from an acoustician. (Letter to the Editor). *Asha*, 19 (1977) 226.

Wendahl, R. W. Some parameters of auditory roughness. *Folia Phoniatrica*, 18 (1966a) 26-32.

Wendahl, R. W. Laryngeal analog synthesis of jitter and shimmer auditory parameters of harshness. *Folia Phoniatrica*, 18 (1966) 98-108.

Wente, E. C., Bedell, E. H., and Swartzel, K. D., Jr. A high speed level recorder for acoustic measurements. *Journal of the Acoustical Society of America*, 6 (1935) 121-129.

Wolf, S. K. and Sette, W. J. Some applications of modern acoustic apparatus. *Journal of the Acoustical Society of America*, 6 (1935) 160-168.

Wolf, S. K., Stanley, D., and Sette, W. J. Quantitative studies on the singing voice. *Journal of the Acoustical Society of America*, 6 (1935) 255-266.

Zaveri, K. Conventional and on-line methods of sound power measurements. *B and K Technical Review*, 3 (1971) 3-27.

CHAPTER **5**

Vocal Fundamental Frequency

There is long-standing and widespread agreement that pitch is an important factor—perhaps etiologically and certainly symptomatically—in vocal disorders (Cooper, 1971; Perkins, 1971a,b; Moore, 1971; Boone, 1971; West and Ansberry, 1968; Brodnitz, 1961; Fairbanks, 1940; Luchsinger and Arnold, 1965; Stone and Sharf, 1973). This vocal attribute has traditionally been evaluated solely according to the therapist's perception and estimate of magnitude, generally on a low to high continuum. The perception then formed the basis of an adequacy judgment: too high, normal, too low, erratic, and so on.

Such methods of assessment are very likely to be inadequate. The descriptive terms are crude and unstandardized. They are also incapable of resolving moderately small differences. Listeners' judgments of pitch have been found to be unreliable (Laguaite and Waldrop, 1964; Montague, Hollien, Hollien, and Wold, 1978). As Brodnitz (1961, p. 51) has pointed out, conclusions about adequacy or acceptability are very likely to be influenced by "personal

tastes, preferences of fashion in voices, . . . and personal identifications." Beyond this lies the very important fact that pitch is not the simple perception of fundamental frequency. Rather, the frequency, intensity, and spectral properties of a sound interact in very complex ways to lead to a given pitch perception (Houtsma and Goldstein, 1972; Goldstein, 1973). Licklider (1951), Fletcher (1934), and Fletcher and Munson (1933) provide good elementary discussions of the basic aspects of the phenomena of pitch perception. The curves of Figure 5-1 (taken from Fletcher, 1934, p. 65) show the intensity effect quite clearly. The perceived pitch of a tone changes as the loudness changes—and the effect is maximal in the expected range of human vocal pitch.

We are led to the conclusion that perceptual judgments alone may well mislead the clinician. Perceived abnormality of pitch may partly reflect the speaker's vocal intensity and vice versa. The judgment of unacceptability may betray clinicians' attitudes as well as patients' deviance. Comparison to a norm requires that both the norm and

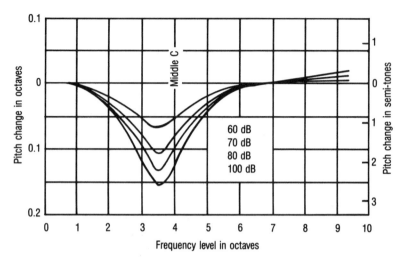

FIGURE 5-1. Changes in the perceived pitch of tones as a function of fundamental frequency and intensity. (From Fletcher, H. Loudness pitch and the timbre of musical tones and their relation to the intensity, the frequency, and the overtone structure. *Journal of the Acoustical Society of America*, 6 (1934) 59-69. Figure 7, p. 65. Reprinted by permission.)

the behavior in question be based on unbiased and objective scales if the factors contributing to the unacceptability of the final vocal product are to be understood and addressed in therapy. So, while it is important for the therapist to judge vocal pitch acceptability, it is vital that the fundamental frequency be measured.

It was not very long ago that fundamental frequency measurements were difficult, time consuming, and often very expensive. This is no longer the case. The instrumentation involved is sometimes complex, but simple methods also exist. As long as the measurement technique and its limitations are well understood, a method can be selected to meet the needs of almost any clinical setting or situation.

GENERAL PHYSICAL PRINCIPLES: UNITS OF MEASUREMENT

The fundamental frequency, denoted F_o, is the rate at which a waveform is repeated per unit time. Older literature states frequency in *cycles per second* (cps), but a special frequency unit has since been almost universally adopted. One hertz (Hz)

is equal to one cycle per second. The *period* (denoted t) is the duration of a single cycle. Frequency and period are therefore mutually reciprocal:

$$t = 1/F_o$$
$$F_o = 1/t$$

Some of the methods to be discussed in this chapter depend on counting the number of cycles per second, that is, they measure frequency in Hz. Others determine the length of the period, generally in milliseconds. To know one value is to know the other.

Fundamental Frequency and Vocal Pitch

In general, pitch (a perceptual attribute of sound) increases with fundamental frequency (a physical parameter of vibration). But the relationship is not linear. The auditory system is more sensitive to some frequency changes than to others (Stevens, Volkmann, and Newman, 1937; Stevens and Volkmann, 1940). In particular, the average listener is more sensitive to changes at lower frequencies: Raising F_o from 100 to 200 Hz results in a much greater change in perceived pitch than going from 3000 to 3100 Hz. The standard musical scale reflects this fact. For example, the frequency of C below middle C is 65.41 Hz, while the D below middle C, perceived to be one note higher, is 73.42 Hz.* A change of one note requires an increase of a bit more than 8 Hz. But going from the C *above* middle C to the D above middle C entails a frequency shift from 261.6 Hz to 293.7 Hz, four times as much. The semitone scale reflects this situation by an exponential growth function.† That is, the difference in semitones between two frequencies grows more slowly as frequency increases. This is graphically illustrated in Figure 5-2.

On the semitone scale, raising a frequency, f_1, by n semitones results in a higher frequency, f_2, according to the relationship

$$f_2 = \left({}^{12}\sqrt{2}\,\right)^n \cdot f_1$$

For example, the frequency 6 semitones above 100 Hz is

$$\begin{aligned}
f_2 &= \left({}^{12}\sqrt{2}\,\right)^6 \cdot 100 \\
f_2 &= (1.059463)^6 \times 100 \\
&= 1.414 \times 100 \\
f_2 &= 141.4 \, \text{Hz}
\end{aligned}$$

The semitone difference, n, between two frequencies, f_1 and f_2 is given by

$$n = \frac{12\,(\log_{10} f_2 - \log_{10} f_1)}{\log_{10} 2}$$

A mathematically equivalent form is

$$n = \frac{12\,\log_{10}\,(f_2/f_1)}{\log_{10} 2}$$

This formula can be made somewhat less intimidating by reducing the constants:

$$\begin{aligned}
\log_{10} 2 \quad &= 0.30103 \quad \text{and} \\
12/\log_{10} 2 &= 39.86.
\end{aligned}$$

---

*Frequency values for the notes of the musical scale are given in Appendix D.

†This is not to say that the semitone values actually scale perceived pitch. The perceptual "mel" scale values can only be derived by asking listeners to assign pitch values to tones. The underlying perceptual processes are too irregular to be expressed in any simple mathematical formula.

Therefore we have

$$\begin{aligned}
&n = 39.86\,(\log_{10} f_2 - \log_{10} f_1) \\
\text{or} \quad &n = 39.86\,\log_{10}(f_2/f_1).
\end{aligned}$$

Thus, for example, the semitone difference between $(f_1 =)$ 200 Hz and $(f_2 =)$ 400 Hz is

$$\begin{aligned}
n &= \frac{12\,(\log_{10} 400 - \log_{10} 200)}{\log_{10} 2} \\[2mm]
&= \frac{12\,(2.6020 - 2.3010)}{0.3010} = \frac{12(0.3010)}{0.3010}
\end{aligned}$$

$n = 12$ semitones.

That is, 400 Hz is 12 semitones higher than 200 Hz. Of course, this is the expected answer: Doubling a frequency is equivalent to raising the tone one octave. There are 12 semitones in an octave.

If the semitone system is to be used for more than frequency comparisons, some frequency must be assigned a semitone value of 0. This done, the scale becomes definite and absolute. Fletcher (1934) proposed that zero semitones be set at 16.35 Hz, which has the effect of making all musical Cs integral multiples of 12 semitones. Also, 16.35 Hz is representative of the lower frequency limit of human hearing.

The semitone scale, then, was devised for much the same reasons as the dB scale, to which it is obviously analogous. Its ability to simplify inter-subject comparisons and its usefulness in quantifying frequency variation, coupled with its foundations in the familiar Western musical scale, have made it quite popular among phonatory researchers. It will be encountered often in the literature of voice production.

HAND MEASUREMENT OF FUNDAMENTAL FREQUENCY

Early methods of determining fundamental frequency did not, of course, rely on electronic counting circuits. The relatively primitive state of electronics often forced the first speech researchers to depend on ingenious, but usually very cumbersome and complex, mechanical means

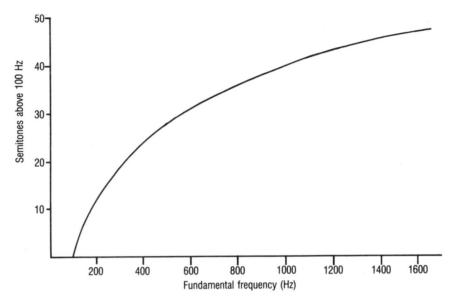

FIGURE 5-2. Relationship of semitones and frequency.

of analysis. The phonodeik (Anderson, 1925), for example, used light reflections from a mirror on a wire made to vibrate by collecting sound power with a diaphragm to produce curves on photographic film. Metfessel (1928) described a system in which the speech signal controlled the flashing of a light that was photographed through a stroboscope disc. The result was a complex pattern of dots and blurred dashes. The position of the rows of dots on the film was indicative of the fundamental frequency. It is an understatement to say that such methods were inconvenient. Metfessel himself described F_o measurement by his method as "an expensive and laborious task, a record of five minutes . . . requiring film costing about fifty dollars with the measuring and graphing of the waves requiring from one hundred to three hundred hours, depending on the desired detail of the measures" (p. 431).

Hand measurement of fundamental frequency is still an alternative. The development of better ways of visualizing the speech waveform has made the task less arduous than the enormous project that confronted Metfessel and his contemporaries. While all-electronic methods are obvi-

ously the fastest and most convenient, hand measurement of F_o is sufficiently easy to be feasible in settings where more sophisticated instrumentation is not available. With just a modicum of care, the results of such an approach need not be any less valid than those produced by more complex means.

Measurement of Graphic Readouts

Fundamental frequency can be determined by measuring the spacing of fundamental periods on a graphic record of the speech signal. This record should, if possible, also include a waveform of precisely known frequency (a 100 Hz square wave serves very well) that can be used as a time scale. If the record is to be made from a tape recording the timing signal ideally should have been recorded on a second tape channel when the voice recording was done. In this way any variations in tape speed will alter the time scale and the speech signal equally and, therefore, not affect the frequency determination.

There are two relatively easy ways of preparing the necessary graphic record. The simpler is to photograph an oscilloscope screen. If a dual-channel oscilloscope is available the speech signal is fed to one channel, and the timing signal to the other (see Figure 5-3). With a single-channel oscilloscope a double exposure may be used to get the speech waveform and timing signal on the same oscillogram, but the precise relationship of simultaneously prerecorded speech and timing waveforms will be lost. The main disadvantage of an oscillogram, of course, is the fact that only a very brief sample can be accommodated. (This may not be a serious limitation for some measures, however.) A chart recorder allows very long samples to be put on paper for later measurement. Unless an optical writing system (Chap. 3) is used, however, a new set of difficulties must be dealt with. The pens of most ink-writing systems are far too sluggish in their response to trace the speech waveform, so their write-out is likely to be little better than a straight line. Also, since most pen recorders have a maximum paper speed on the order of 10 cm/s the spacing of wave peaks might well be too close for accurate resolution. (At a paper speed of 10 cm/s a 200 Hz wave produces peaks spaced only ½ mm apart.)

Successful measurement with a penwriter system depends on deriving the input signal from a recording played at a fraction of the recording speed. If possible, a speed reduction to at least $\frac{1}{16}$ of the recording speed should be used. (A recording

made at 30 inches per second (ips) and played back at $1\frac{7}{8}$ ips provides such a reduction.) One need not be dismayed if a tape recorder with a wide range of speeds is not available, since almost any degree of speed reduction can be achieved by rerecording the original tape with two tape recorders. Suppose, for example, a pair of two-speed machines ($7\frac{1}{2}$ and $3\frac{3}{4}$ ips) is available. The original voice sample is recorded on one of them at $7\frac{1}{2}$ ips. It is then played back at $3\frac{3}{4}$ ips to the other machine, which records the signal at $7\frac{1}{2}$ ips. The new recording is now a half-speed version of the original. When the re-recorded version is played at $3\frac{3}{4}$ ips, the output is a $\frac{1}{4}$ speed version of the original recording. This version can now be tape recorded and played back at half speed, to produce a $\frac{1}{8}$ speed version, and so on. Note, however, that the speed reduction must not be so great as to lower the F_o below the range the tape recorder can reproduce. It is true that re-recording increases noise and signal distortion, but these factors are not of great importance if only the fundamental frequency of the original recording is of interest. More importantly, small irregularities in tape speed may cumulate to produce a significant error in the frequency measurement. However, if the original tape has a timing signal on its second channel its use as the frequency-counting yardstick will preserve measurement accuracy, for the simple reason that any variation of tape speed affects both the speech signal and the timing standard in exactly the same way.

Counting Tape Striations

When absolutely no other means are available, there remains one last-resort option for F_o determination. It is possible to measure the fundamental frequency directly from the surface of the tape itself. Tape recording is based on the creation of magnetized zones in a suitable medium (Chap. 3). Therefore, a recorded tape has sequential regions of strong and weak magnetization whose repetitive spacing is a direct function of the fundamental frequen-

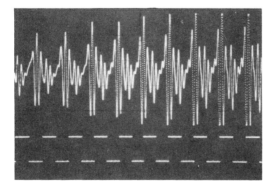

FIGURE 5-3. Oscillogram of a vowel (upper trace) and a simultaneously recorded timing signal (lower trace).

cy. If the areas could be made visible it would be a simple matter to count the number of magnetic "cycles" in a given length of tape and, knowing the tape speed, to derive the fundamental frequency.

Black (1949) used very fine iron filings to visualize the magnetic regions on a tape. When brought into contact with the tape the filings clung only to the strongly magnetized areas, creating a series of striations that could be counted. Leeper and Leeper (1976) have updated this method using a special product called Magna-See® that makes the procedure much more convenient. Magna-See contains microscopic particles of iron material suspended in a volatile liquid. The tape whose recording is to be analyzed is agitated in this suspension for several seconds, allowing the iron particles to adhere to the magnetized regions. When removed from the liquid and dried, striations of iron powder can be clearly seen and counted. The number of striations on a length of tape, divided by the amount of time that length represents, equals the fundamental frequency. If desired, the striations can easily be transferred to the sticky side of cellophane tape and the entire adhesive record can be mounted on a sheet of paper, as shown in Figure 5-4. The 3M Company's magnetic tape viewer (model BX-1022) offers a still more convenient way of observing the magnetic striations (Kelly and Sansone, 1981). When recorded tape is placed in contact with the underside of the viewer, particles of iron in the viewer will, after a few minutes, align themselves with magnetic variations on the tape, permitting counting of striations for F_o estimation. The pattern cannot, however, be permanently stored.

Mueller, Adams, Baehr-Rouse, and Boos (1979) have compared the value of the modal F_o of sustained phonations as determined by visualizing striations to the output of an electronic measurement system. In general, the tape-striation method overestimated the electronic measure by 3 or 4%; the difference between the two was significant for males. It is likely that limitations in measurement of distances accounts for

most of the error. (It should also be noted that the striation method determines mean frequency which, in this study, was compared to an electronically derived modal frequency.) However, the clinician-investigators felt that the error was tolerable for clinical purposes, a conclusion that seems warranted if better methods are not readily accessible.

F_o INSTRUMENTATION: ANALOG ELECTRONICS

Basic Strategies

There are two basic strategies that are most commonly used for electronic extraction of the fundamental frequency or period: peak-picking and zero-crossing detection. The basic conceptual foundation for these will be discussed for sine waves, and then the refinements needed for dealing with real speech signals will be explored.*

Peak-picking

A sine wave has one positive and one negative peak in every cycle. A simple way to determine the fundamental frequency, then, is to count the number of peaks that occur in every second. This is easily accomplished electronically with a circuit known as a *comparator* which produces different outputs depending on whether the signal at its input does or does not exceed a preset threshold. Figure 5-5 shows how this function can be used in measuring F_o. The threshold value for the comparator is set close to the peak voltage of the sine wave. Therefore, the sine wave's voltage exceeds the threshold only during a small portion of the peak in each cycle. This is reflected in the comparator output, whose output is high only for brief intervals. The comparator has, in essence, converted the sine wave signal into a series of pulses, one for each

---

*There are, in fact, several different ways by which these methods are implemented. Any of the electronics texts listed at the end of Chap. 2 can be consulted for alternative techniques.

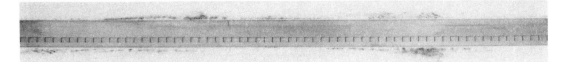

FIGURE 5-4. Tape striations visualized with Magna-See®. (The visualizing material deposited on the tape has been lifted off onto cellophane tape for easier viewing.) The sample was a sustained vowel, recorded at 7.5 ips. This particular tape segment is 5 inches long, representing 5/7.5 = 0.667 s. There are 66 striations on the segment, indicating a fundamental frequency of 66/0.667 = 98.95 Hz.

sine wave peak. The pulses can be applied to an electronic counter which accepts them for a one-second interval. The count at the end of a second is the fundamental frequency, and it can be displayed on some output device. At the end of each one-second counting interval the counter can be immediately reset for another one-second sample, and the counting can be repeated as long as there is an input. This process is schematized in Figure 5-5B. With just a bit more electronic sophistication the time from the start of one peak to the start of the next—the period of the wave—can

also be determined. This measure is not as commonly needed by speech pathologists, however.

Zero-crossing

Not only does every sine wave have two peaks, but its voltage also crosses the zero line twice (once positive-going and once negative-going) in each cycle. If frequency can be counted from the number of peaks per second, it is equally reasonable to assume that it can be counted as the number of times the wave crosses the zero line

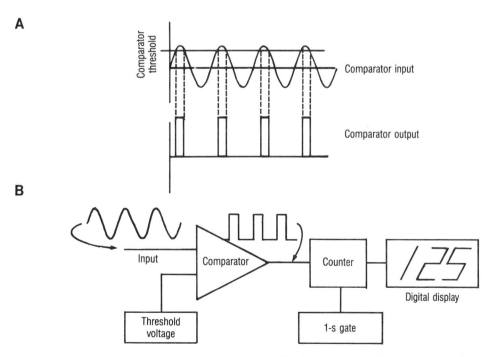

FIGURE 5-5. (A) A comparator produces one pulse for each waveform peak. (B) The comparator output pulses may be counted for successive one-second intervals, and the counts displayed as fundamental frequency readings.

in one direction or the other every second.

A simple method of zero-crossing measurement of F_o is diagrammed in Figure 5-6. The first step is to apply the sine wave input to an amplifier that will purposely distort it by clipping off its peaks, converting it to a series of square waves. A high-pass filter (Chap. 2) is used to block the flat (steady state) parts of the square waves while passing the rapid transition portions. The square waves, which were derived from the original sine waves, are therefore reduced to a series of "spikes." Positive spikes represent the positive-going zero crossings of the original waves; negative spikes are all that remains of negative-going zero crossings. A rectifier (Chap. 2) can eliminate either the positive or negative spikes (the negative ones have been eliminated in Figure 5-6) leaving a single set to be counted in the same way that pulses were counted with peak picking. The number of spikes per second is the fundamental frequency.

Speech waves

Sine waves are the simplest possible signals, so it is easy to apply peak-picking or zero-crossing methods to them. Speech

waves, on the other hand, are extremely complex and their complexity is often of the very sort that most frustrates attempts to use simple methods.

The wave shown in Figure 5-7 is the oscillographic representation of the vowel /ɑ/ spoken by a normal male. Each cycle has two major positive and two major negative peaks (as well as numerous smaller "ripples"). There is also a large number of zero crossings. It is self-evident that simple zero-crossing methods are very likely to produce a F_o reading that is way too high and so are not viable options for analysis. But since one of the peaks is of greater amplitude than the others in the cycle, peak-picking might seem to be possible. The hope, however, is largely illusory.

The difference between the two largest peaks is very small. This implies that a comparator would have to be set very carefully so as to ignore the smaller peak but respond to the larger one. There is so little room for error that failure is almost inevitable: If the amplitude of the entire waveform grows just a little, then both peaks will exceed the comparator's detection threshold. The output of the F_o meter will then be double the true value. On the other hand, if the signal strength falls off just a bit both

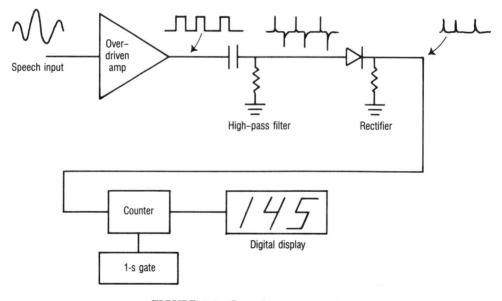

FIGURE 5-6. Counting zero-crossings.

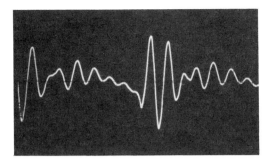

FIGURE 5-7. Waveform of /ɑ/ spoken by a normal male.

peaks might have values below the threshold level, and the comparator will turn out no signal at all. Given the obvious fact that a speech signal is very far from perfectly stable, it is easy to see how a simple F_o meter might almost always produce an incorrect reading. And how would the user know how accurate the measurement is at any given instant?

Filtering

There are several ways of improving the performance of the kind of circuits just discussed. The most obvious is to filter the input signal to eliminate most of the harmonics, leaving a relatively simple waveform for treatment by the rest of the circuit. Unfortunately, the most troublesome harmonics are the ones nearest the fundamental frequency. The filter roll-off (see Chap. 2) must, therefore, be very steep and, if the fundamental frequency changes significantly (as indeed it is likely to during speech), the filter characteristics might be rendered inappropriate. Attempts to circumvent some of these problems by using mechanical analogs of filters (for example, the flap-valve of Smith, 1968) have not met with notable success. In the end, however, it has been the general experience that, with very careful design and sophisticated use of the filter section, it is possible to get sufficient isolation of the fundamental frequency to make peak and zero-crossing detection useful in F_o measurement. While early circuits were often very large and cumbersome

(Obata and Kobayashi, 1938, 1940; Gruenz and Schott, 1949; Dempsey, Draegert, Siskind, and Steer, 1950), compact, lightweight, and efficient modern equivalents are now available commercially. In general, today's instruments provide not only a digital readout of F_o but also a voltage output that can be fed to a strip-chart recorder to obtain a permanent record.

Filters have also been used in more complex ways to improve the reliability of F_o determination. Riesz and Schott (1946), for example, devised an instrument that uses a bandpass filter to analyze the 300–900 Hz frequency band of the input. At any fundamental frequency up to 400 Hz this filtered signal will have at least two harmonics in it. The filtered input is rectified and then low-pass filtered to provide a resultant signal that can be used to generate an output proportional to F_o.

Fundamental Frequency Indicator (FFI)

Sophisticated use of filtering is exemplified by the Fundamental Frequency Indicator (FFI) described in 1965 in an unpublished report by Hollien and Tamburrino. The system is diagrammed in Figure 5-8. Speech input from one channel of a stereophonic tape recorder is applied to a preamplifier that has automatic gain control to compensate for varying amplitude of the speech waveform. The preamplifier feeds the signal to eight parallel low-pass filters whose upper frequency cutoffs are one-half octave apart. This arrangement insures that at least one of the filters will pass the fundamental frequency of the input without any harmonics. The filter outputs are all connected to a special logic unit that finds the lowest filter producing an output. (This will be the one that is devoid of harmonics.) The logic connects this filter output to a circuit that converts the sinusoidal waves to square waves, which are recorded on the second channel of the tape recorder. After being played into the FFI, then, the tape of the speech sample has its original speech track and a new track on which each fundamental period of the speech sig-

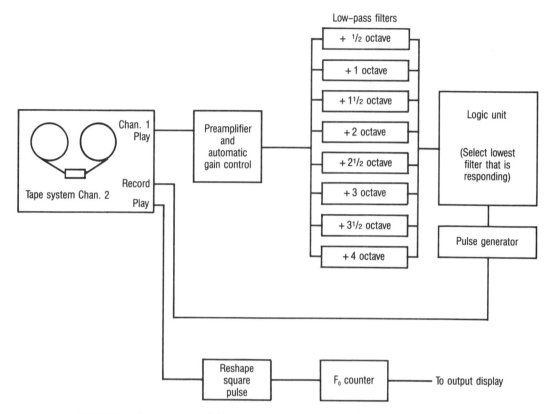

FIGURE 5-8. Functional diagram of the Fundamental Frequency Indicator.

nal is marked by a square pulse. A second playing of the stereo tape is then done at reduced speed. This time the square wave pulses are used to trigger counter circuits that measure the fundamental frequency (Hanley and Peters, 1971). Although a digital indication of F_o can be gotten from the FFI, it has been more commonly used to produce data cards for later computer analysis. Despite its seeming complexity the FFI has been found to be highly reliable and relatively convenient to use in analyzing F_o in modal and loft registers (Saxman and Burk, 1967; Weinberg and Zlatin, 1970; Hollien and Shipp, 1972; Hollien and Jackson 1973). Its 50 Hz lower cutoff frequency, however, severely limits its ability to evaluate pulse register productions (Michel, 1968).

Visi-Pitch®

The Visi-Pitch (Figure 5-9), a relatively recent development of Kay Elemetrics, is a self-contained analog fundamental frequen-

cy analyzer specially designed for ease of use in clinical practice. It provides an oscilloscopic display of both F_o and relative intensity over time, as well as analog voltage outputs of these variables for chart recording. A digital readout is used with a cursor to determine the exact F_o of points on the screen's display. (Horii [1983a] has described a means of interfacing the Visipitch to a microcomputer, and an interface unit is commercially available from Kay Elemetrics Inc.) The Visi-Pitch has achieved widespread acceptance, and its use has become routine in a fairly large number of clinics. The following section describes its functioning in moderate detail for those who might want to take maximal advantage of the possibilities that its circuits offer.

The Visi-Pitch circuit has several novel features that make it quite different from other F_o instruments. The block diagram of Figure 5-10 shows, in a highly simplified way, how the Visi-Pitch functions. Speech input (from a microphone or tape

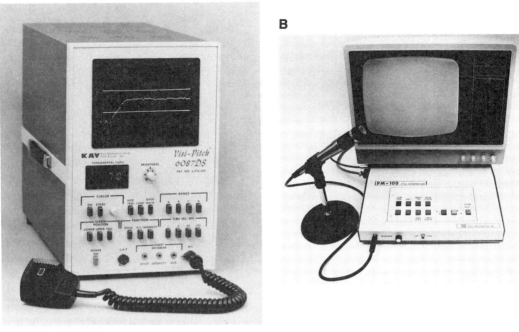

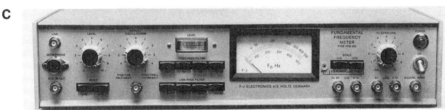

FIGURE 5-9. Fundamental frequency analyzers designed for clinical use. (A) Visi-Pitch (courtesy, Kay Elemetrics, Inc.). (B) PM 100 Pitch Analyzer (courtesy, Voice Identification, Inc.). (C) F-J FFM 650 Fundamental Frequency Analyzer (courtesy, F-J Electronics ApS, Copenhagen, Denmark, and Voice Identification, Inc.).

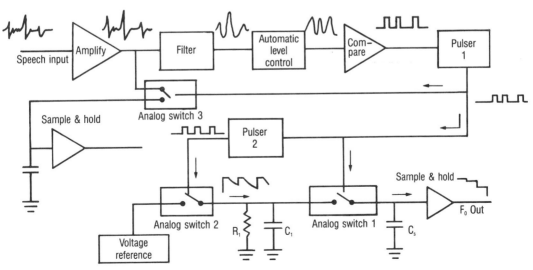

FIGURE 5-10. Functional diagram of the Kay Elemetrics Visi-Pitch.

recording) is first amplified and then low-pass filtered to remove most harmonics. A fast-acting automatic level control then makes the magnitude of all peaks equal and suitable for peak-picking by a comparator (which has a large hysteresis to inhibit detection of any secondary peaks in the waveform). The comparator output (a variable-duration rectangular wave that is also available at a connector on the front panel) is applied to pulse-generator 1, which provides a single, standard-size pulse that activates electronic switch 1, momentarily connecting a "sample-and-hold" amplifier to capacitor C1. When this connection is made, sampling capacitor Cs is charged to the same voltage level as capacitor C1. When, after a very brief interval, the switch opens again, capacitor Cs is left isolated with the charge it acquired. The sample-and-hold amplifier output will show this voltage until the next fundamental period begins, when another pulse is generated that closes switch 1 to update the sample capacitor with a different charge.

If the charge held by capacitor C1 could be made to reflect the duration of the fundamental period, the sample-and-hold amplifier would produce an output that is proportional to the frequency of the last period processed. This can, in fact, be achieved. The end of the pulse from pulse-generator 1 causes the production of another pulse by pulse-generator 2. This one closes electronic switch 2 to connect C1 to a voltage source. After a period of time just long enough to allow C1 to acquire a relatively large charge, the switch opens again, leaving C1 isolated. The charge on C1 will dissipate at a rate determined by the C1R1 combination. Because of this, the voltage across C1 is an accurate (although nonlinear) reflection of how long it has been since it was last recharged. When, at the start of each new fundamental period, pulse-generator 1 causes the sample-and-hold amplifier to "report" the voltage of C1, the output is an analog of the time elapsed since the last charge, which was at the start of the last fundamental period. After being linearized, this output is shown on the oscillo-scope screen. Pulse generator 2 causes C1 to be recharged as soon as its voltage has been transferred to Cs, and the new charge begins to dissipate until it is read by Cs at the start of the next cycle.

The sequence of events in the Visi-Pitch circuit is therefore:

1. A pulse is generated by the peak of every cycle of the input;
2. This pulse causes a "reading" of the voltage on capacitor C1;
3. At the end of the pulse (and hence, of the reading of C1) another pulse causes C1 to be fully charged;
4. The charge on C1 dissipates and its voltage continually diminishes with time;
5. When a new input peak occurs the process repeats from step 1. When sampled at the start of a new cycle, the voltage on C1 is a measure of the time elapsed since the last charge—that is, of the prior fundamental period.

In the Visi-Pitch the pulse that activates switch 1 is also used to momentarily close electronic switch 3. This causes another sample-and-hold amplifier to read the amplitude of the unfiltered input signal at the start of each new cycle. This separate output, representing peak wave amplitude, is used as an intensity measure.

The Visi-Pitch, then, displays the fundamental frequency of each cycle of the speech input, rather than the average F_o of a number of cycles, a very important advantage. The simultaneous display of vocal intensity and provision for determining perturbation (discussed later) greatly enhance this instrument's utility.

PM Pitch Analyzer

The PM Pitch Analyzer, marketed by Voice Identification, Inc., is a measurement system whose zero-crossing detector functions are controlled and enhanced by a built-in microcomputer. Fundamental frequency and intensity curves are shown on a TV-like monitor with a split screen that allows two speech samples (pre- and post-treatment, therapist's model and patient's response, etc.) to be displayed simultaneously. A moveable cursor associated with each trace selects the point whose frequency and/or intensity is numerically indicated at the bottom of the screen. (An analog voltage output is also provided that allows the data to be written by a chart recorder or oscilloscope.) Because the frequency and intensity values of each fundamental period are stored in a digital memory, the user can manipulate the tracing on the screen, for instance, moving one curve left or right so as to line it up with the other.

Operation of the PM Analyzer takes advantage of the interaction of analog circuits and digital processing. The speech signal is input into a bank of bandpass filters with increasing center frequency. The microprocessor rapidly and continuously scans the output of all of the filters and selects the output from the one with the lowest center frequency for further processing. This signal, of course, represents the fundamental frequency with most of its associated harmonics removed. Zero-crossing detection is then performed, and the period of the wave is determined. The microcomputer converts the period to fundamental frequency. The system works so fast that every fundamental period is individually measured. The computer is also programmed to detect very sudden and large jumps in the fundamental frequency. These would most likely be associated with spurious noises or errors in F_o determination. The cycles producing the strange values are rejected by the computer logic.

The PM Analyzer is actually a modular system. Different programs can be plugged into the same housing (much in the way that any microcomputer is expanded) to offer a combination of functions. One such program does statistical analysis of the input. Mean frequency, frequency standard deviation (pitch sigma), cumulative frequency distribution of the pitch periods, and the ratio of voiced to unvoiced time can all be determined and displayed in graphic and digital form. Finally, the average cycle-to-cycle frequency difference (jitter) can also be computed and displayed.

F-J Fundamental Frequency Meter

The fundamental frequency meter (model FFM 650) offered by F-J Electronics is designed to be used with a separate chart recorder or storage oscilloscope. The speech signal (from a microphone or recording) is bandpass filtered to eliminate harmonics. (The filter's upper and lower cutoff frequencies must be set by the user.) The simplified signal is then rectified, reducing it to an approximation of a half sine wave that is applied to a frequency-to-voltage converter. The result is an output voltage proportional to the F_o of the speech signal. The instrument has a calibrated meter on its front panel, but this is of limited use for anything but estimating the frequency of stable, steady-state vowel prolongations. Evaluating frequency contours requires an external display or recording device.

Accelerometry and Glottography

Another way of dealing with the problem of interfering harmonics is to ignore the acoustic speech signal and to analyze instead a correlate of vocal fold activity that has a weak harmonic structure. There are two relatively easy ways of doing this.

Contact microphones and accelerometers (see Chap. 3) are primarily sensitive to body surface vibrations. When placed on the pretracheal surface of the neck their output reflects vocal fold movement and the response of the body wall to the acoustic wave in the trachea. Figure 5-11 shows how much "cleaner" than the oral signal the output of the accelerometer is. Its harmonic content is obviously weaker, and it is also relatively free of articulatory influences, making it much more suitable for F_o extraction (Sugimoto and Hiki, 1962; Koike, 1973; Hencke, 1974a,b; Stevens, Kalikow, and Willemain, 1975; Askenfelt, Gauffin, Sundberg, and Kitzing, 1980).

The electroglottograph (Croatto and Ferrero, 1979; Fourcin, 1974; Fourcin and Abberton, 1972, 1976; Lecluse, Brocaar, and Verschuure, 1975) provides another alternative. The output of this device (discussed more fully in Chap. 6) represents the elec-

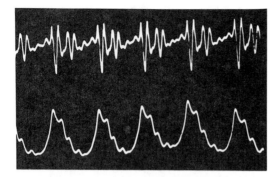

FIGURE 5-11. Simultaneous recordings of /ɑ/ as detected by an accelerometer placed over the trachea (lower trace) and an air microphone (upper trace). The accelerometer signal is relatively free of supraglottal resonance effects.

trical resistance across the larynx, a parameter which changes in a fairly predictable way during the phonatory cycle. Maximal resistance indicates vocal fold separation, while minimal resistance indicates vocal fold closure. There is considerable debate about the precise relationship between the electroglottograph signal and vocal fold behavior, but the periodicity of the fairly simple waveform accurately reflects that of the vocal folds. (Acoustic and electroglottographic waveforms are compared in Figure 5-12.) Although it may be difficult to get a clear electroglottographic trace in some subjects (particularly those with a thick fatty layer over the neck) if a signal can be obtained it represents an optimal choice for F_o measurement. Most electroglottographs therefore include circuitry that produces a voltage analog of the fundamental frequency for chart recording of the F_o pattern. Many also include some form of readout of the instantaneous F_o.

Askenfelt et al. (1980) compared the electroglottographic and accelerometric methods in normal adults and offered the following guidelines for choosing between them:

1. If a clear electroglottographic signal can be obtained from a patient this method should be used. The electroglottograph is even less influenced by articulatory activity than the accelerometer, but the anato-

my of the patient's neck may preclude a clear signal. Furthermore, the electroglottograph output may not accurately reflect F_o if the vocal folds do not contact each other during the glottal cycle (e.g., in cases of paralysis).

2. The accelerometer works on all subjects, but its output is occasionally confounded by articulatory events. It is also more sensitive to changes in vocal intensity than the electroglottograph is.

Therefore, Askenfelt and his colleagues recommend that

for practical use in the phoniatric clinic, it seems that the [electroglottograph] should be preferred as long as it works well, and it should be replaced by the contact microphone for remaining patients. If . . . it is considered important that the same method be used on a great number of subjects, the contact microphone would represent the best choice. (p. 272)

Clinicians will also want to consider the fact that accelerometers are very much less expensive than electroglottographs.

Photoglottography, in which the opening and closing of the glottis modulates a beam of light (Sonesson, 1960; Kitzing and Sonesson, 1974) also provides an electrical signal simple enough for reliable F_o determination (Vallancien, Gautheron, Pasternak, Guisez, and Paley, 1971; Coleman and Wendahl, 1968; Kitzing and Sonesson, 1974; Lisker, Abramson, Cooper, and Schvey, 1966). The technique (discussed more fully in Chap. 6) is somewhat invasive, and therefore is not the method of choice when F_o is the sole variable of interest. But in cases in which glottal activity is under observation, the clinician should bear in mind that the electrical output of the photodetector is more suitable for F_o determination than the vocal signal.

Modifying the Acoustic Signal

Techniques have been devised to modify the vocal signal so as to extract the glottal waveform, free of the effects of articulatory resonances. This can be done mathemat-

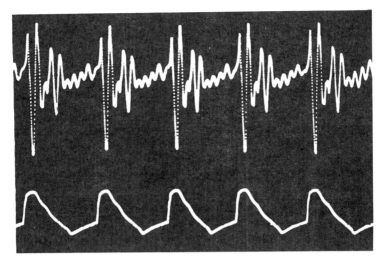

FIGURE 5-12. Electroglottogram (lower trace) and air-microphone (upper trace) records of sustained /ɑ/. The electroglottogram is essentially immune to vocal tract resonances.

ically (with a computer), but it can also be achieved with a special face mask system and filter (Rothenberg, 1973) or with a reflectionless tube fitted to the mouth (Sondhi, 1975). These methods (discussed more fully in Chap. 6) are more encumbering than most of the others considered thus far, but they yield signals of excellent quality for F_o extraction.

Spectrography

A sound spectrogram includes information about the fundamental frequency. Depending on the type of spectrographic display, the information appears in different forms. It is, however, always moderately easy to derive. (Sound spectrography is considered in detail in Chap. 9.)

When the resolving-filter bandwidth is large compared to the fundamental frequency, a "wide-band" spectrogram like the one shown in Figure 5-13 results. The vertical striations represent individual glottal openings. All that need be done to find the fundamental frequency is to count the number of vertical striations between two points along the time axis and divide the number of glottal pulses thus represented by the time-equivalent of the horizontal distance.

That is,

$$F_o = \text{No. of pulses} \div \text{duration of sample.}$$

This procedure has been applied to the spectrogram of Figure 13. In the marked-off interval (the vowel /ou/) there are 15 vertical striations; the interval represents 0.115 s. Therefore, $F_o = 20/0.115 \cong 130$ Hz. The same counting procedure can be applied to every voiced segment. An accurate timing signal is needed to determine the distance-to-time equivalence; the time markers of Figure 5-13 were generated by the spectrograph. A display of a 100 Hz square wave (which has a voltage transition every 0.05 s) would result in the same timing marks.

One caution must be kept in mind when determining F_o in this way: The value obtained is the *average* F_o for the time interval in question. Short-term changes in F_o are not detected. An average F_o is perfectly acceptable if the assumption that F_o is constant during the measurement period is a valid one, or if any shift in F_o during the measurement period is of no consequence.

A resolving filter with a narrow bandwidth generates a spectrogram that shows the vocal harmonics. Since these are at integral multiples of the fundamental frequency, change in the vocal F_o will always produce proportional change in the har-

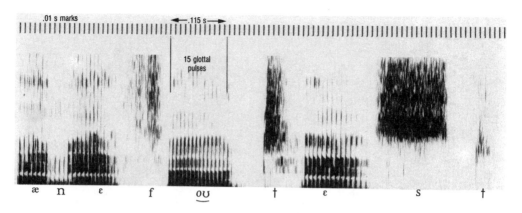

FIGURE 5-13. Sound spectrogram of the utterance "An eff-oh test." Fundamental frequency can be determined by counting the number of vertical striations in a segment and comparing the count to the segment's duration (which, in turn, can be determined from the 0.01 s timing marks at the top). In this case the /oʊ/ diphthong shows 15 glottal striations in 0.115 s. The fundamental frequency was thus 15/0.115 = 130.4 Hz.

monics, making it very easy to see the F_o contour. This can be particularly useful in detecting cyclic variations (tremulous voice) of the fundamental frequency (Lebrun, Devreux, Rousseau, and Dairmont, 1982). If the spectrograph has an adequate scale expander, the fundamental frequency can be read directly from the spectrogram, as in Figure 5-14. In the absence of scale expansion, direct reading is not possible. But because the harmonics bear a simple mathematical relationship to F_o, the fundamental frequency can almost always be determined easily. One need only find the frequency of the nth harmonic and divide it by n. Thus, if the fifth harmonic is at 500 Hz, the fundamental frequency must be 100 Hz.

If higher harmonics are not present, or if the harmonics are very closely spaced, there is a trick that will improve F_o determination. It involves finding the proportionality of the distance between the harmonics and a distance on the vertical axis whose frequency value is known. Figure 5-15 illustrates the technique to be used. Two distances are measured: A is the distance (in millimeters) between two calibrating lines, 2000 Hz apart; B s the distance from the bottom of one harmonic line to the bottom of any other harmonic line, also in millimeters. If n

is the number of harmonic lines traversed in taking measurement B, then the fundamental frequency is

$$F_o = (2000 \times B) \div (A \times n).$$

For the original of Figure 5-15 we have A = 41.5 mm., B = 8.5 mm., and n = 2 harmonic lines. Therefore,

$$F_o = (2000 \times 8.5) \div (41.5 \times 2)$$
$$= 17000/83$$
$$F_o = 204.8 \text{ Hz}.$$

Largely because the distance measurements have limited precision, the F_o calculated by this method is always somewhat approximate. (So are measurements determined from harmonic frequency.) With care, however, the approximation can be very good.

COMPUTER METHODS

The advent of the digital computer opened many new possibilities for fundamental frequency extraction. Some of the its potential has been exploited in implementing previously unheard-of ways of dealing with the vocal signal. The comb-filter method of pitch extraction, for example, was quite exotic until recently, but an application by

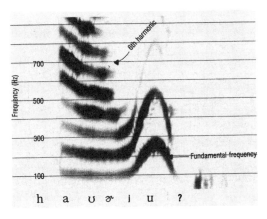

FIGURE 5-14. Narrow band (45 Hz) spectrogram of the utterance "How're you?" with a greatly expanded time scale. The frequency of any harmonic is an integral multiple of the fundamental frequency.

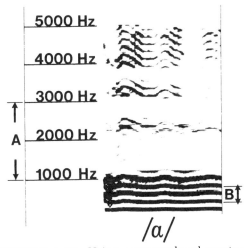

/ɑ/

FIGURE 5-15. Using a narrow band spectrogram to determine fundamental frequency of a sustained vowel. (See accompanying text for method.)

Martin (1981) has already been developed. Primarily, however, the computer has been used to perform formerly impractical analyses. The recent development of the ultra-miniature microcomputer has brought many of these possibilities to clinical facilities. It would be surprising if, in the next several years, computer-based methods were not being used for F_o measurement in many speech clinics.* While a full discussion of mathematical techniques for F_o extraction is well beyond the scope of this book, it may be useful to examine, at least in outline form, some of the ways in which the digital computer can be used for this task.

Analog-derived Methods

Some digital computer techniques are logically lineal descendents of analog electronic methods. That is, they developed out of concepts such as maximum-peak detection or zero-crossing counting. Some, in fact, could be done with analog circuitry (for example, Schroeder, 1968) but digital implementation is more reliable and, in many ways, easier.

*Microcomputers are already capable of implementing some F_o extraction algorithms, but they may not yet be quite good enough for reliable clinical service (Troughear, 1982).

An interesting example of the way in which the digital computer can greatly extend the reliability and validity of F_o determination is provided by Gold and Rabiner (1969). Their method (diagrammed in Figure 5-16) shows clear traces of its analog-analysis heritage, but takes excellent advantage of the unique capabilities of digital processing. The speech input is low-pass filtered to simplify the wave as much as possible. The filtered waveform is then evaluated by a signal-peak processor that converts the input to digital form and uses special algorithms (Gold, 1962) to identify all the waveform peaks. (Recall that there may be more than one set of peaks in each cycle.) The output of this processor is simultaneously applied to six different "estimators" that digitally evaluate the amplitudes of various peaks and troughs (in either absolute or relative terms, as compared to previous peaks). Each estimator uses these data in a different way. The six estimators therefore derive six independent "guesses" of the period. When their work is done, the computer surveys the results and selects the period value that has gotten the most "votes"—that is, the value that has the highest coincidence in the six outputs. This value, which has the greatest

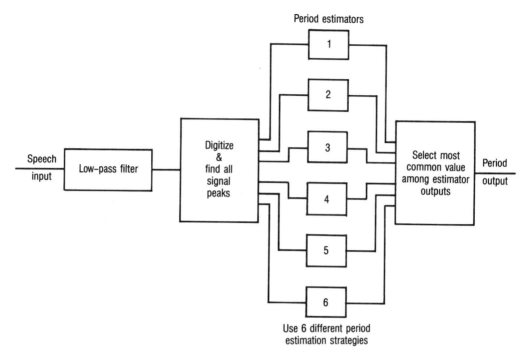

FIGURE 5-16. The period estimation technique of Gold and Rabiner (1969).

probability of being correct, is the final output. The process takes very little time and is repeated as long as a speech signal is present, producing a constantly updated report of F_o over time. The "majority vote" technique improves the validity of the ultimate F_o value reported, which is its prime advantage over those methods that rely on a single estimator. The procedure is fast, but it requires considerable computer capacity, a limitation that becomes less significant as computers mature.

Cepstrum

An extremely powerful method of extracting the fundamental frequency of a speech signal was originally described by Noll (1964). It relies on Fourier analysis of the speech signal and represents a departure from the evolutionary line of analog methods that would not be possible without the high-speed digital processor. The mathematical bases of this technique are, as might be expected, extraordinarily complex. A very cursory outline of what is

involved follows. More complete consideration of the technique (which has become moderately popular) can be found in Wakita (1976. 1977), in Randall and Hee (1981) and in a very clear presentation by Noll (1967).

The vocal signal radiated at the lips represents the characteristics of the glottal source and the action of the vocal tract resonances on the laryngeal pulsations. More formally stated, the voiced speech sound, denoted $f(t)$, is the convolution of a source signal, $s(t)$, and a tract response, $h(t)$. Symbolically,

$$f(t) = s(t)*h(t).$$

"Convolution" (designated by the *) implies an interaction of two sets of spectral properties. The spectrum is represented by the Fourier transform, denoted $\mathbf{F}$. Therefore,

$$\mathbf{F}\,[f(t)] = \mathbf{F}\,[s(t)] \times \mathbf{F}\,[h(t)].$$

That is, the spectrum of the voiced speech signal is the complex product* of the glot-

---

*The term "complex" is used here in its mathematical sense of having both real and imaginary parts.

tal source spectrum and the vocal tract transfer function.

The main problem is finding an efficient way of separating the source and transfer-function characteristics. Now, it is clear from elementary algebra that log(x·y) = log x + log y. Therefore, the logarithm of the spectrum of the vocal signal is equal to the sum of the logarithm of the source spectrum and the logarithm of the transfer function:

$$\log \mathbf{F}\ [f(t)] = \log \mathbf{F}\ [s(t)] + \log \mathbf{F}\ [h(t)].$$

The complex multiplication function is thereby replaced by a simpler additive one, greatly facilitating the ultimate separation of the two spectral responses.

The cepstrum method, flow-charted in Figure 5-17, begins by filtering out the highest frequency components of the speech signal. An analog-to-digital converter is then used to convert the amplitude of every point in the (still quite complex) wave to numerical values at a rate of perhaps 10,000 measurements per second. The wave is then represented by a string of numbers upon which all further operations are done.

The next step is to derive the spectrum of the waveform, that is to discover its frequency components and their amplitudes. Here a problem arises. Clearly, to do the necessary computation one needs to take a string of numbers that represents at least one complete cycle of the speech waveform. But it is not known how long a cycle is. (If the length of the cycle were known, then the frequency would be known, and there would be no need to do a cepstrum analysis!) One can be certain of getting at least one full cycle if a long enough string of numbers is considered. To be absolutely certain, it might be decided to deal with the digital string representing 40 ms of time. (A 40 ms period is equivalent to a frequency of only 25 Hz. Any voiced signal is almost certain to have a higher fundamental, and therefore a shorter period, than that.)

The long sample duration solves one problem but introduces a somewhat more subtle difficulty of its own, illustrated in Figure 5-18. The toptrace is a speech wave

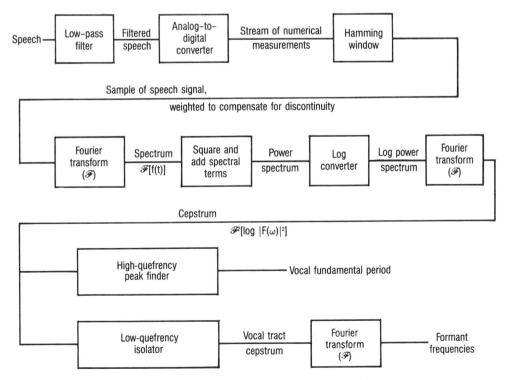

FIGURE 5-17. Flow chart of the cepstrum method of pitch extraction.

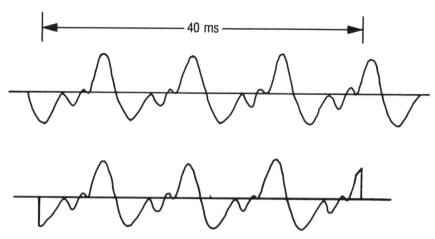

FIGURE 5-18. At the top, a speech wave with a fundamental frequency of about 90 Hz. A 40 ms sample of the wave (bottom) will have sharp discontinuities at either end. These appear to be impulse-like onset and offset phenomena to the computer, which does not "know" that they are a sampling artifact. (In actual practice, the waves are represented by strings of numbers.)

with a F_o of about 90 Hz. When a 40 ms sample of this wave is taken, the computer is given a wave like the one shown at the bottom of the figure. The fact that there is more than one complete cycle is no problem at all: The Fourier analysis takes account of that possibility. The "tags" of partial waves at either end of the sample are a thornier issue. We know that they are parts of waves; the computer does not. It "thinks" that the wave begins and ends at the baseline. The tags are seen as impulse-like onset and offset components. If the Fourier analysis is done using such a wave the spectrum of an impulse (an infinite series of lines spaced across the frequency axis) will be inextricably mixed into the actual spectrum of the real wave. To prevent this artifact, the sample of the digitized wave is put through the digital equivalent of a special filter called a "window" that adjusts the relative importance of terms so that the two ends contribute very little to the final analysis.

The result of processing to this point is a set of weighted measurements of the speech wave. These are now subjected to the Fourier transform to produce a series of real and imaginary terms that represent the frequency, amplitude, and phase relationships of the components of the origi-

nal wave. That is, the frequency spectrum is derived. These real and imaginary terms are squared and added to generate what is known as the "power spectrum" Finally, the logarithm of each of the power-spectrum terms is taken to derive the "logarithm power spectrum" upon which the rest of the analysis is based.

The usefulness of all of this processing becomes more intuitively clear when a logarithm power spectrum, such as the one in Figure 5-19, is examined. Notice that the spectrum is formed of a series of regularly spaced lobes. That is, the spectrum itself shows periodicity, and it turns out that the "period" of this pronounced "ripple" is the same as the period of the glottal pulses. The spectrum also has a lower-frequency (and less regular) undulation to it, emphasized in Figure 5-19 by the dashed line. This feature is due to the vocal tract resonances.

How can the two features of the logarithm power spectrum be separated? Since they represent the simple sum of two functions (rather than complex convolution) the matter is fairly easy. All that is necessary is to handle the logarithm power spectrum as if it were itself a waveform and apply a Fourier analysis to *it*. The Fourier transform of the logarithm power spectrum (formally known as the *inverse Fourier transform*)

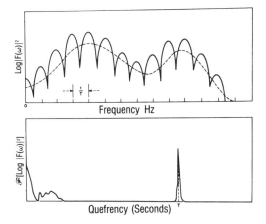

FIGURE 5-19. (A) The logarithm power spectrum of a voiced speech segments. (B) Cepstrum of the power spectrum. (From Noll, A. M. Cepstrum pitch determination. *Journal of the Acoustical Society of America*, 41 (1967) 293-309. Figure 3, p. 296. Reprinted by permission.)

is a new quantity and has been given the name *cepstrum* (a partial reversal of the word spectrum).* The horizontal scale has been assigned the designation *quefrency* to distinguish it from the frequency of a real-time function. Quefrency is measured in seconds and is therefore equivalent to period. Figure 5-19B is the cepstrum that results from a Fourier analysis of the logarithm power spectrum shown in Fig. 19A. The sharp, high-quefrency peak represents the period of the logarithm power spectrum, while the broad, low-quefrency peak represents the factors (vocal tract resonances) that produce the undulations. The fundamental period of the vocal signal is the quefrency peak in the cepstrum; the fundamental frequency is the reciprocal of the quefrency. Once the peak's location is determined (and the fundamental frequency thereby found) the computer can call for another sample of the speech input and repeat the process. The output of the computer is then a data series that shows the fundamental frequency of the speech signal over time.

*Technically the cepstrum results when the inverse Fourier transform is squared, an operation which serves to sharpen the cepstral peaks.

Although not directly relevant to the problem of F_o extraction, it is worth noting that the vocal tract resonance peaks (formants) can be derived from the broad, low-quefrency peak of the cepstrum. One simply treats the cepstrum as an ordinary waveform and subjects it to yet another Fourier analysis! The output of this third spectrum derivation has the unit frequency, and the curve that results is essentially that of the vocal tract transfer function.

The cepstrum method, then, provides a very effective way of deriving vocal F_o and evaluating vocal tract characteristics in a totally noninvasive way (Schafer and Rabiner, 1970). It does, however, require a very powerful computer. When first tried, a two-second sample required more than 45 minutes of computer time. But the creation of the Fast Fourier Transform (Cooley and Tukey, 1965) reduced this very considerably New computer circuit developments have resulted in extremely fast implementation, so that quasi-real time analysis is now possible on only moderately sophisticated computers.

Inverse Filtering

While the cepstrum procedure essentially side-steps the problems caused by convolution of the glottal source and vocal tract transfer characteristics, inverse-filtering methods (first proposed by Miller, 1959) attack these problems head on. It is possible, by very sophisticated techniques, to determine several properties of the vocal tract by mathematical analysis. Fundamental frequency extraction by inverse filtering takes advantage of these techniques in the following way, diagrammed in Figure 5-20.

As with cepstrum analysis, the assumption is made that the acoustic speech signal represents the product of the glottal resonances, vocal tract resonances, and lip radiation characteristics acting on the glottal wave (the pulsatile flow of air through the glottis, called the glottal volume velocity). If the effect of the nonlaryngeal acoustics could be determined, it would be

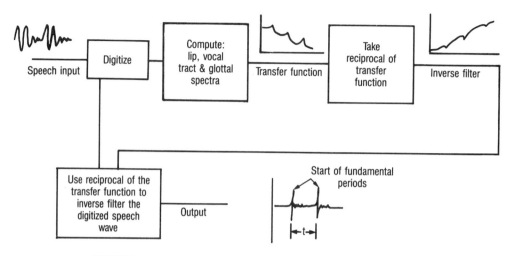

FIGURE 5-20. The general scheme of residue inverse filtering.

possible to subtract them from the radiated acoustic signal, restoring it to a "purer" or simpler form that is more representative of what the larynx itself produced. This, in fact, is what is done in inverse filtering.

First, the speech signal is digitized, and a sample is analyzed to determine the effects of the lip-radiation and vocal tract acoustics on the acoustic wave. In other words, the speaker's nonglottal resonance properties are determined and expressed as a transfer function. (This transfer function is of the kind that speech pathologist have studied in their beginning courses in acoustic phonetics.) The reciprocal of this transfer function is then calculated and is used as a filter through which the speech signal is passed. The result of this inverse-filtering is a relatively simple waveform, the remainder after the vocal tract and lip radiation characteristics are removed. If the process has been done correctly, that remainder could only be the glottal waveform. This form of inverse filtering is therefore called *glottal inverse filtering.*

It is possible to carry the process one step further. The glottal volume velocity wave (which is the exciter of the vocal tract) derives its form from the acoustic characteristics of the glottal space as they interact with pulsatile air bursts. It is possible to estimate the acoustic properties of the glottis and to compensate for them as well as for the vocal tract and lip radiation characteristics. The speech signal can then be filtered to remove essentially everything except for the abrupt pulses of air that are the purest form of vocal system excitation. This more complete filtering process is called *residue inverse filtering.* The residue is, in a sense, a very essence of voice—raw puffs of air with all of the influences of the vocal tract removed. (It is this form of inverse filtering that is schematized in Figure 5-20.) The residue signal has a very sharp pulse at the beginning of every pitch period. It is a fairly simple matter to measure the spacing of the pulses and thereby determine the fundamental frequency of the original signal.

Although residue inverse filtering seems more complicated than glottal inverse filtering (because an additional transfer function must be computed) it turns out, for mathematical and pragmatic reasons, to be somewhat easier to derive. Therefore, even though the residue signal does not directly represent a wave that is actually observable anywhere in the vocal tract, residue inverse filtering is the preferred method for clinical applications.

The conceptual simplicity of inverse filtering obscures the enormous complexity of implementation. More detailed descriptions of inverse filtering and the bases on which it rests are available in Miller (1959), Miller and Mathews (1963), Wakita (1976, 1977), and Davis (1976, 1979). The method is becoming increasingly popular because of its versatility: It evaluates a great many aspects of vocal tract function. Furthermore, Koike and Markel (1975) and Davis (1976) have shown that inverse filtering is a powerful detector of even slight laryngeal dysfunction. Computer programs that implement the method are now commercially available in the ILS® package from Signal Technology, Inc.

FUNDAMENTAL FREQUENCY MEASUREMENTS

A Note on Vocal Registers

Over the years, few issues have been quite so liable to provoke debate (often acrimonious) among the many kinds of vocal specialists as that of vocal registers. Disagreement has characterized almost every aspect of the discussion, and consensus has not yet been achieved on even the most basic points. What is a register? An acoustic attribute of voice? A purely perceptual phenomenon? A product of laryngeal function or of vocal tract characteristics? How many registers are there, and what should they be called? A measure of the confusion is presented by Mörner, Fransson, and Fant (1963) who managed to compile a list of over 100 terms used to describe voice registers. McGlone and Brown (1969) have shown that the cross-over point between different registers is not reliably perceived, a fact that adds to the confusion of categorization.

In a cogent discussion of the register problem, Hollien (1974) attempted to bring a degree of order to the prevailing conceptual and terminological confusion by proposing that a register be defined as a "totally laryngeal unit." That is, in his view a register is the reflection of a specific mode of laryngeal action, rather than of supraglottal resonances. Each register consists of "a

series or range of consecutively phonated frequencies which can be produced with nearly identical vocal quality (p. 125-126)." Ordinarily, adjacent registers have little F_o overlap.

The three registers that can be identified by these criteria have purposely been given new names in order to avoid confusion due to prior—and perhaps confused—usage. Hollien's recommended terminology is summarized below.

Modal register designates the range of fundamental frequencies most commonly used in speaking and singing. (The name is derived from the statistical "mode".) It may include the musical "chest" and "head", or "low," "mid," and "high" registers, depending on how these are defined.
Pulse register describes that phonatory range at the low end of the frequency scale in which the laryngeal output is perceived as pulsatile. (The pulse register has been described more fully in Hollien, Moore, Wendahl, and Michel, 1966; Hollien and Michel, 1968; and Hollien and Wendahl, 1968.) The term is essentially synonymous with "vocal fry," "glottal fry," and the musical "strohbass."
Loft register refers to those frequencies at the upper end of the vocal continuum. It generally corresponds to the older term "falsetto."

In the material that follows, this classification scheme will be used when considering registers.

General Considerations

The vocal fundamental frequency is reflective of the biomechanical characteristics of the vocal folds as they interact with subglottal pressure. The biomechanical properties are determined by laryngeal structure and applied muscle forces. Adjustment of the latter, in turn, is a function of reflexive, affective, and learned voluntary behaviors.

The vocal fundamental frequency provides insight into the adequacy of the interaction of all of those variables that "set" the vocal fold status.* The ability to vary the fundamental frequency demonstrates a great deal about the mechanical adequacy of larygeal structures and about the precision and extent of laryngeal control. The stability of phonatory adjustment is reflected in the amount of shortterm variability (perturbation) of the voice signal. The speech pathologist may therefore be interested in any of several aspects of the voice F_o. A number of different measurements that are likely to be useful are presented in this section.

Speaking Fundamental Frequency (SF_o)

There is an expectation that vocal pitch will be appropriate in some ill-defined way to a speaker's age and sex (Michel and Wendahl, 1971) and perhaps to body type, social situation, and emotional state as well. When the expectation is not realized, further investigation is needed. Evaluation of the fundamental frequencies actually used during speech will show whether a given speaker's vocal signal is really different in frequency from that of comparable speakers or whether the listener's perception of abnormality is based on other aspects of voicing.

Speech is not usually monotonous: The normal speaker uses a range of fundamental frequencies in linguistically prescribed patterns to indicate word and sentence stress, statement form, and affective content. Given this fact, two basic and general properties of the speaking fundamental frequency (SF_o) are of interest: average and variability.

Average SF_o denotes the "average" fundamental frequency value. It seems to be a clear enough term. But there are three different common measures that can, in differ-

ent senses, be considered to be "averages." They will be discussed with reference to the sample set of waveforms shown in Figure 5-21 and tabulated in Table 5-1. The speaker who provided the sample prolonged /a/ at low pitch.

1. Mean F_o is the sum of the frequency measurements divided by the number of waves measured. In other words, it is the parameter most people associate with the word "average." For the sample shown, the mean is

$$\bar{X}_{SF_o} = (f_1 + f_2 + \ldots + f_{24})/24 = 82.21 \text{ Hz}.$$

2. The median SF_o is the fundamental frequency value that marks the 50th percentile of the distribution. That is, half of all the values in the set are greater than the median, and half are smaller than the median. To find the median fundamental frequency for the sample, the individual wave measurements are listed in increasing (or decreasing) order. The number at the middle of the list is the median.* For the sample shown the median is at about 84 Hz.

3. The modal SF_o is the value that occurs most frequently in the list. It is, in other words, the most common entry. For the sample, the modal SF_o is 84.29 Hz.

At this point, the logical question is "If there are three different measures that can be considered to be "averages," which one should be used? The answer, of course, is "That depends . . .": first, on the way in which the values are spread out and second, on what one wants to know.

Irrespective of any other factors, the modal frequency has a certain advantage. By virtue of the fact that it is the most common frequency value in the sample, it is the closest objective approximation of "habitual pitch," considered to be an important speech characteristic by many voice therapists. If, however, the object is to iden-

---

*The importance of subglottal pressure change in the regulation of vocal fundamental frequency has been the subject of some debate (Ladefoged and McKinney, 1963; Lieberman, Knudson, and Mead, 1969) but it is not generally held to be a major contributor in normal speakers (Hixon, Klatt, and Mead, 1971; Shipp, Doherty, and Morrissey, 1979).

---

*If there are an even number of entries the median can be taken as the mean of the two center values. This method works for short lists of numbers, but it is very cumbersome when many waves have been tabulated. Any textbook of elementary statistics gives alternate, more efficient, ways of finding the median.

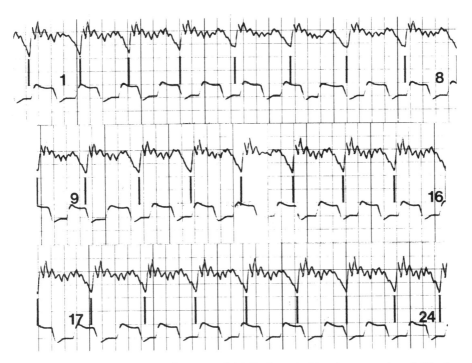

FIGURE 5-21. Pen-recorder output of sustained /ɑ/. Each period has been numbered. The lower (calibrating) wave has a frequency of 100 Hz.

tify a representative vocal fundamental frequency, a value that would represent the "basal" F_o level from which intonational pitch changes are launched, the choice is more difficult.

Whether the median or the mean is more representative depends on the distribution characteristics. Suppose that the frequency of occurrence of F_o values is graphed for two different samples, as in Figure 5-22. (Figure 5-22A is the for the sample shown in Figure 5-21.) In Figure 5-22A, all of the values are arranged with a fair amount of symmetry about a central, quite clearly modal, value. Visual inspection of this graph makes it clear that the median is like-

TABLE 5-1. Fundamental Frequency Values Derived from Figure 5-21

Period No.	Fundamental Frequency	Period No.	Fundamental Frequency
1	84.29	13	82.19
2	86.51	14	84.29
3	84.29	15	82.18
4	76.45	16	80.18
5	76.45	17	78.27
6	74.72	18	76.45
7	73.06	19	86.51
8	78.27	20	82.19
9	88.85	21	84.29
10	80.18	22	86.51
11	82.19	23	86.51
12	84.29	24	93.93

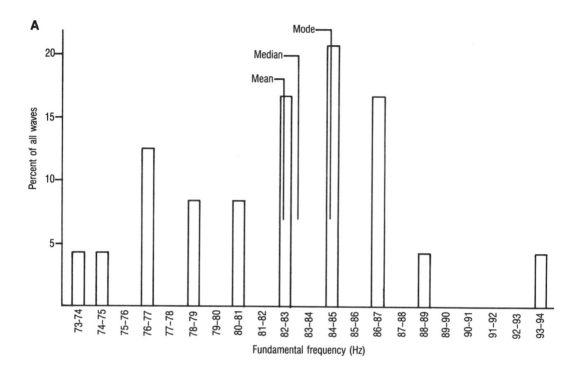

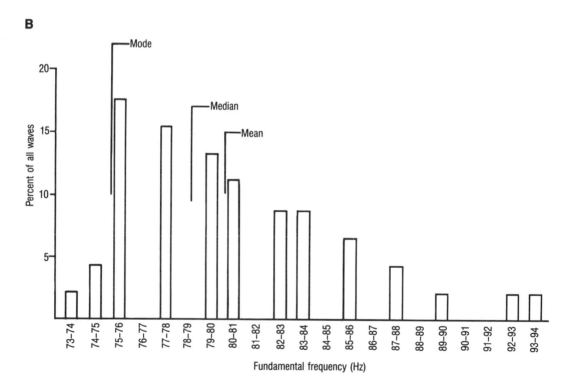

FIGURE 5-22. (A) Distribution of the measured fundamental frequencies in Figure 5-21 and Table 5-1. (B) Distribution of fundamental frequencies for another sample. This distribution is said to be "skewed to the right."

ly to be close to the mode. In this instance, where the distribution approaches what the statistician refers to as "normality," the mean is the best measure of the "average."

The situation is very different for the sample shown in Figure 5-22B, which is said to be *skewed*. The long "tail" to the right of the mode influences the mean and inflates its true value. In this case, the median is more representative of a typical value, and hence is a better "average."

As a general rule, all other things being equal, the mean is a good average value if the distribution is more or less symmetrical; the median is preferable if the distribution is markedly skewed. But in clinical work all other things are rarely equal, especially the all-important question of what the therapist needs to know. As in so many aspects of therapeutics, the decision will have to be made on the basis of the facts of the individual case.

SF$_o$ Variability. Normal speech requires variation in fundamental frequency. Too little or too much variability is undesirable. How may the degree of F_o variation be expressed?

One simple way is to state the SF$_o$ range, which is simply the difference between the highest and lowest F_os found in a sample. (It is common to express the range in semitones.) For the sample of Table 5-1, the range is 20.87 Hz or 4.35 ST. This gives some idea of variability, but it is based on the extremes and thereby may present an inaccurate picture. Notice, for example, that there is a single instance of a high-frequency (93.9 Hz) wave in the sample. It determines the upper limit of the range of observed fundamental frequencies, but it might well have been an accident, a momentary "slip of the larynx." In some ways it is unfair to include it in an estimate of variability; it distorts the overall picture of vocal function. (If it is omitted from the sample, the range diminishes to 3.39 ST.)

A better approach is to use a measure of the average distance of values from the mean as an index of variability. Such a measure, called the "standard deviation," exists. It is defined as the square root of the sum

of the squares of the deviations from the mean.* In algebraic form:

$$S.D. = \sqrt{\sum_{i=1}^{n} (\bar{x} - x_i)^2}$$

The standard deviation is a measure of dispersion that has been quite popular as an index of F_o variability. The symbol for the standard deviation is the Greek letter sigma (σ), and so the standard deviation of the fundamental frequency (often expressed in semitones) has usually been called *pitch sigma*.

By its very nature, pitch sigma is associated with the *mean F$_o$*. Particularly in cases where the median is used as the average, different measures of variability are needed. In these instances it is common to employ the 90% (sometimes 95%) range, which is defined as the frequency values above and below the average between which 90% (or 95%) of the observed frequencies fall. Curry (1940) called the 90% range the *effective range* and felt it to be the best variability measure.

Measuring SF$_o$

Determination of the speaking fundamental frequency requires an adequate speech sample. Two basic decisions about the speech task must be made: Should the patient read a standard test passage or speak spontaneously? How much material must be analyzed to assure a valid measure?

READING VERSUS SPONTANEOUS SPEECH. Using a reading task rather than spontaneous speech has a definite advantage: If the same material is always used it is possible to compare one patient to another. On the other hand, reading ability may affect re-

---

*The complication in getting the average distance is necessary and not due to the whim of statisticians. The square-root-of-the-squares overcomes the problem that the simple sum of the distances of all values from the mean must be zero. If the square root is not taken, the result is S.D.^{2}, which is known as the *variance*. Therefore, S.D. = $\sqrt{variance}$. Textbooks of statistics give more efficient ways of calculating the standard deviation than the one described here.

sults, especially in the case of children (Fairbanks, Wiley, and Lassman, 1949; Fairbanks, Herbert, and Hammond, 1949).

The question of whether the SF_o characteristics of material that is read are different from those of spontaneous speech is pivotal in selecting a sample method (Ramig and Ringel, 1983). Hollien and Jackson (1973), Saxman and Burk (1968), Mysak (1959), and Snidecor (1943) have done studies in which the same research subjects both read and spoke spontaneously. (Snidecor's subjects actually read verbatim transcripts of the extemporaneous speech they had delivered a week earlier.) All found that the mean SF_o during reading was slightly higher than the mean for spontaneous speech. The average differences ranged from 1.78 to 0.47 ST. No large differences were found in F_o variability. Given the small difference between the two tasks, it would seem more efficient to use a reading passage in instances where there is no clinical requirement for a special type of sample and where reading ability is not an issue. Since most research has been done with Fairbank's (1960) "Rainbow Passage" (see Appendix C) this is probably the material most clinicians will want to use.

SAMPLE SIZE. There is a trade-off between the length of the sample analyzed and the accuracy of the SF_o estimate obtained. Shorter samples mean less tedious measurement and easier analysis, but they reflect the actual values of the larger body of speech from which they are drawn less accurately. The problem is to find the shortest possible sample that yields an acceptably accurate measure.

Shipp (1967) cites an unpublished study by the Stanford Speech Research Laboratory that showed that SF_o measures of the second sentence of the Rainbow Passage correlated almost perfectly ($r = .99$) with the same measures of the entire first paragraph. Horii (1975) has done a more extensive investigation of the sampling problem and has come to the following conclusions:

1. For determination of mean SF_o, use of the second or fourth sentences extracted from a reading of the entire first paragraph of the Rainbow Passage is acceptable. This avoids any special effects associated with initial and final sentences and yields an estimate of tolerable accuracy.

2. If analysis of a fixed amount of time (rather than a certain number of linguistic units) is preferred, an accuracy of about ± 3 Hz will require analysis of about 14 s of speech.

3. Using the same sentence, rather than voice samples of equivalent duration, without respect to content, significantly reduces errors of mean SF_o estimates.

4. The low correlation between the SF_o variability of a single sentence and that of the entire passage indicates that significantly longer samples are needed to evaluate this parameter.

Expected Values of SF_o

The literature on SF_o is quite extensive. Vocal pitch is a very prominent feature of speech and has been explored in terms of emotion (Huttar, 1968; Fairbanks, 1940), mental disorder (Saxman and Burk, 1968; Chevrie-Muller, Dodart, Sequier-Dermer, and Salmon, 1971), overall voice quality and effectiveness (Michel, 1968; Snidecor, 1943, 1951), intellectual deficit (Montague, Brown, and Hollien, 1974; Montague, Hollien, Hollien, and Wold, 1978; Michel and Carney, 1964), laryngeal pathology (Murry, 1978), general systemic, neurologic, and endocrine disorders (Weinberg, Dexter, and Horii, 1975; Canter, 1965a; Vuorenkoski, Perheentupa, Vuorenkoski, Lenko, and Tjernlund, 1978), hearing impairment (Gilbert and Campbell, 1980; Boothroyd and Decker, 1972; Martony, 1968), and even sudden infant death syndrome (Colton and Steinschneider, 1980; 1981). It has also been the subject of numerous studies of average normal speakers from birth to old age. Comparability of these studies is often problematic because of differences in sample analysis methods, criteria for subject selection, and the like. This section presents summaries of findings in several categories that are likely to be useful to speech clinicians. Caution in drawing inferences from comparisons of the results of different studies is important.

AVERAGE SF_o—NORMAL ADULTS. Table 5-2 summarizes the findings of several studies that have explored the speaking fundamental frequency level of normal Caucasian adults. Fitch and Holbrook (1970) have provided good data on modal SF_o. They evaluated the "middle 55 words of the Rainbow Passage" as read by 100 men (age 18 to 25.2 years) and 100 women (age 17.75 to 23.5 years). Modal SF_o was determined with a special electronic device, the FLORIDA I. The resultant data, which may be considered normative for this age group, are given in Table 5-3.

The question of possible racial differences in SF_o has been addressed by several investigators. Hollien and Malcik (1962, 1967) and Hollien, Malcik, and Hollien (1965) have found a slightly lower SF_o in young black males as compared to their Caucasian counterparts. Hudson and Holbrook (1981, 1982) found that modal SF_o was somewhat lower for male and female blacks than for Caucasians, and the blacks also had a somewhat greater mean SF_o range. None of these differences, however, was large enough to be clinically meaningful.

AVERAGE SF_o—NORMAL CHILDREN. There have been a number of studies of the SF_o of children, the results of which are summarized in Table 5-4. Hollien and Malcik (1967), and Hollien, Malcik, and Hollien (1965) matched the experimental procedure of Curry (1940) in an attempt to determine the age of vocal maturation in boys. On the basis of their own data and those of comparable studies by others they concluded that vocal mutation

1. appears to occur at less than 14 years of age;
2. occurs at about the same age in Caucasian and black males;
3. is unrelated to climatic differences;
4. may be occurring earlier than in the past.

It should also be noted that SF_o is highly correlated with serum testosterone levels in male adolescents (Pedersen, Kitzing, Krabbe, and Heramb, 1982).

Cross-sectional studies are unfortunately inadequate for assessing vocal maturation. Addressing this problem, Bennett has undertaken a longitudinal study of a group of normal boys and girls, and has published SF_o data for them for ages 8 years 2 months through 11 years 2 months (Bennett, 1983). Her findings, summarized in Table 5-4B, show that SF_o is the same for boys and girls over the age range in question and that SF_o declines across the period. Bennett's study underscores the inadequacy of cross-sectional data for describing age-related changes in children's fundamental frequency.

NORMAL INFANT CRY. The cry of the infant has been the object of considerable research for quite some time (Flatau and Gutzmann, 1906). Two basic interests have motivated this work. First, there has been a persistent conviction that the infant's cry can provide the basis for very early diagnosis of abnormality. This rationale was best exemplified in the work of Karelitz and his associates (Karelitz and Fisichelli, 1962, 1969; Fisichelli, Karelitz, Eichbauer, and Rosenfeld, 1961; Karelitz, Fisichelli, Costa, Karelitz, and Rosenfeld, 1964; Fisichelli, Haber, Davis, and Karelitz, 1966) and in that of Michelsson and Wasz-Höckert (1980). Second, developmental specialists have been concerned with the way in which cry changes with maturation and with its relationship to the ultimate acquisition of speech (Prescott, 1975). A number of findings in this general area may be of interest to speech clinicians.*

The question of whether the infant's cry varies as a function of the provoking stimulus and whether listeners can categorize cries accordingly is a very old one. As opposed to some earlier work (Wasz-Höckert, Partanen, Vuorenkoski, Valanne, and Michelsson, 1964a, 1964b), recent research

---

*Extensive consideration of many aspects of infant cry is provided by Lind (1965) and by Wasz-Höckert, Lind, Vuorenkoski, Partanen, and Valanne (1968).

TABLE 5-2. Speaking Fundamental Frequency of Normal Caucasian Adults*

| Age | | No. of Subj. | Mean SF_o | | | Median SF_o | | S.D.† | Total Range | 90% Range | Source** |
Mean	Range		Hz	ST	Range	Hz	ST	ST	ST	ST	
				MALES							
Spontaneous speech											
"Adult"	—	25	120	34.6	—	—	—	2.64	16.84	—	1
20.3	17.9–25.8	157	123.3	—	90.5–165.2	—	—	3.2	—	—	2
47.9	32 –62	15	100.0	33.0	—	107.9	32.6	—	16.6	9.4	3
73.3	65 –79	12	119.3	34.4	—	120.1	34.3	—	17.0	9.6	3
85.0	80 –92	12	136.2	36.7	—	136.2	36.7	—	19.4	11.4	3
Reading											
"Adult"	—	25	132	36.3	—	129	36.0	3 3	19.78	—	1
"Adult"	—	6	—	—	—	132	36.5	—	—	—	6
Over 18	—	10	110.6	33.0	—	—	—	3.1	—	—	5
47.9	32 –62	15	113.2	33.4	—	110.3	32.9	—	16.79	9.5	3
54.1	26 –79	65	112.5	33.4	84 –151	110.7	33.1	2.41	—	7.95	8
18.1	17.8–18.5	6	—	—	—	137.1	36.8	3.58	—	—	4
20.3	17.9–25.8	157	129.4	35.8	—	—	—	3.2	—	—	2
24.4	20 –29	25	119.5	34.4	—	—	—	—	—	—	7
34.9	30 –39	25	112.2	33.3	—	—	—	—	—	—	7
45.4	40 –49	25	107.1	32.5	—	—	—	—	—	—	7
54.3	50 –59	25	118.4	34.3	—	—	—	—	—	—	7
64.6	60 –69	25	112.2	33.3	—	—	—	—	—	—	7
74.7	70 –79	25	132.1	36.2	—	—	—	—	—	—	7
85.0	80 –92	12	141.0	37.2	—	142.6	37.4	—	19.6	11.2	3
83.6	80 –89	25	146.3	37.9	—	—	—	—	—	—	7

FEMALES

Reading

		N	Mean (Hz)	SD		Range (Hz)								
		6	—				212	44.4	—	—		23.32	9.32	5
"Adult"														
"University students"														
24.6	20 –29	27	199.8	43.3	—	192.2–275.4	201.0	43.4	—	—	3.78	23.32	9.32	10
33.5	30 –40	21	224.3	45.3	—	171.4–221.75	—	—	—	—	2.46	—	—	13
44.4	40 –50	9	196.3	43.0	—	168.5–208.3	—	—	—	—	2.76	—	—	11
46.4	40 –49	9	188.6	42.3	—	189.8–272.9	—	—	—	—	4.00	—	—	11
54.5	—	21	220.8	45.1	—	176.4–241.2	—	—	—	—	4.33	—	—	18
65.8	60 –69	17	199.3	43.3	—	142.8–234.9	—	—	—	—	4.25	—	—	13
72.6	65 –79	15	199.7	43.3	—	154.5–264.6	—	—	—	—	2.96	19.12	9.42	13
75.4	over 70	10	196.6	43.0	—	170.0–248.6	—	—	—	—	4.70	—	—	13
85.0	80 –94	19	202.2	43.5	—	182.9–225.3	—	—	—	—	2.70	17.74	8.56	9
15.5	—	10	199.8	43.3	—	158.6–259.6	—	—	—	—	3.06	—	—	12
16.5	—	89	215.7	44.6	—	153.7–256.4	—	—	—	—	2.96	—	—	12
17.5	—	185	213.9	44.5	—	127.3–263.1	—	—	—	—	3.34	—	—	12
35.4	30 –39	193	211.5	44.3	—	181.0–240.6	—	—	—	—	3.92	—	—	13
		18	213.3	44.5	—		—	—	—	—		—	—	

**Sources:

1. Snidecor, 1943. Impromptu speech followed one week later by reading of verbatim transcript of impromptu statement. Subjects were classed as *superior* speakers by a panel of judges. Hand measurement of mid 23–27 s of samples. Data represent the mean of successive 0.038 s segments.

2. Hollien and Jackson, 1973. Reading of a passage by R. L. Stevenson, as well as extemporaneous speech—about 3 min of each. Analysis by the Fundamental Frequency Indicator (see text).

3. Mysak, 1959. Youngest group are sons of the other two groups. Reading first paragraph of the Rainbow Passage. Analysis by special electronic pitch meter.

4. Curry, 1940. Reading of a 52-word passage. Hand measurement of output. Data represent successive 0.038 s segment means.

5. Michel, 1968. Reading of Rainbow Passage. Analysis by the Fundamental Frequency Indicator (see text). Modal and pulse register studied in the same subjects.

6. Pronovost, 1942, and Snidecor, 1951. Reading of sentences 2–5 of the Rainbow Passage. Speakers were judged superior by a panel of judges. Hand measurement of output. Data represent means of successive 0.038 s intervals. Estimated error about 0.5%.

7. Hollien and Shipp, 1972, and Shipp and Hollien, 1969. Reading first paragraph of the Rainbow Passage. Analysis by the Fundamental Frequency Indicator (see text).

8. Horii, 1975. Reading of first paragraph of the Rainbow Passage. Analysis by a special computer program.

9. McGlone and Hollien, 1963. Reading of first paragraph of the Rainbow Passage, rehearsed. Hand measurement of oscillographic output.

10. Linke, 1973. Test passage unspecified. Subjects represented a range of speaker "effectiveness." Phonellegraphic analysis.

11. Saxman and Burk, 1967. Reading of the Rainbow Passage, rehearsed. Analysis by the Fundamental Frequency Indicator (see text).

12. Hollien and Paul, 1969, and Michel, Hollien, and Moore, 1966. Reading of the Rainbow Passage. Analysis by the Fundamental Frequency Indicator (see text). Note that 307 of the total of 467 subjects were high school cheerleaders, a fact that may have influenced the results.

13. Stoicheff, 1981. Reading of the first paragraph of the Rainbow Passage. Analysis by the Fundamental Frequency Indicator (see text). All subjects were nonsmokers. Older three age groups had significantly lower SF_o than the younger three groups.

*Data in the original sources are presented in semitones (ST) and in Hz. Necessary conversions have been done to present authors' data in both scales for the purposes of this table.
+"Pitch sigma."

155

TABLE 5-3. Modal Speaking Fundamental Frequency: Normal Adults

		SF_o			Range of Modes	
	Mean	Average	Modal	S.D.		
Sex	Age	(Hz)	(ST)*	(ST)	(Hz)	(ST)
Male	19.5	116.65	34.0	2.11	85–155	28.5–38.9
Female	19.5	217.00	44.8	1.70	165–255	40.0–47.5

From Fitch, J. L. and Holbroook, A. Modal fundamental frequency of young adults. *Archives of Otolaryngology,* 92 (1970) 379-382. Table 2, p. 381. Reprinted by permission.
*Computed from authors' data.

TABLE 5-4A. Speaking Fundamental Frequency of Normal Children

AGE		No. of	MEAN F_o*			S.D.†	
Mean	Range	Subj.	Hz	ST	Range	(ST)	Source**
BOYS							
Spontaneous Speech							
4.6		15	252.4	47.4	217.2–292.7		4
6.5		14	247.3	47.0	204.1–274.4		4
Reading							
7.0	6.8– 7.2	15	294	50.0		2.2	2
8.0	7.8– 8.1	15	297	50.2		2.0	2
10.0	9.8–10.2	6	269.7	48.7		2.38	3
14.2	13.9–14.3	6	241.5	46.8		3.40	3
11.2	10 –12	18	226.5	45.5	192.1–268.5	1.51	5
GIRLS							
Spontaneous speech							
5.5		18	247.6	47.0	211.9–295.2		4
6.4		19	247.0	47.0	217.7–274.1		4
Reading							
7.0	6.8– 7.2	15	281	49.2		2.0	1
7.9	7.8– 8.1	15	288	49.6		2.8	1
11.2	10 –12	18	237.5	46.32	198.1–271.1	1.51	5

*Data in original sources is given in either Hz or ST (semitones). Conversions have been done so as to present all data in both scales for the purposes of this table.
†"Pitch sigma."
**Sources:
  1. Fairbanks, Herbert, and Hammond, 1949. Simple 52-word passage embedded in a longer reading selection. Hand measurement of oscillographic readout.
  2. Fairbanks, Wiley, and Lassman, 1949. Same procedure as in note 1.
  3. Curry, 1940. Same procedure as in note 1.
  4. Weinberg and Zlatin, 1970, and Weinberg and Bennet, 1971. Thirty-second sample of elicited spontaneous speech. Compared to Down's syndrome children.
  5. Horii, 1983b. Normal 5th and 6th grade children reading the Rainbow Passage and the Zoo Passage of Fletcher (1971). Computer derivation of data.

TABLE 5-4B. Average SF_o: Development from Ages 8 to 11 (Longitudinal Study)*

Sex	Mean SF_o	S.D.	Range
	Mean age: 8 years 2 months		
Boys	234	19.76	204–270
Girls	235	12.31	221–258
Combined	234	16.88	204–270
	Mean age: 9 years 2 months		
Boys	226	16.42	198–263
Girls	222	8.25	209–236
Combined	224	13.65	198–263
	Mean age: 10 years 2 months		
Boys	224	14.68	208–259
Girls	228	9.37	215–239
Combined	226	12.76	208–259
	Mean age: 11 years 2 months		
Boys	216	15.04	195–259
Girls	221	13.43	200–244
Combined	218	14.57	195–259

From Bennet, S. A 3-year longitudinal study of school-aged children's fundamental frequencies. *Journal of Speech and Hearing Research,* 26 (1983) p. 138 (Table 1). © American Speech-Language-Hearing Association, Rockville, MD. Reprinted by permission.

*15 boys, mean age 8 years 3 months (S.D. 0.48 years) at start; and 10 girls, mean age 8 years 1 month (S.D. 0.41 years) at start. Repetition of "There is a sheet of paper in my coat pocket." Hand measurement of *all* voiced segments on oscillographic readout. Data for each subject is the average of mean frequencies in 50-ms segments.

has tended to cast doubt on the ability of adult listeners to differentiate types of infant cries with certainty, although mothers apparently can reliably judge whether an infant vocalization is a true cry or just "fussing" (Petrovich-Bartell, Cowan, and Morse, 1982). Nor, it seems, can adults reliably identify infant sex on the basis of the fundamental frequency of the cry (Murry, Hollien, and Muller, 1975; Muller, Hollien, and Murry, 1974). The data summarized in Table 5-5, taken from a study by Murry, Amundson, and Hollien (1977) were derived by hand measurement of oscillographic readouts of the first and third 15-s intervals of cry samples of at least 90 s duration. The "pain" stimulus was a rubber band snapped against the baby's foot, while startle was the result of a loud noise. Vocal response to witholding of food was labelled a "hunger" cry.

There is, in these data, a clear tendency

TABLE 5-5. Fundamental Frequency of Infant Distress Cries*

Subjects	Fundamental Frequency (Hz)		
	Pain†	Hunger†	Startle†
Males			
Mean	457.4	451.4	442.2
S.D. of means**	(59.2)	(47.4)	(41.1)
Females			
Mean	424.7	425.7	400.3
S.D. of means**	(47.1)	(52.6)	(24.5)
Overall	441.0	438.5	421.3

From Murry, T., Amundson, P., and Hollien, H. Acoustical characteristics of infant cries: fundamental frequency. *Journal of Child Language,* 4 (1977) 323 (Table 1). Reprinted by permission.

*Four male and 4 female infants. Age 3 months to 6 months. Method: see text.

†See definitions in text.

**Calculated from authors' data.

for males to cry with higher mean F_o than females, a finding in agreement with the results of Sheppard and Lane (1968) who studied two children, but not with those of Colton and Steinschneider (1980) who measured the cries of 66 normal infants. Pain also *seems* to elicit cries with higher F_o than other stimuli do. There is considerable overlap in the data, however. Some females had considerably higher cry fundamental frequencies than some males, and no stimulus condition produced *consistently* higher or lower F_os. The result of the data dispersion is that none of the observed tendencies is statistically significant.

Exploration of developmental changes in cry has been even less complete. Fairbanks (1942) did hand measurement of cry tracings of a single male infant over a period of nine months, but his finding of mean F_os as high as 814 Hz casts doubt on the validity of his methods. More recently Murry, Gracco, and Gracco (1979) have studied the cries of a single female infant from age 2 to 12 weeks. Their data for distress cries are summarized in Table 5-6 along with those of Prescott (1975). Hunger cries consistently had a higher mean F_o than discomfort cries, but no clear developmental trend is apparent.

Spontaneous (nondistress) vocalizations may be more analogous to adult speech than crying is and thus are perhaps of greater interest. They are also harder to study, since they are produced largely at the infant's "whim" and hence cannot be reliably elicited (Keating and Buhr, 1978). Mur-

TABLE 5-6A. Fundamental Frequency of Infant Distress Cries: Development*

Age	F_o (Hz) Mean	F_o (Hz) S.D.	Pitch sigma (Hz)
1–10 days	384	38	32
4–6 weeks	453	67	30†
6–8 weeks	495	53	53†
6–9 months	415	39	53

From Prescott, R. Infant cry sound; developmental features. *Journal of the Acoustical Society of America,* 57 (1975) 1186-1191. Data extracted from Table 1, p. 1189. Reprinted by permission.

*Normal infants, sex unspecified. Spontaneous cries, cause undetermined. Recording in child's normal environment.

†Significantly different (p < .05) and not related to cry duration.

ry, Gracco, and Gracco (1979) evaluated the nondistress (pleasure) vocalizations of the same infant evaluated in Table 5-6 from the age of 8 to 12 weeks. Mean F_o for these sounds was 355.8 Hz—almost exactly the same as that of the child's discomfort cries at the same ages. The average F_o range was considerably smaller, however.

Laufer and Horii (1977) have done a somewhat more extensive exploration of nondistress vocalizations. In a longitudinal study of normal infants (2 males and 2 females) they measured the F_o of utterances of more than 200 ms duration, often resulting from interactions with adults, produced under quasi-naturalistic conditions. Table 5-7A summarizes their findings.

TABLE 5-6B. Fundamental Frequency of Infant Distress Cries: Development in a Single Child*

Age (wks)	Mean F_o (Hz)	Hunger† (Range) (Hz)	Hunger† (Range) (ST)	Pitch sigma (Hz)	Mean F_o (Hz)	Discomfort** (Range) (Hz)	Discomfort** (Range) (ST)	Pitch sigma (Hz)
2	396.5	110–700	32.0	79.9	372.6	80–620	35.5	74.1
4	403.8	80–700	37.6	107.7	341.9	80–680	37.0	115.7
6	449.1	180–740	24.5	80.2	346.7	60–600	39.9	93.1
8	341.3	80–740	38.5	106.9	340.4	40–620	47.4	104.7
10	417.8	100–680	33.2	90.8	380.6	110–560	28.2	88.0
12	427.9	90–680	35.0	93.4	—	—	—	—
Mean	406.1	106.7–706.7	33.5		356.5	74.0–616.0	37.6	
S.D. (Hz)	36.8	37.8–27.3			18.8	26.1–43.4		

From Murry, T., Gracco, V. L., and Gracco, L. C. Infant vocalization during the first twelve weeks. Paper presented at the annual convention of the ASHA, 1979. Also from Murry, T., Hoit-Dalgaard, J. and Gracco, V. Infant vocalization: A longitudinal study of acoustic and temporal parameters. *Folia Phoniatrica,* 35 (1983) 245-253. Reprinted by permission.

*One female infant. Measurement of oscillographic output.

†Food withheld after feeding begun.

**Soiled diaper.

TABLE 5-7A. Fundamental Frequency of Non-Distress Vocalizations by Normal Infants (1−2 weeks)*

Age (weeks)		Average F_o				
		Mean F_o (Hz)	Median F_o (Hz)	Modal F_o (Hz)	S.D. Hz	S.D. ST
1−4	Mean	317	319	329	38.8	2.24
	S.D.	38.2	38.2	48.0	15.2	0.95
5−8	Mean	338	338	344	27.7	1.40
	S.D.	40.8	39.9	43.3	13.5	0.66
9−12	Mean	338	337	346	31.2	1.63
	S.D.	40.1	40.9	43.6	15.2	0.79
13−16	Mean	339	341	346	30.4	1.57
	S.D.	41.7	41.6	44.8	15.5	0.71
17−20	Mean	337	339	349	33.3	1.74
	S.D.	43.3	43.8	50.4	14.5	0.75
21−24	Mean	342	341	356	37.8	1.94
	S.D.	51.5	53.8	62.5	18.0	0.84

Mean Lowest, Mean Highest, and Mean Range
of Fundamental Frequencies within Utterances

Age (weeks)		Mean Lowest (Hz)	Mean Highest (Hz)	Mean 5th%ile (Hz)	Mean 95th%ile (Hz)	Mean 5−95th%ile (Range in ST)
1−4	Mean	217	412	251	372	6.89
	S.D.	62.2	75.9	49.0	54.0	3.15
5−8	Mean	268	408	294	381	4.34
	S.D.	50.0	69.8	40.5	58.5	2.15
9−12	Mean	247	410	285	382	5.07
	S.D.	52.7	63.3	43.6	53.7	2.58
13−16	Mean	252	413	286	283	4.94
	S.D.	48.4	72.9	41.4	56.7	2.34
17−20	Mean	239	423	281	383	5.33
	S.D.	49.7	76.2	44.5	55.8	2.45

From Laufer, M. Z. and Horii, Y. Fundamental frequency characteristics of infant non-distress vocalizations during the first 24 weeks. *Journal of Child Language*, 4 (1977) 171-184. Table 1, p. 175. Reprinted by permission.

Authors cautioned that "individual variation in each of the measures was obscured when averaged as mean data."

*Longitudinal study, 2 male and 2 female normal infants. Spontaneous (sometimes elicited) vocalizations in a quasi-normal environment. Analysis by special computer program.

TABLE 5-7B. Fundamental Frequency of Non-Distress Vocalizations by Normal Infants (11–25 months)*

Age (months)	No. in Group	Mean (Hz)	Range (Hz)	S.D. (Hz)
11–13	2	400	366–435	187
14–16	4	378	305–537	154
17–19	3	363	320–407	68
20–22	2	328	310–362	50
23–25	3	314	269–364	60

From Robb, M. P. and Saxman, J. H. Developmental trends in vocal fundamental frequency of young children. *Journal of Speech and Hearing Research*, 28 (1985) 421-427. Table 4, p. 425. © American Speech-Language Hearing Association, Rockville, MD. Reprinted by permission.

*7 boys, 7 girls. Spontaneous utterances during play. Narrow-band spectrographic measurement. > 70 utterances per child.

There is little variation in average F_o during the period of the study. The average standard deviation of the F_o (pitch sigma), on the other hand, dropped to a low in the 5 to 8 week interval and then tended to increase with age. The mean data obscure individual variations in development that may well be meaningful: Different infants did, in fact, show different patterns of age-related change. This fact underscores the need for caution in dealing with developmental data on young infants. Each one tends to be unique in many ways, and meaningful differences in vocalization can be observed as early as the perinatal period (Ringel and Kluppel, 1964).

Information about the fundamental frequency of utterances during the early stages of language development is provided by the results of Robb and Saxman (1985). They used narrow-band spectrograms (see Chap. 9) to determine the F_o of the vowel segments of at least 70 utterances (spontaneously produced during play with the parents and an examiner) by each child. The data are tabulated in Table 5-7B. There is a clear tendency for fundamental frequency to lower with age, although the high intersubject variability prevented this trend

from reaching statistical significance. The age-related decrease in F_o variability, however, was statistically significant.

MENTAL RETARDATION. There is a considerable body of opinion to the effect that retarded individuals have unusual voices, but there is only a little evidence to support the conclusion that F_o is a distinguishing feature. Neelley, Edison, and Carlile (1968) found that, on the average, a mixed group of retarded young adults had average SF_os 2.7 ST higher than a comparable group of normal speakers, but this small difference is unlikely to be the basis of a perceptual difference.

The vocal characteristics of children with Down's syndrome have perhaps been investigated more fully than those of any other form of mental retardation. Although Benda (1949), for instance, claimed that the low-pitched voices of these children were so typical as to permit diagnosis of the disorder, more recent research has clearly indicated that this is not likely to be due to differences in F_o. Weinberg and Zlatin (1970) found that *higher* SF_o and somewhat greater F_o variability characterized the spontaneous speech of trisomy-21 boys and girls (age 5½ to 6½ years). Michel and Carney (1964), Hollien and Copeland (1965) and Pentz and Gilbert (1983) all failed to find any meaningful differences between the SF_os of mongoloid boys or girls and normals. Montague, Brown, and Hollien (1974) and Montague, Hollien, Hollien, and Wold (1978) have determined that, although the perceived pitch of Down's syndrome children is lower than that of normal children, the actual F_os of the two groups are not meaningfully different. The perception, it was felt, may be due to vocal resonance phenomena. This contention has some support in the research literature (Fisichelli and Karelitz, 1966).

LARYNGEAL PATHOLOGY. Most disorders of the larynx do not, in and of themselves, appear to have a significant influence on the mean SF_o. On the other hand, F_o variability and range do seem to reflect tissue changes, at least in the case of some pathologies. Hecker and Kreul (1971), for example, found that patients with laryngeal cancer had a restricted SF_o range during reading of the second sentence of the Rainbow Passage. They also showed a smaller rate of change of the fundamental frequency. Murry (1978) studied patients with different laryngeal disorders. His data (summarized in Table 5-8) showed that only the standard deviation and range of the SF_o of men with unilateral vocal fold paralysis were different from normal. (His data did tend to support Hecker and Kreul's finding of reduced SF_o range in cases of cancer, however.) Murry was led to conclude that "organically based voice disorders are not characterized by a $[SF_o]$ that is lower than that found in normal voices (p. 378)." Laguaite and Waldrop (1964) and Hufnagle and Hufnagle (1984) have found that fundamental frequency of dysphonic patients does not change significantly as a result of therapy. Vocal fold edema may represent an exception to the general rule. Fritzell, Sundberg and Strange-Ebbesen (1982) found that some women with confirmed edema have

SF_os considerably lower than expected. Further, the SF_o of all their patients rose significantly following surgical stripping of the vocal folds.

STUTTERERS. It is becoming increasingly clear that the fluent speech of stutterers differs from that of normal speakers. An investigation by Healey (1982) measured the F_o characteristics of declarative and interrogative sentences as spoken by adult stutterers and nonstutterers (see Table 5-9). Stutterers had a significantly lower pitch sigma and used a more restricted pitch range. This finding is consistent with the results of earlier work by Travis (1927), Bryngelson (1932), and Schilling and Göler (1961) and argues for a view of stuttering as a problem that extends beyond simple dysfluency.

ESOPHAGEAL PSEUDOPHONATION. Unusual vocal pitch is commonly a hallmark of esophageal voice and is often the object of attempts at therapeutic modification. The data summarized in Table 5-10 provide guidelines of what can be expected of the laryngectomized speaker.*

The relationship between SF_o of esophageal pseudophonation and voice acceptability has been explored by Shipp (1967) who had a very large group of naive listeners rate tape recordings of 33 male esophageal speakers for general speech acceptability. He then compared those with above average ratings to those who were deemed less adequate, and contrasted the six best speakers to the rest. SF_o data were generated by wave-by-wave analysis of the second sentence of the Rainbow Passage. Pitch sigma and the 90% SF_o range had no significant correlation with rated speech acceptability. The relationship of mean SF_o was significant ($p < .05$), but the correlation, at $r = -.35$, was not very strong. It was clear from Shipp's analysis that respiratory noise, duration of the sentence, and percent peri-

TABLE 5-8. Speaking Fundamental Frequency: Laryngeal Pathology*

Group	Mean SF_o (Hz)	SD of SF_o (ST)	Range of SF_o (ST)
Normal	121.9	4.63	10.60
Paralysis	127.0	3.64†	7.55†
Benign mass	133.0	4.34	10.55
Cancer	133.3	3.89	9.04

From Murry, T. Speaking fundamental frequency characteristics associated with voice pathologies. *Journal of Speech and Hearing Disorders*, 43 (1978) 374-379. Table 2, p. 376. © American Speech-Language-Hearing Association, Rockville, MD. Reprinted by permission.

*80 males: 20 normal (mean age 52.5 years; S.D. 11.9); 20 unilateral paralysis (mean age 53.0 years; S.D. 11.35); 20 benign mass (mean age 57.6 years; S.D. 10.05); 20 laryngeal cancer (mean age 60.7 years; S.D. 8.74). Measurement of oscillographic readout of third sentence of Rainbow Passage, extracted from a reading of the entire selection.

†Significantly different from normals.

*Some data for patients with surgically constructed neoglottises are now becoming available. See, for example, Robbins, Fisher, and Logemann (1982).

TABLE 5-9. Variability of the Speaking Fundamental Frequency: Stutterers*

Statistic	Declarative		Interrogative	
	Stutterers	**Normals**	**Stutterers**	**Normals**
Mean SF_o (Hz)	105.65	107.69	113.79	119.25
S.D. of SF_o (ST)	1.35	1.74	1.59	3.19
(pitch sigma)				
Range of SF_o (ST)	5.24	7.28	4.88	8.80

From Healey, E. C. Speaking fundamental frequency characteristics of stutterers and nonstutterers. *Journal of Communication Disorders*, 15 (1982) 21-29. Table 1, p. 27. Copyright 1982 by Elsevier Science Publishing Co., Inc. Reprinted by permission.

Pitch sigma and SF_o range differences between normals and stutterers are significant ($p < .05$).

*10 male stutterers, age 16–52 (mean age 29). 10 normal males, matched to stutterers for age and mean SF_o. Two all-voiced phrases (declarative and interrogative) embedded in a carrier. Hand measurements of oscillographic readout. Only fluent productions analyzed.

odic phonation were more important to the judges.

Esophageal speakers, then, can be expected to have a SF_o about one octave below that of normal speakers (Kyttä, 1964) with variability (in ST) comparable to normal adults. The perceived lack of variability of esophageal pitch probably lies in the nonlinearity of pitch perception at very low frequencies (Stevens and Volkmann, 1940), which has the effect of requiring more F_o change per unit change in pitch. (Clinically significant aspects of the physiology of esophageal pitch variation are considered by van den Berg and Moolenaar-Bijl, 1959).

PULSE REGISTER VERSUS "HARSH" VOICE. It has been shown (Michel and Hollien, 1968) that the "harsh" quality that characterizes some vocal disorders is perceptually distinct from pulse register (vocal fry). The basis for the perception was explored by Michel (1968). Ten normal adult male speakers read the Rainbow Passage using their customary voices and then using continuous pulse register. Another group of ten men whose voices had been judged clinically "harsh" read the same material. SF_o was measured with a phonellograph (pulse register samples) or with the Fundamental Frequency Indicator (normal and harsh voices). Results are summarized in Table 5-11.

It is obvious that pulse register had a much lower mean SF_o than did harsh voic-

es. The measures of variability failed to discriminate between harsh and pulse register voices, although there was considerably greater heterogeneity of the total range of harsh-voice speakers than of pulse-register users. It seems clear that perceptual differentiation of harsh vocal quality from normal pulse register phonation depends heavily on a SF_o discrimination.

Maximum Phonational Frequency Range

Measures of SF_o provide information about how a speaker uses his voice. The *maximum phonational frequency range* (MPFR) says something about his basic vocal ability. It is also likely that the MPFR reflects the physical condition of the phonatory mechanism. Michel and Wendahl (1971, p. 470) are of the opinion that "during speech utilizing a normal phonational mechanism, a certain degree of variability in frequency is expected and indeed deemed necessary. The extent to which the mechanism does not or cannot produce a range of frequencies may be the first indication of non-normal function." "Does not" is in the province of the SF_o; "cannot" may be assessed by the MPFR.

The MPFR may be defined (Hollien, Dew, and Philips, 1971, p. 755) as "that range of vocal frequencies encompassing both the modal and falsetto registers; its extent is from the lowest tone sustainable in the modal register to the highest in falsetto,

TABLE 5-10. Speaking Fundamental Frequency: Esophageal Pseudophonation

No.	Mean SF_o Hz (ST)	Mean SF_o (Range)	S.D. of SF_o Mean Hz (ST)	S.D. of SF_o (Range)	Mean Highest SF_o Hz (ST)	Mean Highest SF_o Range	Mean Lowest SF_o Hz (ST)	Mean Lowest SF_o Range	Source*
Men									
22	65.59 (24.0)	42.92–85.81 (16.7 –28.7)	14.66	7.79–25.00					1
18	57.4 (21.74)		(4.15)						2
6	63.0 (23.2)	50.9 –76.7 (19.4 –26.8)			115.3 (33.7)	95.2–135.5 (30.4–36.6)	25.3 (8.3)	17.2–32.2 (8.0–11.8)	3
15	65.7 (24.1)		(4.12)						4
10	64.6	56.0–104.0							5
15	77.1		22.5		F_o range = 118.1 Hz				6
Women									
15	86.65 (28.87)		(3.94)						2

*Sources:

1. Hoops and Noll, 1969. First paragraph of the Rainbow Passage. Measurement of oscillogram.
2. Weinberg and Bennet, 1971, 1972. Second sentence of Rainbow Passage. Measurement of oscillogram. Poor speakers excluded. Male/female differences are significant ($p < .01$).
3. Curry and Snidecor, 1961; Snidecor and Curry, 1959; Curry, 1962. Six superior speakers. Rainbow passage. Measurement of oscillogram.
4. Torgerson and Martin, 1980. Second sentence of Rainbow Passage. Poor speakers excluded. Measurement of oscillogram. Data are derived from averages of successive 50 ms intervals. Comparison to non-laryngectomee esophageal speakers.
5. Blood, 1984. Second sentence of Rainbow Passage. SF_o derived from contiguous samples by Kay Visi-Pitch.
6. Robbins, Fisher, Blom, and Singer, 1984. Second sentence of Rainbow Passage. Wave-by-wave measurement with interactive computer system.

TABLE 5-11. Speaking Fundamental
Frequency: Pulse Register
and "Harsh" Voices*

Sample	Mean SF_o (Hz)	S.D. of SF_o (ST)	Total Range (ST)	90% Range (ST)
Normal	110.6	3.1		
Pulse				
Mean	36.4†	4.4	25.6	13.5
SD		(0.81)	(2.1)	(2.2)
"Harsh"				
Mean	122.1	3.3	25.6	11.8
SD		(0.86)	(6.4)	(3.9)

From Michel, J. F. Fundamental frequency investigation of vocal fry and harshness. *Journal of Speech
and Hearing Research*, 11 (1968) 590-594. Table 1, p.
593. © American Speech-Language-Hearing Association, Rockville, MD. Reprinted by permission.

*See text for method.

†Mean SF_o of pulse register is significantly different (p < .01) from harsh or normal. Normal and harsh
SF_os are not significantly different from each other.

inclusive." Modal and loft (falsetto) are
both included in the range because of the
difficulty of reliably differentiating them
perceptually. Pulse register is excluded
because it is not normally used continuously for running speech.

Measurement Technique

The MPFR is usually determined using
a pitch-matching procedure. The patient is
asked to sustain a vowel (usually /a/) at the
same pitch as a stimulus tone presented
through an earphone. (A sine-wave oscillator is commonly used to generate the
stimuli.) Beginning at a comfortable fundamental frequency the stimuli are lowered
in pitch (perhaps in 2 ST steps) until the
patient can no longer sustain modal register phonation. Stimulus frequency then
ascends from the comfortable level until loft
register phonation is unsustainable. The
patient's phonations are tape recorded and
later analyzed by any of the F_o-extraction
techniques discussed earlier. Neither the
musical quality of the phonation nor the
accuracy of the pitch match are criteria for
trial acceptability.

Expected Results

NORMAL SPEAKERS. Table 5-12 summarizes the findings of several comparable
studies of the MPFR of normal adults. While
men do not differ from women in the extent of their ranges, it is clear that the older speakers' ranges are restricted by reduced
ability to achieve high vocal F_o. Recently,
Ramig and Ringel (1983) have studied men
in three age groups—25 to 35, 45 to 55,
and 65 to 78. Eight members of each group
were in good physical condition, as estimated by resting heart rate, diastolic and
systolic blood pressure, and forced vital
capacity. The other eight men in each group
were in relatively poor physical condition,
as judged by the same measures. The groups
were not significantly different in terms of
highest or lowest sustainable F_o. Age did
not significantly affect MPFR (which was
measured somewhat differently from the
other studies summarized in Table 5-12),
but physical condition *was* a significant factor. Subjects in good physical condition had
larger phonational ranges than those in
poor condition. It is therefore conceivable
(but not yet proven) that biological aging
(physical condition) is a much more powerful restrictor of MPFR than simple chron-
ological age.

An interesting study by Fishman and
Shipp (1970) evaluated the effect of subject posture on MPFR. Range was determined for each of fifteen males, ages 21 to
33, in standing and supine positions. Data
were derived from a 10 ms segment of each
vowel prolongation. The results (Table
5-13) showed that both upper and lower
fundamental frequency limits are reduced
in the supine position, with a consequent
reduction in the MPFR. Although the difference in the two ranges was statistically
significant (p < .05), it was quite small, sug-
gesting that "unless the absolute limits of
the frequency range are of critical importance, valid vocal range data can be obtained from untrained naive subjects in the
supine position" (Fishman and Shipp,
1970, p. 432). The clinician need not be

TABLE 5-12. Maximum Phonational Frequency Range

Age Mean	Age Range	No. of Subj.	Lowest F_o* Mean	Lowest F_o* Range	Highest F_o* Mean	Highest F_o* Range	MPFR* Mean	MPFR* Range	Note
MEN									
20.3	17.9–25.8	157	79.5 /27.4/	62.0–110.0 /23.1– 33.0/	763.6 /66.5/	392.0–1568.0 /55.0– 79.0/	684.1 /38.8/	/29–54/	3
21.4	18 –36	332	80.1 /27.5/	61.7–123.5 /23 – 35/	674.6 /64.4/	220.0–1567.8 /45 – 79/	594.5 /37.9/	/13–55/	1
Young adult		14	87 /28.9/	69 –110 /24.9– 33.0/	571 /61.5/	440 – 698 /57.0– 65.0/	484 /32.4/	/29–36/	4
27.6	18 –39	31	77.3 /26.9/	—	567.3 /61.4/	—	490 /34.5/	—	2
76.9	68 –89	27	85.3 /28.6/	—	394.2 /55.1/	—	308.9 /26.5/	—	2
56.8†	35.5–75.0	17	80† /27.5†/	40 –120 /15.5– 34.5/	260.0† /47.9†/	190 – 440 /42.5– 57.0/	/22.1†/	/ 8–36/	5
WOMEN									
22.8	18 –36	202	140.2 /37.2/	98 –196 /31 – 43/	1121.5 /73.2/	587.3–2092.8 /62.0– 84.0/	981.3 /37.0/	/23–50/	1
23.5	18 –38	31	134.6 /36.5/	—	895.3 /69.3/	—	760.7 /32.8/	—	2
76.9	66 –93	36	133.8 /36.4/	—	570.6 /61.5/	—	436.8 /25.1/	—	2

Sources:

1. Hollien, Dew, and Philips, 1971.
2. Ptacek, Sander, Maloney, and Jackson, 1966.
3. Hollien and Jackson, 1973. "Extreme intersubject variability." SF_o data are also available for these subjects.
4. Shipp and McGlone, 1971.
5. Canter, 1965A. Research compared normals to Parkinsonian patients.
Data have been converted from Hz to ST, or vice versa, as required.
*Data within slashes (/) are in ST, others in Hz.
†Medians.

overly concerned about patient posture during testing.

PARKINSON'S DISEASE. Canter's (1965a, b) study of the speech of Parkinsonian patients demonstrates the effect that neuropathology may have on laryngeal adjustment capabilities. The data of Table 5-14 show a highly noticeable and statistically significant ($p < .01$) difference in the median lowest frequency attainable by the two groups; highest F_os do not differ significantly, however. The MPFR is accordingly reduced in Parkinson's patients. The inability to achieve a very low F_o is consistent with the increased muscle tone that is characteristic of Parkinson's disease. Other neuropathologies may well influence the MPFR in ways that are consistent with their particular effects on the neuromotor system.

PULSE AND LOFT REGISTERS. Pulse register is, by definition, excluded in the determination of the MPFR; loft register, however, is considered. The limits of F_o adjustment of these registers have been determined separately, however. The data are summarized in Table 5-15, along with findings for the modal register alone.

FREQUENCY PERTURBATION (JITTER)

Definition and Significance

While the MPFR assesses certain aspects of the limits of laryngeal adjustments, and SF_o measures how those adjustments are used in running speech, the degree of frequency perturbation provides an index of the stability of the phonatory system.

Frequency (or *period*) *perturbation*, commonly called *jitter*, is the variability of the fundamental frequency or, reciprocally, of the fundamental period. When measured during running speech, variability is reflected in pitch sigma. Jitter measurements, however, are concerned with *short-term* variation. That is, jitter is a measurement of how much a given period differs from

TABLE 5-13. Maximum Phonational Frequency Range: Effect of Posture*

	Standing		Supine	
	Mean Hz	**Mean†**	**Mean Hz**	**Mean†**
Highest F_o	639.8	63.5	629.1	63.2
Lowest F_o	81.1	27.7	84.2	28.4
MPFR	558.7	35.7	544.9	34.8

From Fishman, B. and Shipp, T. Subject positioning and phonation range measures. *Journal of the Acoustical Society of America*, 48 (1970) 431-432. Table 1, p. 432. Reprinted by permission.
†Computed from authors' data.

the period that immediately follows it, and not how much it differs from a cycle at the other end of the utterance. Jitter, then, is a measure of the frequency variability not accounted for by voluntary changes in F_o. If the phonatory system were an ideal and perfectly stable mechanism, there would be absolutely no difference in fundamental periods except when a speaker purposely changed pitch. Frequency perturbation would be zero. To the extent that jitter is not zero, "perturbation is an acoustic correlate of erratic vibratory patterns" (Beckett, 1969, p. 418) that result from diminished control over the phonatory system (Sorenson, Horii, and Leonard, 1980).

Over fifty years ago Simon (1927, p. 83) concluded that "there are no tones of constant pitch in either vocal or instrumental sounds." The phonatory system is not a perfect machine, and every speaker's vibratory cycles are erratic to some extent. But, on the face of it, one would guess that an abnormal larynx would produce a more erratic voice than a healthy one. On the whole this turns out to be the case. There is by now a considerable body of literature that asserts the usefulness of frequency perturbation measures in evaluation of laryngeal and vocal pathology (Kitajima, Tanabe, and Isshiki, 1975; Davis, 1976; Horii, 1979; Lieberman, 1961, 1963; Hecker and Kreul, 1971; Klingholz and Martin, 1983; Hartmann and von Cramon, 1984; Zyski, Bull,

TABLE 5-14. Maximum Phonational Frequency Range: Parkinson's Disease*

Group	Unit	Lowest F_o Median	Lowest F_o Range	Highest F_o Median	Highest F_o Range	Range in ST† Median	Range in ST† Range
Normal	Hz	80**	40–120	260	190–440		
	ST‡	27.5	15.5–34.5	47.9	42.5–57.0	22.1**	8.0–36.4
Parkinson							
	Hz	100**	80–130	220	140–330		
	ST‡	31.4	27.5–35.9	45.0	37.2–52.0	15.0**	4.0–22.0

From Canter, G. J. Speech characteristics of patients with Parkinson's disease: II. Physiological support for speech. *Journal of Speech and Hearing Disorders*, 30 (1965) 44-49. Table 1, p. 46. © American Speech-Language-Hearing Association, Rockville, MD. Reprinted by permission.

*17 subjects in each group. Age 35.5–75 years; median 56.8; groups matched. Hand measurement of oscillograms.
†Original data in octaves.
**Significant differences: median lowest ($p < .01$), median range ($p < .05$).
‡Computed from author's data.

TABLE 5-15. Maximum Phonational Frequency Range: Pulse and Loft Registers (Young Adults)

No. of Subj.		Lowest F_o Mean	Lowest F_o Range	Highest F_o Mean	Highest F_o Range	MPFR	Source
		PULSE					
Men							
5	Hz	26.8	22–32	80.0	62–92	53.2 Hz	1
	ST	8.4	5.1–11.6	27.3	23.1–29.9	18.9 ST	1
12	Hz	24	—	52	—	28 Hz	2
	ST	6.6	—	20.0	—	13.4 ST	2
Women							
11	Hz	18	—	46	—	28 Hz	2
	ST	1.7	—	17.9	—	16.2 ST	2
		MODAL					
Men							
5	Hz	78.2	65–98	462	330–523	383.8 Hz	1
	ST	26.9	23.9–31.0	57.6	52–60	30.7 ST	1
12	Hz	94	—	287	—	193 Hz	2
	ST	30.3	—	49.6	—	19.4 ST	2
Women							
11	HZ	144	—	538	—	394 Hz	2
	ST	37.7	—	60.5	—	22.8 ST	2
		LOFT					
Men							
12	Hz	275	—	634	—	359 Hz	2
	ST	48.9	—	63.3	—	14.4 ST	2
Women							
11	Hz	495	—	1131	—	636 Hz	2
	ST	59.0	—	73.3	—	14.3 ST	2

Sources:
1. Murry, 1971.
2. Hollien and Michel, 1968.
    Note: Data have been converted to ST if not provided in original.

McDonald, and Johns, 1984).* This should
not be taken to mean that jitter can be used
as the sole diagnostic criterion, or that it
accounts for all of what the listener per-
ceives in the disordered voice. Far from it:
factors such as amplitude perturbation
(Wendahl, 1963, 1966a,b; Takahashi and
Koike, 1975; Horii, 1980), spectral noise
(Emanuel and Austin, 1981; Emanuel, Lively, and McCoy, 1973; Emanuel and Scarinzi,
1979, 1980), and glottal waveform changes (Coleman, 1971) account for a great deal,
perhaps most, of what is heard as abnormality. But frequency perturbation is sufficiently sensitive to pathological changes
in the phonatory process, and perhaps
even to severe respiratory insufficiency
(Gilbert, 1975), to warrant careful consideration here.

*Frequency perturbation may even become a means
of assessing the effects of drugs. See, for example,
Nevlud, Fann, and Falck, (1983).

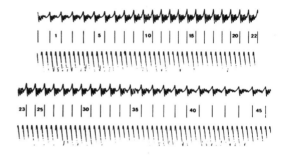

FIGURE 5-23. Oscillogram of a sustained vowel, together with a 200 Hz time-reference wave.
Periods have been numbered successively. This
sample will be used in later jitter determinations.

Measurement Methods

Although frequency perturbation can be
determined from either running speech or
sustained phonation of a vowel, the latter
seems more suitable. In running speech sys-

TABLE 5-16. Data From the Sample of Figure 5-23

Cycle No.	Period* (ms)	F_o† (Hz)	Cycle No.	Period (ms)	F_o (Hz)
1	11.88	84.18	24	9.25	108.11
2	11.75	85.11	25	9.75	102.56
3	11.50	86.96	26	9.63	103.84
4	11.25	88.89	27	9.25	108.11
5	10.88	91.91	28	9.50	105.26
6	10.63	94.07	29	9.74	102.67
7	10.25	97.56	30	10.00	100.00
8	9.75	102.56	31	10.25	97.56
9	9.88	101.21	32	10.25	97.56
10	9.75	102.56	33	10.50	95.24
11	9.50	105.26	34	11.00	90.91
12	9.00	111.11	35	11.25	88.89
13	9.00	111.11	36	11.50	86.96
14	9.25	108.11	37	11.75	85.11
15	9.50	105.26	38	11.88	84.18
16	9.38	106.61	39	12.50	80.00
17	9.25	108.11	40	13.13	76.16
18	9.00	111.11	41	13.75	72.73
19	9.50	105.26	42	13.75	72.73
20	9.75	102.56	43	14.38	69.54
21	8.75	114.29	44	14.38	69.54
22	9.75	102.56	45	15.00	66.67
23	9.38	106.61			

*Mean period: 10.69 ms S.D. = 1.64.
†Mean F_o: 95.50 Hz S.D. = 12.93.

tematic changes in F_o for stress, intonation, and the like are confounded with the unintentional shifts that are of interest. "Sustained vowel phonations," suggests Horii (1979, p. 5), "would seem to be an appropriate phonatory task when more or less random perturbations caused by mechanophysiologic conditions of the vocal folds are in question."

There are many ways of devising an index of frequency perturbation, each with different advantages and drawbacks. Each is cumbersome or tedious in its own way. (The use of a computer or programmable calculator greatly simplifies measurement. Commercial devices are available, and Troughear and Davis [1979] have described a "homebuilt" computer system.) Therapists must therefore decide which method will provide the best evaluation of their patients' vocal attributes with the resources available. The following consideration of the several computational procedures is intended to inform that decision.

Unless a computer is to do *all* of the task, it is assumed that an oscillographic readout of the patient's phonatory waveforms has been prepared. Such a record would be similar to the one shown in Figure 5-23, except that it would be much longer. This record will be used as the example for all of the procedures discussed in this section. While the waveforms and amplitudes in this sample differ from each other, it is only the duration of the cycles that is of concern at the moment.* The successive cycles have been demarcated and numbered consecutively. By referring to the 200 Hz reference signal that was recorded at the same time as the speech sample, the period (*t*) of each wave was determined. The reciprocal of the period is the F_o of the cycle. The measured period and F_o values (given in Table 5-16) will provide the raw data for all further analyses.

Distributions

FUNDAMENTAL FREQUENCY HISTOGRAM. Perhaps the simplest way to analyze the F_o data is to construct a F_o *histogram*, which is nothing more than a bar graph of the occurrences of F_os in the sample. For the example of Figure 5-22 and Table 5-16 the distribution of F_os can be tabled as shown in Table 5-17. The histogram that results from graphing these values is shown in Figure 5-24. (A larger sample would have resulted in a smoother graph.) Schultz-Coulon, Battner, and Fedders (1979) felt that this form of analysis provided the most useful information in voice evaluation, although it does not really measure jitter per se. While it is easy to construct, there is little information about the significance of the histogram's "shape." The method is not currently in general use, although some attempts have been made to relate it to perceptual attributes of abnormal voices (Hammarberg et al, 1980).

DURATIONAL DIFFERENCES HISTOGRAM. Lieberman (1961, 1963) and Iwata and von Leden (1970) have demonstrated the usefulness of examining the distribution of the

TABLE 5-17. Distribution of the Fundamental Frequencies in the Standard Sample

Frequency Interval	Occurences (No.)
65.0– 69.9	3
70.0– 74.9	2
75.0– 79.9	1
80.0– 84.9	3
85.0– 89.9	6
90.0– 94.9	3
95.0– 99.9	4
100.0–104.9	9
105.0–109.9	10
110.0–114.9	4
	45

---

*The specimen sample was specially chosen to have high F_o variability.

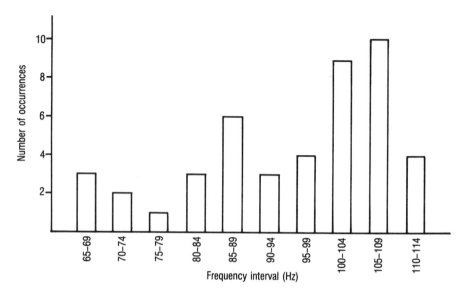

FIGURE 5-24. Frequency histogram for the specimen jitter sample.

magnitude of the differences between adjacent periods. The method requires plotting the percent of occurrence (known in descriptive statistics as the *relative frequency of occurrence*) of the function

$$\Delta t = t_n - t_{n-1}.$$

In descriptive terms, Δt is the absolute difference between the length of period n and the length of the previous period, $n - 1$. The procedure for generating the distribution curve can be illustrated with the data of Table 5-16, as shown in Table 5-18.

First, the several Δts are found by subtracting the period of each wave from the period just before it. (One therefore begins with the second period, and the number of differences will be one less than the number of waves in the sample.) Since only the absolute value of the difference is needed, the sign of the result is ignored. (The Δts are shown in column 3.) Now the number of occurrences in each value interval* is determined (columns 4 and 5), and the percentage of all observations found in each interval is calculated (column 6). In the example at hand, for instance, 4 of the periods

---

*The minimum size of the interval depends on the precision of the original period measurements.

od differences had magnitudes between 0.00 and 0.10 ms. This interval, then, contained 4/44, or 9.1%, of all the differences. The percentages of the distribution are then plotted as in Figure 5-25A.

The distribution shown in Figure 5-25B is taken from Lieberman (1961) and is based on more than 7000 periods produced by six normal male speakers. It shows that most of the differences were very small (< 0.4 ms); perturbations equal to or greater than 0.5 ms account for only about 20% of all observations. (In later work, using more accurate measurement, Lieberman (1963) found that differences > 0.5 ms constituted only about 15% of the total number.) For normal speakers the overall shape of the distribution curve was always the same, although the emotional content of the spoken material did affect the height of the right-hand "shoulder" (Lieberman, 1961; Lieberman and Michaels, 1962). Hoarse speakers had a greater proportion of large differences and, therefore, the "tail" of the curve was elevated in such cases. This fact led to the creation of the "perturbation factor," discussed below. For those willing to go through the trouble of plotting the data (or who have either a computer or an instrument like the PM Analyzer available to do

TABLE 5-18. Generating the Durational Differences Histogram for the Standard Sample

1 Cycle No.	2 Period (ms)	3 $|t_n-t_{n-1}|$ (ms)	1 Cycle No.	2 Period (ms)	3 $|t_n-t_{n-1}|$ (ms)
1	11.88				0.13
		0.13	24	9.25	
2	11.75				0.50
		0.25	25	9.75	
3	11.50				0.12
		0.25	26	9.63	
4	11.25				.38
		0.37	27	9.25	
5	10.88				0.25
		0.25	28	9.50	
6	10.63				0.24
		0.38	29	9.74	
7	10.25				0.26
		0.50	30	10.00	
8	9.75				0.25
		0.13	31	10.25	
9	9.88				0.0
		0.13	32	10.25	
10	9.75				0.25
		0.25	33	10.50	
11	9.50				0.50
		0.50	34	11.00	
12	9.00				0.25
		0.00	35	11.25	
13	9.00				0.25
		0.25	36	11.50	
14	9.25				0.25
		0.25	37	11.75	
15	9.50				0.13
		0.12	38	11.88	
16	9.38				0.62
		0.13	39	12.50	
17	9.25				0.63
		0.25	40	13.13	
18	9.00				0.62
		0.50	41	13.75	
19	9.50				0.00
		0.25	42	13.75	
20	9.75				0.63
		1.00	43	14.38	
21	8.75				0.00
		1.00	44	14.38	
22	9.75				0.62
		0.37	45	15.00	
23	9.38				

TABLE 5-18 *(continued)*

	DISTRIBUTION	
4	5	6
Δt interval	No. of occurrences	Relative frequency (% of occurrences)
0.0 −0.10	4	9.1%
0.11−0.20	8	18.1
0.21−0.30	16	36.4
0.31−0.40	4	9.1
0.41−0.50	5	11.4
0.51−0.60	0	0.0
0.61−0.70	5	11.4
0.71−0.80	0	0.0
0.81−0.90	0	0.0
0.91−1.00	2	4.5
	44	100.0%

it for them) the distribution of the relative frequency of occurrence can provide a "picture" of a patient's vocal perturbation that may be useful in distinguishing among various laryngeal pathologies.

Numerical Indices of Perturbation

In general, one would prefer to generate not a curve, but a "score" that might serve as a perturbation rating. Hopefully, such an index would be reflective of different kinds of disorders and would be sensitive to either improvement or deterioration of the patient's vocal function. A host of approaches to the quantification of frequency perturbation has been created; the more useful of these are considered here.

ABSOLUTE MEASURES. Period perturbation measures that ignore the speaker's F_o can be said to be "absolute." Several such indices have been devised, although none has proven very popular.

Perturbation factor. Lieberman's (1961, 1963) study of frequency perturbation in normal and pathologic voices tended to confirm the observation of von Leden, Moore, and Timcke (1960) that the normal

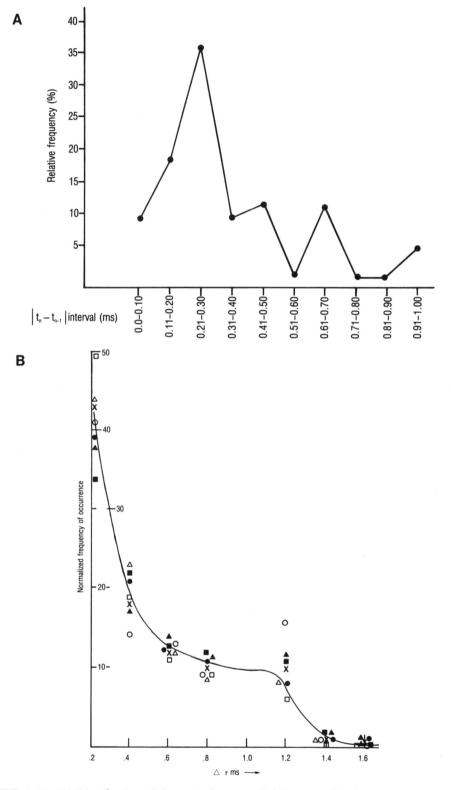

FIGURE 5-25. (A) Distribution of the period-to-period differences for the specimen jitter sample. (B) Distribution of the period-to-period differences in a large sample from 6 speakers. (From Lieberman, P. Perturbations in vocal pitch. *Journal of the Acoustical Society of America,* 33 (1961) 597-603. Figure 4, p. 598. (Reprinted by permission.)

vibratory patterns of the vocal folds are disrupted in the presence of laryngeal pathology and, in particular, that there is a greatly increased tendency for rapid and frequent lapses of vibratory regularity. Specifically, Lieberman (1963) reasoned that frequency perturbations reflect (1) changes in glottal periodicity; (2) alterations of the glottal waveform; and (3) variations of vocal tract configuration that result in phase shifts of the acoustic wave. The first of these (which was of prime interest) was considered to produce cycle-to-cycle period differences greater than 0.5 ms. Lieberman therefore proposed an index that he called the *perturbation factor,* defined as "the integral of the frequency distribution of $\Delta t > 0.5$ ms.'" More simply stated, the perturbation factor is the percentage of all perturbations equal to or greater than a half millisecond. In the data for the specimen sample of Table 5-18, 12 of the 44 period differences are greater than 0.5 ms. The perturbation factor for that sample is therefore $12/44 = 27.3\%$ (a very large perturbation factor indeed).

The perturbation factor may well turn out to be useful as a screening measure for detection of laryngeal disorder, since it

> is sensitive to the size and location of pathologic growths in the speaker's larynx. When growths occur on the speaker's vocal cords, the differences between the perturbation factors of the normal and pathologic larynges are proportional to the size of the pathologic growths as long as the growths do not interfere with normal closure of the vocal cords. . . . Inflammatory conditions and very small nodules . . . have, in general, comparatively small effect on either the perturbation factor or on the acoustic waveform. (Lieberman, 1963, p. 353)

Some validation of these conclusions has been done (Iwata and von Leden, 1970) but more will be needed before the perturbation factor can be widely used in this way.

Directional perturbation factor. A different kind of perturbation measure has been proposed by Hecker and Kreul (1971). Their *directional perturbation factor* (DPF) ignores the *magnitude* of period perturbation;

it is concerned only with the number of times that the frequency change shifts direction. The DPF "takes into account the algebraic sign rather than the magnitude of the difference between adjacent glottal pulse intervals. It was defined as the percentage of the total number of differences for which there is a change in algebraic sign" (Hecker and Kreul, 1971, p. 1279).

The definition is perhaps somewhat confusing but the calculation of the DPF is easily demonstrated by example. Using the data of the specimen sample, Table 5-19 shows how it is done. The period of each cycle is determined (column 2), and the difference between the successive periods is found by subtraction (column 3). For the DPF, however, the sign of the difference is preserved. For example, the difference between cycles 14 and 15 of the sample is *plus* 0.25, but between 15 and 16 it is *minus* 0.12. Now the tabulation of period differences is scanned, and the number of times the sign of the difference *changes* is counted (column 4). The DPF is this sign-change count divided by the total number of differences in the tabulation. In Table 5-19 there are 11 changes of sign among a total of 44 period differences. Therefore, DPF = $11/44 = 25\%$.

Mean directional perturbation factor for older men (age 42 to 75 years, mean age 63.2 years) has been measured at 33.3% (S.D. = 4.2) during reading of a sentence of the Rainbow Passage (Hecker and Kreul, 1971). Izdebski and Murry (1980) found a somewhat higher mean DPF of 58.4% (S.D. = 7.54) for productions of /a/ at comfortable pitch and loudness by 5 normal adults.

Sorensen and Horii (1984) have determined the directional perturbation factor for 20 men and 20 women. Their data (Table 5-20) are so far the most complete available, and may be considered tentative norms for this measure.

F_o-**RELATED MEASURES.** The magnitude of frequency perturbation shows considerable correlation with mean fundamental frequency. A number of researchers (Lieberman, 1963; Beckett, 1969; Koike, 1973; Horii, 1979, 1980) have noted that larger

TABLE 5-19. Computation of the Directional Perturbation Factor for the Standard Sample

1 Cycle No. (i)	2 Period (P_i) (ms)	3 Δt (ms)	4 Sign- change count
1	11.88		
2	11.75	−0.13	
3	11.50	−0.25	
4	11.25	−0.25	
5	10.88	−0.37	
6	10.63	−0.25	
7	10.25	−0.38	
8	0.75	−0.50	
9	9.88	+0.13	1
10	9.75	−0.13	2
11	9.50	−0.25	
12	9.00	−0.50	
13	9.00	0.00	
14	9.25	+0.25	3
15	9.50	+0.25	
16	9.38	−0.12	4
17	9.25	−0.13	
18	9.00	−0.25	
19	9.50	+0.50	5
20	9.75	+0.25	
21	8.75	−1.00	6
22	9.75	+1.00	7
23	9.38	−0.37	8
24	9.25	−0.13	
25	9.75	+0.50	9
26	9.63	−0.12	10
27	9.25	−0.38	
28	9.50	+0.25	11
29	9.74	+0.24	
30	10.00	+0.26	
31	10.25	+0.25	
32	10.25	0.00	
33	10.50	+0.25	
34	11.00	+0.50	
35	11.25	+0.25	
36	11.50	+0.25	
37	11.75	+0.25	
38	11.88	+0.13	
39	12.50	+0.62	
40	13.13	+0.63	
41	13.75	+0.62	
42	13.75	0.00	
43	14.38	+0.63	
44	14.38	0.00	
45	15.00	+0.62	

Computation: 11 changes of sign among 44 differences: DPF = 11/44 = 25%

TABLE 5-20. Directional Perturbation Factor: Normal Adults (Percent Sign Change)*†

Statistic	Vowel		
	/a/	/u/	/i/
Men			
Mean	46.24	49.26	46.37
Range	39.0–52.1	41.0–61.1	34.6–60.3
S.D.	3.59	5.54	6.32
Women			
Mean	48.79	52.77	52.04
Range	39.3–60.0	40.6–62.7	44.7–61.1
S.D.	4.78	6.69	5.23

From Sorensen, D. and Horii, Y. Directional perturbation factors for jitter and for shimmer. *Journal of Communication Disorders*, 16 (1984) 143-151. Table 1, p. 147. © 1984 by Elsevier Science Publishing Co., Inc. Reprinted by permission of the publisher.

*20 men, 20 women (all nonsmokers). Age 25–49 years (mean: males—38.1 years; females 36.4 years). Sustained vowels at 70–80dB SPL for approx. 5 s.

†Amplitude perturbation also assessed for this group. See Chapter 3.

cycle-to-cycle differences are associated with longer fundamental periods. (Reciprocally, higher fundamental frequencies tend to have smaller perturbations.) Horii (1979) had each of six men sustain tones at approximately 2 ST intervals from 98 to 298 Hz and measured the frequency perturbation of each production. The averages for the group are shown in Table 5-21. It is clear that the average perturbation decreases as F_o increases (the correlation is − .95) but the relationship is not monotonic or even invariable.

Analyses by Horii (1979) and by Hollien, Michel, and Doherty (1973) tend to demonstrate that there is no way to compensate exactly for the effect of mean F_o and thereby achieve an "uninfluenced" jitter index. The best compromise is to generate a ratio of some form of mean perturbation to mean period. It is this tack that most jitter indices take. (Honjo and Isshiki (1980) have expressed jitter in semitones, which does make for a frequency-compensated measure. The effectiveness of the correction has not been assessed, however.)

TABLE 5-21. Mean Jitter at Different Fundamental Frequencies*

| | | | | | Semitones Above 98 Hz | | | | | | |
Measures	2	4	6	8	10	12	14	16	18	20	22
Mean Jitter (μs)	51	52	45	41	44	35	30	26	28	28	24
S.D.†	13.7	14.8	14.2	13.1	17.8	10.2	11.9	5.9	9.1	9.0	4.6
Range	38–89	32–79	23–69	24–65	21–77	22–57	17–54	16–38	17–45	16–51	17–32

From Horii, Y. Fundamental frequency perturbation observed in sustained phonation. *Journal of Speech and Hearing Research*, 22 (1979) 5-19. Table 2, p. 11. © American Speech-Language-Hearing Association, Rockville, MD. Reprinted by permission.

*Six men, age 28–43. Sustained /i/, pitch matching, two trials each.

†Computed from author's data.

Jitter ratio and jitter factor. The simplest form of F_0- adjusted perturbation index is the mean perturbation divided by the mean waveform duration. When done in terms of period, the measure is called the *jitter ratio* (Horii, 1979). By definition,

$$\text{Jitter ratio} = \frac{\dfrac{1}{n-1}\left[\displaystyle\sum_{i=1}^{n-1} |P_i - P_{i+1}|\right]}{\dfrac{1}{n}\displaystyle\sum_{i=1}^{n} P_i} \times 1000$$

where p_i = period of the ith cycle, in ms, and N = number of periods in the sample.

For those with little experience in this form of algebraic notation, the mathematics might seem complex. In fact, this is not the case. Put into ordinary language, the numerator is the sum of the absolute values of the differences between successive periods divided by the number of differences measured $(N-1)$. In short, it is the average magnitude of perturbation. The denominator is the sum of the periods divided by the number of periods—that is, it is the mean period. Multiplication by 1000 only serves to make the resultant ratio larger as a matter of convenience.

Table 5-22 uses the specimen sample of Table 5-16 again for the purpose of illustration. As has been done for all the other cases, the periods are tabulated and summed to give

$$\sum_{i=1}^{n} P_i.$$

The absolute value of the difference between each period and its successor, $(|P_i - P_{i+1}|)$ is then determined, and the sum of these values,

$$\sum_{i=1}^{n-1} |P_i - P_{i+1}|,$$

is also taken. The sums are inserted into the formula to find the jitter ratio which, for the specimen sample, turns out to be 30.1.

The frequency-based equivalent of jitter ratio is known as *jitter factor* (Hollien, Michel, and Doherty 1973). That is, jitter factor is the mean difference between the *frequencies* of adjacent cycles divided by the mean *frequency*, multiplied by 100. Formally stated,

$$\text{Jitter factor} = \frac{\dfrac{1}{n-1}\left[\displaystyle\sum_{i=1}^{n-1} |F_i - F_{i+1}|\right]}{\dfrac{1}{n}\displaystyle\sum_{i=1}^{n} F_i} \times 100$$

The jitter factor of the specimen sample, computed in Table 5-23, is 3.128. Typical values of jitter ratio and jitter factor for normal men are shown in Table 5-24.

Period variability index. Deal and Emanuel (1978) have adopted an approach to the quantification of period perturbation that derives from descriptive statistics. Termed the *period variability index* (PVI), it re-

TABLE 5-22. Computation of the Jitter Ratio for the Standard Sample

1 Cycle (i)	2 Period (P_i) (ms)	3 $P_i - P_{i+1}$ (ms)
1	11.88	
2	11.75	0.13
3	11.50	0.25
4	11.25	0.25
5	10.88	0.37
6	10.63	0.25
7	10.25	0.38
8	9.75	0.50
9	9.88	0.13
10	9.75	0.13
11	9.50	0.25
12	9.00	0.50
13	9.00	0.00
14	9.25	0.25
15	9.50	0.25
16	9.38	0.12
17	9.25	0.13
18	9.00	0.25
19	9.50	0.50
20	9.75	0.25
21	8.75	1.00
22	9.75	1.00
23	9.38	0.37
24	9.25	0.13
25	9.75	0.50
26	9.63	0.12
27	9.25	0.38
28	9.50	0.25
29	9.74	0.24
30	10.00	0.26
31	10.25	0.25
32	10.25	0.00
33	10.50	0.25
34	11.00	0.50
35	11.25	0.25
36	11.50	0.25
37	11.75	0.25
38	11.88	0.13
39	12.50	0.62
40	13.13	0.63
41	13.75	0.62
42	13.75	0.00
43	14.38	0.63
44	14.38	0.00
45	15.00	0.62
	480.92	14.14

TABLE 5-22 (continued)

Computation:

$$JR = \frac{\dfrac{1}{n-1}\left[\displaystyle\sum_{i=1}^{n-1}\left|P_i - P_{i+1}\right|\right]}{\dfrac{1}{n}\displaystyle\sum_{i=1}^{n}P_i} \times 1000$$

$$= \frac{\dfrac{1}{45-1}[14.14]}{\dfrac{1}{45}[480.92]} \times 1000 = \frac{0.3214}{10.687} \times 1000$$

$$= 0.0301 \times 1000$$

Jitter ratio $= 30.10$

quires the computation of a coefficient of variation (CV), defined as

$$CV = \frac{\dfrac{1}{n}\left[(P_i - \bar{P})^2\right]}{\bar{P}^2}$$

where p_i = period of the ith cycle

and $\bar{P}$ = mean period

The term $(P_i - \bar{P})$ signifies the difference between the ith period and the mean period. In descriptive terms, then, the coefficient of variation is the mean of the squares of the deviations from the mean divided by the square of the mean. It is akin to the standard deviation of the period, and is not, in actual fact, a true measure of cycle-to-cycle variability. The PVI is the CV times 1000.

In Table 5-25 the PVI is computed for the specimen sample. First, the sum of the periods is divided by the number of periods to find the mean period, $\bar{P}$. Next, the mean period is subtracted from each period value, and the result is squared to provide the series of $(P_i - \bar{P})^2$s in column 3. These values are then added to give

$$\sum_{i=1}^{n}(P_i - \bar{P})^2.$$

TABLE 5-23. Computation of the Jitter Factor for the Standard Sample

1 Cycle No. (i)	2 Freq. (F$_i$) (Hz)	3 F$_i$ − F$_{i+1}$ (Hz)
1	84.18	
2	85.11	0.93
3	86.96	1.85
4	88.89	1.93
5	91.91	3.02
6	94.07	2.16
7	97.56	3.49
8	102.56	5.00
9	101.21	1.35
10	102.56	1.35
11	105.26	2.70
12	111.11	5.85
13	111.11	0.00
14	108.11	3.00
15	105.26	2.85
16	106.61	1.35
17	108.11	1.50
18	111.11	3.00
19	105.26	5.85
20	102.56	2.70
21	114.29	11.73
22	102.56	11.73
23	106.61	4.05
24	108.11	1.50
25	102.56	5.55
26	103.84	1.28
27	108.11	4.27
28	105.26	2.85
29	102.67	2.59
30	100.00	2.67
31	97.56	2.44
32	97.56	0.00
33	95.24	2.32
34	90.91	4.33
35	88.89	2.02
36	86.96	1.93
37	85.11	1.85
38	84.18	0.93
39	80.00	4.18
40	76.16	3.84
41	72.73	3.43
42	72.73	0.00
43	69.54	3.19
44	69.54	0.00
45	66.67	2.87
	4297.30	131.43

TABLE 5-23 (continued)

Computation:

$$JF = \frac{\dfrac{1}{n-1}\left[\displaystyle\sum_{i=1}^{n-1}|F_i - F_{i+1}|\right]}{\dfrac{1}{n}\displaystyle\sum_{i=1}^{n}F_i} \times 100$$

$$= \frac{\dfrac{1}{44}[131.43]}{\dfrac{1}{45}[4297.30]} \times 1000$$

$$= \frac{2.987}{95.496} \times 100$$

$$= 0.03128 \times 100$$

Jitter factor = 3.128

The results of these arithmetic processes are then used according to the formula to derive the coefficient of variation, which is multiplied by 1000 to give the PVI.

The PVI values for normal adult males, shown in Table 5-26, may be used as a basis for comparison with clinical cases seen by speech pathologists.

Relative average perturbation. Changes of fundamental frequency are of two types: relatively slow and steady increases or decreases and abrupt, rapid, quasi-random shifts. The first are, in most cases, related to linguistic variables and hence are volitional. They are best evaluated by measures such as pitch sigma. The sudden, involuntary changes are perturbational. In running speech the two types of fundamental frequency modulation occur simultaneously. Any measure that evaluates one inevitably includes the effects of the other. Even during sustained vowels, F_o may undergo slow changes that are not of interest but that may inflate the measure of jitter. All of the frequency perturbation indices discussed so far, therefore, suffer from a potential problem.

TABLE 5-24. Jitter Ratio and Jitter Factor Values for Normal Males

Age (years)	Subjects (No.)	F_o (Hz)	Absolute Jitter (Mean)	Relative Perturbation Mean	Relative Perturbation Range	Source
Jitter ratio						
28–43	6	98–298			5.3–7.6	1
Jitter factor						
21–37	4	102	0.48	0.47	(0.39–0.54)	2
		142	0.76	0.53	(0.33–0.86)	
		198	0.85	0.43	(0.36–0.52)	
		276	2.67	0.97	(0.77–1.34)	
55–71 (mean 63.8)	5	115.3		0.99	(0.76–1.49)	3

Data from (1) Horri (1979), (2) Hollien, Michel, and Doherty (1973), and (3) Murry and Doherty (1980).

Relative average perturbation (Koike, 1973), also called the *frequency perturbation quotient* (Takahashi and Koike 1975) attempts to mitigate the difficulty by using a form of straightline averaging that greatly reduces the effect of relatively slow changes in F_o. The way it works can be explained with the help of Figure 5-26, in which the periods of successive cycles in a hypothetical sample are plotted. It is obvious that the length of the period is increasing, but the vocal jitter makes the increase erratic. The curve can be smoothed considerably by taking sets of averages. Consider, for example, cycles 6, 7, and 8, which have periods of 7.6, 8.2, and 8.2 ms, respectively. The average of these three periods in 8 ms. This value could be considered to be an estimate of the period that cycle 7, the middle cycle, *should* have had, if there had been no jitter influencing the relatively slow change of period. A measure of the jitter of cycle 7, therefore, would be the difference between its period and the "corrected," or estimated, period. (For cycle 7 in the present example, the jitter would have been 0.2 ms.) The estimated jitter for a single cycle, therefore, is

$$P_i - \left[\frac{P_{i-1} + P_i + P_{i+1}}{3}\right].$$

That is, the difference between its actual period and the mean period for the three cycles of which it is the middle value. The averaging procedure can be used for every set of three cycles in the sample ($P_{1,2,3}$, $P_{2,3,4}$, $P_{3,4,5}$, . . ., $P_{i-1,i,i+1}$) with the result of each averaging considered to be an estimate of the "intended" value of the middle cycle. The plot of these "intended" fundamental periods is shown in Figure 5-26B, together with the original period values. (Notice that, because three periods are used in the averaging, there are two fewer estimates than original period values. The first and last periods are unestimated and cannot be used in the final jitter evaluation.) Average jitter can now be defined as the average difference between period values and their estimates.

The relative average perturbation (RAP) measure performs exactly this process, but without the graphs. The RAP function is defined as

$$RAP = \frac{\dfrac{1}{n-2}\displaystyle\sum_{i=2}^{n-1}\left|\dfrac{P_{i-1} + P_i + P_{i+1}}{3} - P_i\right|}{\dfrac{1}{n}\displaystyle\sum_{i=1}^{n} P_i}$$

The numerator, called the *average absolute perturbation*, should be recognizable as the average difference between actual periods and their three-point estimates.* The de-

*A similar technique that allows any number of periods to be averaged is discussed by Davis (1976, 1979, 1981).

TABLE 5-25. Computation of the Period Variability Index for the Standard Sample

1 Cycle No. (i)	2 Period (P_i) (ms)	3 $(P_i - \bar{P})^2$ (ms)
1	11.88	1.416
2	11.75	1.124
3	11.50	0.656
4	11.25	0.314
5	10.88	0.036
6	10.63	0.004
7	10.25	0.194
8	9.75	0.884
9	9.88	0.656
10	9.75	0.884
11	9.50	1.416
12	9.00	2.856
13	9.00	2.856
14	9.25	2.074
15	9.50	1.416
16	9.38	1.716
17	9.25	2.074
18	9.00	2.856
19	9.50	1.416
20	9.75	0.884
21	8.75	3.764
22	9.75	0.884
23	9.38	1.716
24	9.25	2.074
25	9.75	0.884
26	9.63	1.124
27	9.25	2.074
28	9.50	1.416
29	9.74	0.903
30	10.00	0.476
31	10.25	0.194
32	10.25	0.194
33	10.50	0.036
34	11.00	0.096
35	11.25	0.314
36	11.50	0.656
37	11.75	1.124
38	11.88	1.416
39	12.50	3.276
40	13.13	5.954
41	13.75	9.364
42	13.75	9.364
43	14.38	13.616
44	14.38	13.616
45	15.00	18.576
	480.92	118.84
$\bar{P} =$	10.69	
$\bar{P}^2 =$	114.276	

TABLE 5-25 (continued)

Computation:

$$CV = \frac{\dfrac{1}{n}\left[\displaystyle\sum_{i=1}^{n}(P_i - \bar{P})^2\right]}{\bar{P}^2}$$

$$= \frac{\dfrac{1}{45}[118.84]}{114.276}$$

$$\begin{aligned}
CV &= 2.64 / 114.276 = 0.023 \\
PVI &= CV \times 1000 = 0.023 \times 1000 \\
PVI &= 23.0
\end{aligned}$$

TABLE 5-26. Period Variability Index Values for Normal Males*†

	Period Variability Index	
Vowel	**Mean**	**S.D.**
/u/	0.4451	0.1051
/i/	0.4898	0.1288
/ʌ/	0.4196	0.0979
/a/	0.4412	0.1595
/æ/	0.4951	0.1167

From Deal, R. E. and Emanuel, F. W. Some waveform and spectral features of vowel roughness. *Journal of Speech and Hearing Research,* 21 (1978) 250-264. Table 1, p. 256. © American Speech-Language-Hearing Association, Rockville, MD. Reprinted by permission.
*20 normal adult males. 7 s of phonation at 75 dB SPL. Signal narrow band filtered, analysis of first harmonic.
†Samples originally collected by Sansone and Emanuel, 1970.

nominator, of course, is the mean period, which is included to compensate for the change in mean absolute jitter that occurs with change in F_o.

Table 5-27 generates the RAP for the specimen sample that has served as the example for all the other measures of jitter. Koike (1973) found that the mean frequency RAP for 30 adult speakers of both sexes and various ages was about 0.0046 for the midsection of a sustained /ɑ/. In a later study (with fewer subjects) Takahashi and Koike (1975) obtained the RAP values shown in Table 5-28. Attempts are being

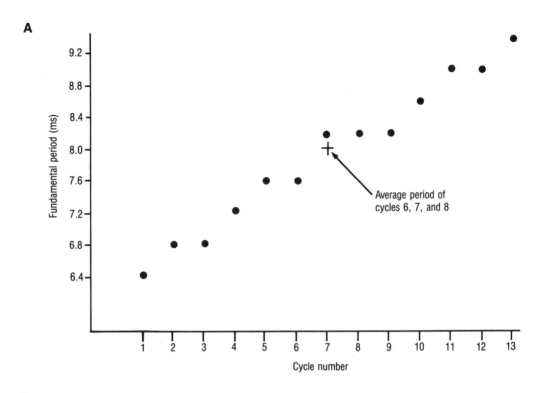

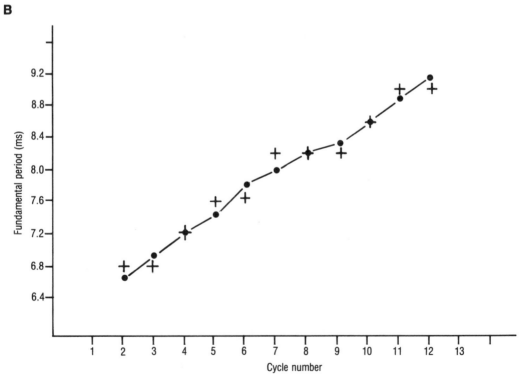

FIGURE 5-26. (A) Plot of the period values of successive cycles in a hypothetical sample. Periods 6, 7, and 8 have been averaged to provide an estimate (+) of cycle 7, as discussed in the text. (B) The three-cycle averages (filled circles, connected by lines) and the original period values (crosses).

TABLE 5-27. Computations of the Relative Average Perturbation for the Standard Sample

1 Cycle No. (i)	2 Period (P_i) (ms)	3 $P_{i-1} + P_i + P_{i+1}$	4 $\dfrac{P_i}{3} - P_i$
1	11.88	—	—
2	11.75	11.71	0.04
3	11.50	11.50	0.00
4	11.25	11.21	0.04
5	10.88	10.92	0.04
6	10.63	10.59	0.04
7	10.25	10.21	0.04
8	9.75	9.96	0.21
9	9.88	9.79	0.09
10	9.75	9.71	0.05
11	9.50	9.42	0.08
12	9.00	9.17	0.17
13	9.00	9.08	0.08
14	9.25	9.25	0.00
15	9.50	9.38	0.12
16	9.38	9.38	0.00
17	9.25	9.21	0.04
18	9.00	9.25	0.25
19	9.50	9.42	0.08
20	9.75	9.33	0.42
21	8.75	9.42	0.67
22	9.75	9.29	0.46
23	9.38	9.46	0.08
24	9.25	9.46	0.21
25	9.75	9.54	0.21
26	9.63	9.54	0.09
27	9.25	9.46	0.21
28	9.50	9.50	0.00
29	9.74	9.75	0.01
30	10.00	10.00	0.00
31	10.25	10.17	0.08
32	10.25	10.33	0.08
33	10.50	10.58	0.08
34	11.00	10.92	0.08
35	11.25	11.25	0.00
36	11.50	11.50	0.00
37	11.75	11.71	0.04
38	11.88	12.04	0.16
39	12.50	12.50	0.00
40	13.13	13.13	0.00
41	13.75	13.54	0.21
42	13.75	13.96	0.21
43	14.38	14.17	0.21
44	14.38	14.59	0.21
45	15.00		
	480.92		5.08

TABLE 5-27 (continued)

Computation:

$$RAP = \frac{\dfrac{1}{n-2} \displaystyle\sum_{i=2}^{n-1} \left| \dfrac{P_{i-1} + P_i + P_{i+1}}{3} - P_i \right|}{\dfrac{1}{n} \displaystyle\sum_{i=1}^{n} P_i}$$

$$= \frac{\dfrac{1}{43}\,(5.08)}{\dfrac{1}{45}\,(480.92)}$$

$$= 1181/10.687$$

$$RAP = 0.011$$

made to establish a mathematical basis for discriminating the data of patients with vocal pathologies from normals (Koike, Takahashi, and Calcaterra, 1977; Davis, 1979, 1981).

Deviation from linear trend. A new measure of frequency perturbation, founded on the same rationale as RAP, has recently been proposed by Ludlow, Coulter, and Gentges (1983). Whereas RAP determines the deviation of a period from the average value of the period and its immediate neighbors, Ludlow and her associates compute a *deviation from linear trend* (DLT) which they define as the difference between a period and the average of the periods two cycles away from it in each direction. The formal definition is

$$DLT_i = \left[\frac{P_{i-2} + P_{i+2}}{2}\right] - P_i$$

The measure of perturbation is the mean DLT,

$$\overline{DLT} = \frac{\displaystyle\sum_{i=a}^{b} |DLT_i|}{b - a}$$

Note that, in its current stage of development, $\overline{DLT}$ evaluates alternate cycles only — P_{i-2}, P_i, and P_{i+2} — which implies that it might not detect perturbation caused by

TABLE 5-28. Relative Average Perturbation Values for Normal Adults

Sex	Subjects (No.)	Mean Age† (years)	Mean F_o (Hz)	Relative Average Perturbation*	
				Mean†	S.D.†
Male	7	27.7	108.1	0.0057	0.00134
Female	2	29.5	206.0	0.0061	0.00056

From Takahashi, H. and Koike, Y. Some perceptual dimensions and acoustical correlates of pathologic voices. *Acta-Otolaryngologica*, Suppl. 338, (1975), 1-24. Table, 1, p.6.
*Also called Frequency Perturbation Quotient.
†Summary data extracted and calculated from authors' table.

a short cycle regularly alternating with a long one, as occurs in pulse register (Cavallo, Baken, and Shaiman, 1984; Hollien, Girard, and Coleman, 1977; Moore and von Leden, 1958; Timcke, von Leden and Moore, 1959; Wendahl, Moore, and Hollien, 1963). Ludlow has proposed that the presence of such alternating waveforms might be shown in a "diplophonia ratio" of DLT to mean absolute perturbation that is very much greater than unity. This suggestion has not been definitively tested, however.

The computation of $\overline{DLT}$ for the standard sample is shown in Table 5-29, while typical $\overline{DLT}$ values are given in Table 5-30.

Factors Influencing Frequency Perturbation

Whatever perturbation measure is chosen, it is likely to be sensitive to a number of jitter-producing phonatory variables. Some of these are normal phenomena of voice production, while others are of pathologic origin.

Normal Phonation

Voice onset and termination characteristically have much greater frequency perturbation that the midsection of a sustained production (Lieberman, 1961; Horii, 1979). Koike (1973) in his study of normal men and women found that, whereas steady-state phonation had a mean relative average perturbation of 0.0046, the first 17 glottal cycles of a normal (soft) vocal initiation had a frequency perturbation of 0.0276 when measured the same way. The rating

for breathy voice onset was 0.0123. Unless voice onset itself is the phenomenon being examincd, clinicians will want to evaluate sustained vowels no less than a half-second or so after voice initiation.

Horii's (1979) data show that dividing absolute frequency perturbation by the mean fundamental frequency tends to overcompensate for the change in jitter with F_o. This is shown in Figure 5-27, in which the positive slope of the regression line for jitter ratio is a measure of the inadequacy of the compensation. Hollien, Michel, and Doherty (1973) have observed the same phenomenon in their jitter factor. There is no reason to believe that it is not the case for other relative measures. Clinicians should therefore expect *relative* perturbation to be somewhat higher in high-frequency voices, while *absolute* jitter magnitude should decrease with increasing F_o.

Vocal intensity may be a factor to be considered. In an unpublished study, (Jacob, 1968, cited by Horii, 1979) it was found that jitter ratio tended to decrease with increasing vocal intensity. This aspect of relative pitch perturbation has not been explored, but it would seem prudent to do all measurements at a standard intensity level.

The question of whether jitter varies systematically across different vowels is as yet unresolved. Wilcox and Horii (1980) and Horii (1980) found that /a/ and /i/ had significantly greater jitter than /u/, whereas Johnson and Michel (1969) observed a tendency for high vowels to show greater jitter than low ones. Further work by Horii (1982) failed to validate any significant difference in mean jitter across 10 English

TABLE 5-29. Computation of the Mean Deviation from Linear Trend (DLT) for the Standard Sample

1 Cycle No. (i)	2 Period (P_i) (ms)	3 $P_{i-2} + P_{i+2}$	4 col. 3 $\times$ P_i (DLT_i)
1	11.88		
2	11.75	11.69	0.06
3	11.50	11.50	0.00
4	11.25	11.19	0.06
5	10.88	10.94	−0.06
6	10.63	10.56	0.07
7	10.25	10.19	0.06
8	9.75	10.06	−0.31
9	9.88	9.75	0.13
10	9.75	9.69	0.06
11	9.50	9.37	0.13
12	9.00	9.25	−0.25
13	9.00	9.12	−0.12
14	9.25	9.25	0.00
15	9.50	9.31	0.19
16	9.38	9.37	0.01
17	9.25	9.19	0.06
18	9.00	9.37	−0.37
19	9.50	9.37	0.13
20	9.75	9.12	0.63
21	8.75	9.75	−1.00
22	9.75	9.06	0.69
23	9.38	9.50	−0.12
24	9.25	9.56	−0.31
25	9.75	9.44	0.31
26	9.63	9.50	0.13
27	9.25	9.56	−0.31
28	9.50	9.49	0.01
29	9.74	9.75	−0.01
30	10.00	9.99	0.01
31	10.25	10.12	0.13
32	10.25	10.37	−0.31
33	10.50	10.62	−0.12
34	11.00	10.87	0.13
35	11.25	11.25	0.00
36	11.50	11.50	0.00
37	11.75	11.69	0.06
38	11.88	12.12	−0.24
39	12.50	12.50	0.00
40	13.13	13.12	0.01
41	13.75	13.44	0.31
42	13.75	14.06	−0.31
43	14.38	14.06	0.32
44	14.38	14.69	−0.31
45	15.00		
			7.85

TABLE 5-29 (continued)

Computation:

$$\overline{DLT} = \frac{\sum_{i=a}^{b} |DLT_i|}{b - a}$$

$$= \frac{7.85}{44 - 2}$$

$$= 7.85 / 42$$

$$\overline{DLT} = 0.187$$

vowels, while Sorensen and Horii (1983) found significantly more jitter for /i/ than for /u/ or /a/ as produced at comfortable pitch and loudness by women. Pending clarification of the issue, it seems obvious that comparisons of jitter values are most safely done only for measurement of the same vowel.

Finally, preliminary evidence (Sorensen and Horii, 1983) points to the possiblity that adult females might normally have more vocal jitter than men, at least for some vowels. Fortunately, the observed sex difference is not great enough to lead to diagnostic error, especially if several different vowels are tested.

Pathology

Studies by a variety of means have shown that frequency perturbation is one of the physical correlates of perceived "hoarseness" or "harshness" (Moore and Thompson, 1965; Lieberman, 1963; Dunker and Schlosshauer, 1961; von Leden, Moore, and Timcke, 1960; Isshiki, Yanagihara, and Morimoto, 1966; Deal and Emanuel, 1978; Bowler, 1964). Wendahl (1966b), using synthetic stimuli, found that jitter of as little as ± 1 Hz around a 100 Hz median F_o was perceived as rough, while increased jitter magnitude was associated with increased perceived roughness. Although frequency perturbation is not the only—and perhaps not even the most important—correlate of hoarseness, it nonetheless seems to be an

TABLE 5-30. DLT Values for Normal Adults

Group*	No.	DLT Mean	DLT S.D.
1	10	21.71	11.99
2	7	38.04	12.28
Overall	17	28.43	

From Ludlow, C., Coulter, D., and Gentges, F. The differential sensitivity of measures of fundamental frequency perturbation to laryngeal neoplasms and neuropathologies. In Bless, D. M. and Abbs, J. H. (Eds.). *Vocal Fold Physiology: Contemporary Research and Clinical Issues.* San Diego: College-Hill, 1983. Tables 33-1 and 33-2, pp. 385, 388. Copyright 1983 by College-Hill Press. Reprinted by permission.

*Subjects: Group 1—6 females, 4 males, 16–72 years (mean ≅ 45). Age and sex matched to a group of subjects with laryngeal neoplasms (see Table 5-31). Group 2—3 females, 4 males, 53–67 years (mean ≅ 60). Age and sex matched to a group of Parkinsonian and a group of Shy-Drager patients. Sustained /a/ after 1 practice trial, "comfortable level." Computer processing of acoustic signal.

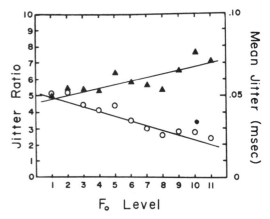

FIGURE 5-27. Mean absolute jitter in milliseconds (circles) and mean jitter ratios (triangles) for six subjects at various frequency levels. For each set of data a straight-line approximation (regression line) has been generated. Mean absolute jitter falls with increasing fundamental frequency, as expected, but mean jitter ratio increases. This indicates that jitter ratio tends to overcorrect for the effect of fundamental frequency. (From Horii, Y. Fundamental frequency perturbation observed in sustained phonation. *Journal of Speech and Hearing Research,* 22 (1979) 5-19. Figure 3, p. 12. © American Speech-Language-Hearing Association, Rockville, MD. Reprinted by permission.)

important concommittant of the laryngeal pathologies that produce the hoarse voice. In this regard it is worth repeating, for instance, that Lieberman (1963) found that while inflammatory and very small growths on the vocal folds only minimally influenced the perturbation factor, larger masses produced increased perturbation in proportion to their size. Koike (1967) has confirmed these findings. Interestingly, Beckett (1969) reported that there was a very significant ($p < .001$) relationship between the degree of F_o perturbation and subjective *vocal constriction* (defined as "the sensation of tightness and/or squeezing in and around the throat that a speaker experiences during phonation"). There is also some preliminary basis for believing that jitter values might differentiate hyper- and hypofunctional voice disorders (Klingholz and Martin, 1985).

The data in Table 5-31 provide some idea of the perturbation values that might be expected in various pathologies. (Values characteristic of normal speakers are included for comparison.) In general, too little work has been done to consider these results as normative. Caution must be exer-

cised in using any of them as a criterion for diagnosis. Because there is significant overlap between perturbation scores of normal and disordered groups (Zyski, Bull, McDonald and Johns, 1984) it is unwise to use perturbation assessment as a screening tool.

Periodicity of Perturbation

Indices of jitter express *average* perturbation, and there is the implication that the period-to-period variability is a random process. But this is not necessarily the case. Various factors could cause the jitter to be regularly altered, resulting in a *cyclic* variation of F_o. An example of such a process in shown (for a simple wave) in Figure 5-28. Technically, the wave is said to be *frequency modulated*. It would be useful to be able to detect any such "periodic-

TABLE 5-31. Frequency Perturbation for Normal and Disordered Voices

Disorder	Measure	Sex	No. of Subj.	Age Mean	Age S.D. or Range	Normal Mean	Normal S.D. or Range	Disorder Mean	Disorder S.D. or Range	Source*
Hoarse	PVI	M	20+20	Adult		0.4807	0.1216	0.8295	0.4783	1
Tumor	DPF	M	5	63.8	55–71	58.5%	45.8–65.3	64.5%	55.4–76.7	3
	DPF	M	5	65.2	61–69					3
	DPF	M	5	63.2	42–75	33.3%	4.2			2
	JF	M	5	63.8	55–71	0.55%	0.76–1.49	3.79%	0.77–9.71	3
	JF	M	5	65.2	61–69					3
	RAP	M	7	27.7		0.0057	0.00134			4
	RAP	M	1	50				0.00687		4
	RAP	F	2	29.5		0.0061	0.00056			4
	RAP	F	1	61				0.2022%		4
Paralysis	RAP	M/F	15?	Adult				0.0176		5
	RAP	M/F	15?	Adult				0.0125		5
	RAP	M	2	49.5				0.0452	0.0537	4
Nodules	RAP	M/F	10	10	6.1–11.5	8.5		0.0123	.0023–.0472	9
	RAP	M	2	54.5				0.0084	0.00049	4
	JR	M/F	10	45.3	16–72	5.00 (μs)	1.78	9.26 (μs)	3.83	8
	DLT	M/F	10	45.3	16–72	21.71 (μs)	11.99	35.76 (μs)	12.55	8
Inflamed	RAP	F	2	36				0.0074	0.00064	4
Esophageal	PF	M	22	58	36–81			41.1%	8.9–66.8	6
	JR	?	9	?				95.47		7

PVI = period variability index, DPF = directional perturbation factor, JF = jitter factor, RAP = relative average perturbation, PF = perturbation factor, JR = jitter ratio, DLT = deviation from linear trend.

*Sources:

1. Deal and Emanuel, 1978. Based on samples collected by Sansone and Emanuel (1970) from normal, and Hanson (1969) from hoarse, speakers. Analysis of narrow-band (10Hz) filtered first harmonic. Normal and hoarse speakers were significantly different, except for /a/.
2. Hecker and Kreul, 1971. One sentence of the Rainbow Passage. Tumors were malignant.
3. Murry and Doherty, 1980. At least 2 s of sustained /a/. DPF was a better discriminator of cancer cases than JF, but the authors caution about generalizing the data.
4. Takahashi and Koike, 1975. Sample of 1.5 s from ost stable portion of sustained /a/ at comfortable pitch and loudness. Mean computed from data processed in article; categories of disorder not as in original publication.
5. Koike, 1973. Thirty-two cycles of steady-state portion of sustained /a/.
6. Hoops and Noll, 1969. Special form of perturbation factor: percentage of observed perturbations greater than *1.0 ms*. First paragraph of Rainbow Passage.
7. Smith, Weinberg, Feth, and Horii, 1978. One s segment of least variable production of /a/ for each subject.
8. Ludlow, Coulter, and Gentges, 1983.
9. Kane and Wellen, 1985. School children. 5 s production of /a/ following two practice trials. Analyzed by protocol of Davis (1976).

185

A

B

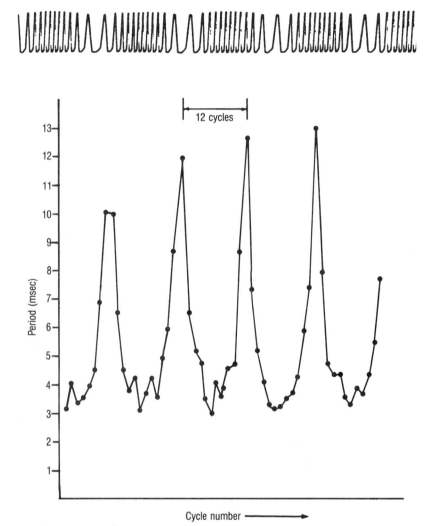

FIGURE 5-28. (A) Cyclic change of fundamental frequency. The perturbing influence changes across an interval of 12 cycles. (B) Period values for the waves of Fig. 5-28A. The plot indicates quite clearly that the perturbation repeats every 12 cycles.

ity of perturbation'' in the jitter data.

A simple way of doing this is to plot the duration of each period, as in Figure 5-28B. It becomes quite clear from the graph that the frequency perturbation varies cyclically over a number of periods. If this were an actual speech signal, one could conclude that there was a regular perturbing influence at work—perhaps a tremor. While graphing periods is a perfectly valid way of probing for perturbational periodicity, it is a tedious and time-consuming process, especially if the cyclicity extends over many fundamental periods. If a programmable calculator or microcomputer is available, serial correlation techniques provide a more sensitive and efficient way.

The *correlation coefficient* is a measure of how precisely the change in one variable mirrors the change in another. A correlation coefficient of 1.00 indicates a perfect relationship, implying that if one factor increases, the other must increase by an exactly proportional amount. If, on the other hand, the correlation coefficient is 0 there is no relationship at all between the two sets of numbers. The correlation coefficient (symbolized r) can be positive, indicating direct proportionality (x ∝ y) or negative, indicating inverse proportionality (x ∝ 1/y). Some feel for the correlation coefficient can be acquired by examining Table 5-32, in which various data on six hypothetical men are correlated. In A, age in years is matched with age in months. Obviously, these two data sets must be perfectly correlated, since age in months is exactly equal to age in years times 12. The perfection of the relationship is shown in the correlation coefficient of + 1.00. Data set B compares heights and weights. One would expect a relationship between the two, but not a perfect one. (Tall men can be very thin and weigh less than their short, fat fellows.) The correlation coefficient of + .90 reflects this. It can be taken to mean that weight is closely, but not perfectly, related to height; other variables enter into the relationship between the two. Lastly, mean SF_o is correlated to bank balance. The correlation coefficient of 0.00 demonstrates a total absence of relationship here.

Another look at Figure 5-28 shows how the correlation coefficient can be of help in finding perturbational periodicity. Because the perturbation pattern repeats (in this case) every 12 cycles, the period of any given wave should more closely match that of a wave 12 cycles (or a multiple of 12 cycles) away than any other. In fact, ideally, the correlation between wave and another one 12 cycles away should be perfect (r = + 1.00), but the correlation should be less with a wave any other distance (not a multiple of 12 waves) away. Therefore, one can determine the correlation of each wave with the one following it (P_i with P_{i+1}), then of each wave with the one two cycles away (P_i with P_{i+2}), then three away (P_i with P_{i+3}), and so on, trying to find the distance at which the correlation coefficient is maximal. The distance between the cycles being correlated is called the *lag*. The lag at which a maximum r is found indicates the number of cycles of the perturbational periodicity. The magnitude of the maximal r shows how much of the perturbation the

TABLE 5-32. Relationships Between Various Sets of Data

Subj. No.	Age (yr)	Age (mo)
1	21.3	255.6
2	37.1	445.2
3	19.8	237.6
4	47.0	564.0
5	33.5	402.0
6	25.8	309.6
Correlation coefficient: r = + 1.00		

Subj. No.	Height (inches)	Weight (lbs)
1	68	157
2	70	155
3	65	135
4	74	167
5	69	151
6	70	161
Correlation coefficient: r = + 0.90		

Subj. No.	SF_o (Hz)	Bank Balance ($)
1	120	1133
2	111	1279
3	106	981
4	115	109
5	98	401
6	107	2521
Correlation coefficient: r = 0.00		

cyclic variation accounts for. The entire process is known as serial correlation, and the change in r across lags is the serial correlation function. The serial correlation technique has been applied to the wave train of Figure 5-28, and the results shown in Figure 5-29. Note how the serial correlation function peaks at a lag of 12.

The calculation of the serial correlation function is done according to the following formulae (Koike, 1969; Iwata, 1972):

$$r_k = \frac{1}{n-k} \sum_{i=1}^{n-k} \frac{P_i P_{i+k} - \bar{P}_1 \bar{P}_2}{S_1 S_2}$$

where: $P_1, P_2, P_3, \ldots, P_i$ = successive period values

n = the number of values in the entire series

k = lag (distance in cycles between waves being correlated)

SELECT BIBLIOGRAPHY

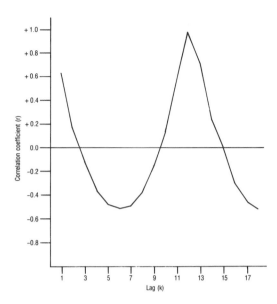

FIGURE 5-29. Serial correlation function for the wavetrain of Figure 5-28.

$$\bar{P}_1 = \sum_{i=1}^{n-k} P_i/(n-k)$$

$$\bar{P}_2 = \sum_{i=k+1}^{n} P_i/(n-k)$$

$$S_1 = \sqrt{\sum_{i=1}^{n-k} \frac{(P_i - \bar{P}_i)^2}{n-k}}$$

$$S_2 = \sqrt{\sum_{i=k+1}^{n} \frac{(P_i - \bar{P}_i)^2}{n-k}}$$

Iwata and von Leden (1970) and Iwata (1972) have presented evidence that different serial correlation functions may be associated with different kinds of laryngeal pathologies, although there are no definitive findings as yet. Koike (1969) also found intensity modulation in pathologic voices.

It is true that determination of the serial correlation function involves a lot of tedious arithmetic. But it is an excellent means of detecting vocal tremor, tissue mass resonance phenomena, and the like. As microcomputers become more widely available to clinicians this technique will have increasing promise. ∎

Anderson, S. H. Design and calibration of a phonodeik. *Journal of the Optical Society of America,* 11 (1925) 31-44.

Askenfelt, A., Gauffin, J., Sundberg, J., and Kitzing, P. A comparison of contact microphone and electroglottograph for the measurement of vocal fundamental frequency. *Journal of Speech and Hearing Research,* 23 (1980) 258-273.

Beckett, R. L. Pitch perturbation as a function of subjective vocal constriction. *Folia Phoniatrica,* 21 (1969) 416-425.

Benda, C. *Mongolism and Cretinism.* New York: Grune and Stratton, 1949.

Bennett, S. A 3-year longitudinal study of school-aged children's fundamental frequencies. *Journal of Speech and Hearing Research,* 26 (1983) 137-142.

Black, J. W. Natural frequency, duration, and intensity of vowels in reading. *Journal of Speech and Hearing Disorders,* 14 (1949) 216-221.

Blood, G. W. Fundamental frequency and intensity measurements in laryngeal and alaryngeal speakers. *Journal of Communication Disorders,* 17 (1984) 319-324.

Boone, D. R. *The Voice and Voice Therapy.* Englewood Cliffs, N. J.: Prentice-Hall, 1971.

Boothroyd, A. and Decker, M. Control of voice pitch by the deaf: an experiment using a visible speech device. *Audiology,* 11 (1972) 343-353.

Bowler, N. W. A fundamental frequency analysis of harsh vocal quality. *Speech Monographs,* 31 (1964) 128-134.

Brodnitz, F. S. *Vocal Rehabilitation.* Rochester, MN: American Academy of Ophthalmology and Otolaryngology, 1961.

Bryngelson, B. A photophonographic analysis of the vocal disturbances in stuttering. *Psychological Monographs,* 43 (1932) 1-30.

Canter, G. J. Speech characteristics of patients with Parkinson's disease: II. Physiological support for speech. *Journal of Speech and Hearing Disorders,* 30 (1965a) 44-49.

Canter, G. J. Speech characteristics of patients with Parkinson's disease: III. Articulation, diadochokinesis, and overall speech adequacy. *Journal of Speech and Hearing Research,* 30 (1965b) 217-224.

Cavallo, S. A., Baken, R. J., and Shaiman, S. Frequency perturbation characteristics of pulse-register phonation. *Journal of Communication Disorders,* 17 (1984) 231-243.

Chevrie-Muller, C., Dodart, F., Sequier-Dermer, N., and Salmon, D. Etudes des paramètres acoustiques de la parole au cours de la schizophrénie de l'adolescent. *Folia Phoniatrica,* 23 (1971) 401-428.

Coleman, R. F. Effect of waveform changes upon roughness perception. *Folia Phoniatrica*, 23 (1971) 314-322.

Coleman, R. F. and Wendahl, R. W. On the validity of laryngeal photosensor monitoring. *Journal of the Acoustical Society of America*, 44 (1968) 1733-1735.

Colton, R. H. and Steinschneider, A. Acoustic relationships of infant cries to the Sudden Infant Death syndrome. In Murry, T. and Murry, J. (Eds.). *Infant Communication: Cry and Early Speech*. Houston: College-Hill, 1980. Pp. 183-208.

Colton, R. H. and Steinschneider, A. The cry characteristics of an infant who died of the Suddent Infant Death syndrome. *Journal of Speech and Hearing Disorders*, 46 (1981) 359-363.

Cooley, J. W. and Tukey, J. W. An algorithm for the machine calculation of complex Fourier series. *Mathematics of Computation*, 19 (1965) 297-301.

Cooper, M. Modern techniques of vocal rehabilitation for functional and organic dysphonias. In Travis, L. E. (Ed.). *Handbook of Speech Pathology and Audiology*. Englewood Cliffs, N. J.: Prentice-Hall, 1971. Chap. 23, pp. 585-616.

Croatto, L. and Ferrero, F. L'esame elettroglottografico applicato ad alcuni case di disodia. *Acta Phoniatrica Latina*, 1 (1979) 247-258.

Curry, E. T. The pitch characteristics of the adolsecent male voice. *Speech Monographs*, 7 (1940) 48-62.

Curry, E. T. Frequency measurement and pitch perception inesophageal speech. In Snidecor, J. C. (Ed.). *Speech Rehabilitation of the Laryngectomized*. Springfield IL: Thomas, 1962. Chap. 5, pp. 85-93.

Curry, E. T. and Snidecor, J. C. Physical measurement and pitch perception in esophageal speech. *Laryngoscope*, 71 (1961) 415-423.

Davis, S. B. Computer evaluation of laryngeal pathology based on inverse filtering of speech. (*SCRL Monograph no. 13*) Santa Barbara, CA: Speech Communications Research Lab, 1976.

Davis, S. B. Acoustic characteristics of normal and pathological voices. In Lass, N. J. (Ed.). *Speech and Language: Advances in Basic Research and Practice*, vol. 1. New York Academic Press, 1979. Pp. 271-335. Reprinted in: Ludlow, C. L. and Hart, M. O. (Eds.). *Proceedings of the Conference on the Assessment of Vocal Pathology*. ASHA Reports, 11 (1981) 97-115.

Deal, R. E. and Emanuel, F. W. Some waveform and spectral features of vowel roughness. *Journal of Speech and Hearing Research*, 21 (1978) 250-264.

Dempsey, M. E., Draegert, G. L., Siskind, R. P., and Steer, M. D. The Purdue pitch meter — a direct-reading fundamental frequency analyzer. *Journal of Speech and Hearing Disorders*, 15 (1950) 135-141.

Dunker, E. and Schlosshauer, B. Unregelmässige Stimmlippenschwingungen bei funktionellen Stimmstörungen. *Zeitschrift für Laryngologie und Rhinologie*, 40 (1961) 919-934.

Emanuel, F. W. and Austin, D. Identification of normal and abnormally rough vowels by spectral noise level measurements. *Journal of Communication Disorders*, 14 (1981) 75-85.

Emanuel, F. W., Lively, M. A., and McCoy, J. F. Spectral noise levels and roughness severity ratings for vowels produced by males and females. *Folia Phoniatrica*, 25 (1973) 110-120.

Emanuel, F. and Scarinzi, A. Vocal register effects on vowel spectral noise and roughness: Findings for adult females. *Journal of Communication Disorders*, 12 (1979) 263-272.

Emanuel, F. and Scarinzi, A. Vocal register effects on vowel spectral noise and roughness: findings for adult males. *Journal of Communication Disorders*, 13 (1980) 121-131.

Fairbanks, G. Recent experimental investigations of vocal pitch in speech. *Journal of the Acoustical Society of America*, 11 (1940) 457-466.

Fairbanks, G. An acoustical study of the pitch of infant hunger wails. *Child Development*, 13 (1942) 227-232.

Fairbanks, G. *Voice and Articulation Drillbook*. New York: Harper and Bros., 1960.

Fairbanks, G., Herbert, E. L., and Hammond, J. M. An acoustical study of vocal pitch in seven- and eight-year-old girls. *Child Development*, 20 (1949) 63-69.

Fairbanks, G., Wiley, John H., and Lassman, F. M. An acoustical study of vocal pitch in seven and eight-year-old boys. *Child Development*, 20 (1949) 63-69.

Fishman, B. V. and Shipp, T. Subject positioning and phonation range measures. *Journal of the Acoustical Society of America*, 48 (1970) 431-432.

Fisichelli, V. R., Haber, A., Davis, J., and Karelitz, S. Audible characteristics of the cries of normal infants and those with Down's syndrome. *Perceptual and Motor Skills*, 23 (1966) 744.

Fisichelli, V. R. and Karelitz, S. Frequency spectra of the cries of normal infants and those with Down's syndrome. *Psychometric Science*, 6 (1966) 195-196.

Fisichelli, V. R., Karelitz, S., Eichbauer, J., and Rosenfeld, L. S. Volume-unit graphs: their production and applicability in studies of infants' cries. *Journal of Psychology*, 52 (1961) 423-427.

Fitch, J. L. and Holbrook, A. Modal vocal fundamental frequency of young adults. *Archives of Otolaryngology*, 92 (1970) 379-382.

Flatau, T. S. and Gutzmann, H. Die Stimme des Säuglings. *Archiv für Laryngologie und Rhinologie*, 18 (1906) 139-151.

Fletcher, H. Loudness, pitch, and the timbre of musical tones and their relation to the intensity, the frequency, and the overtone structure. *Journal of the Acoustical Society of America*, 6 (1934) 59-69.

Fletcher, H. and Munson, W. A. Loudness, its definition, measurement, and calculation. *Journal of the Acoustical Society of America*, 5 (1933) 82-108.

Fletcher, S. G. *Diagnosing Speech Disorders from Cleft Palate*. New York: Grune and Stratton, 1971.

Fourcin, A. J. Laryngographic examination of vocal fold vibration. In Wyke, B. (Ed.). *Ventilatory and Phonatory Control Systems*. New York: Oxford, 1974. Pp. 315-333.

Fourcin, A. J. and Abberton, E. First applications of a new laryngograph. *Medical and Biological Illustration*, 21 (1971) 172-182. Reprinted in: *Volta Review*, 74 (1972) 161-176.

Fourcin, A. J. and Abberton, E. The laryngograph and the voiscope in speech therapy. *Proceedings of the XVI International Congress of Logopedics and Phoniatrics*, 1976. Pp. 116-122.

Fritzell, B., Sundberg, J., and Strange-Ebbesen, A. Pitch change after stripping oedematous vocal folds. *Folia Phoniatrica*, 34 (1982) 29-32.

Gilbert, H. R. Speech characteristics of miners with black lung disease (pneumoconiosis). *Journal of Communication Disorders*, 8 (1975) 129-140.

Gilbert, H. R. and Campbell, M. I. Speaking fundamental frequency in three groups of hearing-impaired individuals. *Journal of Communication Disorders*, 13 (1980) 195-205.

Gold, B. Computer program for pitch extraction. *Journal of the Acoustical Society of America*, 34 (1962) 916-921.

Gold, B. and Rabiner, L. Parallel processing techniques for estimating pitch periods of speech in the time domain. *Journal of the Acoustical Society of America*, 46 (1969) 442-448.

Goldstein, J. L. An optimum processor for the central formation of pitch of complex tones. *Journal of the Acoustical Society of America*, 54 (1973) 1496-1516.

Gruenz, 0. 0., Jr. and Schott, L. 0. Extraction and portrayal of pitch of speech sounds. *Journal of the Acoustical Society of America*, 21 (1949) 487-495.

Hammarberg, B., Fritzell, G., Gauffin, J., Sundberg, J., and Wedin, L. Perceptual and acoustic correlates of abnormal voice qualities. *Acta Otolaryngologica*, 90 (1980) 441-451.

Hanley, T. D. and Peters, R. The speech and hearing laboratory. In Travis, L. E. (Ed.). *Handbook of Speech Pathology and Audiology*. Englewood Cliffs, N.J.: Prentice-Hall, 1971. Chap. 5, pp. 75-140.

Hanson, W. Vowel spectral noise levels and roughness severity ratings for vowels and sentences produced by adult males presenting abnormally rough voice. Unpublished doctoral dissertation, University of Oklahoma, 1969.

Hartmann, E. and von Cramon, D. Acoustic measurement of voice quality in central dysphonia. *Journal of Communication Disorders*, 17 (1984) 425-440.

Healey, E. C. Speaking fundamental frequency characteristics of stutterers and nonstutterers. *Journal of Communication Disorders*, 15 (1982) 21-29.

Hecker, M. H. L. and Kreul, E. J. Descriptions of the speech of patients with cancer of the vocal folds. Part I: measures of fundamental frequency. *Journal of the Acoustical Society of America*, 49 (1971) 1275-1282.

Hencke, W. L. Signals from external accelerometers during phonation: attributes and their internal physical correlates. *MIT Research Laboratory of Electronics Quarterly Progress Report*, 114 (1974a) 224-231.

Hencke, W. L. Display and interpretation of glottal activity as transduced by external accelerometers. *Journal of the Acoustical Society of America*, 55 (1974b) S79A.

Hixon, T. J., Klatt, D. H., and Mead, J. Influence of forced transglottal pressure changes on vocal fundamental frequency. *Journal of the Acoustical Society of America*, 49 (1971) 105.

Hollien, H. On vocal registers. *Journal of Phonetics*, 2 (1974) 125-143.

Hollien, H. and Copeland, R. H. Speaking fundamental frequency (SFF) characteristics of mongoloid girls. *Journal of Speech and Hearing Disorders*, 30 (1965) 344-349.

Hollien, H., Dew, D., and Philips, P. Phonational frequency ranges of adults. *Journal of Speech and Hearing Research*, 14 (1971) 755-760.

Hollien, H., Girard, G. T., and Coleman, R. F. Vocal fold vibratory patterns of pulse register phonation. *Folia Phoniatrica*, 29 (1977) 200-205.

Hollien, H. and Jackson, B. Normative data on the speaking fundamental characteristics of young adult males. *Journal of Phonetics*, 1 (1973) 117-120.

Hollien, H. and Malcik, E. Adolescent voice change in southern Negro males. *Speech Monographs*, 29 (1962) 53-58.

Hollien, H. and Malcik, E. Evaluation of cross-sectional studies of adolescent voice change in males. *Speech Monographs*, 34 (1967) 80-84.

Hollien, H., Malcik, E., and Hollien, B. Adolescent voice change in southern white males. *Speech Monographs*, 32 (1965) 87-90.

Hollien, H. and Michel, J. F. Vocal fry as a phonational register. *Journal of Speech and Hearing Research*. 11 (1968) 600-604.

Hollien, H., Michel, J., and Doherty, E. T. A

method for analyzing vocal jitter in sustained phonation. *Journal of Phonetics*, 1 (1973) 85-91.

Hollien, H., Moore, P., Wendahl, R. W., and Michel, J. F. On the nature of vocal fry. *Journal of Speech and Hearing Research*, 9 (1966) 245-247.

Hollien, H. and Paul, P. A second evaluation of the speaking fundamental frequency characteristics of post-adolescent girls. *Language and Speech*, 12 (1969) 119-124.

Hollien, H. and Shipp, T. Speaking fundamental frequency and chronologic age in males. *Journal of Speech and Hearing Research*, 15 (1972) 155-159.

Hollien, H. and Wendahl, R. W. A perceptual study of vocal fry. *Journal of the Acoustical Society of America*, 43 (1968) 506-509.

Honjo, I. and Isshiki, N. Laryngoscopic and voice characteristics of aged persons. *Archives of Otolaryngology*, 106 (1980) 149-150.

Hoops, H. R. and Noll, J. D. Relationship of selected acoustic variables to judgments of esophageal speech. *Journal of Communication Disorders*, 2 (1969) 1-13.

Horii, Y. Some statistical characteristics of voice fundamental frequency. *Journal of Speech and Hearing Research*, 18 (1975) 192-201.

Horii, Y. Fundamental frequency perturbation observed in sustained phonation. *Journal of Speech and Hearing Research*, 22 (1979) 5-19.

Horii, Y. Vocal shimmer in sustained phonation. *Journal of Speech and Hearing Research*, 23 (1980) 202-209.

Horii, Y. Jitter and shimmer differences among sustained vowel phonations. *Journal of Speech and Hearing Research*, 25 (1982) 12-14.

Horii, Y. Automatic analysis of voice fundamental frequency and intensity using a Visipitch. *Journal of Speech and Hearing Research*, 26 (1983a) 467-471.

Horii, Y. Some acoustic characteristics of oral reading by ten-to twelve-year-old children. *Journal of Communication Disorders*, 16 (1983b) 257-267.

Horii, Y. Jitter and shimmer in sustained vocal fry phonation. *Folia Phoniatrica*, 37 (1985) 81-86.

Houtsma, A. J. and Goldstein, J. L. The central origin of the pitch of complex tones: evidence from musical interval recognition. *Journal of the Acoustical Society of America*, 51 (1972) 520-529.

Hudson, A. and Holbrook, A. A study of the reading fundamental vocal frequency of young adult males. *Journal of Speech and Hearing Research*, 24 (1981) 197-201.

Hudson, A. and Holbrook, A. Fundamental frequency characteristics of young Black adults: spontaneous speaking and oral reading. *Journal of Speech and Hearing Research*, 25 (1982) 25-28.

Hufnagle, J. and Hufnagle, K. An investigation of the relationship between speaking fundamental frequency and vocal quality improvement. *Journal of Communication Disorders*, 17 (1984) 95-100.

Huttar, G. L. Relations between prosodic variables and emotions in normal American English utterances. *Journal of Speech and Hearing Research*, 11 (1968) 481-487.

Isshiki, N., Yanagihara, N., and Morimoto, M. Approach to the objective diagnosis of hoarseness. *Folia Phoniatrica*, 18 (1966) 393-400.

Iwata, S. Periodicities of pitch perturbations in normal and pathologic larynges. *Laryngoscope*, 82 (1972) 87-95.

Iwata, S. and von Leden, H. Pitch perturbations in normal and pathological voices. *Folia Phoniatrica*, 22 (1970) 413-424.

Izdebski, K. and Murry, T. Glottal waveform variability: a preliminary inquiry. In Lawrence, V. and Weinberg, B. (Eds.). *Transcripts of the Ninth Symposium: Care of the Professional Voice*, vol. 1. New York: The Voice Foundation, 1980. Pp. 39-43.

Jacob, L. A normative study of laryngeal jitter. Unpublished masters thesis, University of Kansas, 1968.

Johnson, K. W. and Michel, J. F. The effect of selected vowels on laryngeal jitter. *Asha*, 11 (1969) 96.

Kane, M. and Wellen, C. J. Acoustical measurements and clinical judgments of vocal quality in children with vocal nodules. *Folia Phoniatrica*, 37 (1985) 53-57.

Karelitz, S. and Fisichelli, V. R. The cry thresholds of normal infants and those with brain damage. *Journal of Pediatrics*, 61 (1962) 679-685.

Karelitz, S. and Fisichelli, V. R. Infants' vocalizations and their significance. *Clinical Proceedings of the Children's Hospital*, 25 (1969) 345-361.

Karelitz, S., Fisichelli, V. R., Costa, J., Karelitz, R., and Rosenfeld, L. Relation of crying activity in early infancy to speech and intellectual development at age three years. *Child Development*, 35 (1964) 769-777.

Keating, P. and Buhr, R. Fundamental frequency in the speech of infants and children. *Journal of the Acoustical Society of America*, 63 (1978) 567-571.

Kelly, D. H. and Sansone, F. E. Clinical estimation of fundamental frequency: the 3M plastiform magnetic tape viewer. *Journal of Communication Disorders*, 14 (1981) 123-125.

Kitajima, K., Tanabe, M., and Isshiki, N. Pitch perturbation in normal and pathological voice. *Studia Phonologica*, 9 (1975) 25-32.

Kitzing, P. and Sonesson, B. A photoglottographical study of the female vocal folds during phonation. *Folia Phoniatrica*, 26 (1974) 138-149.

Klingholz, F. and Martin, F. Speech wave aperiodicities at sustained phonation in functional dysphonia. *Folia Phoniatrica*, 35 (1983) 322-327.

Klingholz, F. and Martin, F. Quantitative spectral evaluation of shimmer and jitter. *Journal of Speech and Hearing Research*, 28 (1985) 169-174.

Koike, Y. Application of some acoustic measures for the evaluation of laryngeal dysfunction. *Journal of the Acoustical Society of America*, 42 (1967) 1209.

Koike, Y. Vowel amplitude modulations in patients with laryngeal diseases. *Journal of the Acoustical Society of America*, 45 (1969) 839-844.

Koike, Y. Application of some acoustic measures for the evaluation of laryngeal dysfunction. *Studia Phonologica*, 7 (1973) 17-23.

Koike, Y. and Markel, J. Application of inverse filtering for detecting laryngeal pathology. *Annals of Otology, Rhinology, and Laryngology*, 84 (1975) 117-124.

Koike, Y., Takahashi, H., and Calcaterra, T. C. Acoustic measures for detecting laryngeal pathology. *Acta Otolaryngologica*, 84 (1977) 105-117.

Kyttä, J. Spectrographic studies of the sound quality of oesophageal speech. *Acta Otolaryngologica* Suppl. 188 (1964) 371-377.

Ladefoged, P. and McKinney, N. P. Loudness, sound pressure, and subglottal pressure in speech. *Journal of the Acoustical Society of America*, 35 (1963) 454-460.

Laguaite, J. K. and Waldrop, W. F. Acoustic analysis of fundamental frequency of voices before and after therapy. *Folia Phoniatrica*, 16 (1964) 183-192.

Laufer, M. Z. and Horii, Y. Fundamental frequency characteristics of infant non-distress vocalization during the first twenty-four weeks. *Journal of Child Language*, 4 (1977) 171-184.

Lebrun, Y., Devreux, F., Rousseau, J.-J., and Darimont, P. Tremulous speech: a case report. *Folia Phoniatrica*, 34 (1982) 134-142.

Lecluse, F. L. E., Brocaar, P.M., and Verschuure, J. The electroglottography and its relation to glottal activity. *Folia Phoniatrica*, 27 (1975) 215-224.

Leeper, H. and Leeper, G. Clinical evaluation of the fundamental frequency of normal children and children with vocal nodules employing a striation counting procedure. Paper presented at the annual convention of the ASHA, 1976.

Licklider, J. C. R. Basic correlates of the auditory stimulus. In Stevens, S. S. (Ed.). *Handbook of Experimental Psychology*. New York: Wiley, 1951. Chap. 25, pp. 985-1039.

Lieberman, P. Perturbations in vocal pitch. *Journal of the Acoustical Society of America*, 33 (1961) 597-603.

Lieberman, P. Some acoustic measures of the fundamental periodicity of normal and pathologic larynges. *Journal of the Acoustical Society of America*, 35 (1963) 344-353.

Lieberman, P., Knudson, R. and Mead, J. Determination of the rate of change of fundamental frequency with respect to subglottal pressure during sustained phonation. *Journal of the Acoustical Society of America*, 45 (1969) 1537-1543.

Lieberman, P. and Michaels, S. B. Some aspects of fundamental frequency and envelope amplitude as related to the emotional content of speech. *Journal of the Acoustical Society of America*, 34 (1962) 922-927.

Lind, J. (Ed.). *Newborn Infant Cry*. Uppsala: Almqvist and Wiksells, 1965.

Linke, C. E. A study of pitch characteristics of female voices and their relationship to vocal effectiveness. *Folia Phoniatrica*, 25 (1973) 173-185.

Lisker, L., Abramson, A. S., Cooper, F. S., and Schvey, M. H. Transillumination of the larynx in running speech. *Journal of the Acoustical Society of America*, 45 (1966) 1544-1546.

Luchsinger, R. and Arnold, G. *Voice-Speech-Language*. Belmont, CA: Wadsworth Publishing Co., 1965.

Ludlow, C., Coulter, D., and Gentges, F. The differential sensitivity of measures of fundamental frequency perturbation to laryngeal neoplasms and neuropathologies. In Bless, D. M. and Abbs, J. H. (Eds.). *Vocal Fold Physiology: Contemporary Research and Clinical Issues*. San Diego: College-Hill, 1983. Chap. 33, Pp. 381-392.

Martin, P. Extraction de la fréquence fondamentale par intercorrélation avec une fonction peigne. *Dixièmes Journées d'Etude sur la Parole*, 1981, Pp. 221-232.

Martony, J. On the correction of voice pitch level for severely hard of hearing subjects. *American Annals of the Deaf*, 113 (1968) 195-202.

McGlone, R. E. and Brown, W. S., Jr. Identification of the "shift" between vocal registers. *Journal of the Acoustical Society of America*, 46 (1969) 1033-1036.

McGlone, R. E. and Hollien, H. Vocal pitch characteristics of aged women. *Journal of Speech and Hearing Research*, 6 (1963) 164-170.

Metfessel, M. A photographic method of measuring pitch. *Science*, 68 (1928) 430-432.

Michel, J. F. Fundamental frequency investigation of vocal fry and harshness. *Journal of Speech and Hearing Research*, 11 (1968) 590-594.

Michel, J. F. and Carney, R. J. Pitch characteristics of mongoloid boys. *Journal of Speech and Hearing Disorders*, 29 (1964) 121-125.

Michel, J. F. and Hollien, H. Perceptual differentiation in vocal fry and harshness. *Journal of Speech and Hearing Research*, 11 (1968) 439-443.

Michel, J. F., Hollien, H., and Moore, P. Speaking fundamental frequency characteristics of 15, 16, and 17 year-old girls. *Language and Speech*, 9 (1966) 46-51.

Michel, J. F. and Wendahl, R. Correlates of voice production. In Travis, L. E. (Ed.). *Handbook of Speech Pathology and Audiology*. Englewood Cliffs, NJ: Prentice-Hall, 1971. Chap. 18, pp. 465-480.

Michelsson, K. and Wasz-Höckert, 0. The value of cry analysis in neonatology and early infancy. In Murry, T. and Murry, J. (Eds.). *Infant Communication: Cry and Early Speech*. Houston: College-Hill, 1980. Pp. 152-182.

Miller, R. L. Nature of the vocal cord wave. *Journal of the Acoustical Society of America*, 31 (1959) 667-677.

Miller, J. E. and Mathews, M. V. Investigation of the glottal waveshape by automatic inverse filtering. *Journal of the Acoustical Society of America*, 35 (1963) 1876.

Montague, J. C., Jr., Brown, W. S., Jr., and Hollien, H. Vocal fundamental frequency characteristics of institutionalized Down's syndrome children. *American Journal of Mental Deficiency*, 78 (1974) 414-418.

Montague, J. C., Jr., Hollien, H., Hollien, P. A., and Wold, D. C. Perceived pitch and fundamental frequency comparisons of institutionalized Down's syndrome children. *Folia Phoniatrica*, 30 (1978) 245-256.

Moore, G. P. Voice disorders organically based. In Travis, L. E. (Ed.). *Handbook of Speech Pathology and Audiology*. Englewood Cliffs, NJ: Prentice-Hall, 1971. Chap. 21, pp. 535-569.

Moore, P. and Thompson, C. L. Comments on physiology of hoarseness. *Archives of Otolaryngology*, 81 (1965) 97-102.

Moore, P. and von Leden, H. Dynamic variations of the vibratory pattern in the normal larynx. *Folia Phoniatrica*, 10 (1958) 205-238.

Mörner, M., Fransson, F., and Fant, G. Voice register terminology and standard pitch. *Speech Transmission Laboratory Quarterly Status and Progress Report*, 4/1963, 17-23.

Mueller, P. B., Adams, M., Baehr-Rouse, J., and Boos, D. A. A tape striation counting method for determining fundamental frequency. *Language, Speech, and Hearing Services in Schools*, 10 (1979) 246-248.

Muller, E., Hollien, H., and Murry, T. Perceptual responses to infant crying: identification of cry types. *Journal of Child Language*, 1 (1974) 89-95.

Murry, T. Subglottal pressure and airflow measures during vocal fry phonation. *Journal of Speech and Hearing Research*, 14 (1971) 544-551.

Murry, T. Speaking fundamental frequency characteristics associated with voice pathologies. *Journal of Speech and Hearing Disorders*, 43 (1978) 374-379.

Murry, T., Amundson, P., and Hollien, H. Acoustical characteristics of infant cries: fundamental frequency. *Journal of Child Language*, 4 (1977) 321-328.

Murry, T. and Doherty, E. T. Selected acoustic characteristics of pathologic and normal speakers. *Journal of Speech and Hearing Research*, 23 (1980) 361-369.

Murry, T., Gracco, V. L., and Gracco, L. C. Infant vocalization during the first twelve weeks. Paper presented at the annual convention of the ASHA, 1979.

Murry, T., Hoit-Dalgaard, J., and Gracco, V. Infant vocalization: a longitudinal study of acoustic and temporal parameters. *Folia Phoniatrica*, 35 (1983) 245-253.

Murry, T., Hollien, H., and Muller, E. Perceptual responses to infant crying: maternal recognition and sex judgments. *Journal of Child Language*, 2 (1975) 199-204.

Mysak, E. D. Pitch and duration characteristics of older males. *Journal of Speech and Hearing Research*, 2 (1959) 46-54.

Neelley, J., Edison, S., and Carlile, L. Speaking voice fundamental frequency of mentally retarded adults and normal adults. *American Journal of Mental Deficiency*, 72 (1968) 944-947.

Nevlud, G. N., Fann, W. E., and Falck, F. Acoustic parameters of voice and neuroleptic medication. *Biological Psychiatry*, 18 (1983) 1081-1084.

Noll, A. M. Short-term spectrum and "cepstrum" techniques for vocal pitch detection. *Journal of the Acoustical Society of America*, 36 (1964) 296-302.

Noll, A. M. Cepstrum pitch determination. *Journal of the Acoustical Society of America*, 41 (1967) 293-309.

Obata, J. and Kobayashi, R. An apparatus for direct-recording the pitch and intensity of sound. *Journal of the Acoustical Society of America*, 10 (1938) 147-149.

Obata, J. and Kobayashi, R. Further applications of our direct-reading pitch and intensity recorder. *Journal of the Acoustical Society of America*, 12 (1940) 188-192.

Pedersen, M. F., Kitzing, P., Krabbe, S., and Haremb, S. The change of voice during puberty in 11 to 16 years [sic] old choir singers measured with electroglottographic fundamental frequency analysis and compared to other phenomena of puberty. *Acta Otolaryngologica*, Suppl. 386 (1982) 189-192.

Pentz, A. L. Jr. and Gilbert, H. R. Relation of selected acoustic parameters and perceptual ratings to voice quality of Down syndrome children. *American Journal of Mental Deficiency*, 88 (1983) 203-210.

Petrovich-Bartell, N., Cowan, N., and Morse, P. A. Mothers' perception of infant distress vocalizations. *Journal of Speech and Hearing Research*, 25 (1982) 371-376.

Perkins, W. H. Vocal function: assessment and therapy. In Travis, L. E. (Ed.). *Handbook of Speech Pathology and Audiology*. Englewood Cliffs, NJ: Prentice-Hall, 1971a. Chap. 20, pp. 505-534.

Perkins, W. H. *Speech Pathology*. St. Louis: Mosby, 1971b.

Prescott, R. Infant cry sound: developmental features. *Journal of the Acoustical Society of America*, 57 (1975) 1186-1191.

Pronovost, W. An experimental study of methods for determining the natural and habitual pitch. *Speech Monographs*, 9 (1942) 111-123.

Ptacek, P. H., Sander, E. K., Maloney, W. H., and Jackson, C. C. R. Phonatory and related changes with advanced age. *Journal of Speech and Hearing Research*, 9 (1966) 353-360.

Ramig, L. A. and Ringel, R. L. Effects of physiological aging on selected acoustic characteristics of voice. *Journal of Speech and Hearing Research*, 26 (1983) 22-30.

Randall, R. B. and Hee, J. Cepstrum analysis. *Brüel and Kjaer Technical Review*, 1981 no. 3, 3-40.

Riesz, R. R. and Schott, L. Visible speech cathode-ray translator. *Journal of the Acoustical Society of America*, 18 (1946) 50-61.

Ringel, R. L. and Kluppel, D. D. Neonatal crying: a normative study. *Folia Phoniatrica*, 16 (1964) 1-9.

Robb, M. P. and Saxman, J. H. Developmental trends in vocal fundamental frequency of young children. *Journal of Speech and Hearing Research*, 28 (1985) 421-427.

Robbins, J., Fisher, H., Blom, E., and Singer, M. I. A comparative acoustic study of normal, esophageal, and tracheoesophageal speech production. *Journal of Speech and Hearing Disorders*, 49 (1984) 202-210.

Robbins, J., Fisher, H. B., and Logemann, J. A. Acoustic characteristics of voice production after Staffieri's surgical reconstructive procedure. *Journal of Speech and Hearing Disorders*, 47 (1982) 77-84.

Rothenberg, M. A new inverse-filtering technique for deriving the glottal air flow waveform during voicing. *Journal of the Acoustical Society of America*, 53 (1973) 1632-1645.

Sansone, F. E., jr and Emanuel, F. Spectral noise levels and roughness severity ratings for nor-

mal and simulated rough vowels produced by adult males. *Journal of Speech and Hearing Research*, 13 (1970) 489-502.

Saxman, J. H. and Burk, K. W. Speaking fundamental frequency characteristics of middle-aged females. *Folia Phoniatrica*, 19 (1967) 167-172.

Saxman, J. H. and Burk, K. W. Speaking fundamental frequency and rate characteristics of adult female schizophrenics. *Journal of Speech and Hearing Research*, 11 (1968) 194-203.

Schafer, R. and Rabiner, L. R. System for the automatic formant analysis of voiced speech. *Journal of the Acoustical Society of America*, 47 (1970) 634-648.

Schilling, von A. and Göler, D. V. Zur Frage der Monotonie—Untersuchung beim Stottern. *Folia Phoniatrica*, 13 (1961) 202-218.

Schroeder, M. R. Period histogram and product spectrum: new methods for fundamental frequency measurement. *Journal of the Acoustical Society of America*, 43 (1968) 829-834.

Schultz-Coulon, H.-J., Battmer, R.-D., and Fedders, B. Zur quantitativen Bewertung der Tonhöhenschwankungen Rahmen der Stimmfunktionsprüfung. *Folia Phoniatrica*, 69 (1979) 56-69.

Sheppard, W. C. and Lane, H. L. Development of the prosodic features of infant vocalizing. *Journal of Speech and Hearing Research*, 11 (1968) 94-108.

Shipp, T. Frequency, duration, and perceptual measures in relation to judgments of alaryngeal speech acceptability. *Journal of Speech and Hearing Research*, 10 (1967) 417-427.

Shipp, T. Doherty E. T. and Morrissey, P. Predicting vocal frequency from selected physiologic measures. *Journal of the Acoustical Society of America*, 66 (1979) 678-684.

Shipp, T. and Hollien, H. Perception of the aging male voice. *Journal of Speech and Hearing Research*, 12 (1969) 703-710.

Shipp T. and McGlone R. E. Laryngeal dynamics associated with voice frequency change. *Journal of Speech and Hearing Research*, 14 (1971) 761-768.

Simon, C. The variability of consecutive wavelengths in vocal and instrumental sounds. *Psychological Monographs*, 36 (1927) 41-83.

Smith, B. E., Weinberg, B., Feth, L., and Horii, Y. Vocal roughness and jitter characteristics of vowels produced by esophageal speakers. *Journal of Speech and Hearing Research*, 21 (1978) 240-249.

Smith, S. A valve device for difficult cases of F_o recording. *Folia Phoniatrica*, 20 (1968) 202-206.

Snidecor, J. C. A comparative study of the pitch and duration characteristics of impromptu speaking and oral reading. *Speech Mono-*

graphs, 10 (1943) 50-57.

Snidecor, J. C. The pitch and duration characteristics of superior female speakers during oral reading. *Journal of Speech and Hearing Disorders*, 16 (1951) 44-52.

Snidecor, J. C. and Curry, E. T. Temporal and pitch aspects of superior esophageal speech. *Annals of Otology, Rhinology, and Laryngology*, 68 (1959) 623-629.

Sondhi, M. M. Measurement of the glottal waveform. *Journal of the Acoustical Society of America*, 57 (1975) 228-232.

Sonesson, B. On the anatomy and vibratory pattern of the human vocal folds. *Acta Otolaryngologica*, Suppl. 156 (1960).

Sorensen, D, and Horii, Y. Frequency and amplitude perturbation in the voices of female speakers. *Journal of Communication Disorders*, 16 (1983) 57-61.

Sorensen, D. and Horii, Y. Directional perturbation factors for jitter and for shimmer. *Journal of Communication Disorders*, 17 (1984) 143-151.

Sorensen, D., Horii, Y., and Leonard, R. Effects of laryngeal topical anesthesia on voice fundamental frequency perturbation. *Journal of Speech and Hearing Research*, 23 (1980) 274-283.

Stevens, K. N., Kalikow, D. N., and Willemain, T. R. A miniature accelerometer for detecting glottal waveforms and nasalization. *Journal of Speech and Hearing Research*, 18 (1975) 594-599.

Stevens, S. S. and Volkmann, J. The relation of pitch to frequency: a revised scale. *American Journal of Psychology*, 53 (1940) 329-353.

Stevens, S. S., Volkmann, J., and Newman, E. B. A scale for the measurement of the psychological magnitude pitch. *Journal of the Acoustical Society of America*, 8 (1937) 185-190.

Stoicheff, M. L. Speaking fundamental frequency characteristics of nonsmoking female adults. *Journal of Speech and Hearing Research*, 24 (1981) 437-441.

Stone, R. E., jr and Sharf, D. J. Vocal change associated with the use of atypical pitch and intensity levels. *Folia Phoniatrica*, 25 (1973) 91-103.

Sugimoto, T. and Hiki, S. On the extraction of the pitch signal using the body wall vibration at the throat of the talker. *Proceedings of the Fourth International Congress on Acoustics*, 1962.

Takahashi, H. and Koike, Y. Some perceptual dimensions and acoustical correlates of pathologic voices. *Acta Otolaryngologica*, Suppl. 338 (1975) 1-24.

Timcke, R., von Leden, H., and Moore, P. Laryngeal vibrations: measurements of the glottic wave. Part II: Physiologic variations. *Archives of Otolaryngology*, 69 (1959) 438-444.

Torgerson, J. K. and Martin, D. E. Acoustic and temporal analysis of esophageal speech produced by alaryngeal and laryngeal talkers. *Folia Phoniatrica*, 32 (1980) 315-322.

Travis, L. E. A phono-photographic study of the stutterer's voice and speech. *Psychological Monographs*, 36 (1927) 109-141.

Troughear, R. A note on temporal errors in fundamental frequency perturbation measures for sampled waveforms. *Journal of Speech and Hearing Research*, 25, (1982) 628-630.

Troughear, R. and Davis, P. Real-time microcomputer based voice feature extraction in a speech pathology clinic. *Australian Journal of Human Communication Disorders*, 7 (1979) 4-21.

Vallancien, B. Gautheron, B., Pasternak, L., Guisez, D., and Paley, B. Comparaison des signaux microphoniques, diaphanographiques, et glottographiques, avec application au laryngographe. *Folia Phoniatrica*, 23 (1971) 371-380.

van den Berg, J. and Moolenaar-Bijl, A. J. Cricopharyngeal sphincter, pitch, intensity, and fluency in oesophageal speech. *Practica Oto-Rhino-Laryngologica*, 21 (1959) 298-315.

von Leden, H., Moore, P., and Timcke, R. Laryngeal vibrations: measurements of the glottic wave. Part III: The pathologic larynx. *Archives of Otolaryngology*, 71 (1960) 16-35.

Vuorenkoski, L., Perheentupa, J., Vuorenkoski, V., Lenko, H. L., and Tjernlund, P. Fundamental voice frequency during normal and abnormal growth and after androgen treatment. *Archives of Disease in Childhood*, 53 (1978) 201-209.

Wakita, H. Instrumentation for the study of speech acoustics. In Lass, N. J. (Ed.). *Contemporary Issues in Experimental Phonetics*. New York: Academic Press, 1976. Chap. 1, pp. 3-40.

Wakita, H. Speech analysis and synthesis. In Broad, D. J. (Ed.). *Topics in Speech Science*. Los Angeles: Speech Research Laboratory, 1977. Chap. 3, pp. 69-157.

Wasz-Höckert, O., Lind, J., Vuorenkoski, V., Partanen, T., and Valanne, E. *The Infant Cry: A Spectrographic and Auditory Analysis*. London: Heinemann, 1968.

Wasz-Höckert, O., Partanen, T., Vuorenkoski, V., Valanne, E., and Michelsson, K. Effect of training on the ability to identify specific meanings in newborn and infant vocalizations. *Developmental Medicine and Child Neurology*, 6 (1964a) 393-396.

Wasz-Höckert, O., Partanen, T., Vuorenkoski, V., Valanne, E., and Michelsson, K. The identification of some specific meanings in newborn and infant vocalisation. *Experientia*, 20 (1964b) 154.

Weinberg, B. and Bennett, S. A comparison of the fundamental frequency characteristics of esophageal speech measured on a wave-by-wave and averaging basis. *Journal of Speech and Hearing Research*, 14 (1971) 351-355.

Weinberg, B. and Bennett, S. A study of talker sex identification of esophageal voices. *Journal of Speech and Hearing Research*, 14 (1971) 391-395.

Weinberg, B. and Bennett, S. Selected acoustic characteristics of esophageal speech produced by female laryngectomees. *Journal of Speech and Hearing Research*, 15 (1972) 211-216.

Weinberg, B., Dexter, R., and Horii, Y. Selected speech and fundamental frequency characteristics of patients with acromegaly. *Journal of Speech and Hearing Disorders*, 40 (1975) 253-259.

Weinberg, B. and Zlatin, M. Speaking fundamental frequency characteristics of five- and six-year old children with mongolism. *Journal of Speech and Hearing Research*, 13 (1970) 418-425.

Wendahl, R. W. Laryngeal analog synthesis of harsh voice quality. *Folia Phoniatrica*, 15 (1963) 241-250.

Wendahl, R. W. Some parameters of auditory roughness. *Folia Phoniatrica*, 18 (1966a) 26-32.

Wendahl, R. W. Laryngeal analog synthesis of jitter and shimmer auditory parameters of harshness. *Folia Phoniatrica*, 18 (1966b) 98-108.

Wendahl, R. W., Moore, P., and Hollien, H. Comments on vocal fry. *Folia Phoniatrica*, 15 (1963) 251-255.

West, R. W. and Ansberry, M. *The Rehabilitation of Speech*. New York: Harper and Row, 1968.

Wieser, M. The long-term period measurement, an instrumental method in phoniatry. *Archives of Oto-Rhino-Laryngology*, 226 (1980) 63-72.

Wilcox, K. and Horii, Y. Age and changes in vocal jitter. *Journal of Gerontology*, 35 (1980) 194-198.

Zyski, B. J., Bull, G. L., McDonald, W. E., and Johns, M. E. Perturbation analysis of normal and pathologic larynges. *Folia Phoniatrica*, 36 (1984) 190-198.

CHAPTER **6**

Laryngeal Function

Evaluation of dysphonia and of problems of vocal control must include careful observation of the phonatory actions of the larynx and, in particular, of the vocal folds. Other, more indirect means of assessment, including aerodynamic, spectrographic, and fundamental frequency evaluation provide a great deal of useful information upon which inferences can be based. But in the end the only way to know what the larynx is actually doing is to look at it more or less directly. Laryngeal observation is also the only way to rule out specific structural or functional pathologies.

Typically, this task has been left solely to the laryngologist. Unfortunately, most laryngologists are primarily concerned with tissue pathology or neurological dysfunction The reports they return after laryngeal examination frequently lack clear descriptions of the exact way in which tissue disorders affect vocal fold movement. In cases of "functional" disorder a report of "no visible pathology" is likely to be useless to the vocal rehabilitation specialist. Clearly, in such cases something is not right

about vocal fold action, and it is just that something that the vocal therapist needs to correct.

This is not to denigrate the role of the physician in assessment of vocal disorders. His job is to treat those conditions that require and are amenable to medical or surgical intervention. But it falls to the speech pathologist to remediate abnormal laryngeal functions (perhaps including those that led to tissue pathology in the first place) and, therefore, a separate assessment of laryngeal *behavior* by the vocal therapist is in order. In fact, "brief indirect laryngoscopy without visual documentation [and analysis] is a factor in misdiagnosis of patients with laryngeal disease of central origin" (Ward, Hanson, and Berci, 1981). The need for careful observation is strengthened as our understanding of the relationship of vocal fold action to the final acoustic product improves (Titze and Talkin, 1979; Hirano, 1975; Titze, 1973, 1974; Broad, 1979).

There is a tendency to forego laryngeal observation because of the invasiveness involved. The problems, however, may be overstated. Some procedures are, in fact, invasive and must be performed by a licensed physician. These techniques must nonetheless be well understood by the speech pathologist in order for him or her to be able to interpret the data provided. It is also advisable for the therapist to be present during the laryngeal examination in order to assess for him- or herself any aspects of laryngeal dysfunction that may require correction.

Many examination procedures, however, are not invasive. These can, and should, be part of the vocal therapist's diagnostic armamentarium. What is wanted, in most cases, is an accurate assessment of the behavior of the glottis itself. The needed information can be obtained from what might be termed "glottographic waveforms": changes in any one of a number of variables due to activity at the level of the glottis. Examples of such data include the glottal area function, glottal pressure waveform, glottal volume flow, electrolaryngogram, and vocal fold displacement characteristics. Titze and Talkin (1981) provide a brief, but excellent, overview of the relationships among these.

This chapter explores several techniques currently available for obtaining information about the exact function of the larynx, including photographic, photoelectric, impedance, and acoustic methods. Their value to the therapist lies in their ability to provide a close-up view of the relatively fine details of the movement and contact-patterns of the vocal folds themselves. In other words, these methods offer the means for watching the abnormal activity which, in many cases of dysphonia, is the real target of therapy. For example, in cases of unilateral paralysis the degree to which normal vocal fold is managing compensatory displacement can easily be estimated long before final success results in a clear vocal signal. Thus, progress can be assessed throughout the course of therapy without frequent recourse to a physician. Furthermore, several of the techniques discussed below lend themselves to biofeedback approaches to vocal rehabilitation, and so they can be used as both diagnostic and therapeutic tools.

VISUALIZATION OF VOCAL FOLD MOVEMENT

Ever since Manuel Garcia created the indirect laryngoscope in 1854 visualization of the larynx has been routine. While useful for detecting gross abnormalities of structure and position, simple visual observation of the vocal folds cannot provide much information about vocal fold vibration. At the speeds characteristic of phonation the moving edge of the vocal fold appears as a blur to the unaided eye. There are two fundamentally different ways in which the problem may be solved: high-speed cinematography and stroboscopy. Both approaches, however, require that the larynx be illuminated by a very bright light source and that there be a line-of-sight from the outside to the larynx. That is, before anything else, one must be able to see the larynx, and it must reflect enough light to permit photography.

The basic elements of the simplest system for visualizing the larynx are shown in Figure 6-1. An intense beam of light is reflected by a head mirror onto the laryngeal mirror. The observer (or a motion picture or TV camera) sees the larynx through an aperature in the mirror. Simple light sources tend to produce a great deal of radiation in the infrared region of the spec-

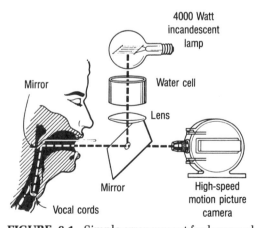

FIGURE 6-1. Simple arrangement for laryngeal photography. (From Fletcher, H. *Speech and Hearing in Communication.* Princeton, NJ: van Nostrand, 1953. Fig. 14, p. 18. Reprinted by permission.)

trum. Some form of filtering must be used to absorb this light, or excessive heating (and possible damage) of the larynx may result. This kind of observation system is inexpensive and quite easy to set up. It is even possible to attach the perforated mirror to the end of the camera lens (Ferguson and Crowder, 1970) to create a very simple photographic system. Sophisticated work, however, will require more complex illumination methods.

Cinematography

Motion pictures of the functioning vocal folds provide an excellent means of evaluating the details of glottal function. Relatively fast filming (about 50 frames per second) provides sufficient "slow motion" to determine the fine points of laryngeal articulatory behavior. Ultrahigh speed (> 4000 frames per second) allows the finer aspects of vocal fold motion during each vibratory cycle to be explored at a speed reduction of 1:250 or more when the film is viewed with a standard projector. The production and analysis of ultrahigh speed films is not easy and requires much more complex instrumentation than the simple system of Figure 6-1. But the extra effort (and expense) may well be justified, particularly in practices that are chiefly concerned with vocal rehabilitation.

There are several different approaches to laryngeal cinematography, each with its advantages and limitations. The clinician will need to select that method which is most likely to provide the needed information with maximal ease and efficiency.

Ultra-high speed photography

Ultra-high speed laryngeal photography, done at an exposure rate of over 4000 frames per second (fps) was developed at Bell Telephone Laboratories (Bell Telephone Laboratories, 1937; Farnsworth, 1940). It was being used to quantify vocal fold movements just a few years later (Brackett, 1948). The technique is expensive, in terms of the requisite equipment and operating costs,

and film analysis is tedious and time-consuming. It may not, therefore, be the preferred approach to the evaluation of most cases. On the other hand,

there is often a puzzling disproportion between subjective symptoms and objective findings during a routine laryngoscopic examination. Many patients with moderate or severe voice changes present little visible evidence in the larynx to explain their vocal abnormalities. In these cases, ultra high speed photography of the larynx often discloses physiologic variations in the vibratory pattern which account for the acoustic manifestations. This diagnostic information has also proved of value in the determination of treatment and in supervision of the indicated therapeutic measures. (Moore, White, and von Leden, 1962, p. 167)

Ordinary camera shutter and transport mechanisms are simply incapable of the speeds required for ultrahigh-speed work. The shutter is therefore replaced by a rotating prism that, as it turns, projects successive images onto the continuously moving film. The very short exposure time requires an extremely bright light source if there is to be adequate exposure of the film. This has required significant improvements in the light source.

Figure 6-2 schematizes a modern sophisticated illumination system developed by Metz, Whitehead, and Peterson (1980). In this arrangement, the light source is a 300 W Xenon arc lamp, equipped with ultraviolet filters, that produces bursts of very intense light, adequate for film speeds up to 6000 fps. On its way to the laryngeal mirror the light beam encounters three special "cold" mirrors that filter out more than 90% of the infrared radiation. The noise of the camera is controlled by locating it in a separate soundproof room and filming through a window.

The advantages gained by the very high frame rate are significant. Consider, for example, a larynx phonating at 100 Hz. Each glottal cycle requires 10 ms. Standard film speed is 16 fps, meaning that 62.5 ms elapses from the start of one frame to the

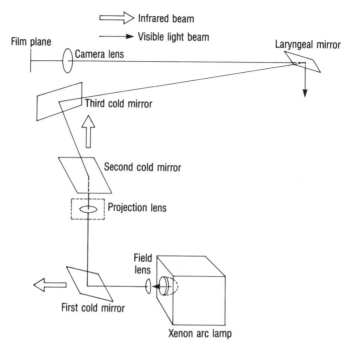

FIGURE 6-2. Improved illumination system for ultrahigh-speed filming of the larynx. (From Metz, D. E., Whitehead, R. L., and Peterson, D. H. An optical illumination system for high-speed laryngeal cinematography. *Journal of the Acoustical Society of America,* 67 (1980) 719-720.Figure 2, p. 719. Reprinted by permission.)

start of the next. In this period, more than six glottal cycles will have occurred. Furthermore, the camera shutter is open for a significant portion of the frame-to-frame period,—certainly long enough for a full glottal cycle to be completed. The record on the standard-speed film will therefore be just as much a smear as the blur seen by the unaided eye.

At 4000 fps, however, the situation is very different. The frame-to-frame interval is only ¼ ms, providing 40 successive exposures during each 10 ms period of the 100 Hz phonation. The high-speed "shutter" is open about 40% of the time, so there is relatively little blurring of the picture. When the film is viewed at the standard projector speed of 16 fps, vocal-fold motion is slowed by a factor of 250. The 10 ms glottal cycle takes 2500 ms (2 ½ s) when projected, and fine details of vocal fold displacements are observable. If the vocal F_o is, let us say, 250 Hz (as for a typical

woman) only 16 exposures will be made during each glottal cycle. This is not as good, although there will still be quite a bit of movement detail. As the F_o rises it may be necessary to increase filming speed. Cameras are available that can expose more than 8000 fps.

Ultra-high speed photography using a laryngeal mirror has proven to be an extraordinary means of getting information about vocal function. Many improvements and modifications of the original technique have been made to overcome limitations or to meet special requirements. Anyone contemplating assembling an ultrahigh-speed filming system might want to consult Moore, White and von Leden (1962), Rubin and LeCover (1960), Metz, Whitehead, and Peterson (1980), Soron (1967), von Leden, LeCover, Ringel, and Isshiki (1966), Hirano, Yoshida, Matsushita, and Nakajima (1974), and Metz and Whitehead (1982).

Endoscopy

The presence of the laryngeal mirror effectively precludes studying laryngeal actions during anything but sustained vowels. Further, it is poorly tolerated by many patients, is difficult to position, and often does not provide an adequate view of the entire length of the vocal folds. These problems have provided the impetus for the development of a number of endoscopic devices—telescopic systems that are inserted into the oral cavity, such as the one shown in Figure 6-3.

Early endoscopes had a light source at the distal end that illuminated the field of view. The optical system, composed of a prism and lenses, provided some magnification. The instrument also generally had some provision for coupling to a camera lens (Taub, 1966a,b; Hahn and Kitzing, 1978). The major problem with these devices was the light source. A bulb bright enough to produce enough light for even moderately fast photography would get very hot and therefore could not be placed in the oropharynx. One could replace the incandescent bulb with a very intense, but relatively cool, electrical discharge flash tube (Bjuggren, 1960), but it requires very high voltages and so exposes the patient to serious electrical risk.

One way out of the dilemma is to use optical fibers to deliver the light (Gould, 1973). The light source itself is located outside of the instrument (where its heat is dissipated) and can be very bright and properly filtered. The optical fibers form a cable that is channelled through the shaft of the endoscope, generally ending in two bundles that project light onto the larynx from either side of the objective lens. The instrument is otherwise conventional. Because of the brilliant illumination, high-speed filming is possible (Gould, Jako, and Tanabe, 1974; Gould, 1977).

Endoscopes with fiber-optic illuminating systems solve the problem of safe and adequate lighting, but they are just as encumbering of the oral cavity as more conventional instruments. A means of circumventing this problem was reported by Sawashima, Hirose, and Fujimura (1967) and Sawashima and Hirose (1968) who designed an endoscope using two fiber-optic bundles forming a single cable. One bundle provides illumination, while the other conveys the image of the larynx back to the eyepiece. (In passing, it should be noted that the fiber bundles must be organized quite differently. The image-carrying fibers must be parallel to each other. If they were randomly organized, the picture at the eyepiece would be a scrambled version of the image entering at the pick-up end. For the illuminating fibers, such "coherence" is immaterial.) The entire fiber cable is only about 5 mm in diameter and is quite flexible. A set of controls in the instrument's handle allows the distal portion of the cable system to be bent and thereby guided into position (Figure 6-4).

The fiberoptic endoscope, commonly called a fiberscope, is inserted through the nasal cavity and, using the positioning controls, is visually guided through the velopharyngeal port, across the oropharynx, and into the hypopharynx. There, the tip is brought to the level of the epiglottis and angled to provide an unobstructed view of the vocal folds, as shown in Figure 6-5. (Sawashima, Abramson, Cooper, and Lisker, 1970; Davidson, Bone, and Nahum, 1974; Saito, Fukuda, Kitahara, and Kokawa,

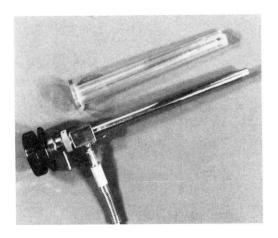

FIGURE 6-3. A simple laryngeal endoscope.

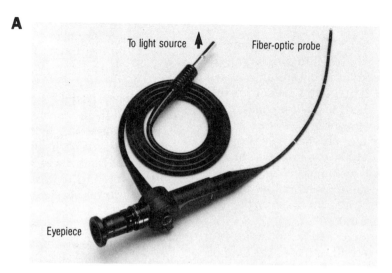

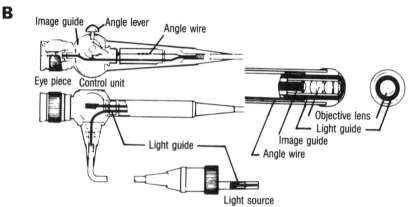

FIGURE 6-4. (A). Fiberoptic laryngeal endoscope ("fiberscope"). (Courtesy of Olympus Corporation, Medical Instrument Division, Lake Success, NY. (B). Organization of the fiberoptic bundles and positioning control of a fiberoptic endoscope. (From Sawashima, M. Fiberoptic observation of the larynx and other speech organs. In Sawashima, M. and Cooper, F. S. (Eds.) *Dynamic Aspects of Speech Production.* Tokyo: University of Tokyo Press, 1977. Pp. 31-46. Figure 1, p. 33. Reprinted by permission.)

1978). The patient does not have to be specially positioned, and so the view is of the functioning larynx in its normal postural relationship to other structures. The fiberscope may also be used to observe velopharyngeal activity (Sawashima and Ushijima, 1972). The ease with which patients tolerate the fiberscope and the excellent view of the larynx that it affords (see Yanagisawa, Strothers, Owens, and Honda, 1983) makes it an instrument of choice in routine clinical assessment of disorders (Brewer and McCall, 1974; Casper, Brew-

er, and Conture, 1982, Gould, 1983; Blaugrund, Gould, Tanaka, and Kitajima, 1983).

The fiberscope does not interfere with oral articulation and does not significantly hinder velar closure. Therefore, it is of enormous value in assessing the articulatory performance of the larynx. It has proven its worth in research in this area that has provided new insights into how the larynx works in concert with the rest of the vocal tract system (Benguerel and Bhatia, 1980; Yoshioka, Löfqvist, and Hirose, 1980; Löfqvist and Yoshioka, 1980; Kagaya, 1974;

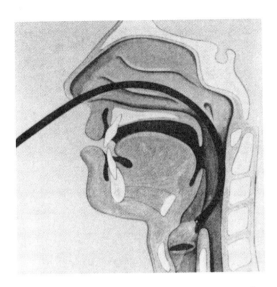

FIGURE 6-5. Position of the fiberscope in the hypopharynx. (Courtesy Machida, Inc.)

Sawashima, 1970; Sawashima, Hirose, and Niimi, 1974). A relatively recent development—a double fiberscope that yields a stereoscopic image—allows vertical movement of laryngeal structures to be quantified, a feat hitherto all but impossible (Niimi and Fujimura, 1976; Fujimura, 1977, 1981; Fujimura, Baer, and Niimi, 1979; Sawashima, Hirose, Honda, and Hibi, 1981). (Other stereoscopic endoscopes, described by Sawashima, Hirose, Honda, Yoshioka, Hibi, Kawase, and Yamada (1983) and by Kakita, Hirano, Kawasaki, and Matsuo (1983) are of the standard telescope type. Since they are not introduced via the nasal passage and do not penetrate into the pharynx, they entail significantly less invasion.) Stereoscopic techniques may ultimately have a major impact on clinical assessment of laryngeal function.

The significant advantages of the fiberscope come at a real price: The transmissive capabilities of the instrument will not permit enough light for high-speed filming. Frame rates are limited to about 50 fps with high-speed (ASA 500) film (Sawashima, 1977; Fujimura, 1981). Articulatory movements may also change the position of the viewing tip, creating ultimate measurement artifacts. Backward motion of the tongue

may interfere with visualization of the glottis. Lastly, the standard method for determining the absolute dimensions of the laryngeal structures cannot be used with the fiberscope. At present there is no convenient way of solving this problem.

Stroboscopy

One can avoid ultrahigh-speed filming, with all of its special illumination and photographic requirements, when the vibratory mode of the vocal folds must be examined. Vocal fold movement can be apparently slowed, or even stopped, through the optical illusion of stroboscopy. (This is the same illusion that makes the blades of a moving electric fan seem to slowly revolve in reverse under certain lighting conditions.) The technique depends on rapidly sampling vocal fold position at selected time intervals. The moving image that is obtained is synthetic in that it is a composite of samples of different cycles. Because of the way in which the illusion is created, it is vitally important that the observer understand the stroboscopic method well. Invalid, misleading, and sometimes foolish conclusions may otherwise be drawn.

Imagine some very rapid event, such as the phonatory opening and closing of the vocal folds, occurring too fast for the eye to follow, in a relatively poorly lit area. Let us assume that the repetition rate is about 100 per second, and each vocal fold cycle is exactly like every other one. Now imagine that the moving vocal folds are suddenly lit with an exceptionally brief burst of light, perhaps lasting only 0.5 ms. The observing eye (or camera) will see a clear image of the structures at a single point in time. Because the light flash was so short, the vocal folds will not have moved an appreciable amount during the time they were lit up, and so the image of them will be sharp. Thanks to persistence of vision, the image will last about a fifth of a second in the observer's eye. Now suppose that the short flashes are repeated at a rate that precisely matches the repetition rate of the vocal fold cycle—that is, 100 flashes per second are produced. Since the flash and repetition rates are exactly matched (and we have already assumed that every vocal fold cycle is precisely like every other one), each flash illuminates the vocal folds at exactly the same point in their cycle. They are always in the same position when the light flash happens. The human eye cannot discriminate separate flashes 1/100 of a second apart, so the observer sees what appears to be constantly lit and *stationary* vocal folds. It seems that the vocal folds have been stopped dead and locked into position at a single point in their vibratory cycle. This is of course not the case, but the illusion offers a fairly good way of getting a clear view of what the folds look like while they are in motion.

The trick can be made a bit more elaborate. Again suppose that the vocal fold cycle repeats at a rate of 100 per second, but this time let the flash rate be only 99 flashes per second. The vocal fold cycle requires 1/100 = 0.01 s, but the flash rate of 99 per second means that the burst of illumination are 1/99 = 0.0101 s apart. Because of this discrepancy each flash is delivered slightly later in the vocal fold cycle than the one before. (In other words, the phase difference between the vocal cycle and the flash cycle steadily increases.) The position of the vocal folds shown by the first flash will not be shown again until the 100th flash. Until then, 100 sucessive positions of the vocal folds will have been seen.

This process is demonstrated in Figure 6-6. At the top, a schematic diagram shows the relationship between "flashes" and positions of a waveform. When the sample points are joined together a slow-motion (or drawn out) version of the sampled wave form is obtained. In the other illustration, the brightness of a tracing of the waveform on an oscilloscope screen has been changed for the duration of each "flash." Notice how, in the oscillogram, the flashes recreate (apparent) cycles at a rate that is very much lower than the real repetition rate. The apparent frequency of the waveform (delta f, or Δf) is equal to the difference

between the vocal fold frequency (f_a) and the flash frequency (f_f):

$$\Delta f = f_a \text{-} f_f.$$

In the examples of Figure 6-6, $\Delta f = 100\text{-}99 = 1$ cycle/s . At this apparent rate, the eye could easily follow (and it would be easy to film) what the vocal folds are doing. But the resulting image would not really be a vocal fold cycle. It would be bits of a hundred such cycles, joined together by persistence of vision. Therein lies a host of potential, and often overlooked, problems.

Figure 6-7 demonstrates some of the pitfalls of stroboscopy that can confound the unwary. Figure 6-7A illustrates what happens if the flash duration is too long. The longer the period of illumination, the more the waveform changes while it is illuminated. The result is exactly analogous to a long-exposure photograph of a moving object: The image is blurred. Obviously the flash duration must be short relative to the speed of the structures being observed.

A more subtle problem is shown in Figure 6-7B. The flash rate is just a bit higher than the waveform repetition rate. The result is that the stroboscopic illumination creates an apparent reversal of the wave. The equation for apparent frequency indicates that this should occur. Suppose the flash rate is 101 per second, while the waveform frequency is 100 per second. Then

$$\Delta f = f_{\text{wave}} \text{-} f_f$$
$$= 100 \text{-} 101$$
$$\Delta f = \text{-}1 \text{ cycles per second.}$$

The negativity of Δf indicates that the apparent movement will be a reversal of the true movement. The experience occurs in everyday life. If an electric fan is turned off there will be a time, as it slows down, when the revolution-per-second rate of the blades is just slightly less than the flicker rate of, say, a fluorescent lamp that illuminates it. At that time the blades will seem to reverse direction and rotate slowly backwards. Under these conditions, the vocal folds might seem to move backwards—opening gestures will be seen as closing movements; surface waves on the vocal folds will

A

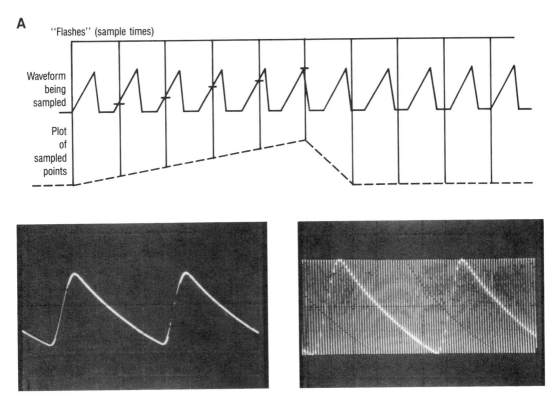

FIGURE 6-6. (A). The principle of stroboscopy. A wavefrom is sampled at a rate slightly lower than its repetition rate. Each sample thus shows the wave at a slightly later point in its cycle than the previous sample. If the sampled points are connected, a "spread-out" representation of the original waveform results. (B). Left: Oscillogram of an asymmetric waveform. Right: In this oscillogram the waveforms are crowded together and almost appear as a background blur. Brief intensifications of the oscilloscope beam at a rate slightly slower than the wave's fundamental frequency create a good expanded representation of the repeating wave. Intensifying the beam for brief intervals is a form of stroboscopy.

seem to move from the sides toward the glottis. The relatively inexperienced examiner might be led to some very strange conclusions indeed.

Figure 6-7C demonstrates an effect that is insidious. In this case the flash rate remains constant, but the waveform repetition rate varies just a bit around the basic 100 per second. The apparent cycle seems to vary in waveform and amplitude, rather than simply in frequency as is really the case. The observer might be led to the conclusion that the movements of the vocal folds varied in extent in an erratic manner from cycle to cycle, when actually only the fundamental frequency was changing.

The reason that this last problem is so serious is that the fundamental frequency of phonation is, in reality, far from perfectly stable. It is, in fact, highly perturbed in patients with many voice disorders (see Chap. 5), and these are the very people on whom stroboscopy is most likely to be done. The possible frequency-perturbation and apparent amplitude deception needs to be dealt with if accurate diagnoses are to be made. This has led to the development of the synchronstroboscope, whose flash rate tracks the patient's fundamental frequency.

The key portion of the synchronstroboscope is a circuit that generates a Δf that is added to the patient's F_o (as transduced by a contact microphone) to produce a stably

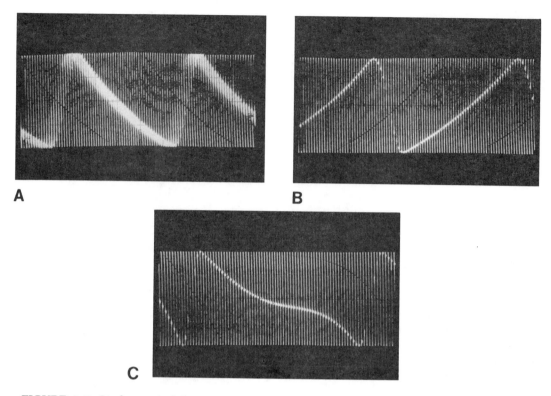

FIGURE 6-7. Stroboscopic defects. (A). Duration of the sampling interval (flash) is too long, resulting in a blurred image. (B). Sampling rate is greater than the wave's fundamental frequency, making the stroboscopic image a reversal of the true waveshape. (A stroboscopic motion picture would appear to run backwards.) (C). If the fundamental frequency of the wave being observed or if the sampling rate is unstable, the stroboscopic representation will be severely distorted.

increasing phase difference between the vocal fold cycle and the flash-triggering point. A number of ways of doing this has been devised (von Leden, 1961; Winckel, 1965). A version produced by van den Berg (1959) includes an adapter that compensates for the frame speed of a motion picture camera so as to permit filming of stroboscopic series. A modern synchron-stroboscope for use with a laryngeal mirror or direct laryngoscope is shown in Figure 6-8. The foot pedal adjusts the magnitude of Δf, thereby changing the rate of apparent motion. It is also possible to trigger the light source of a fiberscope stroboscopically (Saito, Fukuda, Kitahara, and Kokawa, 1978). Given the fiberscope's advantages over standard indirect laryngoscopy this method is likely to grow in popularity.

CORRELATES OF VOCAL FOLD MOTION

While visualization of the larynx is a sine-qua-non of assessing tissue disorders, much useful information is provided by measures that do not reveal what the vocal folds actually look like. An example is the glottal area function (discussed more fully later on), which is the area of the glottal opening as a function of time. In general, these measures can be derived from ultra-high-speed films, and that is the means by which many were originally obtained. But doing so is invasive, tedious, terribly time consuming, and relatively costly. These considerations have motivated a search for simpler methods that rely as much as possible on correlates of vocal fold action that can be easily transduced with a minimum of invasion. None of the techniques dis-

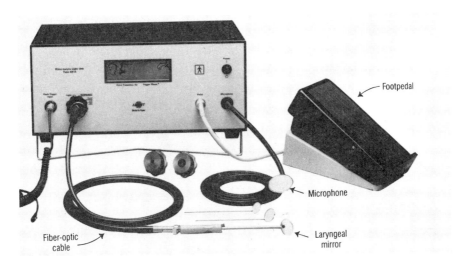

FIGURE 6-8. A synchronstoboscope (Brüel and Kjaer model 4914). The footpedal controls all functions of the instrument. Stroboscopic illumination is delivered to the laryngeal mirror via a fiberoptic cable; a microphone transduces the vocal fundamental frequency. (Courtesy of Brüel and Kjaer, Maerum, Denmark)

cussed below can substitute for good visual assessment of the laryngeal status. But they can generate quantitative and qualitative information that may be equally important to assessment and to the design of a therapeutic regimen.

Photoglottography (PGG)

The principle on which photoglottography rests is simple enough. The glottis is considered as a shutter through which light passes in proportion to the degree of opening. In theory, if a light is made to shine on the glottis, the amount of light passing through is directly proportional to the glottal area. Optoelectronic devices are more than adequate to transduce changes in luminous intensity at the rates typical of laryngeal function. It is possible, therefore, to obtain an electrical voltage proportional to the glottal area—at least in theory. A moment's reflection indicates where the difficulties lie in the conversion of principle to practice: arranging for adequate illumination of the larynx and devising a system to pick up and transduce the transmitted light. Fortunately, current technology has provided several solutions.

Modern photoglottography began with Sonesson (1959, 1960) and has since been modified or combined with other techniques in a number of ways by others (Kitzing, 1977; Kitzing and Löfqvist, 1978; Lisker, Abransom, Cooper, and Schvey, 1966, 1969). A basic photoglottographic setup is shown in Figure 6-9. A bright light source is placed against the neck just below the cricoid cartilage. The lamp causes the subglottal space to be suffused with the light that filters through the tissues of the neck. A pickup probe, either a curved plastic rod or a fiberoptics bundle, transmits any of this light that passes to the pharynx to a photosensor. The result, after amplification, is a voltage that should be proportional to the area of the glottic opening.

It makes no difference what the direction of the light path is, so the light source can be placed on the neck and the illuminator in the oropharynx, or the light can shine from above the larynx and the photosensor can be on the neck. Better yet, illumination can be provided by a fiberscope, passed via the nasal cavity into the hypopharynx. This has the advantage of permitting normal articulatory movements (Lisker, Abramson, Cooper, and Schvey, 1966, 1969).

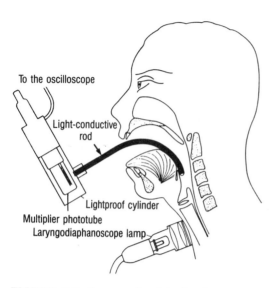

To the oscilloscope

Light-conductive rod

Lightproof cylinder

Multiplier phototube

Laryngodiaphanoscope lamp

FIGURE 6-9. Sonesson's original technique for photoglottography. (From Sonesson, B. On the anatomy and vibratory pattern of the human vocal folds. *Acta Oto-laryngologica*, Suppl. 156 (1960) 1-80. Figure 22, p. 47. Reprinted by permission.)

There are problems with photoglottography, and its validity has been questioned. Specifically, Wendahl and Coleman (1967) and Coleman and Wendahl (1968) reported on simultaneous determinations of the shape of the glottal area curve by ultrahigh- speed filming and photoglottography in four subjects producing sustained vowels. In some cases the curves produced by the two methods were highly congruent, but in many instances they were markedly dissimilar. The discrepancies were particularly serious if the waveforms were used to derive glottal source spectra, as they sometimes have been (Ohala, 1967). The conclusion was that "relating photoglottographic waveforms . . . to glottal area is not only hazardous but invalid in many cases" (Coleman and Wendahl, 1968, p. 1734). But in a more recent study using very similar methods, Harden (1975) obtained completely different results. She found that, for 5 subjects sustaining vowels in each of the three vocal registers, the photoglottograph provided "essentially the same information on glottal area function as that provided by

ultrahigh-speed photography" (Harden, 1975, p. 734). Although the curves generated by the two methods were not identical, the photoelectric method was judged to provide "reasonably approximate information." In another study comparing high-speed filming and photoglottography, Baer, Löfqvist, and McGarr (1983) found that the two methods provide comparable data about peak glottal opening and glottal closure.

There is no clear explanation for the different results of these studies. It is possible, for instance, that some light is transmitted through the greatly thinned edge of the vocal folds under some adjustment conditions. But a number of extrinsic factors do influence the photoglottogram, and the user must keep them in mind in order to control them rigorously. Vallancien, Gautheron, Pasternak, Guisez, and Paley (1971) have summarized them as follows:

1. The amount of light projected on the larynx. This varies with lateral and angular displacement of both the illuminator and the photoelectric transducer. Movements can be produced by activity of the articulators.
2. Changes in light-transmissive characteristics of the neck tissues due to vertical movement of the larynx.
3. Changes in the shape and volume of the hypopharynx caused by tongue retraction during certain productions.

In short, the normal structural displacements of speech may threaten the validity of the measurements. Accordingly, the internal portion of the photoglottograph should be located in such a way as to assure stability. This argues strongly for a per nasal fiberoptic system in that it is least likely to be moved by the tongue and its tip placement, in the laryngeal vestibule, promises a relatively good line of sight to the vocal folds. The fiberscope also has the advantage of allowing the examiner to monitor the adequacy of placement visually and signal any obstruction, such as the epiglottis, that temporarily invalidates the data.

ANALYSIS OF THE GLOTTAL STATUS

Beyond purely qualitative description, high-speed filming and photoglottography can provide quantitative data upon which graphic or numeric analysis of vocal fold function may be performed. This section will discuss some of these.

Vocal Fold Excursion and Glottal Width

A frame-by-frame analysis of the width of the glottis as seen in ultrahigh-speed films is a useful means of quantifying peculiarities of vocal fold movement. The distance of a point along the length of the vocal fold (usually the midpoint) is plotted over time or, equivalently, over frame number. (Note that, as Smith [1954] originally pointed out, complex movements of the *medial* surface of the vocal folds are intermittantly visible in the high-speed films. The most medial point of the vocal fold, as seen in a given frame, may not be on the edge of the superior surface.) If a relative scale is used the distance at maximum opening is usually designated 100% and all other values are scaled accordingly. This technique has been exploited extensively by Timcke, von Leden, and Moore (1958, 1959), von Leden, Moore, and Timcke (1960), and von Leden and Moore (1961). Examples of such analysis (Figure 6-10) show how strikingly it can demonstrate movement abnormality. Trace A shows a normal glottal width function. Opening takes less time than closing, and there is a period of obviously complete closure. The vocal folds move symmetrically. Trace B shows the width function of a patient with a left recurrent nerve paralysis. The paralyzed vocal fold never reaches midline. Its movements, however, seem otherwise fairly normal. The healthy vocal fold passes the midline during what should be the closed phase, but no contact of the vocal folds is achieved. A wider range of abnormal width functions will be considered further on.

Only frame-by-frame analysis of ultrahigh-speed films can provide graphic records like the ones of Figure 6-10 because at the moment no other technique can track each vocal fold separately. Although the information they provide can be of therapeutic value (Fisher and Logemann, 1970), generating these width curves involves an enormous amount of work. It is likely that, except for clinical research, therapists will prefer to rely on stroboscopic observation (filmed, if possible) for documentation of vocal fold movement anomalies.

Glottal Area Function

The glottal area function is the area of the glottal opening plotted over time. It is well correlated to the glottal width function (defined for the present purposes as the distance from the middle of one vocal fold to the middle of the other). Koike and Hirano (1973) computed an average discrepancy between the two of less than 2%. Given this close correspondence the width is often used as an estimate of the relative glottal area, since it is much easier to calculate. If, however, the absolute area is needed, the actual area function must be computed. This can be done mechanically by tracing an outline of the glottis with a planimeter, but even short sequences of film can take hours of measurement time. Efforts have been made to eliminate some of the enormous amount of work entailed through the use of special computer programs and television arrangements (Hayden and Koike, 1972; Childers, Paige, and Moore, 1976; Gould, 1977). This has led to semiautomatic methods, but they are still far too slow, require too much operator intervention, and are far too expensive for routine clinical use. Usually, however, the absolute area is not required. In general it is the *pattern* of area change that is of interest, and for this a relative measure is perfectly adequate.

Parameters of the Area Function

A number of parameters of the area (or glottal width) function have been defined that quantify important aspects of the waveshape. They are based on the durations of various phases of the wave, as shown in Figure 6-11.

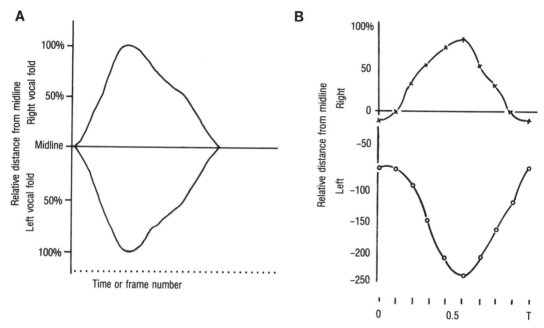

FIGURE 6-10. (A). Normal glottal width function. The distance of the midpoint of each vocal fold from the midline is plotted from successive frames of an ultrahigh speed film. (B). Glottal width function in a case of left recurrent nerve paralysis. The left vocal fold never reaches the midline. Its vibratory excursion is greater than that of the right vocal fold, which crosses the midline slightly, since the paralyzed fold is not there to arrest its medial motion. (From von Leden, H., Moore, P., and Timcke, R. Laryngeal vibrations: Measurements of the glottic wave. Part III: The pathologic larynx. *Archives of Otolaryngology*, 71 (1960) 16-35. Figure 3, p. 19. Reprinted by permission.)

The open phase occupies most of the cycle. It is divided into an opening (closed-to-open; C–O) part and a closing (open-to-closed; O–C) part. The duration of the cycle (its period) is designated T. The durations of these phases are used to compute the following indices.

1. The open quotient (Oq) is the proportion of the period during which the glottis is open:
   Oq = open phase/T.
   When there is no glottal closure,
   Oq = 1.
2. The speed quotient (Sq) measures the symmetry of the opening(C–O) and closing (O–C) parts of the open phase:
   Sq = (C–O)/(O–C).
An Sq of 1 indicates equality of opening and closing times. $Sq < 1$ results when closing takes longer than opening; $Sq > 1$ signals the reverse.

3. The speed index (SI) is another way of describing the symmetry of the opening and closing phases (Hirano, 1981). It is the ratio of the durational difference of the two to the total duration of the open phase. That is,
   $SI = [(C–O) - (O–C)] /$ open time
   $= [(C–O) - (O–C)] / [(C–O) + (O–C)]$.
   This value is related to the speed quotient:
   $SI = [Sq - 1] / [Sq + 1]$.

Figure 6-12 illustrates the relationship of the Sq and SI and what they indicate in terms of waveshape.

The recently proposed speed index has certain advantages over the more firmly entrenched speed quotient. Symmetry of the open phase is indicated by a Sq of 1.00. As the wave is increasingly skewed to the right the Sq decreases to a limit of zero, but the Sq limit for

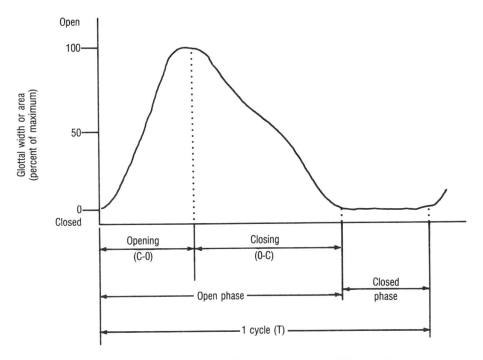

FIGURE 6-11. Divisions of the glottal area or width function.

extreme left-skewing is infinite. Sq grows exponentially as skewness increases to the right. SI, on the other hand, extends from -1 to $+1$ as skewing goes from extreme right to extreme left. Thus a negative value shows a shorter opening than closing part, and a positive value shows a relatively short closing period. Equality of the two is indicated by $SI = 0$. Although the two parameters are mathematically equivalent and interconvertible, SI seems more in keeping with intuitive notions of scaling, and may come to replace Sq.

4. The rate quotient (Rq) is defined as
   $Rq = [\text{closed phase} + (C–O)] / (O–C)$.

It describes the relative duration of the closed and opening phases to the closing interval. Introduced by Kitzing and Sonesson (1974), it has not gained widespread use.

Expected values

NORMAL FUNCTION The variations of several glottographic parameters with changes in F_o and vocal intensity have been systematically studied by ultrahigh-speed filming and photoglottography. Table 6-1 summarizes a set of typical findings obtained photoglottographically. The general accuracy of these data has been confirmed by other photoglottographic studies (Kitzing and Sonesson, 1974) and ultrahigh-speed filming (Moore and von Leden, 1958; von Leden, 1961; Timcke, von Leden and Moore, 1958). Taken together, these investigations support the following generalizations.

1. Open quotient increases with F_o in modal register. At high (loft register) F_o, glottal closure may not occur, so $O_q = 1$. Pulse register has very long closed periods (Hollien, Girard, and Coleman, 1977; Whitehead, Metz, and Whitehead, 1984), so O_q will be very small. O_q varies inversely with vocal intensity.

2. Speed quotient varies directly with vocal intensity. It is essentially unaffected by F_o.

3. The overall pattern of the glottal width

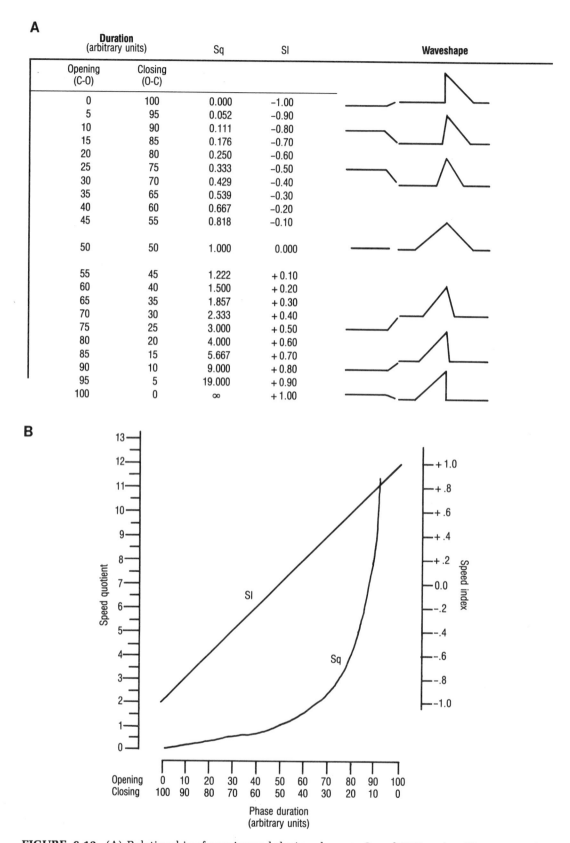

FIGURE 6-12. (A). Relationship of opening and closing phases to S_q and SI (Based on Hirano, 1981.) (B). Comparison of the growth of S_q and SI.

TABLE 6-1. Mean *Oq*, and *SI*: Normal Speakers*

Approx F_o (Hz)	Low Intensity**					
	Oq		*Sq*		*SI†*	
	Mean	Range	Mean	Range	Mean	Range
120	0.57	0.38–0.80	0.92	0.80–1.06	−.04	−.11−+.03
175	0.68	0.49–0.77	0.89	0.72–1.13	−.06	−.16−+.06
225	0.71	0.51–1.00	0.91	0.69–1.18	−.05	−.18−+.08
275	0.80	0.47–1.00	0.85	0.61–1.16	−.08	−.24−+.07
325	0.82	0.54–1.00	0.92	0.59–1.19	−.04	−.25−+.09

Approx F_o (Hz)	High Intensity**					
	Oq		*Sq*		*SI†*	
	Mean	Range	Mean	Range	Mean	Range
120	0.47	0.37–0.58	0.99	0.77–1.44	0.00	−.97−+.19
175	0.58	0.38–0.72	0.99	0.86–1.46	0.00	−.07−+.19
225	0.64	0.49–1.00	0.95	0.59–1.29	−.03	−.26−+.13
275	0.70	0.46–1.00	0.95	0.71–1.18	−.03	−.17−+.08
325	0.77	0.44–1.00	0.97	0.81–1.62	−.01	−.10−+.24

From Sonesson, B. On the anatomy and vibratory pattern of the human vocal folds. *Acta Otolaryngologica*, Suppl. 156 (1960) 1-80. Table 2, p. 62. Reprinted by permission.

*N = 25, age 18–21. Sustained /ɛ/, matching tones. Photoglottography.

**Intensity difference, ~ 6 dB.

†Computed from author's data.

function changes dramatically with register (Fig. 6-13). In fact, the change is part of the definition of register itself (Hollien, 1974).

VOCAL DISORDER Most of the value of the glottal area function in assessment of voice disorders lies in its depiction of possible anomalies of movement of the vocal folds. Obviously, ultrahigh-speed filming or synchronstroboscopy is best for getting this information.

Figure 6-14 illustrates the kinds of glottal width functions that may be encountered in some common pathologies. Failure to achieve glottal closure (6-14A), abnormal excursion of a vocal fold across the midline (6-14B and 6-14C), and phase differences between the displacements of the two folds (6-14B and 6-14C) are typical findings. On the basis of analysis of a great many cases, von Leden, Moore, and Timcke (1960), von Leden and Moore (1961), and Yanagihara (1967) have drawn the following conclusions.

1. Benign lesions do not prevent vibration of the vocal fold on which they are located. Both folds vibrate at the same frequency.

2. In general, abnormal vibration patterns are typical of disease, with the possible exception of very small lesions.

3. The most common (almost ubiquitous) symptom of disease is frequent and rapid changes in vibratory rate. (This can be detected by perturbation analysis. See Chap. 5.)

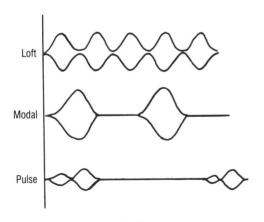

FIGURE 6-13. Vocal fold excursion patterns in the three vocal registers.

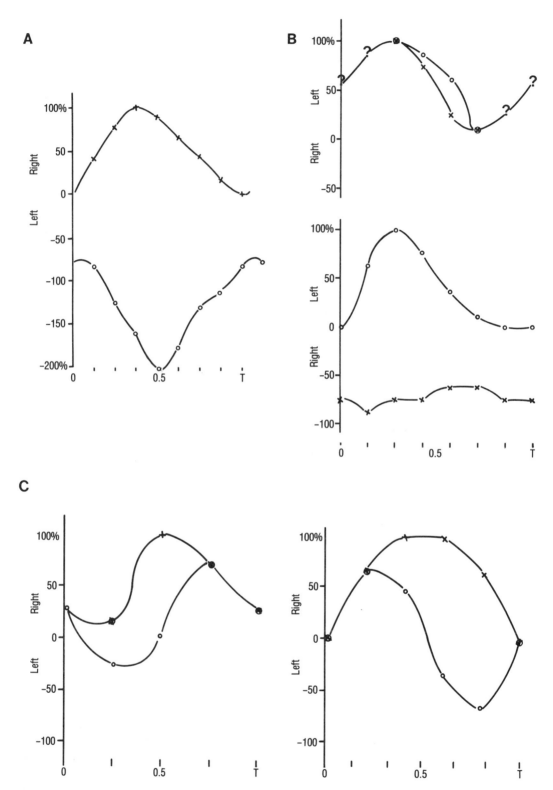

FIGURE 6-14. Vocal fold excursion patterns (glottal width functions) in some common pathologies (A). Left vocal fold paralysis. The paralyzed fold does not come to the midline to effect glottal closure. Its excursion is greater than that of the the healthy fold. (B). Sessile polyp and diffuse edema of

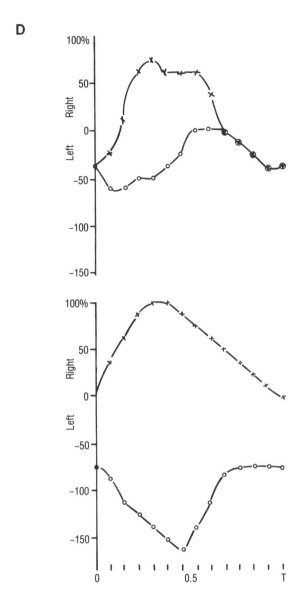

D

the right vocal fold. Upper traces: measurement at the center of the lesion demonstrates how, at this location, the diseased fold follows the movements of the healthy one. Lower traces: width function measured at the posterior end of the membranous folds shows the failure to achieve glottal closure in this area. (C). Left: Fixation of the left cricoarytenoid joint at the midline. There is a constant phase shift of about 90° throughout the cycle. Right: anterior webbing, with a constant phase shift of about 115° (left side lagging). (D). Bilateral polyps, larger on the left. Upper traces: measured in the area of the lesion. Phase shift of about 90° (left side leading) and highly abnormal open phase. Closure is to the left of the midline. Lower traces: measurement posterior to the lesions, showing an abnormal excursion pattern of the left vocal fold and failure to achieve glottal closure in this area. (From von Leden, H., Moore, P. and Timcke, R. Laryngeal vibrations: Measurements of the glottic wave. Part III: The pathologic larynx. *Archives of Otolaryngology*, 71 (1960) 16-35. Figure 5, p. 21; Figure 7, p. 24; Figure 9, p. 27; Figure 12, p. 32. Reprinted by permission.)

4. Damping of vocal fold vibration is caused by all but the very smallest lesions. (Fig. 6-14B)
5. Great increases in excursion are often associated with paralysis. (Fig. 6-14A)
6. There is almost always asynchronism of vibration of the two folds. That is, they will move out of phase.
   a. The phase shift may be constant during the cycle, or it may change. If constant, the open period will show the pattern of Fig. 6-14C.
   b. If the phase shift affects the closed phase, the approximated edges of the vocal folds will deviate from the midline as in Fig. 6-14C.
7. It is common for either the normal or the diseased vocal fold to cross the midline during part of the glottal cycle. (Fig. 6-14C).
8. Projecting soft tumors tend to follow the motions of the opposing healthy vocal fold (Fig. 6-14B). Firm tumors do not.
9. The period of closure is prolonged at the site of a projecting tumor. The projection, however, prevents any approximation in adjoining areas. (Figure 6-14B and 6-14D)
10. The open quotient is often increased.

Hirano, Gould, Lambiase, and Kakita (1981) have confirmed many of these findings in cases of unilateral vocal fold polyps. They have also stressed concurrent changes of the traveling wave of the mucosa. Cycle-to-cycle waveform variability is considerable in many cases of laryngeal pathology. Rapid changes in the glottal waveform contribute significantly to the perception of vocal roughness (Coleman, 1971).

Many of the defects listed above can be seen in, or inferred from, photoglottograms. Unfortunately, the photoglottograph cannot differentiate the action of the two vocal folds, so much information is lost. Attempts to correlate photoglottogram patterns with specific disorders are still at the preliminary stage (Kitzing and Löfqvist, 1979).

Electroglottography (Electrolaryngography, EGG)

Human tissue is a moderately good conductor of electricity. To a fair approximation, bodily structures behave like resistors for which Ohm's law is valid. That is, current through a given structure will be proportional to the applied voltage and inversely proportional to the net resistance. Similarly, if a given current is flowing through a structure, the voltage that is developed will be proportional to the resistance. This concept, discussed more fully by Allison (1970) and by Bagno and Liebman (1959) forms the basis of *electroglottography* (EGG), also known as *electrolaryngography*.

Because it is entirely noninvasive electroglottography has attracted a great deal of interest. It has been used by researchers to probe the function of the normal larynx (Chevrie-Muller, 1967; Reinsch and Gobsch, 1972; Ondráckova, 1972; Kelman, 1981; Rothenberg, 1981), including attempts to confirm the neurochronaxic theory (Chevrie-Muller and Grémy, 1962; van Michel, 1964, 1966; Grémy and Guérin, 1963) or refute it (Decroix and Dujardin, 1958; Lebrun and Hasquin-Deleval, 1971). It is also being used more and more for the diagnosis of pathology (Chevrie-Muller, 1964; van Michel, 1967; Croatto and Ferrero, 1979; Lecluse, Tiwari, and Snow, 1981; Jentzsch, Sasama, and Unger, 1978) and as a tool in vocal therapy (Jentzsch, Unger, and Sasama, 1981; Fourcin, 1974, 1981; Fourcin and Abberton, 1976; Kitzing and Löfqvist, 1979; Reed, 1982). There is every indication that the trend toward increased application of EGG will continue. Since EGG is likely to be increasingly important in vocal rehabilitation, it is considered here in some detail.

Figure 6-15 shows, in a highly schematic way, the form of the laryngeal "resistor" as seen by an electroglottograph. The lines represent paths of current flowing between two electrodes applied to the alae of the thyroid cartilage. In 6-15A, the vocal folds

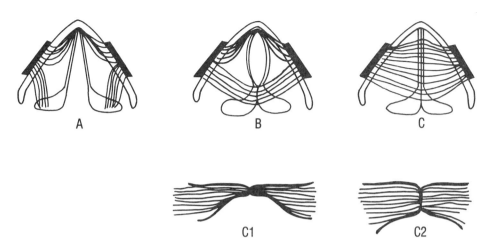

FIGURE 6-15. Current flow (represented by solid lines) between electrodes applied to the thyroid alae. A. Ventilatory position of the folds. B. Open phase of the phonatory cycle. C. Closed phase of the phonatory cycle. C1 and C2. Different degrees of vocal fold contact during the closed phase, seen in coronal section.

are abducted to a nonphonatory position. Air is an excellent electrical insulator and, therefore, the electrical current cannot traverse the glottal space. The current pathways are greatly lengthened as electrons flow (in three dimensions) around the glottis. When the arytenoids adduct and contact each other for phonation (Fig. 6-15B) the current pathway is simplified. Even when the glottis opens during part of the phonatory cycle, there is a moderately good conducting path through the arytenoids (and also a longer path through the perilaryngeal tissues). During the closed phase of vocal fold vibration the electrical pathway is optimized by the contact of the vocal folds. There are, however, degrees of closure. In the closed period of every glottal cycle (at least in modal register) the contact of the vocal folds varies from minimal (Fig. 6-15C1) to maximal (Fig. 6-15C2). Electrical resistance increases with the total length of the current path and decreases with the cross-sectional area of the conducting medium. On this basis, one would expect the trans-laryngeal resistance to constantly (but not linearly) drop as the laryngeal status changed from A to C2. This expectation is borne out in practice, including the change of resistance during the closed phase.

Experimentation has indicated that the resistance sensed by the electroglottograph represents not the area of the glottal opening, but rather the surface area of contact of the (membranous and cartilaginous) vocal folds (van Michel, Pfister, and Luchsinger, 1970; Lecluse, 1974; Fourcin, 1974, 1981; Vallancien, 1972; Kelman, 1981; Lecluse, Brocaar, and Verschuure, 1975; Köster and Smith, 1970). Because the output is not an analog of the glottal area, but respresents instead the status of the larynx as a unit, Fourcin has proposed that the instrument be called an *electrolaryngograph*, rather than an electroglottograph as had been common in the literature (Fourcin, 1981; Fourcin and Abberton, 1976). Unfortunately, while Fourcin's point is well taken, *laryngography* has long been used by radiologists to refer to contrast-medium visualization of the larynx (Landman, 1970). To prevent any confusion it seems wisest to retain the term electroglottography despite its literal inaccuracy. One must also be aware that, irrespective of what name is used, the electroglottograph output is not merely reflective of laryngeal phenomena alone. All structures between the electrodes—and even some quite a distance away—can, and do, interact with the current flow. The output signal is, therefore, not nearly as neat and clean as the naive user might suppose.

The electroglottograph has been improved very significantly since it was developed by Fabre (1957) as an extension of his work on blood flow (Fabre, 1940). What seemed at first so simple and straightforward a procedure needed considerable modification before it was to become a useful clinical tool. The various modifications have led to a number of different varieties of electroglottograph which may, under certain circumstances, produce different outputs for the same event. There is as yet no "standard" electroglottograph, and it is wise to understand the differences among the various devices in order to better judge the validity of findings in the literature and to select for purchase the one most suited to the intended use.

For a number of reasons, both electronic and biological, all electroglottographs work with a high-frequency sinusoidal signal. Clearly the amount of current that can safely be passed through a living subject is small, and all electroglottographs are designed to operate at, and limit current to, safe levels. (Because the subject is, of necessity, part of a live electrical circuit, all electrical safety precautions must be observed during electroglottography. Further, it is extremely unwise to build one's own electroglottograph unless all the necessary safety features can be designed into it.) A problem that all electroglottograph circuits must address is the very small changes in resistance that are produced by changes in vocal fold position. Remembering that the resistance seen by the electroglottograph is that of the entire neck, it is not hard to visualize how small a contribution the larynx makes. Put another way, there is a large volume of tissue to carry current between the electrodes. The addition or loss of the trans-vocal-fold pathway makes little difference compared to the whole. Detecting the laryn-geal contribution may not be quite as hard as finding a needle in a haystack, but it is not so much easier, either. The need to discriminate the appropriate small signal from the background has been a very important factor in all circuit designs.

Early electroglottographs were fairly simple devices using vacuum tubes or just passive elements. They often required a separate highly stable oscillator and an outboard amplifier and demodulator (van Michel, 1967; Vallancien and Faulhaber, 1966). A transistorized device appeared in 1960 (Gougerot, Grémy, and Marstal, 1960; Decroix and Dujardin, 1958). A major advance was the Mark IV Electroglottometer (van Michel and Raskin, 1969), which was quite sensitive and contained all the circuitry (some of it integrated) required to function as a free-standing unit.

Laryngeal resistance changes reflect at least two kinds of events. Relatively slow changes are caused by ventilatory and articulatory adjustments, whereas the vocal fold vibratory cycle generates very rapid resistance changes. The electroglottographs now on the market allow the user to choose whether all resistance changes, or only the fast ones associated with the vocal fold cycle, will be displayed. The most popular electroglottographs commercially available today offer other significant improvements over earlier versions. For instance, they can measure the fundamental frequency or generate pulses for synchronizing a stroboscope.

Commercial instruments

F-J ELECTROGLOTTOGRAPH The F-J Electronics model EG830 (Figure 6-16), designed by Frøkjaer-Jensen and Thorvaldsen (1968) imposes a small voltage (0.5 V) at a frequency of 300 kHz on the neck via two silver electrodes. The transneck resistance is reflected by the current (maximum = 10 mA). Transduction is achieved by a special three-coil transformer, which has the advantage of isolating the electrodes from the current source.

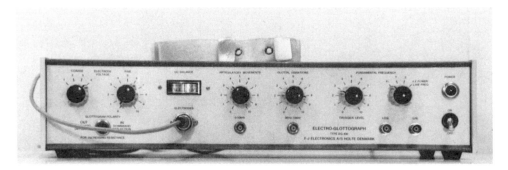

FIGURE 6-16. The F-J Electroglottograph.

The F-J electroglottograph has two separate detector circuits. One is a DC-to-10 kHz amplifier that rectifies and filters the signal to produce an output that includes both slow and rapid (articulatory and phonatory) impedance changes. The other channel is AC coupled; its output frequency range is from 25 to 10 KHz. This circuit is used for observing phonatory cycles. Very slow changes in the baseline resistance of the subject are inevitable and, although they are eliminated from the output of this channel, they change the zero-balance of the system, potentially to the point of distorting the final output. To prevent this the AC channel has circuitry that automatically compensates for very slow changes of the voltage "operating point." Sensitivity of the F-J electroglottograph is 1 V out for a 1% change in resistance between the electrodes.

F-J Electronics also makes a "normalizer" accessory for its electroglottograph. It electrically conditions the EGG wave so that its width and height remain constant on an oscilloscope screen, even when the vocal fundamental frequency and the wave's amplitude are actually changing. This lets the clinician concentrate on the shape of the wave and measure its various phases (Ferrero, Pelamatti, Vagges, and Zovato, 1980). The normalizer provides digital readouts of F_o and of the proportion of each cycle that is occupied by the "opening phase" to facilitate analysis.

VOISCOPE The Voiscope®, developed by Fourcin and his co-workers, is a combined electroglottograph and display system manufactured by Laryngograph Ltd. (Fourcin and Abberton, 1971; Fourcin, 1974, 1981). A constant voltage source provides a 3V, 1 MHz sine wave signal to the neck. Rather than the two electrodes that have typically been used for electroglottography, the Voiscope uses a 3-terminal system. That is, a guard ring connected to ground surrounds each of the electrodes (Figure 6-17). This has the effect of eliminating much of the surface (skin) conduction. Th Voiscope measures the current flowing through the neck from one inner electrode to the other. The current, of course, varies inversely with resistance. As was the case with the F-J electroglottograph, the Voiscope has a circuit that adjusts for slow drift of baseline resistance due to postural change and the like. The time constant of the feedback circuit is such as to minimally affect signals due to glottal vibration or articulatory events. A high-pass (phonatory) and a DC- (all resistance changes) output are provided.

The Voiscope also offers a number of special features. It can be used by two different speakers to produce separate oscilloscope displays that are useful in therapy for getting a patient to match a correct production. The display can also be scrolled across the screen, allowing the therapist to read the record, just as if it were coming

A

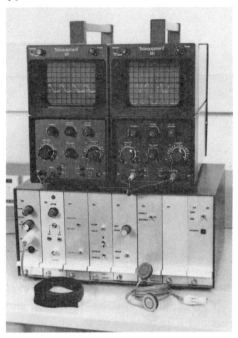

B

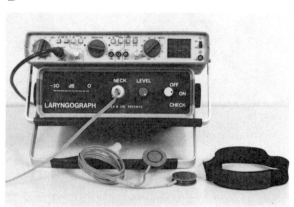

FIGURE 6-17 (A) The Voiscope electroglottograph. (B). The Laryngograph—a smaller, simpler, battery-powered electroglottograph. (Courtesy Laryngograph Ltd, London, England and Kay Elemetrics, Inc.)

from a strip-chart recorder. There is also a provision for transmitting a digital measure of laryngeal period to a computer. The waveform can be normalized to a standard length and amplitude, thereby facilitating comparison of waveform features.

The Voiscope is a modular system to which specialized components, continually being developed, can easily be added. But Laryngograph, Ltd., (the Voiscope's manufacturer) also offers a simple, portable, battery-operated unit, the Laryngograph, for those who require a less elaborate instrument. The Laryngograph can be interfaced to Kay Elemetric's Visi-Pitch (see Chap. 5).

SYNCHROVOICE QUANTITATIVE ELECTRO-GLOTTOGRAPH SynchroVoice, Inc. (Briarcliff Manor, N. Y.) has recently marketed a "quantitative electroglottograph" that has a number of features of clinical value. The instrument passes a 5 mA, 5 MHz current through the neck and detects the neck resistance with a Wheatstone bridge. Three elec-

trodes are used: two lateral to the larynx and one at the midline.

The SynchroVoice unit displays the electroglottogram on a built.in oscilloscope, but there is also an output for use with a chart recorder. A front-panel switch allows the user to select a standard, varying electroglottogram or waveform normalization (maintenance of constant length and height despite changes in the actual waveform parameters). Thanks to a built-in digital memory, the display can be frozen on the screen for careful evaluation.

The Synchrovoice electroglottograph has several digital indicators that are likely to be of particular use to the clinician. In addition to fundamental frequency (or period, depending on the mode selected), there are also readouts of the wave's open quotient (Oq), maximum amplitude and the rate of vocal fold closure (expressed in dB re: maximum per millisecond). A moveable cursor allows selection of specific points in the EGG waveform for quantification.

Electroglottographic Procedures

Although specific details of implementation differ according to the particular electroglottograph being used, the technique of electroglottography is straightforward. The measuring electrodes are attached according to the manufacturer's recommendations. (Some units require that electrode paste be used, other instruments advise against it.) There is no firm rule for the exact location of the electrodes, but in general they should be lateral to the thyroid cartilage at a level that approximates the position of the vocal folds. Positioning is optimized by watching the waveforms generated during trial phonations and moving the electrodes until the best signal is obtained. It should have maximal amplitude, be free of extraneous noise, and have a moderately stable baseline. Although all EGGs have circuitry designed to reject nonphonatory signals and compensate for baseline drift, to some extent they are all still sensitive to movement artifacts. Therefore, the patient should be positioned (preferably with a head support) so as to minimize movement during testing.

Electroglottographic waveforms

The waveform of the glottal cycle (that is, with the slower articulatory and other influences filtered out) has been designated Lx (Fourcin, 1974, 1981). Figure 6-18 shows an example of Lx during sustained /ɑ/ by a normal male. In this particular illustration increasing impedance is downward in the display. Hence, upward movement of the curve indicates more vocal fold contact (closure). There is no agreed upon convention about this, and the literature depicts Lx waveforms with vocal fold opening upward or downward. It is, therefore, important to check the captions in research reports and to indicate the direction of glottal opening and closing on all clinical EGG records.

The Lx waveform is not of interest in itself: Its importance lies in the vocal fold behavior it represents. Considerable re-

search effort has been devoted to establishing what the important features of the waveform are and what they correspond to. As mentioned above, it is very clear that the curve does not reflect glottal size but rather vocal fold contact area. Because of the complex behavior of the free edges of the vocal folds during the phonatory cycle, the contact area function is a very complicated one and is itself not very well understood. It is, therefore, not surprising that the interpretation of Lx is still subject to considerable debate. Both elucidation and revision of currently held views are likely in the future.

Lecluse (1977) and his coworkers (Lecluse, Brocaar, and Verschuure, 1975) have done simultaneous electroglottography and synchronstroboscopy on normal subjects, with results illustrated in Figure 6-19. The overall relationship between the size of the glottic opening and the translaryngeal impedance is apparent but obviously very imperfect. Significant details of vocal fold movement are being missed. Figure 6-20, based on the work of MacCurtain and Fourcin (1982) and of Rothenberg (1981) adds information that clarifies the Lx wave a bit more. An Lx wave is again shown (with decreasing resistance, or glottal closure, upward) but various points are labelled to correspond with positions of the vocal folds as seen in *coronal section*, primarily during the closed phase.

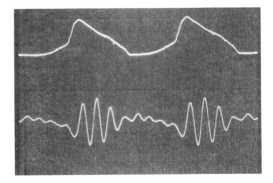

FIGURE 6-18. Lx of modal register phonation at comfortable pitch by a normal adult. Increasing resistance (glottal opening) is downward. The lower trace is the audio wave.

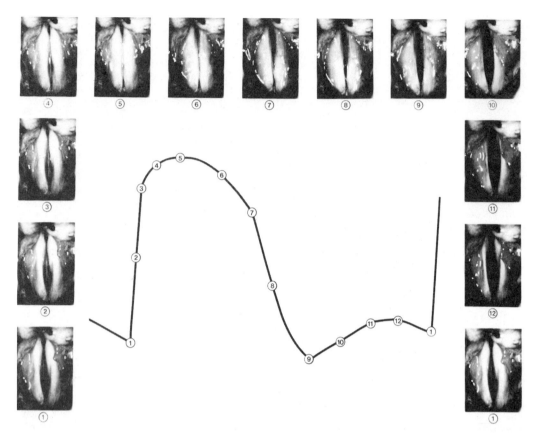

FIGURE 6-19. Lx electroglottogram with simultaneous stroboscopic views of the vocal folds. Photographs correspond to the numbered points in the Lx wave. (Courtesy of F. L. E. Lecluse, ENT Department, Free University Amsterdam, The Netherlands.)

The first thing to note is that the closed phase begins with a very abrupt decrease in translaryngeal impedance. Fourcin (1981) believes that the initial contact between the lower edges of the vocal folds is formed by a mucous bridge between the approaching epithelial covers. The bridge rapidly expands horizontally and is responsible for the very sudden drop in resistance and the very short rise time (points I-II) of the Lx wave. Of course, at the same time the surface area of vocal fold contact is increasing (points II-III), and as it does the Lx curve rises to its peak. As the vertical wave of vocal fold contact continues, the total contact area begins to diminish, and so resistance increases (points III-V) until the vocal folds are separated (point VI).

Rothenberg's (1981) comparison of Lx to the airflow curve has generally confirmed

this interpretation of features of the Lx waveform. He has pointed out, however, that the high-pass filtering that is required for extraction of Lx and the automatic gain control function of the electroglottograph both introduce distortion of the Lx wave. This is seen mostly in the open phase representation, which would be much flatter if there were no filtering. The precise effects of automatic gain control are unfortunately not easily predicted. Similar open-phase distortion has been seen with other instruments (van Michel, Pfister, and Luchsinger, 1970), so the effect is not peculiar to the Fourcin system that Rothenberg used. The significance of irregularities in the open phase of Lx should be interpreted with extreme caution.

The last two figures show that the Lx waveform conveys little information about

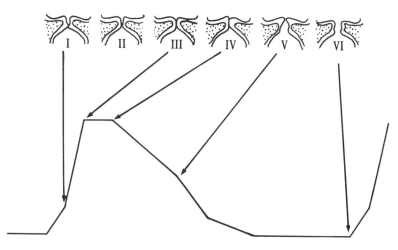

FIGURE 6-20. Relationship of points in the Lx wave to medial contact of the vocal folds. Based on the work of MacCurtain and Fourcin, 1982 and Rothenberg, 1981.

the open phase in any case. It is generally conceded that Lx is useful primarily for its representation of closure events (Fourcin, 1974, 1981; Titze and Talkin, 1981; Croatto, Ferrero, and Arrigoni, 1980; MacCurtain and Fourcin, 1982; Lecluse, Brocaar, and Verschuure, 1975; Fourcin and Abberton, 1976; Hirano, 1981; Childers, et al., 1984) and of the overall duration of the closed phase.

Gx is Fourcin's designation of the unfiltered output of the electroglottograph. Gx shows the large impedance variations associated with any adjustment of the larynx for speech, including positioning of the vocal folds and the setting of their length and tension characteristics before phonation. Figure 6-21 is an example of Gx at the start of the utterance "about" spoken by a middle-aged male. There is no way at present to assess the contributions of the many factors that might influence Gx, and it is therefore of little routine use to the clinician, although attempts to categorize electroglottograms of continuous speech are being made (Chollet and Kahane, 1979).

Validity of electroglottography

The output of the electroglottograph unavoidably represents the sum of an unknown number of unspecified factors in addition to the vocal fold contact area. The question of validity is therefore an important one. If irrelevant variables can be shown to have a merely marginal effect, then validity is only negligibly impaired. But if events beyond the phenomena of interest intervene in a significant way, they must be controlled or the technique is rendered essentially useless.

There is no question that the electroglottograph is a detector of impedance changes. The issue is what the source of those changes might be. Despite the fact that the output curve is not significantly altered by changes in the vowel being produced (Vallancien and Faulhaber, 1967; Fabre, 1958), Smith (1977, 1981) has argued quite forcefully that impedance variations being observed are due to compression of perilaryngeal tissue by acoustic waves. That is, in his view, the electroglottograph really functions as an impedance microphone. In demonstration of his position he has obtained Lx-like waveforms by transducing sound with pieces of meat and wet paper tissue. Even drops of water between the electrodes have provided a fairly good output. He also found that he could produce an Lx-type output by placing both electrodes on one side of the larynx or on a rubber (non-conducting) model of the larynx.

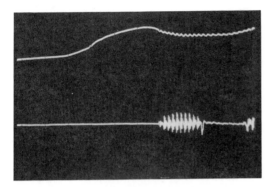

FIGURE 6-21. The top trace shows the Gx (unfiltered) electroglottogram at onset of the word "about." Note the change of baseline resistance, which is very large compared to the minute changes (ripples in the trace) resulting from the vocal fold cycle. Decreasing resistance (glottal closure) is upward. The change at the start of the utterance shows laryngeal preparation—including vocal fold adduction—for phonation. The lower trace is the audio signal.

It is very likely that acoustic waves are, in fact, being transduced by the electroglottograph. But the magnitude of the acoustic contribution to the overall signal is likely to be very small in instruments currently in use. If so, then validity of the waveform is not harmed. A complete assessment of the situation, however, has yet to be undertaken.

The preponderance of opinion seems to favor the basic theoretical reality of the vocal fold contact area assumption. There are, however, threats to validity in the application of the technique that must be taken into account and controlled for.

1. Electrode placement. Lecluse, Brocaar, and Verschuure (1975) have found (in a study using excised larynges) that signal to noise ratio is optimized when the electrodes are positioned at the level of the vocal folds.

2. Skin-electrode resistance. There is some impedance introduced at the electrode-skin interface. If the electrode impedance remains constant it constitutes no problem. Slow drift will be filtered out by the high-pass characteristics of the Lx

mode, but will alter the Gx trace. Relatively fast changes of electrode resistance, however, will introduce artifacts into the data. Consequently, electrodes must be clean and firmly fixed at a properly prepared site.

3. Fat tissue is a very poor conductor. A substantial fatty layer under the skin can degrade the Lx signal badly. The presence of significant fat may explain why electroglottography has not been particularly successful with very young children, although other factors may also be responsible (Holm, 1971).

4. Vertical larynx height changes for different articulations and phonational qualities, especially for F_o (Ewan and Krones, 1974; Shipp, 1975, 1979; Shipp and Izdebski, 1975). This results in a change in the relationship of the electrodes to the vocal folds and thereby influences the electroglottographic waveform. If phonations at different pitches are to be compared, caution in interpretation is advisable.

5. Head movement alters the relationship of neck structures and may compromise the data output. The high-pass filtering of Lx will eliminate much of the baseline shift, but some artifact may remain. It is important that the subject's head be stabilized with a headrest.

If the Gx waveform is being evaluated, another factor becomes potentially important:

6. High pressure in the pharynx, typical of plosives and fricatives, enlarges the pharynx with consequent compression of peripharyngeal tissue. This will cause a noticeable shift in the Gx baseline value.

One final caution needs emphasis. It is entirely possible to tape record the Lx wave for future reference and evaluation. The ordinary tape recorder uses direct recording, so very low frequencies are lost. The flat, or nearly flat, portions of the Lx wave represent low-frequency or DC- components. Unless an FM recorder is used distortion will occur in the recording process, making the data of dubious value on playback.

Summary

What, then, can be said about the electroglottogram? The following conclusions seem justified in light of our present understanding:

1. It provides far more information about the closed phase of the glottal cycle than about the open phase and, in particular, it provides some level of insight about vertical contact changes.
2. It is not possible to determine the exact instant of opening or closing of the vocal folds (Köster and Smith, 1970). It is clear, however, that a minimum-resistance peak represents maximal closure, while the opposite peak shows a point in the open phase. The slopes between the peaks do correspond, at least grossly, to opening and closure phases. Onset of closure is usually signaled by a rapid fall of resistance, with a "knee" in the closing portion of the wave (Childers, Naik, Larar, Krishnamurthy, and Moore, 1983; Childers, Smith, and Moore, 1984).
3. Quantification of phases of the vocal fold cycle on the basis of Lx is of questionable validity, although quantitative measures of Lx may be relevant to evaluation of vocal disorder. (See, for example, Dejonckere and Lebacq [1985].)
4. Lx may permit qualitative descriptions of laryngeal actions, especially when used in conjunction with other types of measures (Hirano, 1981; Vallancien, Gautheron, Pasternak, Guisez, and Paley, 1971; Titze and Talkin, 1981; Kitzing, 1982; Baer, Titze, and Yoshioka, 1983).

Voice quality and Lx

Lx and acoustic waveforms for sustained /ɑ/ with different vocal qualities are shown in Figure 6-22. All productions are by the same normal male; increasing resistance (less contact, greater opening) is downward in each case. Trace A is normal modal register. Glottal closure is marked by a sharp rise of the waveform (sudden increase in vocal fold contact) while the opening phase is more gradual, with a more moderate slope. There is a distinct "knee" in the waveform during the opening phase (arrow) that has been found to correspond to the onset of glottal airflow (Fourcin, 1981). The vocal folds therefore must have begun to separate at this point in the Lx cycle. The relatively flat segment of the wave signifies an open glottis. Note that the closing phase is associated with the largest peak of the acoustic waveform. This is as it should be, since it is closure of the glottis that provides the major excitation of the vocal tract.

Breathy voice (Trace B) is signaled by a very long open phase, shown as a prolongation of the relatively flat bottom of the waveform. It is possible, of course, to produce extremely breathy voice with almost no vocal fold contact. The clearly indicated sharp drop in resistance (upward excursion) of the waveform shows that this was not the case for the production illustrated. The audio trace again shows that the sudden glottal closure provides the acoustic excitation of the tract. Pulse register (vocal fry) phonation is characterized by irregularity of vocal fold vibration, shown in Trace C. In this example, the open phase is fairly long compared to the closed phase, which is not necessarily typical of phonation in this register. Note that the audio signal shows two instances of doubled waves—a weak excitation followed very quickly by a stronger one (arrows). In each case the excitations correspond to sudden changes in Lx. Loft (falsetto) register (Trace D) presents significant problems. The Lx wave characteristically is very small, and sinusoidal in appearance (Fabre, 1958; Gougerot, Grémy, and Marstal, 1960). This reflects the thinning of the vocal folds and possible failure to achieve full closure that is characteristic of loft register.

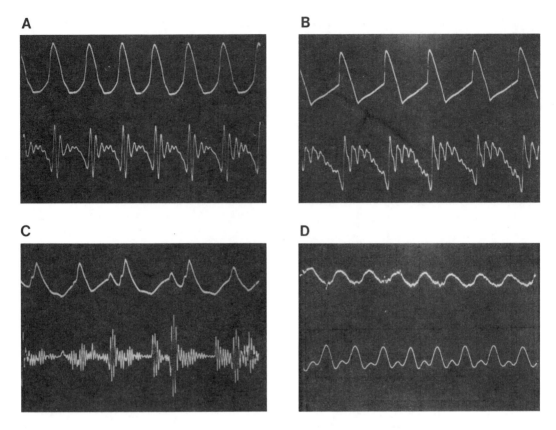

FIGURE 6-22. Lx for different voice qualities. Increased resistance (glottal opening, less vocal fold contact) is downward. The lower trace in each pair is the audio wave. (A). Modal register, normal phonation. (B).Modal register, breathy voice. (C). Pulse register. (D). Loft register.

Electroglottography has attracted a great deal of interest and has been used as a method to probe the function of the normal larynx (Chevrie-Muller, 1967; Reinsch and Gobsch, 1972; Ondráckova, 1972; Kelman, 1981; Rothenberg, 1981), including attempts to confirm the neurochronaxic theory (Chevrie-Muller and Grémy, 1962; van Michel, 1964, 1966; Grémy and Guérin, 1963) or refute it (Decroix and Dujardin, 1958; Lebrun and Hasquin-Deleval, 1971). It is also being used for the diagnosis of pathology (Chevrie-Muller, 1964; van Michel, 1967; Croatto and Ferrero, 1979; Lecluse, Tiwari, and Snow, 1981; Jentzsch, Sasama, and Unger, 1978) and as a tool in vocal therapy (Jentzsch, Unger, and Sasama, 1981; Fourcin, 1974, 1981; Fourcin and Abberton, 1976; Kitzing and Löfqvist, 1979; Reed, 1982).

Quantitative aspects of Lx

The same indices that are applied to the glottal area function can be computed from the Lx waveform. Because Lx does not represent glottal area, however, the resulting numbers are very different.

Reinsch and Gobsch (1972) calculated an Oq of 0.85 ± 10% in modal register at moderate intensity from the Lx traces of 23 young adult men and women. Unger, Unger, and Tietze (1981) found an Oq of approximately 0.81 and a figure of about 0.89 can be calculated from the data of Kelman (1981). It seems, then, that the Oq of Lx is higher than the one derived from the glottal area function. Since the exact correspondence between Lx and vocal fold actions remains obscure there is no way to explain this at the moment. (It is possible that the time constants of the electrolaryngograph play a role, however.)

On a less rigorously quantified level, Lx can be "read" to provide an estimate of normality. Fourcin (1981), Kelman (1981), MacCurtain and Fourcin (1982), and Reed (1982) make the following points:

1. Uniformity of Lx amplitude is associated with low perturbation.
2. A rapid and sharply defined closing phase indicates good vocal tract acoustic excitation and efficient vocal production.
3. The closing phase takes less time than the opening phase.
4. Long closure duration is correlated with relatively undamped spectral peaks.

Lx in pathology

Lx often shows pathology by the absence of normal features or by their modification rather than by clear-cut pathologic signs. Although the search for pathognomonic features continues, no abnormal features have yet been found that can be said to be reliably diagnostic of a given vocal condition (Hanson, Gerratt, and Ward, 1983; Rambaud-Pistone, 1984; Childers, Smith, and Moore, 1984; Dejonckere and Lebacq, 1985). There may be a decrease in the Lx-derived Oq. Unger, Unger, and Tietze (1981), for example, found that the mean Oq in several cases of functional voice disorder was 0.74, while mean Oq was 0.80 in uncompensated, and 0.76 in compensated, recurrent paralysis. The high variability associated with the data did not allow Oq to differentiate between normal and dysphonic speakers.

On the whole, Lx is evaluated qualitatively. It is best used together with other glottographic signals to provide a picture of what the vocal folds are doing, particularly in terms of their closure patterns.* The electroglottogram, displayed on an oscilloscope

---

*Lx can be particularly useful as a diagnostic tool when combined with xeroradiography (Berry, Epstein, Fourcin, Freeman, MacCurtain, and Noscoe, 1982; Berry, Epstein, Freeman, MacCurtain, and Noscoe, 1982; Noscoe, 1982).

screen, has also been found to be useful as a biofeedback tool in therapeutic management of many types of dysphonia.

Ultrasound

The ultrasound techniques discussed in Chap. 11 can also be used for observation of the larynx. The size of the vocal folds, their location, the complexity of their movements, and the small distances they traverse during phonation create very special difficulties in adapting ultrasound for laryngeal examination.

Since the edges of the vocal folds constitute a very small target, the ultrasonic beam must be very narrow and well defined. The laws of physics conspire to make such a beam very difficult to obtain. A small ultrasound transmitter crystal produces a small beam, but the angle of divergence increases with decreasing crystal size. At the depth of the vocal folds, the beam will likely have enlarged too much. A large crystal produces a less diverging beam, but one that is too large to be optimal in the first place. Higher frequency is associated with less beam spread, but absorption by intervening tissue is increased. Final design of the transducer system has to represent a compromise that balances all of these factors. Optimization must be undertaken with an eye to the specific measures to be obtained, which explains the very different designs that have been proposed. Typically, transducers range from 5 to 18 mm (circular or rectangular) in size, and frequencies are commonly in the range of 1 to 5 MHz (Holmer, Kitzing, and Linström, 1973; Hertz, Lindström and Sonesson, 1970; Hamlet, 1980, 1981).

Two resolution factors are of vital importance in examining the larynx. When transducers are placed on the side of the neck, opening and closing of the glottis represents a change of the axial distance of the edge of the vocal fold. Resolution in this dimension is theoretically limited to ½ the ultrasound wavelength. If, for instance, the speed of ultrasound in muscle is about 1500 m/s. a 2.5 MHz wave has a wavelength of

0.6 mm. The best resolution attainable would be to 0.3 mm. No system comes close to the theoretical limit of resolution and, therefore, fine detail of glottal opening and closing displacements cannot be discriminated with certainty. Lateral resolution, on the other hand, depends on the size of the beam at the target. It is clear from the earlier discussion of beam size that fine lateral resolution is exceptionally difficult to achieve. Details of vertical motions at the edge of the vocal folds still lie beyond the resolving power of ultrasound instrumentation.

Echoglottography

Vocal fold position can be tracked using the same principles as SONAR. The process is called echoglottography. During phonation, the velocity of the edges of the vocal folds is moderately great. Tracking them adequately requires that the ultrasound pulses be very short and their repetition rate high. Generally, medical ultrasound reflectoscopes are inadequate with respect to these requirements, and special instruments have been designed (Holmer, Kitzing, and Lindström, 1973; Hertz, Lindström and Sonesson, 1970) that provide up to 10,000 pulses per second and offer better characteristics for time-motion displays.

Echoglottography has successfully shown glottal motion in the form of an undulating echo curve in the T-M mode (Figure 6-23). While the opening and closing phases are discernible, the closed and open intervals are not well demonstrated. Hertz, Linström and Sonesson (1970) have measured vocal fold excursions on the order of 1 mm with their system and have been able to calculate approximate open and speed quotients. Kaneko, Uchida, Suzuki, et al. (1981) have used two probes to view both vocal folds simultaneously, permitting evaluation of the symmetry of their motion. They have also been able to resolve lateral and vertical displacements of a single vocal-fold edge using their dual-probe system.

Unfortunately, the edge of the vocal fold does not move as a single flat reflecting plane (Saito, Fukuda, Isogai, and Ono, 1981). The complexity of the changes in its shape creates very confusing echoes, as shown in Figure 6-23B through 6-23E. When the vocal folds are in position A the ultrasound beam encounters only one reflecting surface. The A-mode representation is as in Figure 6-23C. But when the vocal folds are configured like position B, the beam is reflected from two tissue-air interfaces, one at the upper surface of the fold and the other, a bit further away, at the edge. The resulting A-mode display (Figure 6-23D) therefore has two peaks. In the T-M mode the multiple-echo pattern fades in and out (Fig. 6-23E) as the folds change shape. Clearly, interpretation of the echoglottogram is not likely to be a simple matter.

On the other hand, the echoglottograph can provide relatively clear-cut data (within the limits of its resolution) if the actual movement pattern of the vocal folds is not at issue. Hamlet (1972b), for instance, used simple A-mode displays to show that the glottis is narrower during whispered /a/ than during whispered /s/, while Munhall and Ostry (1983) have successfully timed laryngeal articulatory behaviors.

Finally, it is important to remember that ultrasonic scanning techniques are relatively new and are still in a rapidly evolving stage of development. Improvements in transducers, such as scanned arrays (Zagzebski, Bless, and Ewanowski, 1983; Kaneko, Suzuki, Uchida, Kanesaka, Komatsu, and Shimada, 1983; Zagzebski and Bless, 1983) and in support electronics bode well for future importance.

Continuous wave

Ultrasonic waves can be constantly applied to the neck, and the magnitude of the transmission from one side to the other determined. Such a *continuous wave* (CW) technique is analogous to electroglottography. Air is an extremely poor ultrasound transmission medium. Therefore, if an ultrasound beam is projected across the larynx from one side of the neck, it

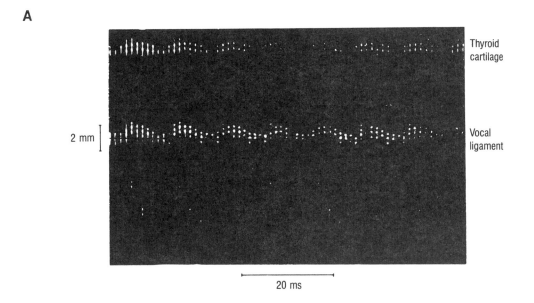

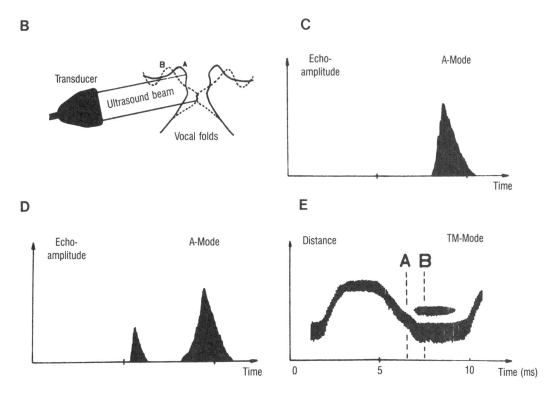

FIGURE 6-23. Ultrasonic scans of the vocal folds. (A). T-M display during phonation. (From Hertz, C.H., Lindström, K., and Sonesson, B. Ultrasonic recording of the vibrating vocal folds. *Acta Otolaryngologica*, 69 (1970) 223-230. Fig. 4, p. 228. Reprinted by permission.) (B–E) Relationship of the ultrasonic beam to the vocal folds. The complex movements of the free edge of the vocal fold (points A and B) produce A-mode displays of C and D, while the T-M mode pattern may resemble that of E. (From Holmer, N.-G., Kitzing, P., and Lindström, K. Echo glottography. *Acta Otolaryngologica*, 75 (1973) 454-463. Figure 8, p. 461. Reprinted by permission.)

will be interrupted by the air in the open glottis, and a receiver on the other side will pick up no signal. When the vocal folds are in contact, however, a transmission path exists. Continuous waveglottography should show an "on-off" pattern that corresponds to the closed and open phases, respectively. The technique was first used by Bordone-Sacerdote and Sacerdote (1965) and has been more fully developed and exploited by Hamlet. She has shown, for instance, that the open quotient varies with vowel nasalization (Hamlet, 1973), and she has also explored laryngeal excitation of the vocal tract (Hamlet, 1971). Holmer and Rundqvist 1975) have used CW ultrasound to obtain a simple waveform for the extraction of F_o

One would expect that the amplitude of the transmitted CW signal would increase in rough proportion to the degree of vocal fold contact. That is, (again analogous to electroglottography) changing vocal fold contact area should result in amplitude modulation of the ultrasonic carrier. Hamlet and Palmer (1974) have shown this to be the case. She has also demonstrated (Hamlet, 1980) that a demodulated waveform can even show features suggestive of the vertical phase difference in the movements of the edge of the vocal fold.

This degree of resolution requires a very narrow ultrasound beam (Hamlet, 1972a). Such a beam is very sensitive to changes in the position of the larynx in the neck. If the larynx moves either up or down, the transmission bridge across the airway—the vocal folds—moves out of the path and transmission is lost. Therefore, narrow-beam CW ultrasound can be used to determine the exact level of the vocal folds. Their position when adducted is betrayed by a maximum-amplitude ultrasound signal when the transducers are moved along the neck. Hamlet (1980) has used this fact to confirm the findings of Shipp (1975) on vertical larynx height. Use of ultrasound *arrays*, with a row of transducers excited in very rapid sequence, may provide a means of continuously tracking larynx height in the future (Hamlet, 1981; Hamlet and Reid, 1972).

Combined Echo and Transmission

In an attempt to extract maximum information from ultrasonic probing of the larynx Kaneko, Kobayashi, et al. (1976) created a new technique. Adopting the premise that laryngeal behavior can best be evaluated only when the glottal area and the movement pattern of the vocal folds are both known, they combined the CW and pulse-echo techniqes and did simultaneous measures of the subglottal pressure. While a great deal of information is obtained this way, the method is complex and does not seem to offer greater insight than can be attained by other means.

Doppler-effect monitoring

Attempts have been made to use the Doppler frequency shift of the ultrasound echos to determine the actual velocity of the edge of the vocal folds during phonation. The method was first tried in a series of pilot studies by Minifie, Kelsey, and Hixon (1968) that were soon followed by comparisons of the ultrasound data to simultaneous ultrahigh-speed films (Beach and Kelsey, 1969). While the procedure has intuitive appeal, the experimental results were disappointing. Ultrasound-based velocities and displacements (found by integrating the velocity data) differed from those found by measurement of the films in timing, magnitude, and overall patterns. There was also significant ambiguity and inconsistency in the ultrasound data. This is not surprising: The movement of the edge of the vocal folds is nonuniform and complex, and the returned echos probably represent different motions occurring at the same time in different places. The researchers were forced to conclude that the quality of the data made "positive identification of a particular type of vocal fold motion by inspection of the associated Doppler signal impossible" (Beach and Kelsey, 1969, p. 1047).

Ultrasound nonetheless holds promise as a noninvasive means of laryngeal monitoring, all of its current problems notwithstanding. Studies of the last several years have confirmed its potential and pointed the way to needed improvements.

Acoustic Extraction of the Glottal Wave

The glottal wave may be defined as the pattern of the glottal volume velocity—the changes in glottal airflow with time. There are two reasons why this waveform is of interest. First, it constitutes the vocal tract excitation. It is, in the purest sense of the word, the voice. Anything heard by a listener is the product of this voice excitation and the vocal tract's acoustic characteristics. If it can be extracted the glottal wave can be acoustically analyzed to provide significant information about the vocal component of speech.

Second, and more germane to the present topic, the glottal wave is an indicator of the size of the glottis. That is, it serves as a good estimator of the glottal area function. While the glottal wave can be, and classically has been, determined from the glottal area function as measured from ultrahigh-speed films, it is also possible to derive it acoustically. Two different approaches are readily applicable: neutralization of vocal tract characteristics by a reflectionless tube and inverse filtering.

Reflectionless (Sondhi) Tube

Vocal tract modification of the glottal waveform into the final voice signal is achieved through the effect of nonuniformities of the vocal tract diameter (creating resonant spaces) and, more important, the sudden change at the lips from a small diameter system to the infinite diameter of the free space outside the mouth. Any sudden change in the size of a tube implies a discontinuity in its acoustic impedance, and at any such impedance shift some of the signal is transmitted, but the rest is reflected back toward the source. The discontinuity of the vocal tract at the lips creates a very sudden and exceptionally large change in acoustic impedance, called the lip-radiation impedance. A significant portion of the egressive speech signal is, therefore, reflected from the lips back toward the larynx. The glottal waveform interacts with its own reflections in the resonant spaces of the vocal tract to produce the signal heard by the listener as a distinctive speech sound. If the vocal tract could be made fairly uniform in its cross-sectional shape, and if the lip radiation impedance could be eliminated, the emergent signal would be the unaltered glottal wave itself.

Sondhi (1975) proposed a conceptually simple way of achieving the necessary modifications of a speaker's vocal tract. Uniformity of the tube is approximated during production of a neutral, schwa-like vowel. The elimination of the radiation impedance is trickier. For this a special metal tube is needed (Figure 6-24), about 2 m in length with a diameter that approximates that of the speaker's vocal tract, between 2 and 2 3/4 cm. The speaker seals his lips around the open end of the tube and phonates a neutral vowel with good velopharyngeal closure. The signal is picked up by a precision miniature microphone inserted through the tube wall.

What makes the system work is a long (1 = m) wedge of sound-absorbent material that closes the distal end of the tube. If properly shaped this will soak up essentially all of the impinging sound energy and, therefore, none will be reflected back into the vocal tract. Such a (quasi-) reflectionless tube essentially extends the acoustic length of the vocal tract to the functional equivalent of infinity and eliminates the radiation impedance.

If the system were sealed, with no way for the expired air to escape, the pressure inside the tube would quickly rise to the level of the subglottal pressure, and in the resultant absence of a transglottal pressure drop phonation would cease. Therefore, provision must be made for venting the tube to the outside. The way in which this is done is important. If the vent is not large enough, air pressure in the Sondhi tube will rise, and laryngeal behavior may be changed in compensation. On the other hand, the vent must be small enough, and so placed, as to avoid creating reflections that defeat the purpose of the system. Hill-

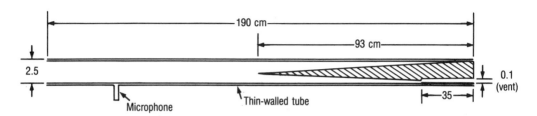

FIGURE 6-24. Design of a reflectionless (Sondhi) tube. (Dimensions in cm).

man and Weinberg (1981) have evaluated different venting methods; Figure 6-24 incorporates their recommendations. While Sondhi's original device used fiberglass as the absorbent material, polyurethane foam is now the material of choice. Details for constructing a reflectionless tube system have been published by Monsen and Engebretson (1977), Monsen (1981), and Hillman and Weinberg (1981a). The construction itself is not difficult, but the system must then be tested to verify its lack of resonances across a sufficiently broad bandwidth. This requires coupling sinusoidal signals across the frequency spectrum to the mouth end of the tube and measuring the amplitude and phase-shift of the tube's response to the injected signals. Details of the calibration procedure are given by Hillman, Weinberg, and Tree (1978).

SONDHI-TUBE GLOTTAL WAVEFORM. Examples of waveforms sensed in a Sondhi-tube at different loudness levels are shown in Figure 6-25. High pressure is upwards and corresponds to increased glottal opening. The wave has a simple shape that is, in fact, similar to that of the glottal area function as measured from ultrahigh-speed films. There is, however, a disturbing difference. In most cases, there is a distinct closed phase during the glottal cycle. During this period the vocal folds are in medial contact, there is no glottal opening, and airflow must be zero. The closed phase takes a significant amount of time—on the order of 1/3 of the glottal cycle. Furthermore, as will be discussed later, the relative duration of the closed phase increases with vocal intensity.

Except for a momentary minimum, the glottal waves of Figure 6-25 fail to show such a closed phase. The problem is not unique to Monsen's data. Other researchers (Sondhi, 1975; Tanabe, Isshiki, and Kitajima, 1978) have published similar traces. Hillman and Weinberg (1981b) have explored the causes of imperfections in the Sondhi-tube representation of the glottal volume velocity and have concluded that the closed-phase problem is caused by the influence of the first formant. The Sondhi tube's validity rests on the assumption that the vocal tract being tested has a uniform diameter. This is obviously not the case with a real human structure, so the uniform-diameter assumption is never met in practice. Apparently, the deviation of the real from the ideal is sufficiently great to produce the closed-phase distortion that is so commonly seen. The Sondhi-tube is imperfect in other ways, too. Clearly, no real tube is absolutely without reflections, and it is unlikely that the tube diameter actually matches (and is therefore a good extension of) the cross-sectional diameter of the speaker's vocal tract. Despite the designer's best efforts, there is likely to remain a sudden change in the system diameter where the Sondhi tube meets the lips. The net result of any of these deviations from the assumptions of the rationale is the occurrence of resonances that distort the glottal waveform.

If it is the examiner's intention to quantify important aspects of the glottal waveform for comparison to normative data generated by other means, the reflectionless tube is probably not the best method to use. Under laboratory conditions the tube's out-

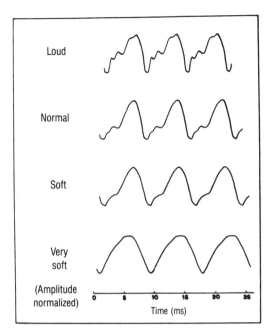

Loud

Normal

Soft

Very
soft

(Amplitude
normalized)

Time (ms)

FIGURE 6-25. Glottal waves sensed by a reflectionless tube. (From Monsen, R. B. The use of a reflectionless tube to assess vocal function. In Ludlow, C. L. and Hart, M. 0. (Eds.) *Proceedings of the Conference on the Assessment of Vocal Pathology.* ASHA Reports No. 11 (1981) 141-150. Figure 8, p. 145. Reprinted by permission.)

put can approximate synthetic waves generated by a mathematical vocal-fold model (Monsen, Engebretson, and Vemula, 1978). It is also recognized that the waveform does show abnormalities in cases of confirmed vocal disorder (Tanabe, Isshiki, and Kitajima, 1978). But, given the poorly understood distortions produced by the measurement system, it is not really possible to relate waveform irregularities back to distinct aberrations of laryngeal function, and not enough research on the waveform differences—whatever they may represent—has been done to allow their use for differential diagnosis of dysphonia.

Inverse filtering

The idea of inverse filtering is to derive the vocal tract transfer function and construct a filter that is its inverse. If the

(voiced) speech signal is subjected to such a filter, the acoustic effects of the vocal tract are negated, and the original glottal waveform is restored. The method was first proposed by Miller (1959) who initially implemented it with analog filter circuits. It has since become more common to use a digital computer to generate inverse-filter equations (Miller and Mathews, 1963).

More recently Rothenberg (1973, 1977, 1981) has described a method that returns to the use of analog filtering, but with the difference that the input is the volume-velocity (flow) waveform radiated from the mouth, rather than the radiated pressure wave sensed by a microphone. The volume-velocity wave is transduced using the principle of the pneumotachograph (see Chap. 8) in a special modification. The primary transducer in Rothenberg's system (Figure 6-26) is a face mask circumferentially vented by relatively large holes covered by fine-mesh wire screening. These serve as resistive elements across which a pressure proportional to the flow is developed. Whereas the frequency response of a pneumotachograph is very poor, the mask system has a time resolution of less than ½ ms. Therefore, very rapid changes in airflow can be transduced. The total resistance of the screen elements is very small, keeping pressure inside the mask under 0.3 cm $H_2O/L/s$. The pressure difference across the screen elements that is created by the airflow is sensed by a pair of specially modified microphones connected to a differential amplifier that outputs a voltage proportional to the instantaneous airflow.

The inverse filter network is a special circuit with essentially no phase shift to distort the signal. The filter characteristics are initially set on the basis of spectrographic analysis of the oral flow waveform. They are then adjusted to produce a final glottal waveform with minimal evidence of vocal-tract formants. The final output resembles waves derived from ultrahigh-speed films and photoglottographs quite closely.

The waveforms obtained from either of these acoustic techniques can be tape re-

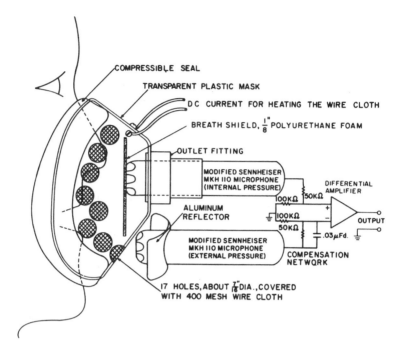

FIGURE 6-26. Circumferentially-vented mask system for transduction of instantaneous airflow. The output signal is inverse-filtered for extraction of the glottal wave. (From Rothenberg, M. A new inverse-filtering technique for deriving the glottal air flow waveform during voicing. *Journal of the Acoustical Society of America*, 53 (1973) 1632-1645. Figure 2, p. 1634. Reprinted by permission.)

corded if an FM recorder is available. Both methods require a considerable amount of user adjustment and neither can analyze continuous speech. ∎

SELECT BIBLIOGRAPHY

Allison, R. D. Bioelectric impedance measurements—introduction to basic factors in impedance plethysmography. In Allison, R. D. (Ed.) *Basic Factors in Bioelectric Impedance Measurements*. Pittsburgh: Instrument Society of America, 1970.pp. 1-70.

Baer, T., Löfqvist, A., and McGarr, N. S. Laryngeal vibrations: a comparison between high-speed filming and glottographic techniques. *Haskins Laboratories Status Report on Speech Research*, SR-73 (1983) 283-291.

Baer, T., Titze, R., and Yoshioka, H. Multiple simultaneous measures of vocal fold activity. In Bless, D. M. and Abbs, J. H. (Eds.). *Vocal Fold Physiology: Contemporary Research and Clinical Issues*. San Diego: College-Hill, 1983. Chap. 19, pp. 227-237.

Bagno, S. and Liebman, F. M. Impedance measurements of living tissue. *Electronics*, 32 (1959) 62-63.

Beach, J. L. and Kelsey, C. A. Ultrasonic doppler monitoring of vocal-fold velocity and displacement. *Journal of the Acoustical Society of America* 46 (1969) 1045-1047.

Bell Telephone Laboratories. High speed motion pictures of the vocal cords. (Motion picture) New York: Bell Telephone Laboratories Bureau of Publications, 1937.

Benguerel, A.-P. and Bhatia, T. K. Hindi stop consonants: an acoustic and fiberoptic study. *Phonetica* 37 (1980) 134-148.

Berry, R. J., Epstein, R., Fourcin, A. J., Freeman, M., MacCurtain, F., and Noscoe, N. An objective analysis of voice disorder: Part one. *British Journal of Disorders of Communicaton*, 17 (1982) 67-76.

Berry, R. J., Epstein, R., Freeman, M., MacCurtain, F., and Noscoe, N. An objective analysis of voice disorders: Part two. *British Journal of Disorders of Communication*, 17 (1982) 77-85.

Bjuggren, G. Device for laryngeal phase-determinable flash photography. *Folia Phoniatrica* 12 (1960) 36-41.

Blaugrund, S. M., Gould, W. J., Tanaka, S., and Kitajima, K. The fiberscope: analysis and function of laryngeal reconstruction. In Titze, I. R. and Scherer, R. C. (Eds.), *Vocal Fold Physiology: Biomechanics, Acoustics, and Phonatray Control*. Denver: Denver Center for the Performing Arts, 1983. Chap. 22., pp. 252-255.

Bordone-Sacerdote, C. and Sacerdote, G. Investigations on the movement of the glottis by ultrasound. *Proceedings of the Fifth International Congress on Acoustics* (Liege, Belgium), 1965.

Brackett, I.P. The vibration of vocal folds at selected frequencies. *Annals of Otology, Rhinology, and Laryngology* 57 (1948) 556-558.

Brewer, D. W. and McCall, G. Visible laryngeal changes during voice therapy: fiberoptic study. *Annals of Otolgy, Rhinology, and Laryngology* 83 (1974) 423-427.

Broad, D. J. The new theories of vocal fold vibration. In Lass, Norman J. (Ed.) *Speech and Language: Advances in Basic Research and Practice*, vol. 2. New York: Academic Press, 1979. Pp. 203-257.

Casper, J., Brewer, D. W., and Conture, E. G. Speech therapy patient evaluation techniques with the fiberscope. In Lawrence, V (Ed.) *Transcripts of the Tenth Symposium on care of the Professional Voice*. New York: The Voice Foundation, 1982. Part II, pp. 136-140.

Chevrie-Muller, C. Etude de fonctionnnement laryngé chez les bègues par la méthode glottographique. *Revue da Laryngologie* 85 (1964) 763-774.

Chevrie- Muller, C. Contribution à l'étude des traces glottographiques chez l'adulte normal. *Revue de Laryngologie* 88 (1967) 227-244.

Chevrie-Muller, C. and Grémy, F. Etude de l'électro-glottogramme et du phonogramme en période de "mue vocale". *Annales d'Oto-Laryngologie* 79 (1962) 1035-1044.

Childers, D. G., Paige, A. and Moore, G. P. Laryngeal vibration patterns: machine-aided measurements from high-speed film. *Archives of Otolaryngology* 102 (1976) 407-410.

Childers, D. G., Naik, J. M., Larar, J. N., Krishnamurthy, A K., and Moore, G. P. Electroglottography, speech and ultra-high speed cinematography. In Titze, L. R. and Scherer, R. C. (Eds.), *Vocal Fold Physiology: Biomechanics, Acoustics, and Phonatory Control*. Denver: Denver Center for the Performing Arts, 1983. Chap. 17.

Childers, D. G., Smith, A. M., and Moore, G. P. Relationships between electroglottograph, speech, and vocal cord contact. *Folia Phoniatrica* 36 (1984) 105-118.

Chollet, G. F. and Kahane, J. C. Laryngeal patterns of consonant productions in sentences observed with an impedance glottograph. In Hollien, H. and Hollien, P. (Eds.) *Currents Is-*sues in the Phonetic Sciences*. Amsterdam: John Benjamins B.V., 1979. Pp. 119-128.

Coleman, R. F. Effect of waveform changes upon roughness perception. *Folia Phoniatrica* 23 1971 314-322.

Coleman, R. F. and Wendahl, R. W. 0n the validity of laryngeal photosensor monitoring. *Journal of the Acoustical Society of America* 44 (1968) 1733-1735.

Croatto, L. and Ferrero, F. L'esame elettroglottografico applicato ad alcuni casi di disodia. *Acta Phoniatrica Latina* 1 (1979) 247-258.

Croatto, L., Ferrero, F. E., and Arrigoni, L. Comparazione fra segnale elettroglottografico e sengale fotoelettroglottografico: primi risulti. *Acta Phoniatrica Latina* 2 (1980) 213-224.

Davidson, T. M., Bone, R. C., and Nahum, L. M. Flexible fiberoptic laryngobronchoscopy. *Laryngoscope* 84 (1974) 1876-1882.

Decroix, G. and Dujardin, J. Etude des accolements glottiques au cours de la phonation par la glottographie de haute fréquence. *Journal Français d'Oto-Rhino-Laryngologie* 7 (1958) 493-499.

Dejonckere, P. H. and Lebacq, J. Electroglottography and vocal nodules: An attempt to quantify the shape of the signal. *Folia Phoniatrica* 37 (1985) 195-200.

Ewan, W. G. and Krones, R. Measuring larynx movement using the thyroumbrometer. *Journal of Phonetics* 2 (1974) 327-335.

Fabre, P. Sphygmographie par simple contact d'électrodes cutanées introduisant dans l'artère de faibles courants de haute fréquence détecteurs de ses variations volumétriques. *Comptes Rendus de la Société de Biologie* 133 (1940) 639-641.

Fabre, P. Un procédé électrique percutané d'inscription de l'accolement glottique au cours de la phonation: glottographie de haute fréquence. Premiers résultats. *Bulletin de l'Académie Nationale de Médecine* 141 (1957) 66-69.

Fabre, P. Etude comparée des glottogrammes et des phonogrammes de la voix humaine. *Annales d'Oto-Laryngologie* 75 (1958) 767-775.

Fabre, P. Glottographie respiratoire, appareillage et premiers résultats. *Comptes Rendus de l'Académie des Sciences* 252 (1961a) 1386.

Fabre, P. Glottographie respiratoire. *Annales d'Oto-Laryngologie* 78 (1961b) 814-824.

Farnsworth, D. W. High-speed motion pictures of the human vocal cords. *Bell Laboratories Record* 18 (1940) 203-208.

Ferguson, G. B. and Crowder, W. J. A simple method of laryngeal and other cavity photography. *Archives of Otolaryngology* 92 (1970) 201-203.

Ferrero, F., Pelamatti, G. M., Vagges, K., and Zovato, S. Normalizzazione temporale e spettrale del segnale elettro-glottografico (per uno studio sistematico delle disfonie). *Acta Phoniatrica Latina* 2 (1980) 225-234.

Fisher, H. B. and Logemann, J. A. Objective evaluation of therapy for vocal nodules: a case report. *Journal of Speech and Hearing Disorders* 35 (1970) 277-285.

Fourcin, A. J. Laryngographic examination of vocal fold vibration. In Wyke, B. (Ed.) *Ventilatory and Phonatory Control Systems.* New York: Oxford University Press, 1974. Pp. 315-333.

Fourcin, A. J. Laryngographic assessment of phonatory function. In Ludlow, C. L. and Hart, M. 0. (Eds.) *Proceedings of the Conference on the Assessment of Vocal Pathology, ASHA Reports,* 11 (1981). Pp. 116-127.

Fourcin, A. J. and Abberton, E. First applications of a new laryngograph. *Medical and Biological Illustration* 21 (1971) 172-182.
Reprinted in: *Volta Review* 74 (1972) 161-176.
Reprinted in: Levitt, J. M. and Houde, R. A. (Eds.) *Sensory Aids for the Hearing Impaired.* N.Y.: John Wiley, 1980. Pp. 376-386.

Fourcin, A. J. and Abberton, E. The laryngograph and the Voiscope in speech therapy. *Proceedings of the 16 International Congress of Logopedics and Phoniatrics,* 1976. Pp. 116-122.

Frøkjaer-Jensen, B. and Thorvaldsen, P. Construction of a Fabre of glottograph. *Annual Report of the Institute of Phonetics of the University of Copenhagen,* 3 (1968) 1-8.

Fujimura, O. Stereo-fiberscope. In Sawashima, M. and Cooper, F. S. (Eds.) *Dynamic Aspects of Speech Production.* Tokyo: University of Tokyo Press, 1977. Pp. 133-137.

Fujimura, O. Fiberoptic observation and measurement of vocal fold movement. In Ludlow, Christy L. and Hart, Molly O. (Eds.) *Proceedings of the Conference on the Assessment of Vocal Pathology, ASHA reports* 11 (1981). Pp.59-69

Fujimura, O., Baer, T., and Niimi, S. A stereofiberscope with a magnetic interlens bridge for laryngeal observation. *Journal of the Acoustical Society of America* 65 (1979) 478-480.

Gilbert, H. R., Potter, C. R., and Hoodin, R. Laryngograph as a measure of vocal fold contact area. *Journal of Speech and Hearing Research* 27 (1984) 178-182.

Gougerot, L., Grémy, F., and Marstal, N. Glottographie à large bande passante. Application à l'étude de la voix de fausset. *Journal de Physiologie* 52 (1960) 823-832.

Gould, W. J. The Gould laryngoscope. *Transactions of the American Academy of Opthalmology and Otolaryngology* 77 (1973) 139-141.

Gould, W. J. Newer aspects of high-speed photography of the vocal folds. In Sawashima, Masayuki and Cooper, Franklin S. *Dynamic*

Aspects of Sppech Production. Tokyo Press, 1977. Pp. 139-144.

Gould, W. J. The fiberscope: flexible and rigid for laryngeal function evaluation. In Titze, I. R. and Scherer, R. C. (Eds.), *Vocal Fold Physiology: Biomechanics, Acoustics, and Phonatory Control.* Denver: Denver Center for the Performing Arts, 1983. Chap. 21, pp. 249-251.

Gould, W. J., Jako, G. J., and Tanabe, M. Advances in high-speed motion picture photography of the larynx. *Transactions of the American Academy of Opthalmology and Otolaryngology,* 78 (1974) 276-278.

Grémy, F. and Guérin, C. Etude du glottogramme chez l'enfant sourd en cours de rééducation vocale. *Annales d'Oto-Laryngologie* 80 (1963) 803-815.

Hahn, C. and Kitzing, P. Indirect endoscopic photography of the larynx. *Journal of Audiovisual Media in Medicine* 1 (1978) 121-130.

Hamlet, S. L. Location of slope discontinuities in glottal pulse shapes during vocal fry. *Journal of the Acoustical Society of America.* 50 (1971) 1561-1562.

Hamlet, S. L. Interpretation of ultrasonic signals in terms of phase difference of vocal fold vibration. *Journal of the Acoustical Society of America* 51 (1972a) 90-91.

Hamlet, S. L. Vocal fold articulatory activity during whispered sibilants. *Archives of Otolaryngology* 95 (1972b) 211-213.

Hamlet, S. L. Vocal compensation: an ultrasonic study of vocal fold vibration in normal and nasal vowels. *Cleft Palate Journal* 10 (1973) 267-285.

Hamlet, S. L. Ultrasonic measurement of larynx height and vocal vibratory pattern. *Journal of the Acoustical Society of America* 68 (1980) 121-126.

Hamlet, S. L. Ultrasound assessment of phonatory function. In Ludlow, C. L. and Hart, M. O. (Eds.) *Proceedings of the Conference on the Assessment of Vocal Pathology. ASHA Reports* 11 (1981) Pp. 128-140

Hamlet, S. L. and Palmer, J. M. Investigation of laryngeal trills using the transmission of ultrasound through the larynx. *Folia Phoniatrica* 26 (1974) 362-377.

Hamlet, S. L. and Reid, J. M. Transmission of ultrasound through the larynx as a means of determining vocal-fold activity. *IEEE Transactions on Biomedical Engineering* BME-19 (1972) 34-37.

Hanson, D. G., Gerratt, B. R., and Ward, P. H. Glottographic measurement of vocal dysfunction: A preliminary report. *Annals of Otology, Rhinolgy, and Laryngology,* 92 (1983) 413-420.

Harden, R. J. Comparison of glottal area changes as measured from ultrahigh-speed photographs and photoelectric glottographs. *Journal of Speech and Hearing Research* 18 (1975) 728-738.

Hayden, E. H. and Koike, Y. A data processing scheme for frame by frame film analysis. *Folia Phoniatrica* 24 (1972) 169-181.

Hertz, C. H., Lindström, K., and Sonesson, B. Ultrasonic recording of the vibrating vocal folds. *Acta Otolaryngologica* 69 (1970) 223-230.

Hillman, R. E. and Weinberg, B. A new procedure for venting a reflectionless tube. *Journal of the Acoustical Society of America* 69 (1981A) 1449-1451.

Hillman, R. E. and Weinberg, B. Estimation of glottal volume velocity waveform properties: a review and study of some methodological assumptions. In Lass, Norman J. (Ed.), *Speech and Language: Advances in Basic Research and Practice*, vol. 6. New York: Academic Press, 1981B, pp. 411-473.

Hillman, R. E., Weinberg, B. and Tree, D. Glottal waveform measurement: equipment, calibration, and application. Paper presented at the 1978 Convention of the American Speech and Hearing Association.

Hirano, M. Phonosurgery: basic and clinical investigations. *Otologia* (Fukuoka) 21 (1975) 239-440.

Hirano, M. *Clinical Examination of Voice.* New York: Springer-Verlag, 1981.

Hirano, M., Gould, W. J., Lambiase, A., and Kakita, Y. Vibratory behavior of the vocal folds in a case of a unilateral polyp. *Folia Phoniatrica* 33 (1981) 275-284.

Hirano, M., Yoshida, Y., Matsushita, H., and Nakajima, T. An apparatus for ultra highspeed cinematography of the vocal cords. *Annals of Otology, Rhinology, and Laryngology* 83 1974 12-18.

Hollien, H. On vocal registers. *Journal of Phonetics* 2 (1974) 125.143.

Hollien, H., Girard, G. T., and Coleman, R. F. Vocal fold vibratory patterns of pusle register. *Folia Phoniatrica* 29 (1977) 200-205.

Holm, C. L'évolution de la phonation de la première enfance à la puberté: une étude électroglottographique. *Journal Français d'Oto-Rhino-Laryngologie* 20 (1971) 437-440.

Holmer, N.-G., Kitzing, P., and Lindström, K. Echo glottography. *Acta Otolaryngologica* 75 (1973) 454-463.

Holmer, N.-G. and Rundqvist, H. E. Ultrasonic registration of the fundamental frequency of a voice during normal speech. *Journal of the Acoustical Society of America* 58 (1975) 1073-1077.

Jentzsch, H., Sasama, R., and Unger, E. Elektroglottographische Untersuchungen zur Problematik des Stimmeinsatzes bei zusammen-hängenden Sprechen. *Folia Phoniatrica* 30 (1978) 59-66.

Jentzsch, H., Unger, E., and Sasama, R. Elektroglottographische Verlaufskontrollen bei Patienten mit funktionellen Stimmstörungen. *Folia Phoniatrica* 33 (1981) 234-241.

Kagaya, R. A fiberoptic and acoustic study of the Korean stops, affricates, and fricatives. *Journal of Phonetics* 2 (1974) 161-180.

Kakita, Y., Hirano, M., Kawasaki, H., and Matsuo, K. Stereolaryngoscopy: a new method to extract vertical movement of the vocal fold during vibration. In Titze, I. R. and Scherer, R. C. (Eds), *Vocal Fold Physiology: Biomechanics, Acoustics, and Phonatary Control.* Denver: Denver Center for the Performing Arts, 1983. Chap. 16, pp. 191-201.

Kaneko, T., Kobayashi, N., Tachibana, M., Naito, J., Hayawaki, K., Uchida, K., Yoshioka, T., and Suzuki, H. L'ultrasonoglottographie; l'aire neutre glottique et la vibration de la corde vocale. *Revue de Laryngologie* 97 (1976) 363-369.

Kaneko, T., Uchida, K., Suzuki, H., Komatsu, K., Kanesaka, T., Kobayashi, N., and Naito, J. Ultransonic observations of vocal fold vibration. In Stevens, K. N. and Hirano, M. (Eds.) *Vocal Fold Physiology.* Tokyo: University of Tokyo, 1981. Pp. 107-117.

Kaneko, T., Suzuki, H., Uchida, K., Kanesaka, T., Komatsu, K., and Shimada, A. The movement of the inner layers of the vocal fold during phonation—observation by ultrasonic method. In Bless, D. M. and Abbs, J. H. (Eds.). *Vocal Fold Physiology: Comtemporary Research and Clinical Issues.* San Diego: College-Hill, 1983. Chap. 18, pp. 223-237.

Kelman, A. W. Vibratory pattern of the vocal folds. *Folia Phoniatrica* 33 (1981) 73-99.

Kitzing, P. Methode zur kombinierten photo- und elektroglotto-graphischen Registrierung von Stimmlippenschwingungen. *Folia Phoniatrica* 29 (1977) 249-260.

Kitzing, P. Photo- and electroglottographical recording of the laryngeal vibratory pattern during different registers. *Folia Phoniatrica* 34 (1982) 234-241.

Kitzing, P. and Löfqvist, A. Clinical application of combined electro- and photoglottography. *Proceedings of the 17th Congress of Logopedics and Phoniatrics*, 1978.

Kitzing, P. and Löfqvist, A. Evaluation of voice therapy by means of photoglottography. *Folia Phoniatrica* 31 (1979) 103-109.

Kitzing, P. and Sonesson, B. A photoglottographical study of the female vocal folds during phonation. *Folia Phoniatrica* 26 (1974) 138-149.

Koike, Y. and Hirano, M. Glottal-area time function and subglottal pressure variation. *Jour-*

nal of the Acoustical Society of America 54 (1973) 1618-1627.

Köster, J.P. and Smith, S. Zur Interpretation elektrischer und photoelektrischer Glottogramme. Folia Phoniatrica 22 (1970) 9299.

Landman, G. H. M. Laryngography and Cinelaryngography. Baltimore: Williams and Wilkins, 1970.

Lebrun, Y. and Hasquin-Deleval, J. On the socalled ‚dissociations' between electroglottogram and phonogram. Folia Phoniatrica 23 (1971) 225-227.

Lecluse, F. L. E. Laboratory investigations in electroglottography. Proceedings of the 16 International Congress of Logopedics and Phoniatrics, 1974, Pp. 294-296.

Lecluse, F. L. E. Elektroglottographie. Utrecht Drukkerijelinkwijk, B. V., 1977

Lecluse, F. L. E., Brocaar, M. P., and Verschurre, J. The electroglottography and its relation to glottal activity. Folia Phoniatrica, 27 (1975) 215-224.

Lecluse, F. L., Tiwari, R. M., and Snow, G. B. Electroglottographic studies of Staffieri neoglottis. Laryngoscope 91 (1981) 971-975.

Lisker, L., Abramson, A. S., Cooper, F. S., and Schvey, M. H. Transillumination of the larynx in running speech. Journal of the Acoustical Society of America 39 (1966) 1218.

Lisker, L., Abramson, A. S., Cooper, F. S., and Schvey, M. H. Transillumination of the larynx in running speech. Journal of the Acoustical Society of America 45 (1969) 1554-1546.

Löfqvist, A. and Yoshioka, H. Laryngeal activity in Icelandic obstruent production. Haskins Laboratories Status Report on Speech Research SR63/64 (1980) 275-292.

MacCurtain, F. and Fourcin, A. J. Applications of the electro-laryngograph wave form display. ln Lawrence, Van L. (Ed.) Transcripts of the Tenth Symposium on Care of the Professional Voice. New York: The Voice Foundation, 1982. Part II pp. 51-57.

Metz, D. E. and Whitehead, R. L. Simultaneous collection of multiple physiologic data with high speed laryngeal film data. In Lawrence, V. L. (Ed.) Transcripts of the Tenth Symposium on Care of the Professional Voice. New York: The Voice Foundation, 1982. Part II pp. 73-77.

Metz, D. E., Whitehead, R. L., and Peterson, D. H. An optical-illumination system for highspeed laryngeal cinematography. Journal of the Acoustical Society of America 67 (1980) 719-720.

Miller, J. E. and Mathews, M. V. Investigation of the glottal waveshape by automatic inverse filtering. Journal of the Acoustical Society of America 35 (1963) 1876.

Miller, R. L. Nature of the vocal cord wave. Journal of the Acoustical Society of America 31 (1959) 667-677.

Minifie, F. D., Kelsey, C. A., and Hixon, T. J. Measurement of vocal fold motion using an ultrasonic Doppler velocity monitor. Journal of the Acoustical Society of America 43 (1968) 1165-1169.

Monsen, R. B. The use of a reflectionless tube to assess vocal function. In Ludlow, C. L. and Hart, M. 0. (Eds.) Proceedings of the Conference on the Assessment of Vocal Pathology. ASHA Reports 11 (1981) Pp. 141-150.

Monsen, R. B. and Engebretson, A. M. Study of variations in the male and female glottal wave. Journal of the Acoustical Society of America 62 (1977) 981-993.

Monsen, R. B., Engebretson, A. M. and Vemula, N. R. Indirect assessment of the contribution of subglotal air pressure and vocal-fold tension to changes of fundamental frequency in English. Journal of the Acoustical Society of America 64 (1978) 65-80.

Moore, P. and von Leden, H. Dynamic variations of the vibratory pattern in the normal larynx. Folia Phoniatrica 10 (1958) 205-238.

Moore, G. P., White, F. D., and von Leden, H. Ultra high speed photography in laryngeal physiology. Journal of Speech and Hearing Disorders 27 (1962) 165-171.

Munhall, K. G., and Ostry, D. J. Ultrasonic measurement of laryngeal kinematics. In Titze, I. R. and Scherer, R. C. (Eds.), Vocal Fold Physiology: Biomechanics, Acoustics, and Phonatary Control. Denver: Denver Center for the Performing Arts, 1983. Chap. 12.

Niimi, S. and Fujimura, O. Stereo-fiberscope investigation of the larynx. Paper presented at the Conference on the Care of the Professional Voice, New York, 1976.

Noscoe, N. J., High definition radiographic analysis of voice and its disorders Radiography, 48 (1982) 147-150.

Ohala, J. Studies of variations in glottal aperature using photoelectric glottography. Journal of the Acoustical Society of America 41 (1967) 1613.

Ondráckova, J. Vocal chord activity. Its dynamics and role in speech production. Folia Phoniatrica 24 (1972) 405-419.

Rambaud-Pistone, E. Place de l'étude instrumentale dans le bilan vocal. Bulletin d'Audiophonologie 17 (1984) 43-58.

Reed, V. W. The electroglottograph in voice teaching. In Lawrence, V. L. (Ed.) Transcripts of the Tenth Symposium on Care of the Professional Voice. New York: The Voice Foundation, 1982. Pp. 58-65.

Reinsch, M. and Gobsch, H. Zur quantitativen Auswertung elektroglottographischer Kurven bei Normalpersonen. Folia Phoniatrica 24 (1972) 1-6.

Rothenberg, M. A new inverse-filtering technique for deriving the glottal air flow waveform during voicing. Journal of the Acoustical

Society of America 53 (1973) 1632-1645.

Rothenberg, M. Measurement of airflow in speech. Journal of Speech and Hearing Research 20 (1977) 155-176.

Rothenberg, M. Some relations between glottal air flow and vocal fold contact area. In Ludlow, Christy L. and Hart, Molly O. (Eds.) Proceedings of the Conference on the Assessment of Vocal Pathology. ASHA Reports 11 (1981). Pp. 88-96.

Rubin, H. J. and LeCover, M. Technique of high-speed photography of the larynx. Annals of Otology, Rhinology, and Laryngology 69 (1960) 1072-1083.

Saito, S., Fukuda, H., Isogai, Y., and Ono, H. Xray stroboscopy. In Stevens, K. N. and Hirano, M. (Eds.). Vocal Fold Physiology. Tokyo: University of Tokyo, 1981. Pp. 107-117.

Saito, S., Fukuda, H., Kitahara, S., and Kokawa, N. Stroboscopic observation of vocal fold vibration with fiberoptics. Folia Phoniatrica 30 (1978) 241-244.

Sawashima, M. Glottal adjustments for English obstruents. Haskins Laboratories Status Report on Speech Research SR21/22 (1970) 180-200.

Sawashima, M. Fiberoptic observation of the larynx and other speech organs. In Sawashima, M. and Cooper, F. S. (Eds.) Dynamic Aspects of Speech Production. Tokyo: University of Tokyo Press, 1977. Pp. 31-46.

Sawashima, M., Abramson, A. S., Cooper, F. S., and Lisker, L. Observing laryngeal adjustments during running speech by use of a fiberoptics system. Phonetica 22 (1970) 193-201.

Sawashima, M. and Hirose, H. A new laryngoscopic technique by use of fiberoptics. Journal of the Acoustical Society of America 43 (1968) 168-169.

Sawashima, M., Hirose, H., and Fujimura, O. Observation of the larynx by a fiberscope inserted through the nose. Journal of the Acoustical Society of Amercia 42 (1967) 1208.

Sawashima, M., Hirose, H., Honda, K., Yoshioka, H., Hibi, S. R., Kawase, N., and Yamada, M. Stereoscopic measurement of the laryngeal structure. In Bless, D. M. and Abbs, J. H. (Eds.). Vocal Fold Physiology: Contemporary Research and Clinical Issues. San Diego: College-Hill 1983 Chap. 22 pp. 265-276

Sawashima, M., Hirose, H., Honda, K., and Hibi, S. Measurement of the laryngeal structures by use of a stereoendoscope. Proceedings of the Conference on Vocal Fold Physiology, Madison, WI 1981. Pp. 96-101.

Sawashima, M., Hirose, H. and Niimi, S. Glottal conditions in articulation of Japanese voiceless consonants. Proceedings of the 16 International Congress of Logopedics and Phoniatrics. Basel: S. Karger, 1974. Pp. 409-414.

Sawashima, M. and Ushijima, T. The use of fiberscope in speech research. In Hirschberg, J., Szèpe, Gy., and Vass-Kovács, E. (Eds.) Papers in Interdisciplinary Speech Research. Budapest: Akadèmiai Kiadö 1972. Pp. 229-231

Shipp, T. Vertical laryngeal position during continuous and discrete vocal frequency change. Journal of Speech and Hearing Research 18 (1975) 707-718.

Shipp, T. Vertical larynx position in singers with jaw stabilized. In Lawrence, V. (Ed.) Transcripts of the Seventh Symposium on Care of the Professional Voice. New York: The Voice Foundation, 1979. Part I. pp. 44-77.

Shipp, T. and Izdebski, K. Vocal frequency and vertical larynx positioning by singers and nonsingers. Journal of the Acoustical Society of America 58 (1975) 1104-1106.

Smith, S. Remarks on the physiology of the vibrations of the vocal cords. Folia Phoniatrica 6 (1954) 166-178.

Smith, S. Electroglottography. Proceedings of the 17 International Congress of Logopedics and Phoniatrics, 1977.

Smith, S. Research on the principle of electroglottography. Folia Phoniatrica 33 (1981) 1-10.

Sondhi, M. M. Measurement of the glottal waveform. Journal of the Acoustical Society of America 57 (1975) 228-232.

Sonesson, B. A method for studying the vibratory movements of the vocal folds. Journal of Laryngology and Otology 73 (1959) 732-737.

Sonesson, B. On the anatomy and vibratory pattern of the human vocal folds. Acta Otolaryngologica, suppl. 156 (1960) 1-80.

Soron, H. 1. High-speed photography in speech research. Journal of Speech and Hearing Research 10 (1967) 768-776.

Tanabe, M., Isshiki, N. and Kitajima, K. Application of reflectionless acoustic tube for extraction of the glottal waveform. Studia Phonologica 12 (1978) 31-38.

Taub, S. The Taub oral panendoscope: a new technique. Cleft Palate Journal 3 (1966a) 328-346.

Taub, S. Oral panendoscope for direct observation and audiovisual recording of velopharyngeal areas during phonation. Transactions of the American Academy of Ophthalmology and Otolaryngology(1966b) 855-857.

Timcke, R., von Leden, H., and Moore, P. Laryngeal vibrations: measurements of the glottic wave. Part 1. The normal vibratory cycle. Archives of Otolaryngology 68 (1958) 1-19.

Timcke, R., von Leden, H., and Moore, P. Laryngeal vibrations: measurements of the glottic wave. Part II: Physiologic variations. Archives of Otolaryngology 69 (1959) 438-444.

Titze, I. R. The human vocal cords: a mathematical model. Part I. Phonetica 28 (1973) 129-170.

Titze, I. R. The human vocal cords: a mathematical model. Part II. *Phonetica* 29 (1974) 1-21.

Titze, I. R. and Talkin, D. T. A theoretical study of the affects of various laryngeal configurations on the acoustics of phonation. *Journal of the Acoustical Society of America* 66 (1979) 60-74.

Titze, I. and Talkin, D. Simulation and interpretation of glottographic waveforms. In Ludlow, C. L. and Hart, M. 0. (Eds.) *Proceedings of the Conference on the Assessment of Vocal Pathology. ASHA Reports* 11 (1981) 48-55

Unger, E., Unger, H. and Tietze, G. Stimmuntersuchungen mittels der elektroglottographischen Einzelkurven. *Folia Phoniatrica* 33 (1981) 168-180.

Vallancien, B. Nouvelles recherches sur le mécanisme vibratoire du larynx. *Acta Oto-rhino-laryngologica* 26 (1972) 725-740.

Vallancien, B. and Faulhaber, J. Causes d'erreurs en glottographie. *Journal Français d'Otorhinolaryngologie* 15 (1966) 383-394.

Vallancien, B. and Faulhaber, J. What to think of glottography. *Folia Phoniatrica* 19 (1967) 39-44.

Vallancien, B., Gautheron, B., Pasternak, L. Guisez, D., and Paley, B. Comparaison des signaux microphoniques, diaphanographiques et glottographiques avec application au laryngographe. *Folia Phoniatrica* 23 (1971) 371-380.

van den Berg, J. A Δf-generator and movie-adapter unit for laryngo-stroboscopy. *Practica Oto-rhino-laryngologica* 21 (1959) 355-363.

van Michel, Cl. Etude, par la méthode électroglottographique, des comportements glottiques de type phonatoire en dehors de toute émission sonore. *Revue de Laryngologie* 7-8 (1964) 469-475.

van Michel, Cl. Mouvements glottiques phonatoires sans émission sonore: étude électroglottographique. *Folia Phoniatrica* 18 (1966) 1-18.

van Michel, C. Morphologie de la courbe glottographique dans certains troubles fonctionnels du larynx. *Folia Phoniatrica* 19 (1967) 192-202.

van Michel, Cl., Pfister, K. A., and Luchsinger, R. Electroglottographie et cinématographie laryngée ultra-rapide: comparaison des résultats. *Folia Phoniatrica* 22 (1970) 81-91.

van Michel, Cl. and Raskin, L. L'électroglottomètre Mark 4, son principe, ses possibilités. *Folia Phoniatrica* 21 (1969) 145-157.

von Leden, H. The electronic synchron-stroboscope. *Annals of Otology, Rhinology, and Laryngology* 70 (1961) 881-893.

von Leden, H., LeCover, M., Ringel, R. L., and Isshiki, N. Improvements in laryngeal cinematography. *Archives of Otolaryngology* 83 (1966) 482-487.

von Leden, H., and Moore, P. Vibratory pattern of the vocal cords in unilateral laryngeal paralysis. *Acta Oto-laryngologica* 53 (1961) 493-506.

von Leden, H., Moore, P., and Timcke, R. Laryngeal vibrations: measurements of the glottic wave. Part III: the pathologic larynx. *Archives of Otolaryngology* 71 (1960) 16-35.

Ward, P. H., Hanson, D. G., and Berci, G. Photographic studies of the larynx in central laryngeal paresis and paralysis. *Acta Oto-laryngologica* 91 (1981) 353-367.

Wendahl, R. W., and Coleman, R. F. Vocal cord spectra derived from glottal-area waveforms and subglottal photocell monitoring. *Journal of the Acoustical Society of America* 41 (1967) 1613A.

Whitehead, R. L., Metz, D. E., and Whitehead, B. H. Vibratory patterns of the vocal folds during pulse register phonation. *Journal of the Acoustical Society of America* 75 (1984) 1293-1297

Winckel, F. Phoniatric acoustics. In Luchsinger, R. L. and Arnold, G. E. (Eds.) *Voice-Speech-Language.* Belmont, CA: Wadsworth, 1965. Pp. 24-55.

Yanagihara, N. Hoarseness: investigation of the physiological mechanisms. *Annals of Otorhinolaryngology* 76 (1967) 472-488.

Yanagisawa, E., Strothers, G., Owens, T., and Honda, K. Videolaryngoscopy: a comparison of fiberscopic and telescopic documentation. *Annals of Otology, Rhinology, and Laryngology* 92 (1983) 430-436.

Yoshioka, H., Löfqvist, A., and Hirose, H. Laryngeal adjustments in Japanese voiceless sound production. *Haskins Laboratories Status Report on Speech Research* SR63/64 (1980) 293-308.

Zagzebski, J. A. and Bless, D. M. Correspondence of ultrasonic and stroboscopic visualization of vocal folds. ln Titze, I. R. and Scherer, R. C. (Eds.), *Vocal Fold Physiology: Biomechanics, Acoustics, and Phonatory Control.* Denver: Denver Center for the Performing Arts, 1983. Chap. 13, pp. 163-168.

Zagzebski, J. A., Bless, D. M., and Ewanowski, S. J. Pulse echo imaging of the larynx using rapid ultrasonic scanners. In Bless, D. M. and Abbs, J. H. (Eds.). *Vocal Fold Physiology: Contemporary Research and Clinical Issues.* San Diego: College-Hill, 1983. Chap. 17 pp. 210-222.

CHAPTER 7

Air Pressure

The sounds of speech are the product of careful and precise use of the air pressure generated by the respiratory system. It is frequently useful to know what the air pressure is in a given region of the vocal tract (especially as compared to the pressure at some other location) and, often more important, to observe changes in air pressure values that result from speech activity. Such observations, coupled with an understanding of vocal tract structure and function, permit the clinician to infer a great deal about the nature and degree of speech abnormality. The importance of such air pressure measures has motivated the development of numerous measurement instruments and techniques. The most useful of these will be discussed in this section.

GENERAL PHYSICAL PRINCIPLES

Definition and Units of Measurement

Pressure is defined as the force per unit area acting perpendicular to a surface. Both the unit of force and the area may be selected to suit the application. One would not, for example, find it convenient to measure the pressure in a child's balloon in tons per square yard nor the pressure at the depths of the ocean in grams per square millimeter. In the field of speech and hearing the most common force unit has been the dyne (d) and the area most frequently used has been the square centimeter (cm²). Recent revisions of the international system of weights and measures have given more currency to a pressure unit called the *pascal*. One pascal (Pa) is equivalent to a force of one newton acting on a surface of one square meter. (The pascal is the exact equivalent of the *torr*, an older term which is still in frequent use.)

Important as it is to know and understand these units of measurement, they are not often encountered in descriptions of speech behavior. Rather, a simpler and more direct yardstick is usually applied. Its basis is exemplified by the U-tube manometer (shown in Figure 7-1) which is a simple tube partially filled with a liquid. When both ends of the tube are open the level of the liquid will be same in both sides. As excess pressure is applied to the column of liquid on one side, it forces fluid out, causing the column of liquid on the other side to rise. The applied pressure can be described in terms

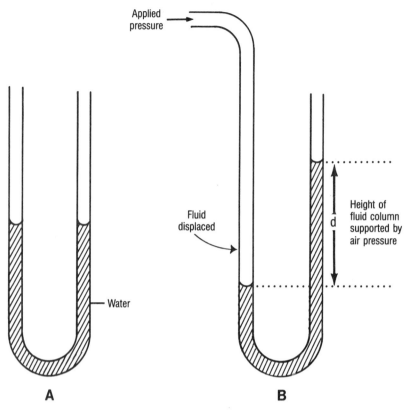

FIGURE 7-1. The U-tube manometer (A) is simply a glass tube filled with water. Pressure applied to one arm of the tube, as in B, causes the water to rise in the other arm. The difference in the level of water in the two arms is a measure of the applied pressure.

of the height of the column of liquid it is supporting—that is, as the vertical distance between the two liquid levels. To say, for example, that a person's subglottal pressure for speech is 7 cm H_2O is to indicate that the air below the larynx exerts enough force to hold up a column of water 7 cm high.

Common units of measurement that will be encountered in the current speech and hearing literature include centimeters of water (cm H_2O), millimeters of mercury (mm Hg, also called *torrs* or *pascals*) and dynes per square centimeter (d/cm²), mentioned above. Older literature may refer to ounces per square inch (oz/in²) and an occasional instrument (for example the Hunter oral manometer, which is still found in many clinics) may be calibrated this way. Conversion from one pressure unit to an-

other is straightforward; the necessary information is provided in Appendix A.

The height of the column of liquid in the U-tube manometer is really a function of *two* opposing forces: the air pressure applied to one side of the U-tube and whatever pressure might be acting on the other side. In Figure 7-1, while the pressure to be measured is applied to one side, the other is left open to the atmosphere. But the atmosphere itself exerts pressure (that is what a barometer measures), and this acts on the open side of the U-tube. The resultant height of the fluid column, therefore, represents not simply the applied air pressure, but rather the difference between it and the pressure of the atmosphere. The height of the fluid column in Figure 7-1 really should be said to be "d" units greater than atmospheric pressure. Engineers refer to this kind of measure as *gauge pressure.* It is also possible to measure pressure as compared to a vacuum *(absolute pressure)* or as compared to some other pressure *(differential pressure).* Absolute pressure is clearly of little value to the speech clinician, and it will not generally be encountered. All three types of pressure measures are schematized in Figure 7-2.

Influence of Flow on Pressure Measurement

If the air whose pressure is to be determined is not moving (as when maximum sustainable oral air pressure is to be assessed), its pressure is the same in all directions and the spatial orientation of the tube through which the pressure is sampled is irrelevant. The situation is very different if pressure must be measured during an air flow (as during speech). The force exerted against a surface by a stream of air is the result of two factors: the static air pressure (which is the component of interest) and the *kinetic energy pressure* (common-

ly called the *stagnation pressure)* which is a result of the momentum of the air molecules. The latter is due to the speed of air movement rather than to the driving pressure itself. It must not be allowed to exert an influence on the pressure measurement.

Figure 7-3 shows how the kinetic energy pressure alters the air pressure measurement. When the pressure-sampling tube faces into the airflow (points upstream, Figure 7-3A) both the static and kinetic energy pressures impinge on the measurement system, giving a spuriously high reading. When the tube faces away from the air flow (points downstream, Figure 7-3B) the observed pressure is the static pressure *minus* the kinetic energy pressure, a value significantly below the static pressure alone. The solution to the measurement problem lies in orienting the probe tube so that its opening is perpendicular to the flow, as in Figure 7-3C. This orientation is more easily described than achieved with precision, but incorrect placement of the probe tube is a major threat to validity, so at least an approximation of perpendicularity must be

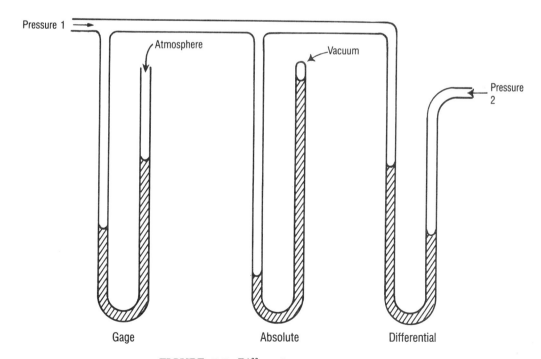

FIGURE 7-2. Different pressure measures.

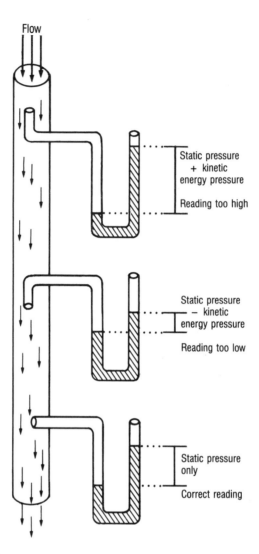

FIGURE 7-3. Effect on the pressure reading of different orientations of the sensing tube in a flow. If the sensing tube faces into the flow, the reading represents static *plus* kinetic pressures. If it faces away from the flow, the reading is of the static pressure *minus* the kinetic pressure. Only when the sensing tube faces perpendicular to the flow does the reading reflect the static pressure alone.

obtained if useful pressure measures are to be taken. An interesting example of grossly inflated pressure values, no doubt due to stagnation pressure effects, may be seen in the intraoral pressure values obtained by Black (1950) and analyzed by Hardy (1965).

Static and Dynamic Measures

The choice of a measurement technique is very strongly influenced by whether the pressure to be observed is static (relatively stable) or dynamic (characterized by fairly rapid change). For example, the determination of maximum oral breath pressure involves observation of a static pressure: The client maintains an intraoral pressure for a relatively long time. On the other hand, determination of intraoral air pressure during /p/ in running speech involves a dynamic pressure: The air pressure rises rapidly, is sustained for only a fraction of a second, and then is released. Static pressures are equivalent to DC electrical signals, while dynamic pressures represent AC events (see Chap. 2). Accurate recording of dynamic pressures will require instrumentation capable of faithfully reproducing even the fastest fluctuations. More precisely stated, the measurement system must have an adequate frequency response. The emphasis here is on the response of the *system*, the combination of transducer, amplifier, and readout device.* Since most transducers are too big to be placed directly into the vocal tract where pressure is to be measured, a sensing probe tube of some sort will almost always be needed. This tube can and does limit the frequency response of the system, and its effects should be considered when interpreting results. Sensing tubes are described in greater detail with specific instruments in the discussion that follows.

For precise measurement of dynamic pressures it is important that the transducer neither expand nor contract as the pressure inside it changes. It should not, in other words, behave like an elastic balloon. If it does fluctuate in size, air will flow into the tube and transducer, from the region in which the sensing tube lies, as pressure rises, and it will flow back out as pressure falls. These volumetric reactions reduce the amount of pressure change by the pneumatic equivalent of electronic integration. A system that smooths out the very pressure changes it should be detecting is said to be excessively compliant. Most electronic pressure transducers will not present the clinician with this problem: The volumetric displacement of a typical unit is on the order of 0.01 ml. But simpler devices, such as a U-tube manometer, may have a displacement of several milliliters at typical vocal tract pressures, making them useless for dynamic measurements even if their other limitations could be remedied.

PRESSURE INSTRUMENTATION

Sensing Tube

As a rule, pressure transducers are located externally and are coupled to the vocal tract region in which pressure is to

be observed by a probe or sensing tube. When measuring quasi-static pressures, or when the probe's interference with speech behavior is not a concern, the tube can be of any convenient type. Standard laboratory rubber tubing, for example, is commonly used with oral manometers and is suitable for use with other devices of this category.

Dynamic pressure measurements confront the clinician with more complex problems. The sensing tube will frequently have to be placed where the lip or tongue may jostle it as they move, so the sensing tube and the means of fastening it in place should ideally be as small and unobtrusive as possible. Any reduction of the tube's diameter, or increase in its length, increases its impedance, which limits frequency response and may interfere with measurement validity. Hardy (1965) felt that curvature of the sensing tube also affects system response, although this has not been borne out in tests conducted by Edmonds et al. (1971). All of these problems become more acute as the pressure fluctuations become more rapid (that is, there is progressive high-frequency loss). The choice of a sensing tube must, therefore, represent a compromise between the minimization of deleterious factors and the important requirement that the measurement process not disrupt speech activity.

For most applications, a polyethylene tube having an internal diameter of 1.4 to 1.6 mm is used. This size will fit on a 17-gauge hypodermic needle, which is used to couple it to the fitting used on many pressure transducers. Shaping the tube for specific applications is accomplished by inserting a length of relatively thick copper wire or solder into it and bending the tube-cum-wire to the desired shape. With the wire serving as the form, the tube is immersed in boiling water until softened, then it is removed and allowed to cool. The wire is then pulled out, leaving the sensing tube shaped as needed. To keep the length of the sensing tube to a minimum (no more than 15 cm, if at all possible) the pressure transducer should be located very close to the client's face.

---

*The influence of various system characteristics on measurement accuracy is analyzed by Fry (1960).

U-Tube Manometer

Construction and Physical Principles

An extremely simple device, the U-tube manometer is available to any clinical facility. Although a U-tube can be bought, one is easily made in just a few minutes by mounting a bent section of laboratory glass tubing on a vertical surface. (If glass-bending skills or facilities are not available, two straight tubes can be connected at the bottom with rubber or plastic tubing.) The mounted tube is filled to half its height with water to which a very small amount of detergent is added to reduce surface-tension effects. Care must be taken to avoid trapping air bubbles in the tube during the filling operation. The sensing tube is attached to one arm and the device is ready for use.

The functioning of the U-tube manometer rests on fundamental physical principles; it is therefore inherently calibrated. Readings are taken of the difference between the heights of the liquid columns. This distance is itself the pressure measurement. The choice of fluid for filling the U-tube is governed by the expected magnitude of the pressure to be measured. The denser the liquid the less displacement of the column per unit of force. That is, sensitivity diminishes with increased fluid density. The two substances most commonly used are water (for relatively low pressures) and mercury (for higher pressures). Other fluids with densities less that that of water could serve in cases where still greater sensitivity is needed. Measurement validity is dependent, at least in part, on the purity of the liquid used. For clinical purposes ordinary clean mercury or tap water will suffice.

Implementation

Because it requires the movement of a large mass over a significant distance, the response of the U-tube manometer is inherently slow. Accordingly, it is useful only for static pressures. It is also difficult to read accurately with any speed. While schemes for electronically transducing the height of the column have been worked out, they are hardly worth the significant investment required. Obviously, it would be better to purchase an electronic transduction system in the first place. The U-tube, then, cannot generate a permanent record.

DETERMINATION OF STATIC PRESSURE. The U-tube manometer is most commonly used to measure static oral or nasal pressure. All that is required is that the sensing tube be fitted with a suitable mouthpiece (a short length of fire-polished glass tubing will do in many instances) or with a nasal olive. (If the latter is not available a substitute may be made by molding ear-mold plastic around the end of a glass tube.) The sensing tube is then simply held in the mouth or fitted to a naris.

CALIBRATION OF OTHER PRESSURE TRANSDUCERS. Because it is inherently calibrated the U-tube manometer is often used to calibrate other pressure transducers. It is this purpose, in fact, that the U-tube most commonly serves. Figure 7-4 shows how the U-tube and the device to be calibrated are connected in parallel to a source of air pressure (in this case, a hypodermic syringe). The air pressure acts equally on both devices, and thus the output of the device being calibrated represents the pressure shown by the U-tube.

Bourdon Tube

Construction and Physical Principles

The device used in most dial-type pressure gauges is the Bourdon tube, which is one type of "elastic" pressure transducer. The Bourdon tube itself is a thin-walled metal tube whose cross section is a flattened circle (Figure 7-5A). Increased pressure within the tube causes it to bend outward: Its cross section becomes more nearly circular. The resulting stress forces the free end of the tube to be displaced. The direction of this movement depends on the

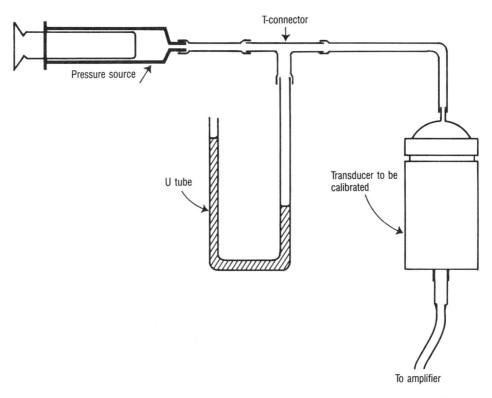

FIGURE 7-4. Connection of a U-tube manometer for calibrating a pressure transducer.

shape of the tube; the "C" form, shown in Figure 7-5B is common. The movement of the free end of the Bourdon tube is used to drive a dial pointer via a mechanical linkage to permit pressure to be read directly. In cases where an electronic output is desirable the movement of the tube can be transduced in a number of ways, for example by linkage to a special transformer called a *linear variable differential transformer* (LVDT) or by having it move a shutter to vary the amount of light that shines on a photocell (as in some pressure transducers marketed by Narco Biosystems, Inc.) These schemes, however, require considerable mechanical structure, which is likely to reduce reliability, frequency response, and overall ruggedness. Despite its very real limitations in terms of resolution and frequency response, the Bourdon-type oral manometer (such as the one produced by Hunter) can be "a useful clinical tool when it is used properly and when the obtained

results are interpreted in ways which are consistent with our current knowledge of it" (Morris, 1966, p. 362).

Strain Gauge Pressure Transducers

Physical principles and construction

Strain gauges are transduucers that exhibit a change of some electrical property (most commonly resistance) when they are deformed (strained) by some external force (stress). Strain gauge pressure transducers take advantage of this property. The pressure sensing tube is connected to a dome-shaped cavity whose floor is a relatively flexible diaphragm. The floor is deformed by the air pressure inside the dome. It is this deformation (strain) that the system actually measures. Strain gauge pressure transducers thus contain a primary transducer (the diaphragm) and a second-

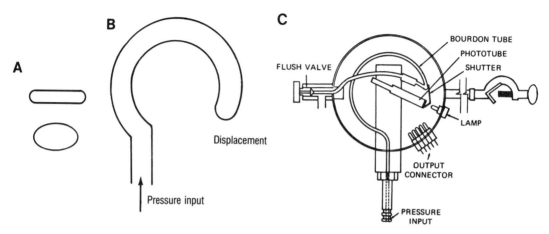

FIGURE 7-5. (A) Cross-section of a Bourdon tube when its internal (relative) pressure is zero (top), and when its internal pressure is high (bottom). (B). C-form Bourdon tube. When the cross-section shape changes, the resulting strain produces an overall opening of the C. Motion of the free end can move a dial pointer.

ary transducer (the strain gauges mounted on the diaphragm). In general, these transducers will contain four strain gauges wired in a Wheatstone bridge configuration (see Chap. 2). A typical strain gauge transducer is shown in Figure 7-6.

Unbonded strain gauge transducers are generally of the form shown in Figure 7-7. Movement of the diaphragm changes the amount of stretch of the gauge wires attached to it. This produces a change in the wires' resistances that is sensed by appropriate external circuitry. This type of transducer is very popular and widely available. It has good sensitivity and excellent reliability. It is, however, somewhat less rugged than some of the other transducer types and may be damaged by severe physical shock (for example, being dropped) or by even moderately forceful contact with the diaphragm.

In the *bonded strain gauge transducer* the elements that sense diaphragm movement are either bonded directly to the diaphragm or are special semiconductor elements that are actually part of it. Bonded strain gauge transducers are more rugged than unbonded types and their response is mostly dependent on inherent properties of the semiconductor elements which makes them more sensitive. They are also less affected by vibration in use.

Implementation

All strain gauge transducers require both an excitation voltage and an amplifier to track the bridge output (see Figure 7-8). Since the gauge system is resistive, the excitation voltage may be either DC or AC at any convenient frequency. It is very important that the bridge supply be very stable: Any change in excitation will result in a proportional change in the bridge output, an artifact that will confound the pressure measurement. Although the necessary excitation source and amplifier are generally purchased ready-made, highly miniaturized hybrid circuits are now available (for example, from Analog Devices, Inc.) that make it fairly easy and very cheap to assemble one's own precision system for use in a clinic.

During use, the pressure gauge is clamped to a solid support, and the open end of the sensing tube is positioned in the region of the vocal tract whose pressure is to be observed.

Calibration of pressure gauges

Manufacturers generally provide calibration data for the individual pressure gauges they sell. There are two common formats in which this information may appear.

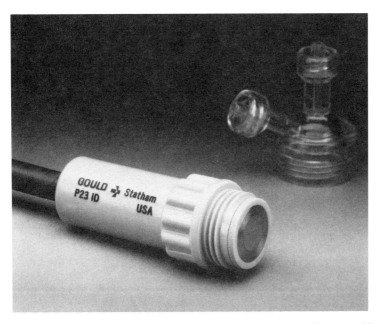

FIGURE 7-6. A typical resistive strain-gauge pressure transducer, the Statham P23. (Courtesy, Gould Inc., Cardiovascular Products Division, 1900 Williams Drive, Oxnard, CA 93030, manufacturers of Statham transducers)

1. Volts output per volt excitation per unit pressure. A Statham model P23BB unbonded pressure gauge, for example, has a stated calibration factor of 268.7 μV/V/cm Hg. This indicates that for each volt of bridge excitation the gauge produces 0.0002687 volts for each centimeter of mercury of applied pressure. If an excitation voltage of 12 V is used and the gauge is sensing an air pressure of 2 cm Hg, the amplifier at the bridge output will receive an input of 0.00645 V (.0002687 x 12 V x 2 cm Hg).

2. Volts output per volt excitation, full scale. This description indicates the voltage output for each volt of excitation at the maximum pressure for which the gauge is rated. Thus, a pressure gauge with a stated sensitivity of 5 mV/V full scale that can transduce pressures up to 25 cm H_2O would be expected to output 0.2 mV per volt of excitation per centimeter of water pressure (5 mV/25 cm H_2O = 0.2 mV/V/cm H_2O). With an excitation of 20 V the output would be 4 mV per cm H_2O (0.2 mV x 20 V = 4 mV).

Aside from providing a description of the overall sensitivity of the transducer, the manufacturer's calibration data are not really very useful. In the first place, the calibration of any device may change with time and use. Second, the final output of the transduction system also depends on the gain of the amplifiers to which the transducer is connected, and the gauge manufacturer cannot know what the user's amplifier is like. Fortunately, using a U-tube to calibrate a pressure transducer is so simple that it is easy to calibrate a pressure measurement system right in the setting in which it will be used.

Calibration requires that the pressure source, gauge, and U-tube be set up as in Figure 7-4. Pressures are generated over the entire range to which the gauge is sensitive, and readings of the amplifier's output voltage are taken at every pressure level. A table is then constructed that shows the relationship of voltage output for pressure input. Enough different pressures within the gauge's range should be tested to provide a good basis for estimating the system's linearity. Obviously, the excitation voltage or gain setting of the amplifier must not be changed between calibration and use. Cal-

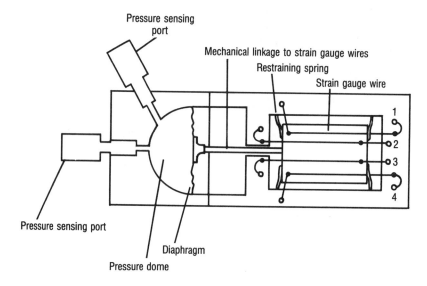

FIGURE 7-7. Cutaway schematic of a typical unbonded strain gauge transducer. Note that whenever wires 2 and 3 are stretched wires 1 and 4 are shortened. The restraining springs protect the wires from overload.

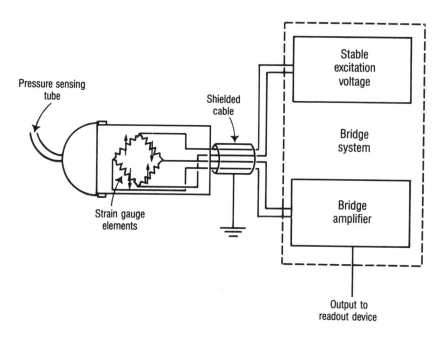

FIGURE 7-8. Block diagram of a strain-gauge transducer system.

ibration should be repeated every time the system is set up or after it is altered in any way.

Reactance-Based Pressure Transducers

Pressure may also be sensed by causing it to alter the reactance of a capacitor or inductor (see Chap. 2). Variable capacitance transducers used for work in speech and hearing are generally confined to the role of condenser microphones for recording of speech signals. (However, Fischer-Jørgenson and Hansen (1959) have described a capacitative pressure transducer.) On the other hand, inductive transducers have achieved moderate popularity in recent years and, therefore, warrant separate consideration.

Variable Inductance Transducers

PHYSICAL PRINCIPLES AND CONSTRUCTION. The inductance of a coil can be made to vary in a number of ways under the influence of changing air pressure. One of these is exemplified by a variable-reluctance pressure gauge made by Validyne. (Reluctance is the magnetic equivalent of impedance.) It uses two inductors in series, and is diagrammed in Figure 7-9. In this system a diaphragm of a magnetically permeable material (stainless steel) is positioned so as to divide a small cavity into two equal and separate spaces, each of which can serve as a pressure chamber. In the wall of each of the cavities is a toroidal inductive coil (shown in section in Figure 7-9A). As the pressure in one chamber rises, the diaphragm is deflected (Figure 7-9B), moving away from the coil on the high-pressure side and toward the coil in the low-pressure chamber. Because the diaphragm has high magnetic permeability, the inductance of one coil increases as the diaphragm moves closer to it, while the inductance of the other decreases as the diaphragm moves away.

The advantages of the two-coil arrange-

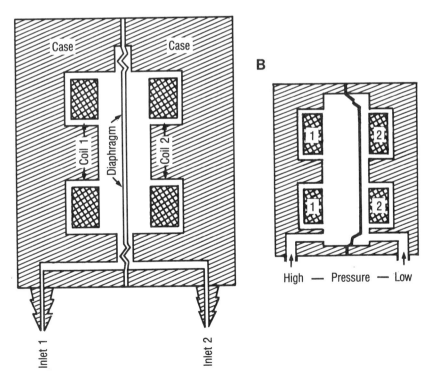

FIGURE 7-9. (A). Section through a variable-reluctance pressure transducer. (B). When pressure on one side of the diaphragm is higher than the pressure on the other side, the diaphragm is pushed to the low-pressure side. This changes the inductive balance of the coils.

ment are significant. From an electrical point of view, half of a bridge circuit has been formed, with benefits similar to those of resistive bridges: greatly improved sensitivity and inherent temperature compensation. Other benefits are gained as well. The transducer is quite rugged and will withstand considerable mechanical shock. In addition, it is fairly tolerant of serious overpressure, greatly reducing the possibility that it will be damaged by application of pressures beyond its operating range. Frequency response is also very good. Variable reluctance transducers, however, require AC excitation (since the reactance at DC for any inductor is zero), and thus a carrier amplifier system (Chap. 3) will be needed. These transducers are also susceptible to the presence of stray magnetic fields, which could be a problem (although not very serious) if they are used in conjunction with devices such as magnetometers (Chap. 11). Their price is comparable to resistive strain gauge units.

IMPLEMENTATION. Variable reluctance transducers are used in exactly the same way as the resistive strain gauge devices already discussed. The inductive transducers, however, require somewhat different support electronics, schematized in Figure 7-10.

Because transduction depends on variations of inductive reactance, the excitation must be a sine wave. This is provided by the carrier oscillator, shown on the left in Figure 7-10. It is critical that the amplitude of the excitation waveform be stable, and so a feedback loop is incorporated into the oscillator to control its output. The gauge itself contains only half of a bridge circuit, and thus the excitation is provided through a transformer in the carrier amplifier whose secondary winding provides the two fixed inductors needed to complete the bridge. The output of the bridge is amplified and demodulated to provide a voltage analog of the air pressure acting on the diaphragm within the transducer. Excitation and demodulation systems (carrier amplifiers) are generally available from the transducer manufacturer. A system such as the one shown requires only minor modification to permit it to be used with resistive strain gauge transducers as well.

CALIBRATION. Variable reluctance transducers have very good sensitivity. The Validyne MP45-871, for example, has a nominal output of 25 mV/V full scale. With the recommended 5 V excitation voltage at a frequency of 5000 Hz its output would be 0.125 V at maximal transducible pressure. Exact calibration of the output voltage is achieved using a U-tube in the way described previously.

Other Transducers

Recent advances in electronic technology have led to the development of new techniques or significant improvement in existing methods. Miniaturization has progressed impressively. While much of this progress has not yet "trickled down" to the clinical area, it may represent the wave of the future and therefore merits some discussion.

Miniaturized pressure transducers

The enormous advances in miniaturization are beginning to have repercussions in the design of pressure transducers. Hixon (1972), for instance, described transducers small enough to be placed in the esophagus and stomach for determination of transdiaphragmatic pressure. Koike and Perkins (1968) also discuss a transducer—a semiconductor bonded resistive type, cylindrical in form, 3 mm in diameter and 4 mm long—that can be introduced into almost any space in the vocal tract. Aside from the convenience afforded by these instruments, they have the advantages of relatively high sensitivity and excellent frequency response. Calibration, however, is more difficult than in the case of more conventional devices. Certain types also seem to be prone to excessive temperature sensitivity or unexplained drift (see Subtelny, Worth, and Sakuda (1966) and Hardy's (1967) critique of their instrumentation).

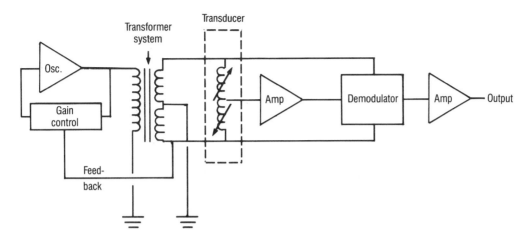

FIGURE 7-10. Block diagram of a carrier oscillator system for a variable reluctance transducer.

Integrated circuit technology has made it possible to fabricate a semiconductor bonded strain gauge transducer together with all of its associated excitation and output electronics in a single miniature package. Transduction systems of this sort, available from National Semiconductor Corp., come in sizes as small as 0.80 × 0.75 inches, and generate as much as 12 V of output, ready for display by a readout device without further processing. While not yet in routine use in speech pathology, transducers of this type are bound to earn a place in clinics in the near future.

Table 7-1 summarizes important characteristics of the various pressure transducers available as an aid to selecting the device most suitable in a given setting.

AIR PRESSURE MEASUREMENTS

Maximum Intraoral Air Pressure

The purpose of this non-speech measurement is to assess a patient's ability to generate air pressure on demand. The test rests on the assumption that the pressure measured in the mouth is generated by the respiratory system (and special precaution must be taken to assure that this is the case). Since there is very little or no air flow and the glottis is open during the test, intraoral pressure is equal to lung pressure.

Technique

INSTRUMENTATION. Traditionally maximum intraoral air pressure is evaluated with a U-tube or a Bourdon-type oral manometer. Any other pressure transducer with an adequate maximum-pressure rating can be used, however.

METHOD. The test requires that the patient blow into the sensing tube with as much force as possible. It is important that there is a tight lip seal around the sensing tube and that there is no nasal air leakage. Hardy (1961) suggests that if there is lip paresis (for example, in cases of cerebral palsy) a face mask might be required. In fact, a mask should be considered in any case of facial muscle weakness. A nose clip should be used to prevent nasal airflow. When the clinician is satisfied that the patient is producing maximal expiratory efforts the highest pressure reading shown on the gauge, even momentarily, is recorded as the test result.

This test is intended to evaluate a capability of the respiratory system. But intraoral air pressure can also be produced by sealing the oral cavity off from the pharynx with a linguavelar contact and using oral movement (buccal contraction) to compress the intraoral air. The resulting pressure is not the measure of interest in this test. To prevent this action a "bleed valve"

TABLE 7–1. Summary of Pressure Transducers

Type	Sensitivity	Frequency Response	Excitation	Support Electronics	Ruggedness	Remarks
U-tube	Varies	Exceptionally poor	None	None	Good	Cannot be read with precision. Limited to static measures. No permanent record.
Bourdon type	Moderate	Poor	None	None—mechanical	Moderate	Static measures only. No permanent record.
Strain gauge Unbonded	Low	Good	AC or DC	Bridge excitation and instrumentation amplifier	Poor–moderate	Sensitive to vibration
Bonded	Low	Good			moderate	
Semiconductor	Very good	Good			Good Good	
Inductive	Very good	Excellent	AC only	Carrier amplifier	Excellent	

is placed in the measurement system. This represents a shunt by which air is allowed to escape from the oral cavity. If pressure is being produced by oral valving, the loss of air will quickly cause the pressure to fall dramatically. Only if the air is constantly replenished from the lungs will it be possible for the patient to maintain a high intraoral pressure for a significant period of time. A bleed valve is built into commercially available Bourdon-type manometers. In other systems a T-tube with a very narrow opening in its side arm may be connected to the sensing tube to achieve the same effect. This arrangement is diagrammed in the section on "Subglottal Pressure," Figure 7-14. For the purposes of the present test, however, the opening of the bleed tube should be smaller than the one shown there.

Advantages and limitations

This test is extremely simple and requires minimal instrumentation. It does not, however, evaluate speech performance. Therefore, it is difficult to draw inferences from the results beyond the conclusion that adequate pressure for speech is at least possible.

Expected results

The data in Table 7-2 represent the means of the highest pressures (not necessarily sustained) achieved in two trials following a practice effort by normal subjects. Measurement was done with a U-tube manometer.

Data of this type should be interpreted with extreme caution. Morris (1966) quite correctly points out that manometric results are not measures of intraoral breath pressure for speech. The absolute values themselves have no utility since there is no criterion for "adequate," and normal speakers differ radically in their performance on this task—a fact demonstrated by the wide ranges cited in the table. The usefulness of breath pressure measures lies almost exclusively in the generation of breath pressure ratios from them. These are discussed in Chapter 10.

Dynamic Intraoral Pressure

The intraoral air pressures that accompany speech provide insight into the function of the entire speech system. Abnormal pressure values might reflect inadequate or unstable ventilatory support. But they may

TABLE 7–2. Mean Maximum Intraoral Air Pressure

No. of Subjects	Age Range	Maximum Pressure* (cm H$_2$O) Mean	SD	Pressure Range* (cm H$_2$O)
Males				
31	18–39	166.9	37.3	96–244
27	68–89	123.7	42.9	36–198
Females				
31	18–38	121.4	23.6	81–178
35	66–93	87.6	36.6	25–188

From Ptacek, P. H., Sander, E. K., Maloney, W. H., and Jackson, C. C. Phonatory and related changes with advanced age. *Journal of Speech and Hearing Research*, 9 (1966) 353–360. Tables 3 and 4, p. 357. ©American Speech-Language-Hearing Association, Rockville, MD. Reprinted by permission.

*Data converted from inches of water.

also indicate inappropriate velopharyngeal status or abnormality in the degree, location, or timing of vocal tract constrictions. There is some evidence that intraoral air pressure is a key articulatory variable. That is, it is possible that speakers adjust other physiologic parameters (such as air flow) to maintain specific air pressures, at least for some consonants (Warren, Hall, and Davis, 1981).

Technique

Sensing Tube and Pressure Gauge. Generally, intraoral pressure is measured with a sensing tube placed in the posterior oral cavity or in the oropharynx. There are two common means of achieving this, each having its own disadvantages. The tube may be passed through the nasal cavity until its tip hangs somewhat below the velum. Since the end of such a nasal tube points into the airstream it is important that the tip be closed and that the tube walls be perforated near the tip region to provide sensing ports opening perpendicular to the flow (see previous section on "Influence of Flow on Pressure Measurement.") The advantage of the nasal tube placement is that there is no interference

with movement of the articulators, nor will vigorous tongue or lip activity displace the sensing tube. Velar movement does not seem to compromise the measurement significantly, nor is velopharyngeal closure measurably affected, provided the tube is thin enough. Polyethylene tubing with an outer diameter of about 2 mm works quite well.

Some patients may have trouble tolerating a nasal approach. In these cases a sensing tube may be molded to lie in the buccogingival sulcus and curve around the last molar so that the opening of the tube is approximately at the midline and oriented perpendicular to the airflow. It can be anchored in place by tying it to a molar with dental floss. The tube leaves the oral cavity at the corner of the lips. (This tube placement is illustrated in Figure 7-11A.) While easy to implement and less invasive than nasal placement, this method leaves the tube more prone to displacement by tongue, cheek, and labial movements.

With either sensing-tube placement, the free end of the tube is connected to an external pressure transducer located close to the patient (Figure 7-11B). The oral end of the tube is likely to fill with saliva, which interferes with accurate measurement. Therefore, it is advisable to connect the sensing tube to the pressure gauge via a three-way stopcock, as in Figure 7-11B. A large hypodermic syringe connected to the stopcock assembly can be used to inject a blast of air into the sensing tube to clear it when necessary.

Intraoral Transducers. Pressure gauges small enough to fit within the oral cavity have been designed. Subtelny, Worth, and Sakuda (1966), for instance, used a special semiconductor strain gauge device (manufactured for them by the General Electric Company) that was about 10 mm in diameter and about 3 mm thick. This was pasted to the palate to sense intraoral pressure during running speech. Unfortunately, the transducer's output tended to drift significantly in a way that was highly suggestive of sensitivity to the temperature difference of

A

B

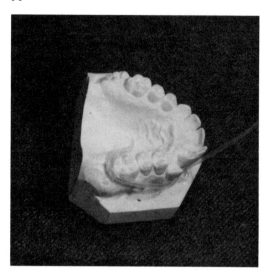

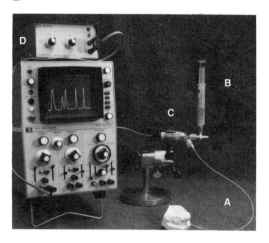

FIGURE 7-11. (A). Placement of a sensing tube around the last molar. The tube lies in the bucco-gingival sulcus and exits at the corner of the mouth. Note that the open end of the tube is perpendicular to the direction of airflow. (B). Set up for intraoral pressure measurement. A. sensing tube; B. hypodermic syringe mounted on a three-way stopcock; C. pressure transducer; D. carrier amplifier.

the egressive and ingressive tidal air flow. This, of course, casts doubt on the validity of the measurement (see the critique of the method by Hardy, 1967) and illustrates the kind of problems that may well arise as efforts are made to improve transduction techniques. Intraoral devices are probably no less encumbering of articulation than a sensing tube, and the electrical connections to intraoral gauges must pass the lips just as a sensing tube would. It is clear, then, that they offer little advantage over a standard pressure gauge, which is also usable for other kinds of measures.

Method

Intraoral air pressure may be examined during running speech, but this procedure leaves too many potentially confounding variables uncontrolled. Variability of peak pressure for the same phoneme spoken by a given speaker is much greater during or-dinary speech than during repetition of carefully specified test utterances (Miller and Daniloff, 1977). For this reason testing usually involves having the patient repeat

selected utterances—generally of the CVC or VCV type—a number of times. Usually it is the peak air pressure attained during the consonant that is of interest. To con-trol testing further, the test utterances are commonly embedded in a carrier phrase, such as "It's a _____ again," and subjects are instructed to speak at a standard effort level. Often the patient is asked to talk so that the pointer of a sound level or VU-meter is deflected to within a few units of some preselected reading (perhaps repre-senting 70 dBSPL). Several repetitions of each phoneme being tested are needed be-cause the mean pressure and its variabili-ty (in the form of the standard deviation) are both important.

Data are commonly derived from a pen writer or oscilloscope display of the trans-ducer output. (The raw signals can also be stored on an FM tape system for later anal-ysis if desired). Such a readout is shown in Figure 7-12. When possible, the audio waveform should appear with the pressure record in order to align the acoustic and pressure events in time. (By using special circuitry, such as the Kay Elemetrics Agnel-

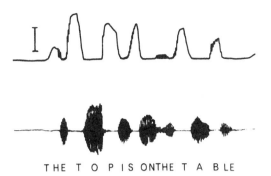

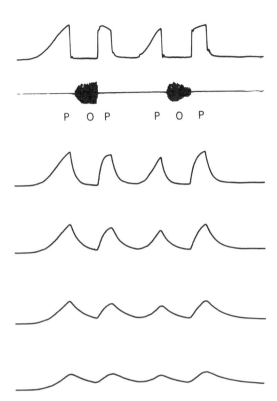

FIGURE 7-12. Pressure events during the utterance "The top is on the table." Top: intraoral pressure sensed by nasal catheter and resistive strain gauge transducer. Bottom: audio record. The calibration line accompanying the pressure trace represents 6 cm H_2O.

lograph (Karnell and Willis (1982b), the pressure trace can be put onto a spectrogram of the utterance.) Interpretation of the pressure record is discussed in more detail in the next section.

Expected results

The Output Record. Figure 7-12 shows intraoral pressure as measured via a nasal catheter and strain gauge transducer while the patient said "the top is on the table" at moderate loudness. This output is typical of a normal speaker. The calibration mark accompanying the pressure trace equals 6 cm H_2O. Peaks indicate the consonants; during full vowels the intraoral pressure is essentially zero. The audio trace is used to identify the location of each phoneme whose pressure is determined from the height of the pressure peak. Thus the intraoral pressure during the first /t/ was about 12 cm H_2O, while the /t/ in "table" was produced with about 10 cm H_2O pressure. The /p/ had a peak pressure of around 9 cm H_2O, compared to 5 cm H_2O for the postvocalic /b/. The relative uniformity of the durations of the pressure peaks is consistent with the nature of the utterance and may be considered an indicator of speech-timing stability.

The shape of the pressure peaks for the

FIGURE 7-13. Effect of frequency response on a pressure record. At the top is an adequate recording of the pressure events and audio signal of the utterance "pop pop." The lower traces show the effects of increasingly poor frequency response on the pressure record.

plosives is significant for two reasons.* The sharp fall in intraoral pressure coincident with the audio-record's plosive burst shows normal function: If the plosive release had been sluggish the pressure record would show it. Equally important is the fact that a sharp fall of the pressure traces demonstrates the adequacy of the measuring system's frequency response. Figure 7-13 shows how pressure peaks change as the frequency response of the measurement system falls off—that is, as the system becomes more sluggish. Notice that the pressure peaks become less distinct, broader, more smoothly rounded, and merge with

---

*Pressure-peak shapes and their relation to articulatory functioning is explored by Müller and Brown (1980).

TABLE 7–3. Mean Peak Intraoral Pressure in cm H₂O*

Phoneme	Males Mean	SD	Females Mean	SD	Children Mean	SD
p	6.43	1.07	7.52	2.17	9.66	3.34
b	4.37	1.42	6.05	1.82	6.57	1.97
t	6.18	1.29	7.44	1.92	9.35	2.76
d	4.52	1.60	6.67	1.91	6.78	1.73
s	5.69	1.14	6.41	2.64	7.95	2.13
z	4.30	1.18	5.23	1.77	5.91	1.52
f	5.80	0.65	6.34	2.95	7.95	2.93
v	3.82	0.53	4.37	0.86	5.13	2.44
tʃ	6.77	1.01	7.32	2.28	10.48	3.64
dʒ	5.92	1.28	6.72	1.77	9.83	2.65
l	1.09	0.62	1.39	0.25	0.68	0.53
r	0.99	0.57	2.01	0.96	1.93	1.48
w	0.78	0.66	1.54	0.96	2.01	0.98
m	0.22	0.47	0.60	1.05	0.00	0.00
n	0.43	0.70	0.45	0.68	0.00	0.00

From Subtelny, J. D., Worth, J. H., and Sakuda, M. Intraoral pressure and rate of flow during speech. *Journal of Speech and Hearing Research*, 9 (1966) 498–518. Table 1, p. 505. ©American Speech-Language-Hearing Association, Rockville, MD. Reprinted by permission.

*Based on 10 adult males, 10 adult females, and 10 children (age 6–10). VCV syllables, with V constant. Special intraoral transducer.

TABLE 7–4. Mean Peak Intraoral Pressure in Children (cm H₂O)

Phoneme	Prevocalic	Inter-vocalic	Post-vocalic
p	6.69	8.23	6.24
b	3.14	4.05	2.57
t	6.64	8.34	6.26
d	2.91	3.76	2.69
ʃ	6.25	7.18	5.22
ʒ	3.87	4.38	3.10
θ	5.77	6.62	5.15
ð	3.79	4.09	2.92
s	5.74	6.91	5.32
z	3.57	3.99	3.21
f	5.56	6.45	5.13
v	3.15	3.60	2.58

From Arkebauer, H. J., Hixon, T. J., and Hardy, J. C. Peak intraoral air pressures during speech. *Journal of Speech and Hearing Research*, 10 (1967) 196–208. Table 1, page 200. ©American Speech-Language-Hearing Association, Rockville, MD. Reprinted by permission.

*6 males, 4 females; age 8 years 2 months - 12 years 2 months (mean 10 years 0 months); /CΛC/ or /ΛCΛ/, three repetitions per phoneme; Normal pitch and loudness; post-molar sensing tube, strain-gauge transducer.

TABLE 7–5. Pressure Change with Age—/p/ and /b/*

Group	/p/ Mean†	SD	/b/ Mean†	SD
Children	7.1	1.7	5.4	1.7
Youth	7.7	1.5	4.7	1.5
Adult	6.0	1.0	3.3	1.4

From Bernthal, J. E. and Beukelman, D. R. Intraoral air pressure during the production of /p/ and /b/ by children, youths, and adults. *Journal of Speech and Hearing Research*, 21 (1978) 361–371. Table 2, p. 368. ©American Speech-Language-Hearing Association, Rockville, MD. Reprinted by permission.

*6 males and 6 females in each group: Children: 4 years 6 months to 6 years 9 months (mean: 5 years 10 months). Youth: 10 years 0 months to 12 years 10 months (mean: 11 years 7 months). Adults: 19 years 6 months to 46 years 2 months (mean: 30 years 3 months). Plosive in 12 monosyllabic words, pre- and post-vocalic (carrier: "Buy a . . ."). Comfortable loudness. Postmolar sensing tube; strain gauge transducer.

†Prevocalic and intervocalic combined. For /p/ children and youth significantly higher than adult; For /b/ all differences are significant.

TABLE 7–6. Mean Peak Intraoral Pressure of CVC Syllables versus Spontaneous Speech (cm H_2O)*

Phoneme	/CʌC/ syllable		Monologue	
	Mean†	Range of Means	Mean†	Range of Means
p	5.5	4.2–6.7	4.6	3.4–6.0
b	3.0	2.7–3.4	2.9	2.5–3.5
t	5.1	4.7–5.8	4.9	3.5–5.9
d	3.5	2.5–4.4	2.5	1.6–3.0
k	5.2	5.0–5.5	5.1	3.5–6.2
g	3.6	2.8–4.4	3.1	2.2–4.0

From Miller, C. J. and Daniloff, R. Aerodynamics of stops in continuous speech. *Journal of Phonetics*, 5 (1977) 351–360. Table 1, p. 356. With permission from the *Journal of Phonetics*, copyright 1977 by Academic Press Inc. (London) Ltd.

*Three adult "phonetically trained" males. Five repetitions each of /CʌC/ words; 5 min monologue. Nasal catheter and resistive strain gauge.

†Pre- and postvocalic combined. Note: "Individuals differed with respect to mean values and with respect to the two speaking contexts" (p. 357). "Variability for monologue items is much greater" (p. 354).

each other to create an erroneous impression of serious speech abnormality. The importance of verifying response adequacy of the system being used is apparent. The stability of the pressure baseline (the absence of drift) and the resolution of small pressure changes (for example during /-ɑnðe/ and /-bl-/) are also important indicators of measurement accuracy and should be checked in any system before use.

Pressure Values. Data on a wide range of phonemes measured under the same conditions in children and adults are scarce.* Tables 7-3 and 7-4, however, can serve as a general guide for comparison of test results. The data in Table 7-3 were obtained with a special intraoral transducer and may be less than optimally valid (see "Intraoral Transducers" section, this chapter). Consequently these data should be compared to those of other research, such as the data in Tables 7-5 and 7-6.

Malécot (1966a, 1968) also presents peak intraoral air pressure values for many of the phonemes listed in the two preceding

---

*A special note of caution is in order. Counihan (1972, p. 184) reminds us that "the use of sensitive instruments to measure oral and nasal air pressure and airflow . . . is relatively recent. Problems related to differences in instrumentation and . . . methods of measurement make direct comparison of results in different studies difficult."

tables. His values, however, are consistently —and often significantly— higher than those presented above. This may be due, at least in part, to the loudness level ("one which is appropriate for talking to a person 4 feet away under ideal acoustic conditions") used by his subjects.

The question of why intraoral pressure changes with age is currently unresolved. Although studies such as those of Stathopoulos and Weismer (1985) and of Bernthal and Beukelman (1978), summarized in Table 7-5, show that children use higher intraoral pressures than older speakers, at least one investigation (Stathopoulos, 1986) indicates that the difference may only reflect the fact that children speak more loudly (Table 7-7).

Hixon et al. (1967) have determined that vocal intensity level is approximately proportional to the 1.3 power of intraoral air pressure. That is,

$$SPL \propto P_{io}{}^{\sim 1.3}.$$

This relationship has been essentially confirmed by Ringel et al (1967) and by Leeper and Noll (1972).

Consistency of Intraoral Air Pressure Measures. Brown and McGlone (1969b) determined that, under controlled conditions of voice fundamental frequency and intensity, adult speakers varied their peak intraoral

TABLE 7–7.   Relationship of Mean Peak
             Intraoral Air Pressure to Effort
             or Intensity (cm H_2O)*

Phoneme	Conver- sational	Effort Level Greater	Much greater
ʃ	4.48	7.28	10.76
s	4.34	7.20	10.45
Mean†	4.41	7.24	10.61

From Hixon, T. J. Turbulent noise sources for speech. *Folia Phoniatrica,* 19 (1966) 168–182. Table 1, p. 177. Reprinted by permission.

*Nine adult males; 10 repetitions of each phoneme at each effort level; postmolar sensing tube; resistive strain gauge.

†derived from data; not in original table.

pressures for /t ʌ/ very little, even when repetitions over a period of 5 days were compared. Brown and Shearer (1970) found similar constancy for /s, z, p, and w/. Hence, when controlled testing conditions are used, high intrasubject variability over time should be viewed as clinically suspect. Note, however, that esophageal speakers routinely have high intraoral pressure variability (Murry and Brown, 1975).

Influences on intraoral air pressure

It is clear that the intraoral air pressures observed during speech vary as a function of a large number of variables. Most of these have not been fully explored. Table 7-8 summarizes these influences in cases where there are enough data to warrant at least a tentative judgment.

Subglottal Pressure (P_s)

The subglottal pressure represents the energy immediately available for creation of the acoustic signals of speech. It should be of appropriate magnitude and, perhaps even more important, it should be well regulated—that is, stable.

Inappropriate levels of subglottal pressure or inadequate pressure regulation can cause abnormal speech intensity levels or (to a lesser extent) sudden shifts in vocal fundamental frequency (Baken and Orlikoff, 1986; Baken and Orlikoff, in press;

Hixon, Klatt, and Mead, 1971; Ladefoged and McKinney, 1963; Lieberman, Knudson, and Mead, 1969; Rothenberg and Mahshie, 1977; van den Berg, 1958). Subglottal pressure may be adversely affected by problems of neuromuscular control of the chest wall (for example, athetosis or lower motoneuron paresis), by disorders which result in unacceptable vocal tract impedances (e.g., vocal fold paralysis) or by severe ventilatory incompetence (such as advanced emphysema). Measurement of the subglottal pressure is, therefore, potentially of great diagnostic and therapeutic value in a range of speech disorders. Clinical interpretation of findings requires a firm knowledge of the respiratory mechanics of speech. Good reviews of the rather complex interactions involved are provided in Mead, Bouhuys, and Proctor (1968), Hixon, Mead, and Goldman (1976) and Minifie, Hixon, and Williams (1973).

While it is an easy matter to obtain a nonspeech estimate of the subglottal pressure likely to be used by a patient for speech, there is unfortunately no simple, direct, and convenient technique for actually measuring subglottal pressure during speech. Essentially three useful methods have been developed, but each has very significant disadvantages or limitations. These three different methods are discussed separately below.

Non-speech estimates of P_s

Hixon and his coworkers, using the simplest possible instrumentation, have developed two methods of obtaining estimates of a patient's ability to generate and sustain subglottal pressure.

The first method (described by Netsell and Hixon, 1978) is diagrammed in Figure 17-14A. Essentially it places the equivalent of a normal glottal resistance outside of the vocal tract. If the patient blows air through this artificial resistance with about the same effort as would be used for speech, the intraoral pressure will approximate a speech subglottal pressure quite closely. One has only to measure the static intra-

TABLE 7–8. Summary of Influences on Peak Intraoral Pressure

Higher Pressure Associated with:	Lower Pressure Associated with:	According to:
Voiceless plosives	Voiced plosives	Arkebauer et al. (1967) Lisker (1970)* Lubker & Parris (1970) Miller & Daniloff (1977) Netsell (1969) Slis (1970) Karnell & Willis (1982a) Stathopoulos (1984) Stathopoulos & Weismer (1985) Stathopoulos (1986)
Voiceless plosives	Voiceless fricatives	Arkebauer et al. (1967)
Voiceless fricatives	Voiced fricatives	Arkebauer et al. (1967) Slis (1970) Subtelny et al. (1966) Scully (1971) Stathopoulos (1984)†
Intervocalic plosive	Prevocalic plosive	Arkebauer et al. (1967) Brown & Ruder (1972)
Prevocalic plosive	Postvocalic plosive	Bernthal & Beukelman (1978) Brown et al. (1970) Malécot (1968) Stathopoulos & Weismer (1985) Stathopoulos (1986)
High effort or SPL	Low effort or SPL	Brown & Brandt (1971) Brown & McGlone (1974) Hixon (1966) Hixon et al. (1967) Leeper & Noll (1972) Ringel et al. (1967) Slis (1970) Klich (1982) Stathopoulos (1986)
Children**	Adult**	Bernthal & Beukelman (1978) Subtelny et al. (1966) Stathopoulos & Weismer (1985) Stathopoulos (1986)
Syllable stress‡		Flege (1983) Brown & McGlone (1974) Netsell (1970)
Syllable repetition rate‡		Hixon (1966)

*With qualifications.
†Findings contrary to effect described.
**Probably due to the fact that children tend to speak at higher SPL than adults. See Stathopolous (1986).
‡No consistent effect.

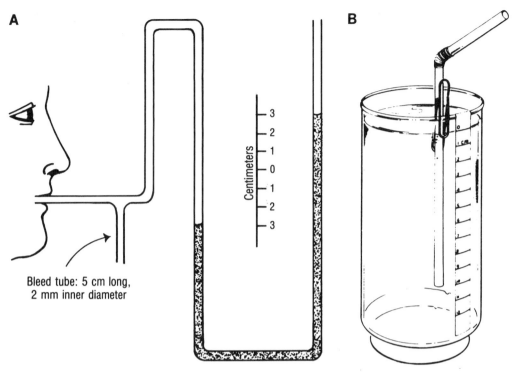

FIGURE 7-14. (A). A method of estimating ability to generate P_s. The bleed tube has a resistance of about 75 cm H_2O/L/sec. (B.) Apparatus for P_s estimation constructed of housefold objects (From Hixon, T. J., Hawley, L. L., and Wilson, K. J. An around-the-house device for the clinical determination of respiratory driving pressure: A note on making simple even simpler. *Journal of Speech and Hearing Disorders*, 47 (1982) 413-415. Figure 1, p. 414. ©American Speech-Language-Hearing Association, Rockville, MD. (Reprinted by permission.)

oral pressure to obtain a good estimate of the patient's ability to generate subglottal pressure.

The artificial glottal resistance is formed by a *leak-* or *bleed-tube* in the measurement system. Originally, Netsell and Hixon suggested that the bleed tube have a resistance of 75 cm H_2O/L/s, which would be approximated by a glass tube 5 cm long having an internal diameter of 2 mm. Later research (Smitheran and Hixon, 1981) indicated that this resistance might more appropriately be in the range of 35 cm H_2O/L/s. Therefore, a tube of the same length with an internal diameter of about 2.75 cm would perhaps be more suitable as a substitute for the glottal resistance. A U-tube manometer is adequate for the measurement of the intraoral air pressure.

To obtain the P_s estimate the patient is instructed to blow into the tube and maintain a fixed level of pressure for a specified amount of time. Failure to achieve and hold adequate velopharyngeal closure, or a good lip seal to the inlet, violates the assumptions on which the test is based and, hence, will compromise validity of the results. It is also important that there be an air flow out of the leak tube at the instant of measurement.

The other method (Hixon, Hawley, and Wilson, 1982) involves extremely simple materials that are likely to be available around the house. The "instrument" (shown in Figure 7-14B) is made from a tall (at least 12 cm) jar or water glass. A centimeter ruler is attached vertically to the jar's outer surface. (Alternatively, a strip of adhesive tape can be marked at half-centimeter intervals and fixed to the jar.) A paper clip holds an ordinary drinking straw (the kind with an accordion pleat, which allows bending, is best) upright just inside the jar near the ruler. The jar is filled with water exactly to the level of the ruler's zero marking. The pressure at any given point in the water is determined by the point's depth below the surface. (In essence, the system is a functionally inverted version of a U-tube.) If a patient can blow air out of the straw, his breath pressure must be greater than the pressure pushing water into the straw. That pressure is directly measured by the depth of the straw's open end.

The patient is asked to blow into the straw using an amount of effort that is comparable to speech. The straw is moved up or down until its open end is just at the depth at which bubbles are created and rise to the surface of the water. The oral breath pressure in cm H_2O is then just a bit greater than the depth of the open end of straw (which can be read from the ruler). The patient must produce bubbles continuously for five seconds before the pressure reading is considered an indication of sustainable P_s. The same precautions that were associated with the leak-tube estimate apply in this case: There must be a good lip seal to the straw and velopharyngeal closure must be maintained. Because the patient is producing bubbles, air is being lost from the system, and so a separate bleed valve to guard against oral valving is not really needed. However, it is probably wise to include a separate bleed resistance (in the form of the glass tube discussed above) if possible.

Advantages and Limitations. These techniques are extremely simple, inexpensive, and non-threatening to the patient. They are valuable both for screening patients' performances and for providing feedback during the course of therapeutic management. Their chief limitation, of course, is that the measurements are not obtained during speech and, especially in the case of the straw and bubble technique, are somewhat approximate. Nonetheless, these methods

are likely to be very useful in case management (for an example, see Netsell and Daniel, 1979).

Expected Results. Netsell and Hixon (1978) have found, after evaluating more than 120 dysarthric patients, that the ability to sustain a subglottal pressure of 5 cm H_2O for 5 s is a rule-of-thumb minimum for adequately meeting speech requirements.

Speech measurements: Direct methods

The most straightforward way of observing any pressure is to place the sensing tube right into the region where the pressure is. For the subglottic region this may be accomplished via the pharynx either with a specially configured sensing tube (van den Berg, 1956) or with a special ultraminiature pressure transducer (Koike and Perkins, 1968; Perkins and Koike, 1969; Kitzing and Löfqvist, 1975; Koike 1981; Kitzing, Carlborg, and Löfqvist, 1982). Unfortunately these methods require that a tube remain between the vocal folds and, despite reports that this does not interfere with phonation, intubation techniques for direct evaluation of P_s have not been widely accepted by speech professionals. The currently common practice involves puncturing the trachea with a large-bore hypodermic needle. This can be left in place and the sensing tube attached to it, or it can be used as a sleeve through which a sensing tube is introduced into the trachea (the needle itself is then withdrawn). Netsell (1969), for example, reports using a needle about 4 cm long with an inner diameter of 0.055 cm inserted between the first and second tracheal rings. The needle is attached to the pressure transducer with a polyethylene tube. The same instrumentation considerations previously discussed under dynamic intraoral pressure measurement apply in the case of direct measurement of P_s.

ADVANTAGES AND LIMITATIONS. The prime advantage of the tracheal-puncture technique is its directness. In contrast to other methods that rely on observation of a correlate of P_s, this procedure requires no special calibration aside from that of the pressure transducer itself. All other factors being equal, it yields an inherently accurate measure. The drawbacks of the method, however, are obvious and significant. While not particularly painful, the procedure is very likely to provoke considerable patient anxiety. Technically a surgical procedure, placement of the sensing tube must be done by a physician and is attended by some risk of damage or bleeding. In extreme instances a painful subdermal air bubble can accidentally be produced. These problems have motivated the development of more innocuous indirect approaches.

Speech measurements: Indirect methods

Indirect measurement entails the determination of a pressure that is analogous, or closely related, to the subglottal pressure. Indirect pressure may be estimated from intraesophageal pressure or from the pressure in a sealed body plethysmograph. While neither method yields results as accurate as those obtained from an intratracheal probe, the fact that neither requires surgical placement of the sensing tube makes them more suitable for clinical use. Finally, it is also possible to obtain a somewhat more approximate and discontinuous estimate of P_s from the oral pressure during specially designed speech tasks.

ESOPHAGEAL PRESSURE. The esophagus passes through the thorax and hence is influenced by the intrathoracic pressure. It also lies against the membranous, relatively compliant, posterior portion of the trachea. Thus, it is reasonable to assume that the pressure of a bolus of air in the esophagus (P_E) might accurately reflect the tracheal (that is, the subglottal) pressure (P_s).

While this reasoning is intuitively appealing it overlooks a number of important factors. (They are considered in some detail by Bouhuys, Proctor, and Mead [1966], Lieberman [1968] and van den Berg [1956].)

The most significant problems arise from the fact that, while the esophagus runs through the thorax it lies outside the lungs in the pleural space. Recall that the pressure in this region is always lower than the pressure in the lungs. It is not surprising, therefore, that P_E does not equal P_s. Another consequence of the pleural location of the esophagus is that the lung recoil forces act in opposite directions on the alveolar air and on the esophagus. For example, at the lung volumes typical of speech, lung stretch causes an inward recoil of the lung membranes. That is, the lungs act like blown-up balloons and tend to shrink back toward their uninflated size. This diminishes their volume, and compresses the air in them, raising its pressure. At the same time, however, shrinkage of the lungs increases the volume of the pleural space, lowering the pleural pressure. The degree to which the subglottal pressure is affected by lung recoil forces (and the extent to which esophageal pressure is changed in the opposite direction) varies with the lung volume. Therefore, a lung-volume-correction factor must be applied to P_E before it can serve as an estimate of P_s.

There are two problems inherent in achieving the necessary correction. First, the actual recoil-induced pressure at any given lung volume is different in different people, and there is no way of predicting it *a priori*. Second, while the recoil pressure varies with lung volume in a fairly linear way in the mid-region of the vital capacity range, as one approaches the extremes of lung volume the relationship becomes markedly nonlinear, again in essentially unpredictable ways. This might not be a catastrophic problem in normal speakers, but patients in rehabilitation programs cannot be so categorized, and they are more likely to use lung volumes near the extremes of their vital capacities. For these reasons, different calibration techniques have been devised to delineate and compensate for the change in P_E due solely to change in lung volume in the specific patient being evaluated. (These calibrations are discussed in the "Method" section.) One of these calibration procedures *must* be applied if the measurements are to be of any use.

Instrumentation. Aside from the standard pressure transducer, the main item of instrumentation required for measurement of intraesophageal pressure is a long sensing tube ending in a thin-walled rubber balloon. Several different designs have been tested; they vary primarily in the length of the balloon itself (Fry, Stead, Ebert, Lubin, and Wells, 1952; Lieberman, 1968; Milic-Emili, Mead, Turner and Glauser, 1964); van den Berg, 1956).

The design proposed by van den Berg (1956), shown in Figure 7-15, is typical of those in current use. It is mounted at the end of a long (> 50 cm) polyethylene tube having a 2 mm diameter and a 1.5 mm bore. The balloon itself is 11.5 cm long and 1 cm in diameter, made of very thin rubber. The catheter is perforated with 2 holes of 1.4 mm diameter for every centimeter of length enclosed by the balloon; its transducer end is, of course, fitted with an appropriate connector. Subjects quickly learn to swallow the balloon with ease, especially if aided by sips of water.

Method. Measuring esophageal pressure is a difficult procedure that will require the skills of a physician or similarly trained individual. The two critical aspects are placing the balloon and calibrating the output.

Balloon Placement. The empty balloon is inserted via the nasal cavity into the esoph-

agus. The catheter may simply be advanced either a fixed distance or it can be inserted to the level of some anatomical reference point. Draper, Ladefoged, and Whitteridge (1960) recommend a balloon placement 34 cm from the nares with a balloon 2.5 cm long, while Fry et al. (1952) placed their 18 cm long balloon 42 cm from the nares. Ladefoged (1963) placed his balloon at the presumed level of the tracheal bifurcation. Since the optimal location of the balloon is the one that results in the smallest artifacts (for instance, cardiac pulses) with the best pressure sample, it seems best to adjust the balloon's position for each client, rather than to depend on a fixed (and perhaps arbitrary) distance. The placement technique described by Lieberman (1968) seems well suited to clinical work. The empty balloon is passed into the upper portion of the esophagus and then filled with a small amount of air. (The air merely serves as a bolus whose pressure can be sensed. The quantity of air should not be more than 1 or 2 mL. Under no circumstances should the balloon be filled to the point at which it is at all stretched, or accuracy will be severely compromised.) While monitoring transducer output on an oscilloscope the position of the balloon is adjusted until tracheal movement artifacts are observed; the balloon is then lowered about 1 cm. This procedure reportedly provides readings that are relatively free of cardiac pulses, although peristaltic waves in the esophagus will still be apparent.

Calibration. While the pressure transducer itself may be calibrated against a U-tube

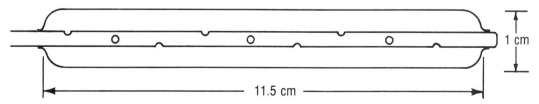

FIGURE 7-15. The intraesophageal pressure probe described by van den Berg (1956). The thin-walled balloon is formed around the end of a long polyethylene sensing tube.

manometer, the strong influence of lung volume on esophageal pressure makes it imperative that an additional calibration of the entire system be done at different lung volumes for each subject. There are several ways of going about this.

Ladefoged (1964) and Ladefoged and McKinney (1963) propose a calibration method that rests on the following principle. If the glottis remains open and the velopharyngeal port closed, the intraoral air pressure must be the same as the tracheal pressure when one exhales against a resistance. Calibration for changes of esophageal pressure thus requires that intraoral air pressure be monitored along with esophageal pressure as the client blows against an oral obstruction with different amounts of effort. Each esophageal pressure reading obtained can be equated with a measured intraoral air pressure to generate a table of equivalents. This procedure is repeated at several lung volumes. A sample oscillographic record of the results of this maneuver at a single lung volume is shown in Figure 7-16. The obviously nonlinear esophageal pressure scale can be drawn onto a separate sheet to be used as a template in reading pressures at this lung volume from the pen-recorder output of the actual evaluation tasks. Note that the procedure requires a second pressure-measuring system (for intraoral air pressure) and a means of monitoring lung volume.

Lieberman (1968) has used a calibration technique which is simpler to implement. While not as accurate as Ladefoged's method, it gives results which are sufficiently valid for everyday clinical use. It assumes that (1) the recoil pressure generated in the lungs is essentially a linear function of the lung volume for the duration of an utterance of 2 or 3 s and (2) that the decrease in lung volume proceeds at a steady rate during speech. (The second assumption ignores phonetic variations in flow, but it is a usable approximation from the point of view of the length of the entire utterance.) Now, if the airway is unobstructed by glottal closure or oral constriction, the trache-

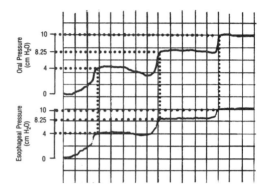

FIGURE 7-16. Calibration of the esophageal pressure according to the method recommmended by Ladefoged and McKinney (1963). Known intraoral pressures are used to determine esophageal pressure equivalents. The P_e scale (bottom) is assigned values of the P_{oral} pressures. Note that the P_e scale is nonlinear.

al pressure must be zero when there is no airflow. During speech this condition is met at every transition from inspiration to expiration or vice versa. During the speech task, therefore, airflow is simultaneously recorded and is read out along with the esophageal pressure in the final oscillographic or pen-recorder record. A sample of such an output showing how the calibration is handled is presented in Figure 7-17. Every point in the esophageal pressure record that corresponds to a point of ventilatory phase transition (as shown by the flow record) is considered to represent $P_s = 0$ and is so marked. These zero points are connected together to form a series of "zero-pressure lines." The subglottal pressure at any point in the record is read as the distance of the esophageal pressure trace (expressed in terms of the calibration of the transducer originally done with a U-tube) above the zero pressure baseline just below it. In essence, construction of the deduced base lines subtracts out the lung-volume error. Since each breath-group begins and ends with a ventilatory phase transition, each has its own (approximate) correction factor. (Sample records using a variation of this baseline correction method are provided in

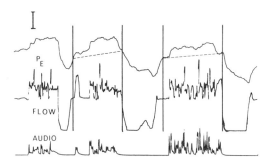

FIGURE 7-17. Calibration of an esophageal pressure record according to Lieberman's (1968) method. Respiratory phase transitions (shown in the flow record) are delineated by vertical lines. They are used to define points in the record when the tracheal pressure must be zero. For each breath-group the beginning and ending zero-pressure points are connected to form a pressure base-line (dashed lines). Pressure measures are then made in terms of the height of the trace above the pressure base-line. The calibration line accompanying the pressure trace equals 10 cm H_2O.

Lagefoged, 1968.) Lieberman (1968) has found that this calibration results in estimates of P_s that are accurate within about 1 cm H_2O, provided that the speaker does not use lung volumes near the extremes of his vital capacity.

Advantages and Limitations. Using an esophageal balloon to sense a correlate of subglottal pressure has the obvious advantage of avoiding tracheal puncture, with its attendant risks, pain, and client anxiety. It must be recognized, however, that this method is not altogether anxiety-free either, and since it is itself somewhat invasive its implementation is accompanied by reduced, but none the less real, risk. Clearly, the esophageal balloon should be inserted by a physician.

The question of the validity of the resultant data has been debated at some length in the technical literature. While van den Berg (1956), for example, concluded that esophageal estimates were generally accurate within 10%, McGlone (1967) found rea-

son to reject the method, as did Rubin, LeCover, and Vennard (1967). Kunze (1964) has published a carefully considered review of direct and indirect subglottal pressure measurement techniques and found esophageal pressure measures wanting. Some of the problems he identified are addressed by Ladefoged (1964). Detailed consideration of means of improving validity is also provided in the other articles cited in the reference list.

While the theoretical issues and practical problems discussed in these assessments certainly merit consideration, the clinician should bear in mind that the researchers participating in the published debate had measurement objectives very different from those that guide clinical rehabilitation. That is, the purpose behind development of various subglottal pressure measurement procedures is the generation of highly accurate data that will permit testing hypotheses resulting from various physiological theories. In the research laboratory uncertainty of measurement often proves fatal to hypothesis confirmation. The clinician's objectives are very different, in that it is rare for small differences in P_s to be of clinical importance. In general the speech pathologist will be more interested in the client's ability to generate subglottal pressures that at least fall into the usable range, to vary the pressure voluntarily, and, perhaps of supreme importance, to maintain the stability of whatever pressure is being used. With reasonable care, the accuracy of esophageal pressure measurements will be adequate for the purposes of the clinical rehabilitation specialist even if they are not sufficiently precise to satisfy the speech scientist.

Plethysmography

Hixon (1972) and Warren (1976) have described a method for evaluating P_s using a body plethysmograph (described in Chap. 8). For this measurement a dome is hermetically clamped to the top of the body box, enclosing the client's head (see Figure 7-18). In this arrangement the plethysmograph forms a quasi-closed system with the client inside, breathing to and from the space within the box. As the client inhales (increasing his lung volume) the increase in the size of his body causes the amount of free space inside the box to diminish; the reverse is true on expiration. In short, the closed system has a constant volume—an increase in the volume of one part (for instance, the lungs) will be exactly matched by a decrease in the volume of the other part (the free space within the box) if all other factors are constant.

Determination of P_s rests on the fact that at least one of the other factors does *not* remain constant. Any change in lung volume occurs together with (and, indeed, is produced by) a change in alveolar pressure. Boyle's law states that the volume of a gas is inversely proportional to its pressure:

$$V \propto 1/P.$$

If alveolar pressure increases somewhat, the volume of the lungs will diminish a little, and vice versa. This change of volume does *not* result in movement of air from one part of the closed system to the other and, therefore, the pressure in the space surrounding the client will change by a proportional amount in the opposite direction.

A simple example may clarify the reasons for this. Increased pressure within the lungs implies that the gas molecules already present are forced to occupy less space (thus, the pressure increase is proportional to the lung volume decrease). If the lungs (and hence the chest as a whole) take up less volume, then the surrounding space within the box must be increased. If no molecules move from the lungs to the outside, then the enlargement of the space around the body within the box means that the molecules there have a little *more* space in which they can move around, which is another way of saying that the pressure of the surrounding air drops. Hence, in this configuration of the body plethysmograph, any change in the pressure within the box should be due to compressional effects

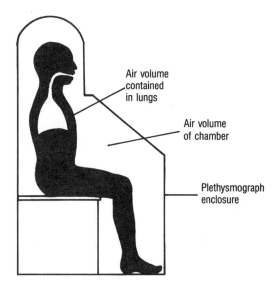

FIGURE 7-18. The body plethysmograph. When completely sealed within the box the subject's lungs and the surrounding space constitute two parts of a single volume of air. Assuming that the pressure inside the box does not change, expansion of one part of the air volume must be at the expense of the other part of the volume, since the total air volume in the box must remain constant.

only—that is, it should reflect lung pressure. Because there is only a negligible difference between lung and subglottal pressures, the air pressure of the plethysmograph is an index of P_s.

Unfortunately, the lung volume is very different from the volume of the air surrounding the subject and, therefore, the magnitude of the box pressure change is proportional to, *but not equal to*, the change in P_s. This means that the method requires special calibration procedures, similar to those used for esophageal pressure estimates.

Instrumentation. The actual setup required is diagrammed in Figure 7-19. The client normally breathes into the space within the chamber. There is, however, a special tube, closed at one end, mounted just in front of the client's mouth. A pressure transducer is connected to measure

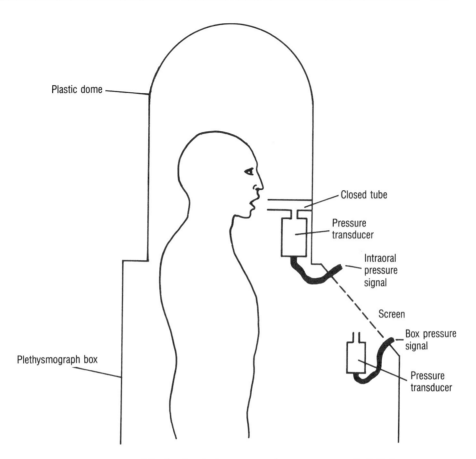

FIGURE 7-19. Use of the body plethysmograph to measure subglottal pressure.

pressure in this tube during calibration. Measurement of the box pressure, the correlate of P_s, is accomplished with another pressure transducer that senses the pressure just inside of a screened opening in the box wall. The screen provides a moderately high resistance to the flow of air, across which the pressure appears. The opening allows slow changes in pressure (equivalent to DC voltage) to be equalized, while allowing comparatively rapid (AC-type) changes to be measured. Functionally, then, the box can be considered to be sealed for high-frequency AC signals, but fully vented for DC.

Calibration. The system is calibrated by having the client seal his lips around the mouth tube and, keeping his glottis open, compress and expand the gas in his lungs by attempting to "pant" into it. The pressure transducer attached to the mouth tube records the intraoral pressure during this maneuver. Since the glottis is open, this matches the lung pressure quite closely. The intraoral pressures are then used to calibrate the box pressures that were simultaneously recorded.

Since the calibration thus obtained is valid only for the lung volume at which the calibrating maneuver was performed, the client is usually asked to do the calibrating task, come off the mouth tube, and immediately speak the test utterances with no intervening inspiration or expiration. If the lung volume changes significantly during the utterance (because of its length or because of excessive air usage), a second calibration will be required at its end. In this case the client is asked to hold his breath at the postsample lung volume and perform the "panting" maneuver into the mouth tube again. The change in calibration factor due to lung volume change can thereby be accounted for. A single calibration suffices for short utterances if air usage is essentially normal.

Advantages and limitations. The prime advantage of the plethysmographic method of estimating subglottal pressure is the fact that it is completely noninvasive. Not only does this eliminate risk, but it makes the measurement procedure far more acceptable to the client. In fact, this method may be the only way to obtain P_s measures during speech in young children, for whom the plethysmograph may be decorated as a "space ship," and the measurement procedure made part of an appropriate game. While frequent calibrations are required, the technique is based on fairly straightforward and well understood physical principles. With a modicum of care, measures of exceptional precision and unquestionable validity are possible. The cost of a body plethysmograph is relatively high, but since it may also be used for airflow and lung volume measurements, its versatility permits the higher capital investment to be amortized over greater use.

ORAL PRESSURE DURING PLOSIVES. When the vocal folds are abducted and the oral airway closed during the production of a voiceless plosive, the intraoral air pressure rises to the value of the tracheal pressure. The two are, in fact, essentially equal when the intraoral pressure reaches its maximum (Netsell, 1969; Shipp, 1973). The oral pressure peak during plosive production can be considered, therefore, to be a good estimate of the subglottic pressure if the speech task is carefully constructed.

Method. Smitheran and Hixon (1981) have taken advantage of this situation in their procedure for assessing laryngeal re-

sistance. While subject to certain limitations and problems (Rothenberg, 1982; Smitheran and Hixon, 1981), the method is likely to be very useful to clinicians. The protocol requires the subject to produce 7 repetitions of the syllable /pi/ at a rate of 1.5 syllables per second. Intraoral pressure is sensed by a polyethylene tube and pressure transducer. The client is required to produce the syllable train, after an inhalation to twice normal depth, on a single continuous expiration. Normal pitch and loudness are used, and the syllables should all receive equal stress. The peak intraoral pressures are considered to equal the subglottal pressure.

If oral air flow measures are taken simultaneously, the flow during the vowel may be used to estimate the laryngeal resistance. Dividing the pressure (in cm H_2O) by the flow (in liters per second) provides the laryngeal resistance in cm $H_2O/L/s$ *if* the velopharyngeal port is tightly sealed during the syllable and *if* the oropharyngeal resistance is close to zero.

Advantages and Limitations. This method has the advantage of being very simple to use. It entails no significant invasiveness, requires only simple instrumentation, and involves a speech task that is within the competence of most clients. On the other hand, the measure is based on discontinuous estimates of both pressure and flow, and the two quantities are never sampled at the same time. There is continuing controversy about the validity of estimating P_s in this way. However, Löfqvist, Carlborg, and Kitzing (1982) have shown that an acceptable estimate results if the oral pressure is taken at the midpoint of a line connecting two successive pressure peaks. But, since a number of factors can influence oral pressure, caution should be exercised in interpreting the data in special cases.

ORAL PRESSURE DURING AIRWAY INTERRUPTION. Another way to force the oral air pressure to approximate P_s is to suddenly block the airway during speech. This can be accomplished by closing a valve at the outlet of the face mask that the speaker wears. In essence, the valve closure constitutes an artificial plosive articulation.

Method. Sawashima and his coworkers (Sawashima, Kiritani, Sekimoto, Horiguchi, Okafuji, and Shirai, 1983; Sawashima, Honda, Kiritani, Sekimoto, Ogawa, and Shirai, 1984) implement this technique with a specially made, electrically operated valve that achieves rapid and complete closure when the tester pushes a button. It takes up to 200 ms for the oral pressure to rise to the magnitude of the subglottal pressure. Since ventilatory and vocal tract adjustments can change the pressure if the closure persists (Baken and Orlikoff, in press) the valve must not be kept closed too long. Sawashima and his colleagues recommend that closure be limited by an electronic timer to a maximum of 400 ms. The estimate of subglottal pressure is represented by the height of a pressure trace (on a graphic readout) at the point where the trace just levels off after valve closure.

Advantages and Limitations. The advantages that derive from the noninvasiveness of this method are offset by the relative complexity and expense of the valve system and its electronic control system. Care must be taken to ensure that the valve closure does not cause a subject reaction that, by changing the subglottal pressure, would result in an invalid measure. Finally, the valve closure is likely to be quite disruptive of speech and might cause the speaker to use abnormal or compensatory behaviors after the first trial.

Expected Results

MINIMUM P_s FOR SPEECH. Initiation of phonation requires a transglottal pressure drop of 2 to 4 cm H_2O. A pressure 1 or 2 cm H_2O lower is sufficient to sustain phonation already under way (Lieberman et al., 1969; Draper et al., 1960). A conservative clinical rule of thumb, therefore, is that minimally adequate speech requires that the client be able to sustain a subglottal pressure of no less than 5 cm H_2O for at least 5 s (Netsell and Hixon, 1978; Netsell and Daniel, 1979).

STABILITY OF P_s. When speaking with uniform loudness the mean tracheal pressure is kept "remarkably constant" by a normal speaker (Draper et al., 1960). Small variations due to sudden vocal tract impedance changes will occur, however. For example, Netsell (1969) measured P_s during production of /t/ and /d/ in the syllables /ʌ:tʌ/ and /ʌ:dʌ/ and found that the only observable difference between the pattern of P_s during the two was a sudden, but small, decrease of pressure during the plosive phase of /t/. The drop in pressure terminated with a return to the preplosive value when voicing resumed. A similar tendency is apparent for both /p/ and /b/ in the data of McGlone and Shipp (1972) and Murry and Brown (1979) as well as Slis (1970), who found that P_s dropped during /h/, a phoneme produced with very low vocal tract impedance. This kind of pressure drop is due to the sudden loss of significant vocal tract obstruction and is not a reflection of change in the generation of P_s. Also, of course, the subglottal pressure rises and falls slightly across the glottal cycle (Koike and Hirano, 1973). Aside from this kind of transient phenomenon, instability of subglottal pressure in the absence of intentional loudness changes or word stress should be seen as abnormal and clinically suspect.

TYPICAL VALUES OF P_s. The subglottal pressures presented in Table 7-9 were measured by tracheal puncture in 9 young adult males producing 2 s of steady state phonation at comfortable pitch and loudness in pulse (glottal fry) register and at 10% pitch and 25 and 75% intensity levels in modal register. Differences between the vocal registers were not significant for this sustained-phonation task. Murry (1971) reported that P_s was higher during pulse- than during modal-register phonation. However, the

TABLE 7–9. Mean Subglottal Pressure in Pulse and Modal Registers During Sustained Phonation*

Register	F_o (Hz) Mean	F_o (Hz) Range	P_s (cm H$_2$O) Mean	P_s (cm H$_2$O) Range
Pulse	34	18–65	5.3	2.5–7.6
Modal	108	87–117	5.0†	2.8–7.0†

From McGlone, R. E. and Shipp, T. Some physiologic correlates of vocal fry phonation. *Journal of Speech and Hearing Research*, 14 (1971) 769–775. Table 1, p. 772. ©American Speech-Language-Hearing Association, Rockville, MD. Reprinted by permission.

*Nine men, young adults; 2-s phonations; pulse: comfortable pitch and loudness; modal: 10% pitch levels; 25 and 75% intensity levels. Tracheal puncture.

†The 25 and 75% intensity levels combined; differences between vocal registers not significant.

TABLE 7–10. Subglottal Pressure at Different Loudness Levels

Condition	Mean P_s (cm H$_2$O)* Consonants	Mean P_s (cm H$_2$O)* /h/
Whisper	10.0	6.5
Normally loud	11.5	8.5
Shout	19.0	19.5

From Slis, I.H. Articulatory measurements on voiced, voiceless, and nasal consonants. *Phonetica*, 21 (1970) 193-210. Reprinted by permission.

*Data derived from author's tabulation; rounded to nearest 0.5.

pulse register phonation that normally occurs during terminal syllables in running speech seems to be characterized by a P_s that is considerably *lower* than that of the modal phonation that preceded it (Murry and Brown, 1971b).

RELATIONSHIP OF P_s TO VOCAL INTENSITY. Subglottal pressure varies directly with vocal intensity. The exact relationship is not linear, and it appears to differ quantitatively among individuals. Isshiki (1964) found (in a single male subject) that P_s, measured by tracheal puncture, varied from 3 to 25 cm H$_2$O as intensity increased from 65 to 95 dB SPL. The approximate relationship was

$$SPL \propto P_s^{3.3 \pm 0.7}.$$

Considering only the middle loudness range, where P_s was between 10 and 30 cm H$_2$O, Ladefoged and McKinney (1963, p. 456) found that "peak subglottal pressure was proportional to the 0.6 power of the peak [rms] sound pressure." That is,

$$P_s \propto dB\ SPL^{0.6}.$$

The relationship of P_s and intensity is well illustrated in Table 7-10, which is de-

rived from data presented by Slis (1970), who measured esophageal pressure during consonants in the syllables /bɔCoet/ and /bɔCɔ/ as produced by Dutch speakers.

RELATIONSHIP OF P_s TO WORD STRESS. Stress, or "prominencing" of syllables, can be divided into two types: sentence-level and lexical stress. Lexical stress clarifies grammatical function, as in the words *import* (noun) versus *import* (verb). In sentence-level stress one word is chosen, for semantic or pragmatic reasons, as the focus of the sentence (as in "*She* did it," in which "she" is the stressed element). Sentence-level stress is almost always heavily marked for prominence, while, in conversation, lexical stress may be essentially unmarked. Only in careful, "citational" pronunciation is it the case that, as Ladefoged (1968, p. 143) notes, "accompanying every stressed syllable there is always an increase in the subglottal pressure." This observation receives support in the data of McGlone and Shipp (1972) who contrasted P_s during production of /p/ and /b/ in stressed (/ɔpa/, /ɔba/) and unstressed (/ɑpɔ/, /ɑbɔ/) positions. P_s for the stressed productions of their 10 subjects was somewhat higher on the average. The relationship between stress and P_s, however, is extremely complex. Because of the multiple cuing for word stress (of which subglottal pressure change is only a part), it is only partially understood. ■

Select Bibliography

Anonymous *Introduction to Transducers for Instrumentation*. Oxnard, CA: Gould, Inc., Statham Instruments Division, 1966.

Arkebauer, H. J., Hixon, T. J., and Hardy, J. C. Peak intraoral air pressures during speech. *Journal of Speech and Hearing Research*, 10, (1967) 196-208.

Baken, R. J. and Orlikoff, R. F. Phonatory response to step-function changes in supraglottal pressure. In Harris, K. S., Baer, T., and Sasaki, C. (Eds.) *Vocal Fold Physiology: Laryngeal Function in Phonation and Respiration*. San Diego, CA: College-Hill, in press.

Baken, R. J. and Orlikoff, R. F. Perturbation of vocal fundamental frequency during voiced fricatives. Presentation at the International Conference on Voice, Kurume, Japan, 1986.

Bernthal, J. E. and Beukelman, D. R. Intraoral air pressure during the production of /p/ and /b/ by children, youths, and adults. *Journal of Speech and Hearing Research*, 21 (1978) 361-371.

Black, J. W. The pressure component in the production of consonants. *Journal of Speech Disorders*, 15 (1950) 207-210.

Bouhuys, A., Proctor, D. F., and Mead, J. Kinetic aspects of singing. *Journal of Applied Physiology*, 21 (1966) 483-496.

Brown, W. S., jr. and Brandt, J. F. Effects of auditory masking on vocal intensity and intraoral air pressure during sentence production. *Journal of the Acoustical Society of America*, 49 (1971) 1903-1905.

Brown, W. S., jr. and McGlone, R. E. Relation of intraoral air pressure to oral cavity size. *Folia Phoniatrica*, 21 (1969a) 321-331.

Brown, W. S., jr. and McGlone, R. E. Constancy of intraoral air pressure. *Folia Phoniatrica*, 21 (1969b) 332-339.

Brown, W. S., jr. and McGlone, R. E. Aerodynamic and acoustic study of stress in sentence productions. *Journal of the Acoustical Society of America*, 56 (1974) 971-974.

Brown, W. S., jr., McGlone, R. E., Tarlow, A. and Shipp, T. Intraoral air pressures associated with specific phonetic positions. *Phonetica*, 22 (1970) 202-212.

Brown, W. S., jr. and Ruder, K. F. Phonetic factors affecting intraoral air pressure associated with stop consonants. In Rigault, A. and Charbonneau, R. (Eds.). *Proceedings of the Seventh International Congress of Phonetic Sciences*. The Hague: Mouton, 1972. Pp. 294-299.

Brown, W. S., jr. and Shearer, W. M. Constancy of intraoral air pressure related to integrated pressure-time measures. *Folia Phoniatrica*, 22 (1970) 49-57.

Counihan, Donald T. Oral and nasal air flow and air pressure measures. In Bzoch, K. R. Ed.). *Communicative Disorders Related to Cleft Lip and Cleft Palate*. Boston: Little, Brown, and Co., 1972. Pp. 178-185.

Draper, M. H., Ladefoged, P., and Whitteridge, D. Expiratory pressures and air flow during speech. *British Medical Journal*, 18 (1960) 1837-1843.

Edmonds, T. D., Lilly, D. J., and Hardy, J. C. Dynamic characteristics of air-pressure measuring systems used in speech research. *Journal of the Acoustical Society of America*, 50 (1971) 1051-1057.

Fischer-Jørgensen, E. and Hansen, A. T. An electrical manometer and its use in phonetic research. *Phonetica*, 4 (1959) 43-53.

Flege, J. E. The influence of stress, position, and utterance length on the pressure characteristics of English /p/ and /b/. *Journal of Speech and Hearing Research*, 26 (1983) 111-118.

Fry, D. L. Physiologic recording by modern instruments with particular reference to pressure recording. *Physiological Reviews*, 40 (1960) 753-787.

Fry, D. L., Stead, W. W., Ebert, R. V., Lubin, R. I., and Wells, H. S. The measurement of intraesophageal pressure and its relationship to intrathoracic pressure. *Laboratory and Clinical Medicine*, 40 (1952) 664-673.

Hanson, M. L. A study of velopharyngeal competence in children with repaired cleft palates. *Cleft Palate Journal*, 1 (1964) 217-231.

Hardy, J. C. Intraoral breath pressure in cerebral palsy. *Journal of Speech and Hearing Disorders*, 26 (1961) 309-319.

Hardy, J. C. Air flow and air pressure studies. *ASHA Reports*, 1 (1965) 141-152.

Hardy, J. C. Techniques of measuring intraoral air pressure and rate of air flow. *Journal of Speech and Hearing Research*, 10 (1967) 650-654.

Hixon, T. J. Turbulent noise sources for speech. *Folia Phoniatrica*, 19 (1966) 168-182.

Hixon, T. J. Some new techniques for measuring the biomechanical events of speech production: one laboratory's experiences. *ASHA Reports*, 7 (1972) 68-103.

Hixon, T. J., Klatt, D. H., and Mead, J. Influence of forced transglottal pressure changes on vocal fundamental frequency. *Journal of the Acoustical Society of America*, 49 (1971) 105.

Hixon, T. J., Hawley, J. L., and Wilson, K. J. An around-the-house device for the clinical determination of respiratory driving pressure: A note on making simple even simpler. *Journal of Speech and Hearing Disorders*, 47 (1982) 413-415.

Hixon, T. J., Mead, J., and Goldman, M. Dynamics of the chest wall during speech production: Function of the rib cage, diaphragm, and abdomen. *Journal of Speech and Hearing Research*, 19 (1976) 297-356.

Hixon, T. J., Minifie, F. D., and Tait, C. A. Correlates of turbulent noise production for speech. *Journal of Speech and Hearing Research*, 10 (1967) 133-140.

Hixon, T. J. and Smitheran, J. R. A reply to Rothenberg. *Journal of Speech and Hearing Disorders*, 47 (1982) 220-223.

Isshiki, N. Regulatory mechanism of voice intensity variation. *Journal of Speech and Hearing Research*, 7 (1964) 17-29.

Kantner, C. E. The rational of blowing exercises for patients with reparied cleft palates. *Journal of Speech Disorders*, 12 (1947) 281-286.

Karnell, M. P. and Willis, C. R. The effect of vowel context on consonantal intraoral air pressure. *Folia Phoniatrica*, 34 (1982a) 1-8.

Karnell, M. P. and Willis, C. R. The reliability of the Kay Agnellograph pressure translator in the study of consonantal intraoral air pressure. *Folia Phoniatrica*, 34 (1982b) 53-56.

Kitzing, P, Carlborg, B. and Löfqvist, A. Aerodynamic and glottographic studies of the laryngeal vibratory cycle. *Folia Phoniatrica*, 34 (1982) 216-224.

Kitzing, P., and Löfqvist, A. Subglottal and oral air pressures during phonation — preliminary investigation using a miniature transducer system. *Medical and Biological Engineering,*, 13 (1975) 644-648.

Klich, R. J. Effects of speech level and vowel context on intraoral air pressure in vocal and whispered speech. *Folia Phoniatrica*, 34 (1982) 33-40.

Koike, Y. Sub- and supraglottal pressure variation during phonation. In Stevens, K. N. and Hirano, M. (Eds.) *Vocal Fold Physiology*. Tokyo: University of Tokyo Press, 1981. Chap. 14, pp. 181-192.

Koike, Y. and Hirano, M. Glottal-area time function and subglottal pressure variation. *Journal of the Acoustical Society of America* 54 (1973) 1618-1627.

Koike, Y. and Perkins, W. H. Application of a miniaturized pressure transducer for experimental speech research. *Folia Phoniatrica*, 20 (1968) 360-368.

Kunze, L. H. Evaluation of methods of estimating subglottal air pressure. *Journal of Speech and Hearing Research*, 7 (1964) 151-164.

Ladefoged, P. Some physiological parameters in speech. *Language and Speech* 6 (1963) 109-119.

Ladefoged, P. Comment on 'Evaluation of methods of estimating sub-glottal air pressure' *Journal of Speech and Hearing Research*, (1964) 291-292.

Ladefoged, P. Linguistic aspects of respiratory phenomena. In Bouhuys, A. (Ed.). *Sound Pro-duction in Man. (Annals of the New York Academy of Sciences*, vol. 155). New York: New York Academy of Sciences, 1968. Pp. 141-151.

Ladefoged, P. and McKinney, N. P. Loudness, sound pressure, and subglottal pressure in speech. *Journal of the Acoustical Society of America*, 35 (1963) 454-460.

Leeper, H. A. and Noll, J. D. Pressure measurements of articulatory behavior during alterations of vocal effort. *Journal of the Acoustical Society of America*, 51 (1972) 1291-1295.

Lieberman, P. Direct comparison of subglottal and esophageal pressure during speech. *Journal of the Acoustical Society of America*, 43 (1968) 1157-1164.

Lieberman, P., Knudson, R., and Mead, J. Determination of the rate of change of fundamental frequency with respect to subglottal air pressure during sustained phonation. *Journal of the Acoustical Society of America*, 45 (1969) 1537-1543.

Lisker, L. Supraglottal air pressure in the production of English stops. *Language and Speech*, 13 (1970) 215-230.

Löfqvist, A., Carlborg, B. and Kitzing, P. Initial validation of an indirect measure of subglottal pressure during vowels. *Journal of the Acoustical Society of America*, 72 (1982) 633-635.

Lubker, J. F. and Parris, P. J. Simultaneous measurements of intraoral pressure, force of labial contact, and labial electromyography during production of the stop consonant cognates /p/ and /b/. *Journal of the Acoustical Society of America*, 47 (1970) 625-633.

Malécot, A. The effectiveness of intra-oral air pressure-pulse parameters in distinguishing between stop cognates. *Phonetica*, 14 (1966) 65-81.

Malécot, A. The force of articulation of American stops and fricatives as a function of position. *Phonetica*, 18 (1968) 95-102.

McGlone, R. E. Intraesophageal pressure during syllable repetition. *Journal of the Acoustical Society of America*, 42 (1967) 1208.

McGlone, R. E. and Shipp, T. Some physiologic correlates of vocal fry phonation. *Journal of Speech and Hearing Research*, 14 (1971) 769-775.

McGlone, R. E. and Shipp, T. Comparison of subglottal air pressures associated with /p/ and /b/. *Journal of the Acoustical Society of America*, 51 (1972) 664-665.

McWilliams, B. J. and Bradley, D. P. Ratings of velopharyngeal closure during blowing and speech. *Cleft Palate Journal*, 2 (1965) 46-55.

Mead, J., Bouhuys, A., and Proctor, D. F. Mechanisms generating subglottic pressure. In Bouhuys, A. (Ed.). *Sound Production in Man (Annals of the New York Academy of Sciences*, vol. 155). New York: New York Academy of

Sciences, 1968. Pp. 177-181.

Milic-Emili, J., Mead, J., Turner, J. M., and Glauser, E. M. Improved technique for estimating pleural pressure from esophageal balloons. *Journal of Applied Physiology,* 18 (1964) 208-211.

Miller, C. J. and Daniloff, R. Aerodynamics of stops in continuous speech. *Journal of Phonetics,* 5 (1977) 351-360.

Minifie, F. D., Hixon, T. J., and Williams, F. (Eds.). *Normal Aspects of Speech, Hearing, and Language.* Englewood Cliffs, N.J.: Prentice-Hall, 1973.

Morris, H. L. The oral manometer as a diagnostic tool in clinical speech pathology. *Journal of Speech and Hearing Disorders,* 31 (1966) 362-369.

Morris, H. L. and Smith, J. K. A multiple approach for evaluating velopharyngeal competency. *Journal of Speech and Hearing Disorders,* 27 (1962) 218-226.

Müller, E. M. and Brown, W. S., jr. Variations in the supraglottal air pressure and their articulatory interpretation. In Lass, N. J. (Ed.). *Speech and Language: Advances in Basic Research and Practice.* New York: Academic Press, 1980. Pp. 317-389.

Murry, T. Subglottal pressure and airflow measures during vocal fry phonation. *Journal of Speech and Hearing Research* 14 (1971) 544-551.

Murry, T. and Brown, W. S., jr. Intraoral air pressure variability in esophageal speakers. *Folia Phoniatrica,* 27 (1975) 237-249.

Murry, T. and Brown, W. S., jr. Regulation of vocal intensity during vocal fry phonation. *Journal of the Acoustical Society of America,* 49 (1971a) 1905-1907.

Murry, T. and Brown, W. S., jr. Subglottal air pressure during two types of vocal activity: vocal fry and modal phonation. *Folia Phoniatrica,* 23 (1971b) 440-449.

Murry, T. and Brown, W. S., jr. Aerodynamic interactions associated with voiced-voiceless stop consonants. *Folia Phoniatrica,* 31 (1979) 82-88.

Netsell, R. Subglottal and intraoral air pressures during the intervocalic contrast of /t/ and /d/. *Phonetica,* 20 (1969) 68-73.

Netsell, R. Underlying physiological mechanisms of syllable stress. *Journal of the Acoustical Society of America,* 47 (1970) 103.

Netsell, R. and Daniel, B. Dysarthria in adults: physiologic approach to rehabilitation. *Archives of Physical Medicine and Rehabilitation,* 60 (1979) 502-508.

Netsell, R. and Hixon, T. J. A noninvasive method for clinically estimating subglottal air pressure. *Journal of Speech and Hearing Disorders,* 43 (1978) 326-330.

Perkins, W. H. and Koike, Y. Patterns of sub-

glottal pressure variations during phonation: a preliminary report. *Folia Phoniatrica,* 21 (1969) 1-8.

Pitzner, J. C. and Morris, H. L. Articulation skills and adequacy of breath pressure ratios of children with cleft palate. *Journal of Speech and Hearing Disorders,* 31 (1966) 26-40.

Ptacek, P. H., Sander, E. K., Maloney, W. H., and Jackson, C. C. R. Phonatory and related changes with advanced age. *Journal of Speech and Hearing Research,* 9 (1966) 353-360.

Ringel, R. L., House, A. S., and Montgomery, A. H. Scaling articulatory behavior: intraoral air pressure. *Journal of the Acoustical Society of America,* 42 (1967) 1209.

Rothenberg, M. Interpolating subglottal pressure from oral pressure. *Journal of Speech and Hearing Disorders,* 47 (1982) 219-220.

Rothenberg, M. and Mahshie, J. Induced transglottal pressure variations during voicing. *Journal of the Acoustical Society of America,* 62 (1977) S14A.

Rubin, H. J., LeCover, M., and Vennard, W. Vocal intensity, subglottic pressure, and air flow relationships in singers. *Folia Phoniatrica,* 19 (1967) 393-413.

Sawashima, M., Honda, K., Kiritani, S., Sekimoto, S., Ogawa, S., and Shirai, K. Further works on the airway interruption method of measuring expiratory air pressure during phonation. *Annual Bulletin of the Research Institute for Logopedics and Phoniatrics,* 18 (1984) 19-26.

Sawashima, M., Kiritani, S., Sekimoto, S., Horiguchi, S., Okafuji, K., and Shirai, K. The airway interruption technique for measuring expiratory air pressure during phonation. *Annual Bulletin of the Research Institute for Logopedics and Phoniatrics,* 17 (1983) 23-32.

Scully, C. A comparison of /s/ and /z/ for an English speaker. *Language and Speech,* 14 (1971) 187-200.

Shelton, R. L., Jr., Brooks, A., and Youngstrom, K. A. Clinical assessment of palatopharyngeal closure. *Journal of Speech and Hearing Disorders,* 30 (1965) 37-43.

Shipp, T. Intraoral air pressure and lip occlusion in midvocalic stop consonant production. *Journal of Phonetics,* 1 (1973) 167-170.

Slis, I. H. Articulatory measurements on voiced, voiceless, and nasal consonants. *Phonetica,* 21 (1970) 193-210.

Smitheran, J. R. and Hixon, T. J. A clinical method for estimating laryngeal airway resistance during vowel production. *Journal of Speech and Hearing Disorders,* 46 (1981) 138-146.

Spriestersbach, D. C. and Powers, G. R. Articulation skills, velopharyngeal closure, and oral breath pressure of children with cleft palates. *Journal of Speech and Hearing Research,* 2 (1959) 318-325.

Stathopoulos, E. T. Oral air flow during vowel production of children and adults. *Cleft Palate Journal*, 21 (1984) 277-285.

Stathopoulos, E. T. Relationship between intraoral air pressure and vocal intensity in children and adults. *Journal of Speech and Hearing Research*, 29 (1986) 71-74.

Stathopoulos, E. T. and Weismer, G. Oral airflow and air pressure during speech production: a comparative study of children, youths, and adults. *Folia Phoniatrica*, 37 (1985) 152-159.

Subtelny, J. D., Worth, J. H., and Sakuda, M. Intraoral pressure and rate of flow during speech. *Journal of Speech and Hearing Research*, 9 (1966) 498-518.

van den Berg, Jw. Direct and indirect determination of the mean subglottic pressure. *Folia Phoniatrica*, 8 (1956) 1-24.

van den Berg, Jw. Myoelastic-aerodynamic theory of voice production. *Journal of Speech and Hearing Research*, 1 (1958) 227-244.

Warren, D. W. Aerodynamics of speech production. In Lass, N. J. (Ed.). *Contemporary Issues in Experimental Phonetics*. New York: Academic Press, 1976. Pp. 105-137.

Warren, D. W., Hall, D. J., and Davis, J. Oral port constriction and pressure-airflow relationships during sibilant productions. *Folia Phoniatrica*, 33 (1981) 380-394.

CHAPTER 8

Airflow and Volume

The vocal tract is an *aerodynamic* sound generator and resonator system. Variations in the flow of air through it reflect changes in the "manner" of consonant and vowel articulations. Evaluation of air flow, then, can provide considerable insight into speech system dysfunction and efficiency. The data can be of great assistance in improving the precision of initial diagnosis, documenting change during therapy, and providing biofeedback to patients with voice or articulation pathologies (Gordon, Morton, and Simpson, 1978; Amerman and Williams, 1979; Bastian, Unger, and Sasama, 1981).

GENERAL PHYSICAL PRINCIPLES

Good discussions of airflow phenomena and air volume characteristics of speech can be found in almost any elementary textbook of speech physiology or phonetics. This section will present a summary of pertinent information that will be important in applying or interpreting airflow or air volume measurements.

Airflow

Flow is the term used to describe the movement of a quantity of gas through a given area in a unit of time. (The rate of flow is also referred to as the *volume velocity*.) As in the case of air pressure, several different units may serve to quantify a given flow. Liters or milliliters per second or per minute are the most common, the choice being made to suit the specific situation. Table 8-1 provides the required conversion factors for changing from one set of units to another.

Flow-pressure relationship

When a gas flows its molecules are being driven from a region of relatively high pressure to one where the pressure is lower. The pressure difference between the two areas is called the *driving pressure*. The rate of flow of a gas is directly proportional to the driving pressure and inversely proportional to the resistance of the conduit through which the gas is moving.

TABLE 8–1. Conversion Factors for Flow Units.

	Milliliters* per second (mL/s)	Liters* per second (L/s)
Liters† per minute (L/min)	0.06	60
Milliliters† per minute	60	60,000

*To convert a value at the top to one at the side, *multiply* by the number in the appropriate box.
Example:
  100mL/sec = ? L/min = 100 × 0.06 = 6 L/min
  †To convert a value at the side to one at the top, *divide* by the number in the appropriate box.

That is,

$$U = P/Z \qquad (1)$$

where U = flow (volume velocity)
  P = driving pressure
  Z = impedance (resistance) of the pathway

This is simply a pneumatic version of Ohm's Law (see Chap. 2), and it may be rearranged in the same ways. Therefore,

$$Z = P/U \qquad (2)$$

and

$$P = U \times Z. \qquad (3)$$

These restatements of the flow-pressure-impedance relationship are particularly important. Equation 2 implies that the impedance of a system (for instance, the vocal tract) can be expressed in terms of flow through it and the driving pressure. In fact, impedance is often quantified in just such terms. One might, for example, describe a vocal tract as having an impedance of 70 cm of water per liter per second (70 $cmH_2O/L/s$), meaning that its impedance is high enough to produce a pressure drop of 70 cmH_2O for each liter per second of flow through it. (This does *not* mean that the flow ever actually has to be 1 L/s. A driving pressure of 7 cmH_2O at a flow of 0.1 L/s, for instance, represents an impedance

of 70 $cmH_2O/L/s$. An impedance of this magnitude is normal for voicing. A much smaller figure might be indicative of laryngeal adductor paralysis, while a larger value might characterize hyperadduction.)

The other alternative form of the relationship, $P = U \times Z$ (Equation 3), states the principle upon which the most common method of measuring airflow is based. In simple terms, it says that the pressure difference (P) between two points along an air stream is a function of the flow (U) and of the system's impedance between those points (Z). It also implies something: A pressure difference will be created across any impedance placed in an airflow. This statement is important and must be kept in mind whenever one deals with air flow measurement. It will explain many of the phenomena to be discussed later.

Laminar and turbulent flow

When a sizable pressure forces a gas through a tube of relatively large diameter the molecules all tend to move at the same speed along straight parallel paths. Pressure characteristics are stable and orderly. This kind of flow is described as *laminar*. It is the quiet flow of a large deep river between wide banks. If the tube becomes narrower (that is, if its impedance rises) or if the rate of flow becomes significantly greater, the flow pattern tends to change. The paths of the gas molecules become less universally parallel, and local velocity variations are produced. Irregularities of flow (eddy currents) appear, and there are small and random pressure fluctuations from point to point. The flow is said to be *turbulent*. It resembles the flow in a river as it becomes overswollen with too much rain. Turbulent air flow is characteristic of speech sounds (such as fricatives) that are produced by the high impedance of a tight vocal-tract constriction.* The degree of turbulence of an airflow is often significant. Some flow

---

*The generation of vocal tract air turbulence and its acoustic properties are analyzed by Stevens (1971) and Catford (1977).

transducers—particularly the warm-wire types, will yield inaccurate measures in the presence of a lot of turbulence, and certain measurement rationales are based on the assumption of laminar flow. In effect, turbulence represents pressure-flow noise, and its reduction may be important.

Air Volume

All of the air used for speech by a normal speaker is drawn from the same reservoir: the lungs. Therefore, air volumes used in speaking represent a change in lung volume, and some techniques for determining air usage actually monitor lung inflation status, instead of metering air passing out of the vocal tract. In general, the speech pathologist will be more interested in volume change than in lung volume itself. For example, we are almost never concerned with the actual volume of the lungs (including, for example, the dead space) but rather with the level to which the lungs are inflated before, or deflated during, speech. To say that a patient used 1 L of air for a phonatory task is to indicate that the lung volume diminished by that amount. The variable of primary interest in this chapter is not how much air is in storage, but how much is moved in accomplishing a speech task. Colloquially speaking, the bank balance is of less interest than the size of the withdrawals.

Flow-volume relationship

Flow is the rate of change of volume. To return to the phonating patient just mentioned, if the one liter volume change occured in 10 s of voice production, then it is apparent that the *mean* flow (volume velocity, U) was 100 mL/s. That is,

$$U = \Delta V/\Delta t, \qquad (4)$$

flow is equal to the volume change (ΔV) divided by the time over which the change occurred (Δt). In our example, therefore, U = 1 L/10 s, which is 0.1 L (or 100 mL) per second. Thus, if one is interested in the average flow during some period of time,

one need only divide the volume of air used by the amount of time in question.

All of this really means that the volume change per unit of time is the *slope* of the volume line on a graph, such as that shown in Figure 8-1A. Mathematically, the slope of the volume line is $\Delta V/\Delta t$. Figure 8-1 illustrates a major problem with using a simple averaging technique. Both of the graphs shown represent 1 L of air being used in 10 s. Therefore, the average flow for both recordings is 100 mL/s. In 1A, however, air usage is relatively steady, and the average flow for the 10 s is a good indicator of the actual flow at any point in time during the task. In 8-1B, however, the situation is very different. The rate at which the volume increases (that is, the slope of the line) fluctuates significantly. A liter of air has indeed been used in 10 s, but this average does not provide a good estimate of what the flow is likely to be at any given instant.

Clearly, what is needed is a way of expressing the average change of volume during successive, but exceptionally short, intervals of time. The shorter the time interval, the more accurate the representation of the real flow. In fact, it would be ideal if the change of volume could be computed for time intervals so short that they are zero seconds long. Then one could be sure that the actual flow *at every instant* was observed.

While it might seem a bit strange, there is a way to find the slope of a line at a single point (that is, when $\Delta t = 0$). Such a measure is, in fact, one of the bases of the calculus. It is called the *derivative*. (The process of determining the derivative is known as *differentiation*.) Flow, then, is the rate of change of the volume at every point in time. It is, in the language of the calculus, the derivative of the volume. The mathematical notation for this is

$$\text{Flow} = dV/dt.^* \qquad (5)$$

It is common to denote this function as $\dot{V}$, where the dot indicates *derivative*. (Indeed,

---

*The notation dV/dt is to be read as a symbol. It does not represent a fraction.

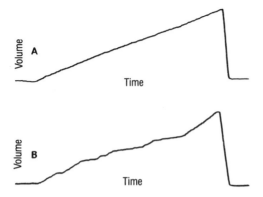

FIGURE 8–1. Each of the traces represents 1 L of air expired over a period of 10 s. Trace A, however, shows a fairly uniform flow rate, while the varying slope of trace B indicates variations in flow rate.

$\dot{V}$ is a standard symbol for flow in the physiological literature.) Figure 8-2 shows the same volume trace as in Figure 8-1B, but with the inclusion of a line representing dV/dt—the derivative of the volume, or the flow, at every point in time. Note that the changes in flow from instant to instant are dramatic.

Fortunately, one need not master the calculus to generate a flow line from volume data. It is easily done with an electronic circuit called a *differentiator*. What is important is to bear in mind that flow data can be derived from volume data. The average flow can be calculated if one knows only how much air was used in a certain amount of time, or the instantaneous flow can be derived if the volume at every point in time is available. Both measures have their uses.

If the flow rate can be computed from the volume change, it is reasonable to assume that the process might be reversible. Given a flow, one should be able to find the volume change. It is indeed possible although, in cases where the flow changes very rapidly, it may be difficult. Volume is the product of flow and time:

$$V = U \times t. \tag{6}$$

If a steady flow persists for a known interval of time, determination of the volume

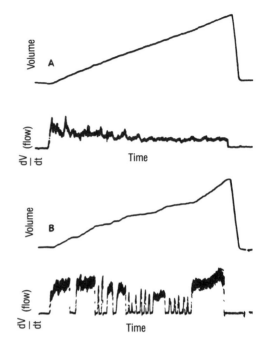

FIGURE 8–2. Same volume records as in Figure 8-1, but with the addition of a trace indicating the derivative of volume (that is, the *flow*) associated with each.

of air moved is simple and direct. For example, if a patient phonated for 10 s using a (remarkably steady) flow of 150 m L/ s, he must have used 150 mL × 10 s = 1500 mL = 1.5 L of air. A flow-versus-time graph of such rock-steady phonation is shown in Figure 8-3. This graphic representation illustrates an important fact. Multiplying flow by time gives the area enclosed by the flow trace. Volume, then, could be defined as the area under the line on a readout of flow data. Figure 8-4A demonstrates the obvious problem in applying this concept: How does one compute the actual area under this highly irregular line? Again, the calculus provides a way in the form of the *integral*. In the present discussion the *integral* can be described as the cumulative area under the flow curve. (The notation for the integral of the flow is ∫ V; the process is called *integration*.) Calculation of the integral can be very difficult. However, as was the case with the derivative, one need not

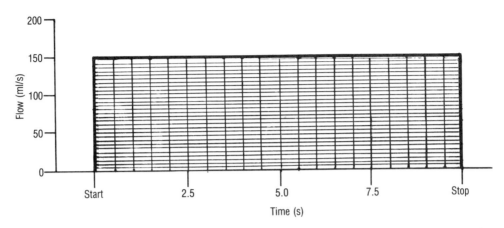

FIGURE 8–3. Graph of 10 s of phonation at an exceptionally constant flow of 150 mL/s. The air volume used is equal to flow x time, and is represented by the *area* under the flow line.

bother. There are simple and readily available electronic circuits that provide an output equal to the integral of the input. If supplied with an electrical signal representing flow, they produce an output representing the cumulative volume. Figure 8-4B shows the integral of flow resulting from the trace of Figure 8-4A. (A relatively simple do-it-yourself integrator circuit for use in speech work has been described by Hardy and Edmonds, 1968).

SUMMARY. Flow is the rate of change of volume. It is expressed as the *derivative* of volume. Volume is the product of flow and time. It is the *integral* of flow.

The foregoing discussion leads to the conclusion that flow and volume change are essentially two sides of the same coin and that instrumentation to measure one can often be used to determine the other. This is shown schematically in Figure 8-5, in which both flow and volume are derived from a single measurement device. The flow signal can be integrated to produce a volume output, or a volume signal can be differentiated to produce a flow signal.

In this chapter instruments are categorized as either volume- or flow-measuring systems according to their primary output.

But an integrator or differentiator can be added to that output to produce the complementary measure.

The Gas Laws

To a much greater extent than solids or liquids, the volume of a gas is affected by its pressure and temperature.* Increasing the pressure diminishes gas volume very significantly. (A small SCUBA tank of highly-compressed air can, therefore, contain enough gas to sustain a diver for a long time.) Conversely, increasing temperature causes a gas to expand. These effects are of more than academic interest when it comes to measuring speech or lung volumes. The air in the lungs during speech is pressurized and is at body temperature (about 37°C). However, in a collecting device such as a spirometer that same air is at close to atmospheric pressure (0 cmH$_2$O) and at room temperature (about 20°C). Therefore, the volume of the air in the spirometer is not the same as the volume the same air occupied when it was still in the respiratory system.

Fortunately, under ordinary circum-

---

*More complete discussions of the gas laws can be found in Peters (1969), Comroe, Forster, DuBois, Briscoe, and Carlsen (1962), or any elementary physics text.

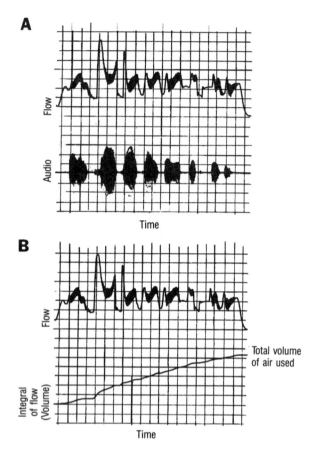

FIGURE 8–4. (A) Airflow during counting from one to seven. (B) The bottom trace shows the integral of the flow (that is, the expired *volume*).

stances pressure and temperature differences are not so large as to create a clinically meaningful difference in air volume. For everyday clinical purposes, then, they can probably be safely ignored, especially if the values result from the same testing procedure, applied under essentially the same conditions.

It is nonetheless wise to be aware of the principles that govern gas volumes, especially when comparing the results of different studies in the literature (in which correction factors may be used) or when designing clinical research studies. The most important "gas laws" that quantify volume changes are summarized below.

Pressure: Boyle's law

The effect of pressure on a gas is expressed by Boyle's law, which states that (if temperature does not change) the product of volume and pressure is constant. That is,

$$P_1V_1 = P_2V_2$$

where the subscript 1 denotes the original value, and 2 indicates the new quantity. Rearranging, the new volume of a gas after a change in pressure is

$$V_2 = V_1(P_1/P_2).$$

Put into words, Boyle's law says that the volume of a gas after a pressure change is

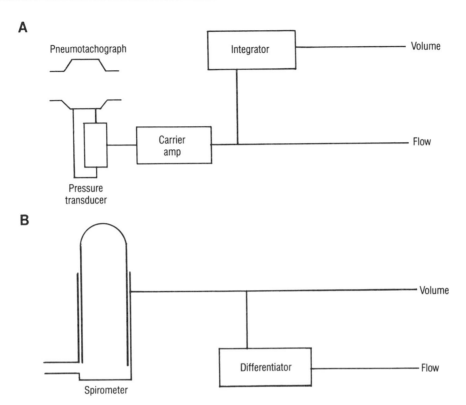

FIGURE 8–5. Alternative methods of deriving flow and volume from a single transducer: (A) By integration of the output of a flow transducer (e.g., a pneumotachograph); (B) by differentiation of the output of a volumetric device (such as a spirometer).

equal to its former volume times the ratio of the original and new pressures.

Temperature: Charles' law

Charles' law states that the volume of a gas varies directly with temperature (assuming that pressure remains constant). Therefore, volume change with temperature can be calculated as

$$V_2 = V_1(T_1/T_2)$$

where, as before, the subscripts denote original (1) and new (2) conditions. T, the temperature, must be expressed in absolute terms, as degrees *Kelvin* (°K). Zero degrees Kelvin equals $-273°C$.

Combined pressure and temperature

Obviously, Boyle's and Charle's laws can be combined to a single volume-cor-

rection equation. Simple algebraic manipulation gives

$$V_2 = V_1 (T_2/T_1) (P_1/P_2).$$

Water vapor

Each gas that makes up the mixture called air accounts for part of the air's total pressure. Dalton's law states that each gas makes an *independent* contribution to the total. Therefore, if one of the gases in the air mixture should be lost, the total pressure would diminish. The other gases would not "compensate" for the loss. As air cools after exhalation, part of the water vapor in the air condenses. This represents a loss of some of the pressure contribution made by the water vapor and, therefore, a change in the volume of the gas. Hence, another correction factor is needed. Unfortunately, the "partial pressure" of water at different temperatures is not easily calculated: It must be found in a table of partial pressures.

BTPS

From all the above, it becomes clear that different volume data can be compared with precision only if the temperature, pressure, and water-saturation conditions under which they were obtained are known. Rather than make the user of data perform the necessary calculations, it is common in the research literature to report volume data already converted to a set of standard conditions. These are body temperature, atmospheric pressure, and saturated with water vapor. The label *BTPS* is used to denote the fact that the volume being reported has been corrected to the standard conditions. BTPS values can be compared across test conditions, across subjects, or across research studies without further manipulation.

AIRFLOW

Instrumentation

Face masks

Evaluation of airflow requires that all of the air to be measured, and only the air to be measured, pass through the flow transducers. For evaluation of speech behavior it is important that the channeling of air be done in a way that does not alter articulatory performance.

In general these requirements are met by attaching the flow transducer to the outlet of an anestheia-type face mask, like the one shown in Figure 8-6. This solution is not ideal, however, and a number of precautions must be taken and some compromises accepted.

It is vitally important that the face mask not leak around the edges, allowing air to escape without passing through the transducer. Although cushioning around the mask's periphery helps minimize this prob-

lem, it is still necessary to use a substantial harness around the head to keep the edges of the mask tightly pressed against the face. Lubker and Moll (1965) found that this had definite effects on labial and mandibular motion, and it lowered the maximal rate of syllable production (but not so much that conversational speech rate was affected). Their subjects did not perceive a need to use greater effort for speech, but the possibility other speakers might perceive this need cannot be completely ignored.

The problem of contact with the articulators can be alleviated by using a very large mask that encloses the entire face (like a baseball catcher's mask) as described, for instance, by Klatt, Stevens, and Mead (1968). Alternatively, a "space helmet" type of arrangement could be used, thereby completely eliminating contact with the face. This type of solution exacerbates another difficulty of mask-type arrangements. Any air collector represents a volume added to the vocal tract that increases the ventilatory dead space through which the patient must breathe. Tidal breathing patterns will change to accommodate to this ventilatory situation. The volume of an adult-size mask is only about 150 mL when in place, but even that may be enough to cause noticeable ventilatory adaptation. While a small change in tidal breathing does not in itself have a meaningful impact on speech behavior, it is sometimes enough to frighten a patient sufficiently to cause his speech to be abnormal in some way. With very large face masks and helmet arrangements the degradation of ventilatory conditions may have a more deleterious effect on speech than the restriction of articulatory movement that they are designed to avoid (Hardy, 1965).

The dead space problem can be solved by providing a *bias airflow* (Hixon, 1972). That is, a pump can be used to force a constant and steady flow of fresh air into the mask at a known rate. The fresh air leaves the mask via the flow transducer together with the ventilatory airflow. The magnitude of the bias flow is then subtracted from the

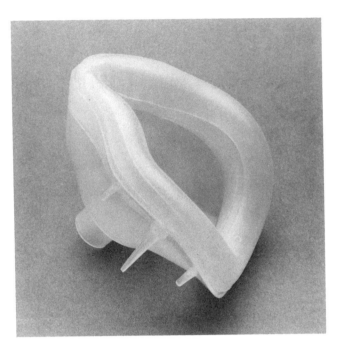

FIGURE 8–6. Anesthesia-type face mask. (Courtesy of Puritan-Bennett Corp., Overland Park, KS)

flow measurement, leaving a remainder that represents vocal tract flow alone. In most cases the use of an ordinary small face mask will be acceptable for clinical evaluation. But, despite its added complexity, the bias flow system is advantageous in those cases (for example, very young children, highly anxious or cerebral palsied patients) where a small, confining mask is poorly tolerated.

SEPARATING ORAL AND NASAL FLOW. The interior of the mask can be divided in order to channel oral and nasal flows through different outlets, to either or both of which a flow transducer can be connected. Lubker and Moll (1965) used a plexiglass diaphragm, edged with a bumper of ¼ inch rubber tubing, to divide the interior of a face mask into two chambers, each provided with an outlet port. Similar arrangements are described by Hixon (1966), Quigley, Webster, Coffey, Kelleher, and Grant (1963), Quigley, Shiere, Webster, and Cobb (1964), and Hixon, Saxman, and McQueen (1967).

Airflow Transducers

Many different means, ranging from pinwheel rotors to ultra-sonic detectors (Collatina, Barone, Monini, and Bolasco, 1980), can be used to transduce an airflow into an appropriate electrical signal. The various methods have been applied in a very wide variety of devices. Only a few, however, are suitable to the needs of speech clinicians. The discussion to follow, therefore, will be limited to the pneumotachograph, warm-wire anemometer, plethysmograph, and electro-aerometer.

Pneumotachograph

PHYSICAL PRINCIPLES AND CONSTRUCTION. Broadly speaking, a pneumotachograph (Figure 8-7) is any primary transducer that takes advantage of one of the airflow principles discussed earlier: A pressure drop occurs across any resistance introduced into an airstream. The pneumotachograph generates a pressure proportional to flow,

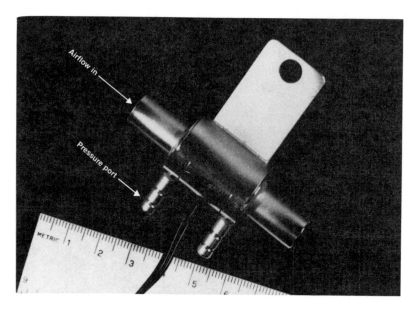

FIGURE 8–7. Fleisch pneumotachograph.

and this pressure must then be transduced (by a secondary transducer) to provide a proportional electrical signal. The pneumotachograph's resistance to airflow is created in one of two ways. Either a fine wire-mesh screen is used, or else the air is channeled through a series of narrow tubes. In the former case, the resistance is a function of the wire mesh—the more wires per square centimeter of screening, the higher the resistance. The tube-type system, called a Fleisch pneumotachograph, has an impedance (Z) whose magnitude is governed by Poiseuille's law,

$$Z = \frac{8\,\mu l}{\pi r^4}$$

where μ = gas viscosity
       l = tube length
       r = tube radius

Therefore, the longer the tubes and the smaller their radius, the greater the resistance to airflow. Irrespective of specific construction, however, all pneumotachographs have sensing ports on either side of the resistive element. Through these the pressure drop created by the resistance is sampled. This pressure difference is the output of the pneumotachograph.*

The magnitude of the pressure drop within the pneumotachograph is governed by the aerodynamic principles discussed earlier: $P = U \times Z$. For a given airflow, U, the pressure drop, P, can be increased (making the pneumotachograph more sensitive) by increasing the impedance, Z. But higher impedance disrupts breathing more. (Try breathing through a soda straw, which represents a very high impedance.) For minimal interference with normal ventilatory (including speech) behavior, the transducer should have negligible impedance. But this, in a pneumotachograph, means low sensitivity. One is trapped between two conflicting requirements. The nature of the dilemma indicates that a single transducer will not be suitable for a wide range of rates of flow and, therefore, pneumotachographs are offered in different "sizes." Those intended for measuring low flow rates have higher impedances than those designed for larger flows. When doing flow measurement it is important to select a unit

---

*The physics of pneumotachographs has been experimentally investigated by Fry, Hyatt, McCall, and Mallos (1957).

with enough impedance to get adequate measures, but not enough to interfere with the airflows being observed. Table 8-2 shows the characteristics of several sizes of pneumotachographs offered by OEM, a major distributor of Fleisch pneumotachographs. Under ordinary conditions of use the pneumotachograph will be much cooler than the expiratory flow through it, and, because air coming from the lungs is saturated with water vapor, condensation will occur within it. As water droplets form on the resistive element they tend to block the small openings, raising the impedance, playing havoc with the device's calibration. To prevent this a small current is passed through the resistive element; the resultant heating eliminates the condensation problem. (A heater-current supply can be purchased from the transducer manufacturer, but simple transformers providing 6.3 VAC and having a current capability of about 2 A serve quite nicely and are available at electronics supply stores.)

Despite the fact that it requires a face mask and imposes extra equipment requirements (i.e., a secondary pressure transducer, appropriate amplifier, and current for the heater), the pneumotachograph has several features that make it the instrument of choice for airflow evaluation (van den Berg, 1962; Hardy, 1967; Lubker, 1970). It is highly reliable and, because of its comparatively uncomplicated structure, relatively inexpensive. It is also rugged—virtually immune to mishandling—and easy to maintain. Its output is linear over the range for which it is designed, making it easy to calibrate, and it holds its calibration very well over time. It also differentiates between egressive and ingressive airflows, a feature not characteristic of all flow systems.

Variations on the Pneumotachograph Principle. The basic principle of the pneumotachograph (the imposition of a impedance to produce a measurable pressure drop proportional to flow) has been incorporated into a number of special face-mask designs that provide special advantages. Klatt, Stevens, and Mead (1968) have used a very large mask that encloses the entire face, minimizing articulatory loading. A wire screen in the front of the mask serves as the resistive element. The difference between the pressure inside the mask and atmospheric pressure is, therefore, proportional to flow. Rothenberg (1973, 1977) has constructed screen-vented face masks that, when used with special pressure sensors, provide excellent frequency response; so good, in fact, that the individual glottal pulses are essentially undistorted. (His articles also present an excellent discussion of the theoretical bases of flow measurement with this kind of system.)

IMPLEMENTATION. A block diagram of a typical pneumotachograph system is shown in Figure 8-8. A mask is fitted snugly to the patient's face with the pneumotachograph attached to its outlet. It is important that the mask not leak; this should be checked carefully. If the mask outlet is closed off, the patient should be able to blow quite forcefully, generating a large positive pressure inside the mask, before air leakage occurs. The pneumotachograph's output is the pressure drop across its resistive element. This is sensed by attaching a *differential* pressure transducer (see Chap. 7) to its pressure ports by means of rubber or plastic tubing. The transducer's output is

TABLE 8–2. Characteristics of Typical Fleisch Pneumotachographs

Transducer Size	Useful Maximum Flow (L/s)	Resistance (cm H$_2$O/L/s)	Dead Space (mL)
0000	0.02	75	1.7
000	0.05	30	1.7
00*	0.10	15	1.7
0*	0.30	5	4.7
1*	1.00	1.5	15.
2	3.00	0.5	40.
3	6.00	0.25	92.
4	14.00	0.11	200.

Data are for transducers by OEM, Inc.
*Units most useful for speech work.

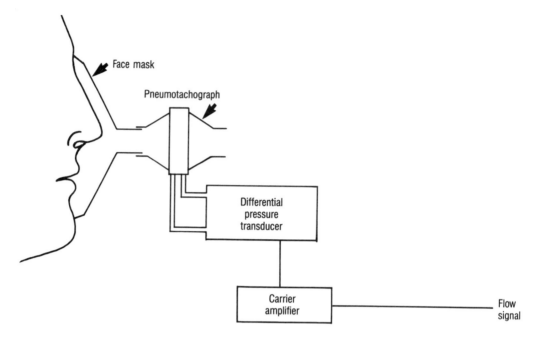

FIGURE 8–8. Block diagram of a typical pneumotachograph system.

the electrical analog of airflow. Because the impedance of the pneumotachograph must be kept low, the pressure difference to be measured will be quite small, probably far less than 1 cmH$_2$O. The pressure transducer must, therefore, be as sensitive as possible. The pneumotachograph's heater current is turned on, and the device allowed to warm up before use.

Warm-wire anemometer

PHYSICAL BASES AND CONSTRUCTION. The electrical resistance of any material changes in known ways with termperature. This fact is the basis for measurement of airflow by the warm-wire anemometer. When a ventilatory or speech airflow passes over it, an electrically heated wire will be cooled significantly. The consequent change of the wire's resistance can be measured; it serves as an index of the magnitude of the flow.

There are a number of different ways in which this basic principle is actually exploited. In the simplest case (diagrammed in Figure 8-9A) a constant current is passed through a wire having a relatively high resistance. Doing this causes the wire to dissipate power as heat. (Power in watts is equal to the resistance times the square of the current.) The temperature of the wire therefore rises. Ohm's Law (see Chap. 7) states that $E = IR$. That is, if current, I, passes through a resistance, R, a voltage difference, E, is produced across the resistance. If the current is constant, then any change in the resistance will show up as an equivalent change in the voltage difference. The resistance of the wire changes with temperature, and the temperature of a heated wire will change with alterations in the amount of air flowing past it. The reason for the latter effect is simple enough. Any flow of air past the wire carries heat away with it, thereby lowering the wire's temperature. The greater the airflow, the faster heat is lost, and the cooler the wire becomes. So the resistance of the wire should mirror the airflow. The resistance, in turn, can be tracked by monitoring the voltage drop across the wire.

There are a number of important problems with this simple system. Most signif-

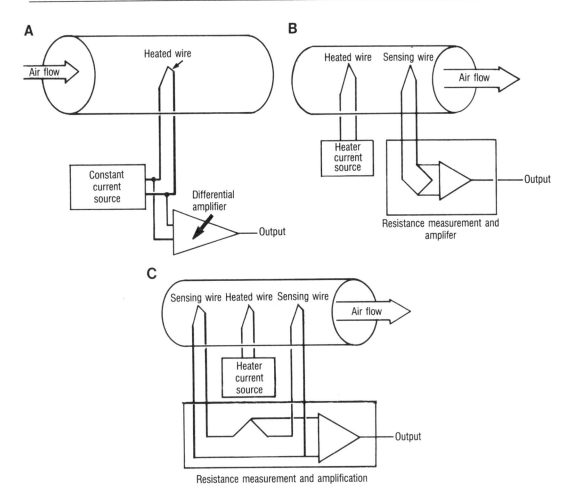

FIGURE 8–9. (A) A simple warm-wire anemometer. The sensing wire is heated by a constant current. The voltage drop across it is proportional to its resistance, which is in turn related to its temperature. The differential amplifier senses the voltage drop, and its output, therefore, indicates the flow rate. (B) Two-wire anemometer system. (C) Directionally sensitive warm-wire anemometer. Heat is transferred from the central heated element to one or the other of the sensing wires, depending on the direction of air flow. The resulting changes in resistance are sensed and are converted to an analog voltage representing the magnitude and direction of airflow.

icant is its nonlinearity. For a number of reasons the voltage drop changes in an irregular way as the flow changes. Either complex calibrating scales or, when possible, special electronic linearizing circuits are required. Beyond this is the fact that egressive air (essentially at body temperature) is considerably warmer than ingressive air (at room temperature) and, therefore, cools the wire less for the same rate of flow. Transducer sensitivity, in other words, differs with flow direction.

The latter problem has been addressed by Quigley, Shiere, Webster, and Cobb (1964) in a way diagrammed in Figure 8-9B. In this system two wire filaments are used. One is unheated and senses any change in temperature of the passing air. A special electronic circuit provides just enough current to heat the other filament to an absolute temperature of about 120% of the unheated reference wire. The greater the airflow the faster the heated wire cools, and thus more current is required to keep it heated to the proper level. The magnitude of the heater current is an analog of airflow, irrespective of the temperature of the flowing air. This transduction scheme represents an improvement over the single heated wire, but it does not provide for discrimination of the direction of airflow. This is not a trivial problem, since small ingressive flows occur during speech articulation (Isshiki and Ringel, 1964; Lubker and Moll, 1965) and their detection is all but impossible in the absence of flow direction sensitivity.

It is possible, with relatively simple electronic circuitry, to use two heated wires to detect only the direction of airflow, without determining its magnitude (Micco, 1973). But, on the whole, it would obviously be better to determine magnitude and direction from a single instrument. A hot-wire flow meter that can achieve this has been created by Yoshiya, Nakajima, Nagai, and Jitsukawa (1975). It is schematized in Figure 8-9C. A platinum wire within the transducer is maintained at a temperature of about 375°C. A short distance away, in front of and behind this heated element, are two other unheated sensing wires. Air flowing through the transducer passes over all three wire elements in series. In the absence of any airflow, the heated wire warms its vicinity and the two sensing wires are at the same temperature. As air flows, however, the upstream wire is cooled somewhat, and the air is then heated by the hot wire before passing to the second sensing element, whose temperature it raises. An airflow thus produces a significant temperature (and hence resistance) difference between the two sensing elements. The resistance change is monitoried by appropriate circuitry that produces the final analog output voltage. If the direction of the airstream changes, the resistance difference between the two sensing wires reverses, and the polarity of the voltage output switches.

Despite the ingenious steps taken to minimize their deficiencies, warm-wire anemometers exhibit a number of limitations that remain significant (see Hardy, 1967; van den Berg, 1962; and Lubker, 1970). Because they all depend on relatively slow temperature change, their frequency response is limited. Rapid changes of flow are likely to be distorted in the output, and very brief events might not appear at all. Some modern anemometers, however, have response characteristics that can be considered adequate if visualization of laryngeal chopping of the airstream is not required (Hardy, 1965). A careful check of specifications is, therefore, desirable before any purchase. As mentioned above, the relationship between airflow and wire resistance is by no means linear. While special electronics can handle this difficulty to some extent, it is generally necessary to generate special calibration tables for each transducer. This is a tedious and inconvenient process at best, and it may seriously inhibit collection of adequate data (van Hattum and Worth, 1967).

Finally, there remains a problem that is somewhat more subtle than those just reviewed, but potentially of great impact. The warm-wire system is really only sensitive to flow in the immediate vicinity of the sensing element. Since the wire itself occupies only a small fraction of the cross-sectional area of the tube, the transducer actually dtermines the flow of that small sample of the total stream that happens to pass near its sensing element. This sample is valid only to the extent that the flow is laminar. As turbulence increases, random eddy currents and local flow variations increase, making it more likely that the wire will be influenced by them. The result may be a measurement that represents the significant perturbations of a limited region within the airstream, rather than the more stable average magnitude of the entire flow. Laminar flow cannot be guaranteed under all circumstance and, unfortunately, there is no easy way to determine the extent to which turbulence may have confounded the system output.

IMPLEMENTATION. The warm-wire ane-mometer, witn its associated electronics, represents a complete transducer. No secondary transducer is required, as with the pneumotachograph. Attempts have been made (Subtelny et al., 1966, 1969) to place an array of anemometer wires in front of the mouth in order to eliminate the need for a face mask. The resulting measures, however, have very dubious validity, and so it is best to use one of the air-collecting systems described earlier.

While the warm-wire anemometer offers the advantage of a relatively simple setup compared to other flow-measuring systems, its problems and limitations outweigh this one benefit. Consequently, most clinicians, given a choice, will prefer an alternative method for evaluating airflow.

Body plethysmograph

The body plethysmograph, described by Mead (1960) can be modified to measure airflow (Hixon, 1972; Warren, 1976). This may be accomplished in two ways, illustrated in Figure 8-10.

In the first method (Figure 8-10A) the patient's body is enclosed within the plethysmograph. A special collar forms an airtight seal around the neck. During inspiration and expiration the volume of the body increases and decreases, compressing and rarefying the air within the box. The pressure change causes air to flow through a screen in the wall of the box that serves as a resistance. The screen, therefore, functions like the resistive element of a pneumotachograph, so the pressure difference across it is proportional to the flow of air in or out of the lungs. In this case, of course, a differential pressure transducer is not needed, since it is *gauge pressure* that is being measured (see introduction to Chap. 7). It should be clear that inspiration causes air to flow out of the plethysmograph (as the lungs enlarge, taking up more space in the box), while expiration results in an airflow into the box. In this sense the transducer

flow is an *inverse* of the lung volume change.

What the plethysmograph actually measures is change in lung volume. Strictly speaking, this is not the same as flow. The reason is that the lung volume is altered by two effects. First, air is moved in or out of the ventilatory system: *This* is the phenomenon of interest. But the lung volume also changes as a function of changes in alveolar pressure, and this also contributes to the flow across the plethysmograph's resistive element.* The two components of the transducer output signal—lung volume change and alveolar pressure change—cannot be separated with the arrangement shown in Figure 8-10A, but the magnitude of the error is small and can be ignored for most clinical purposes. (Hixon [1972] describes a more elaborate plethysmographic arrangement that provides for separate measures of transglottal flow and alveolar pressure.)

Figure 8-10B shows how a plethysmograph can be used to measure flow alone. The box itself remains open, but the patient's head is enclosed in the plethysmograph dome. The collar is again used to form an airtight seal around the neck. As is the case when the body box is used, a screen (this time in the dome) serves as the resistance across which a pressure proportional to the flow is measured. This method actually uses the plethysmograph as a rather special modification of a face-mask and pneumotachograph system. In essence, the patient is placed inside the flow transducer. While one would not want to purchase a plethysmograph in order to be able to implement this technique, it is a good method to use if a plethysmograph is on hand.

Electro-aerometer

The electro-aerometer (Smith, 1960; van den Berg, 1962) represents a very different

---

*This phenomenon is discussed more fully under "Subglottal pressure" in Chap. 7.

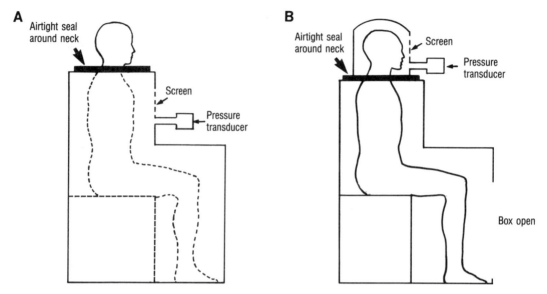

FIGURE 8–10. Using the body plethysmograph for flow measurement. (A) The flow signal from the body portion of the box represents airflow *and* intrathoracic pressure changes. (B) Measuring pressure from the dome eliminates the influence of lung pressure.

approach to the transduction of air flow. The primary transducer is a rubber flap valve through which the airstream must pass. The valve has a resistance of between 1.25 and 3.0 $cmH_2O/L/s$ that produces a pressure drop in the air flowing through it. This pressure causes the valve's two rubber flaps to separate. A light beam is directed through the valve to be sensed by a photodiode (the secondary transducer). The amount of light transmitted is proportional to the area of the valve opening, which is in turn proportional to the pressure drop and, therefore, to the airflow. The output of the photodiode is an analog of flow rate. Each flap valve is a one-way device: One is required for ingressive, and another for egressive, air.

In the commercial version of this instrument the valves are mounted as part of the face-mask assembly. Manufacturer's specifications indicate a range of 0-1600 mL/s (with linearity best in the 0-1000 mL/s range) and a frequency response of DC to 200 Hz. Systems can be configured to measure oral and nasal airflow simultaneously. There are not yet enough reports on this instrument to evaluate its performance in routine use.

Summary of flow transducers

The various flow transducers discussed in this section are compared in Table 8-3.

Calibration of Flow Systems

Flow measuring systems are calibrated by observing the system output when airflows of precisely known magnitude are passed through the transducer. Calibration requires a source of compressed air and a precision metering device to monitor the flow rate.

Rotameter (flow meter)

Metering of airflow is most easily done with a *rotameter* also known as a *flow meter*). This simple, reliable, and relatively inexpensive device works on a variable-area principle. As indicated in Figure 8-11, the rotameter consists of a glass tube, a small and precisely machined ball, and a

TABLE 8–3. Summary of Flow Transducers

Transducer	Additional Equipment Required	Frequency Response	Linearity	Notes
Pneumo-tachograph	Differential pressure transducer system Heater current supply	Good	Excellent	Preferred method; stable, reliable rugged
Warm-wire anemometer	None. Complete system.	Poor	Very poor	Usually insensitive to direction of flow
Plethysmo-graph	Pressure transducer system	Good	Good-to-Excellent	Large, expensive, but useful for other measures
Electro-aerometer	None. Complete system.	Moderate	Fair	Relatively recent arrival

measurement scale. The tube widens uniformly from bottom to top, while the ball within it has a diameter very nearly identical to the inner diameter of the tube's lower end. When a stream of air is introduced into the inlet, the ball (resting at the bottom) presents a very high resistance to the flow (since it effectively blocks the passage completely). A relatively high pressure develops beneath it, forcing the ball upward. Since the tube grows wider from bottom to top, there is an ever-growing gap between the ball (known as the *float*) and the tube walls as the ball rises. Air can, therefore, escape more easily around the ball as it rises. In other words, as the ball moves upward it represents a constantly smaller resistance, so the pressure under it will fall to a point that is just sufficient to keep it suspended in the airstream. Clearly, the height at which this happens is directly related to the flow rate, and thus the height of the ball can be read from the rotameter scale as a flow rate value.

The sensitivity and range of the rotameter depend on the material of which the float is made (less dense materials yield greater sensitivity) and the taper of the tube (greater tapers provide extended ranges). Manufacturers offer rotameters of many sensitivities, and the clinician should select one appropriate to the sensitivity of the transducers to be calibrated. It should have

a range that is not too wide (smaller ranges generally provide more accurate readings) and that is centered on a value within the range of actual airflows that will be measured in practice.

Compressed air source

Accurate calibration demands that the calibrating airstream be free of observable fluctuations and that it not change slowly during the calibration period. The best source of an airstream is a large tank of compressed air (a SCUBA tank is sufficient). Gases other than air can be used, but inaccuracy will be introduced into the calibration to the extent that the density of the gas differs from that of air. Obviously, flammable gases should never be used, nor should oxygen, which also presents a fire hazard. The tank of compressed air should be fitted with a regulator so that the flow can be controlled. A good quality air compressor can be used to provide an airstream, but it must be fitted with a filter if there is any danger of it spraying oil, which will gum up the rotameter and the transducer.

A vacuum cleaner can serve as the compressor if it has an air-outlet connection, as many tank-types do. A filter of lightly-packed glass wool should be placed in the hose line between the vacuum cleaner and the transducer, and a valve should be added

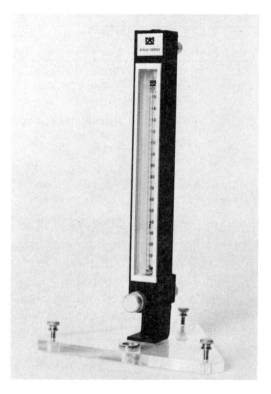

FIGURE 8–11. The rotameter consists of a tapered glass tube with a spherical float. Airflow from the bottom to top causes the float to rise to a level proportional to the flow rate. (Courtesy of Matheson Gas Products, Secaucus, NJ)

to the line to control airflow. The vacuum side of the vacuum cleaner can also be used as a "negative" airflow for calibration if the connections to the rotatmeter are reversed. That is, the vacuum line should be connected to what is normally the rotameter's output connection, while the transducer, through which the air will pass before going to the rotameter, is connected to the inlet connection.

Calibration method

Figure 8-12 shows how a calibrating setup is arranged. The rotameter and flow transducer are connected in series, the airstream passing first through one and then the other. The airflow is adjusted at the tank to some convenient value, and the voltage

output of the transducer system is noted. Airflow is then changed to a new value, and a new reading of the output is taken. This process is repeated at several different flow rates over the range of the system, generating a table of correspondence between flow and transducer output. If the transduction system is a highly stable one (such as a pneumotachograph) this calibration need be done only occasionally. It must, of course, be repeated whenever any system characteristic or component is changed.

It is exceptionally difficult to measure the frequency response of an airflow system, and for this reason the adequacy of the response is best estimated by evaluating the quality of the system output when measures are done on a normal speaker. (Examples of such records are provided for several of the measurements discussed below.) Alternatively, good approximations of a "step function" (or very sudden change) in airflow through the system can be achieved by attaching a balloon to the outlet of the flow transducer and blowing it up by coupling a relatively high-pressure air supply to the inlet. After the balloon has achieved maximal size it is punctured, causing a sudden onset of airflow through the transducer. The readout of the flow reveals how quickly the system responds to a dramatic and almost instantaneous change.

AIR FLOW MEASUREMENTS

If driving pressure is adequate and constant, then airflow measurements reflect on the integrity of the vocal tract. Increased flow must indicate a more dilated constriction and reduced airway resistance since, as pointed out earlier, air-path diameter and air-path impedance are inversely proportional to each other. The record of a dynamic airflow also indicates the time relationship of impedance changes, an important consideration in many speech disorders.

Broadly speaking, there are three categories of airflow that are of maximal interest

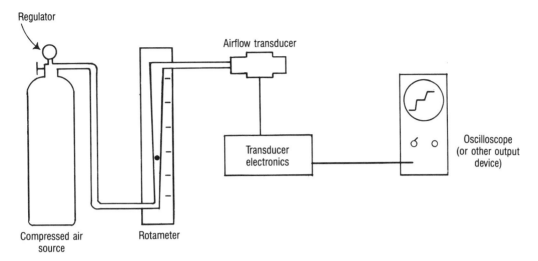

FIGURE 8–12. Set-up for calibration of a flow measurement system.

to the speech pathologist: (1) flow associated with consonants; (2) airflow during sustained phonation; and (3) nasal airflow. The first evaluates oral articulatory events, while the second is an indicator of the functional efficiency of the laryngeal system. Nasal flow is primarily of use in assessing velopharyngeal function and is, therefore, discussed in Chapter 10, which deals with those issues.

Consonants: Mean Peak Airflow

Technique

Most frequently this measurement is obtained using test syllables of the CV or VC type, perhaps in a carrier phrase. The variable of interest is the *maximum flow* observed during the consonant (or vowel) being examined. Multiple repetitions are gathered, and the mean and standard deviation of the flow maxima are computed. High variability (large standard deviation) is as significant a finding as an abnormal mean.

Measurement requires a face mask or other air-collecting arrangement and a flow transducer with appropriate support electronics. If significant nasal escape of air is likely, it is best to use a modified face mask to collect only oral airflow, unless the total vocal tract flow is of interest. Nasal consonants, of course, will show predominantly nasal air emission.

Peak airflow varies as a function of speech intensity. It is, therefore, of some importance that speech itensity be controlled during testing. Although Brown, Murry, and Hughes (1976) suggested that visual feedback to the patient (via a VU meter, for example) should be used to minimize intensity variations, recent research by Stathopoulos (1985) has shown that simply instructing the subject to maintain a comfortable speech loudness is just as effective in controlling vocal variability.

Expected results

OUTPUT RECORD. Flow traces obtained with a pneumotachograph during production of /saɪ saɪ/ and /aɪs aɪs/ are shown in Figure 8-13. During the vocalic portion of each syllable the expiratory airflow is "chopped" by the action of the vocal folds; this is reflected in the flow trace whenever there is voicing. Flow shows a clear peak during /s/. In the present instance it is the height of this peak that is measured.

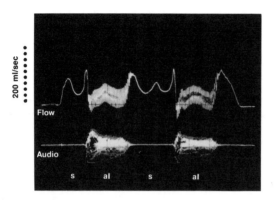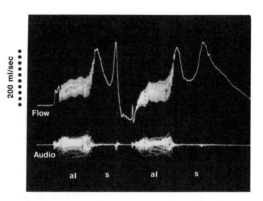

FIGURE 8–13. Flow records: (A) /saɪ/ and (B) /aɪs/. The dotted lines to the right of the flow traces indicate 0.2 L/s.

Evaluation of peak airflow requires that the frequency response of the instrumentation system be adequate. Figure 8-14 demonstrates quite clearly how the airflow peaks are flattened when this requirement is not met. Note also how the pulsatile character of voicing disappears from the trace as the frequency response falls off. This is a sure sign of inadequacy.

TYPICAL VALUES.   Table 8-4 gives typical adult values for peak airflow and Tables 8-5 through 8-7 demonstrate how these values may be expected to change with varying conditions.

Data for children are very sparse. Trullinger and Emanuel (1983) have shown that peak airflows for the six English plosives tend to increase across the 8- to 10-year-old range they studied. Further, their findings show that peak airflows of the children's productions of the several plosives follow essentially the same rank order as adult plosive productions. As with adults, higher airflows are associated with the children's voiceless plosives.

Continuous Speech

Technique

While observation of airflow for isolated phonemes provides valuable informa-

tion about specific articulatory acts, it is very often desirable to obtain airflow records for running speech. During ongoing utterances, cognition, coarticulation, syntactic and semantic planning, and suprasegmental organization all conspire to make speech more difficult to control and more likely to show breakdown. It is possible to construct stimuli that will facilitate evaluation of specific aspects of speech performance. For example, sentences can be loaded with voiced phonemes, with high-impedance sounds, and the like. It may also be useful to compare the aerodynamic characteristics of a phoneme when spoken in an isolated syllable to those of the same phoneme produced in the context of a longer utterance.

The average airflow over the duration of a relatively long spoken passage might also be of use to the clinician—particularly for establishing a baseline against which the effect of therapy can be judged. From the data presented in the preceding tables it is clear that the mean flow will be strongly influenced by the content of the spoken material. To assure comparability of trials, most clinicians will wish to select some piece of prose to use as a standard. Over the years the Rainbow Passage (Fairbanks, 1960) has generally come to fill this need. Its full text, together with a partial analysis of its content, is given in Appendix C.

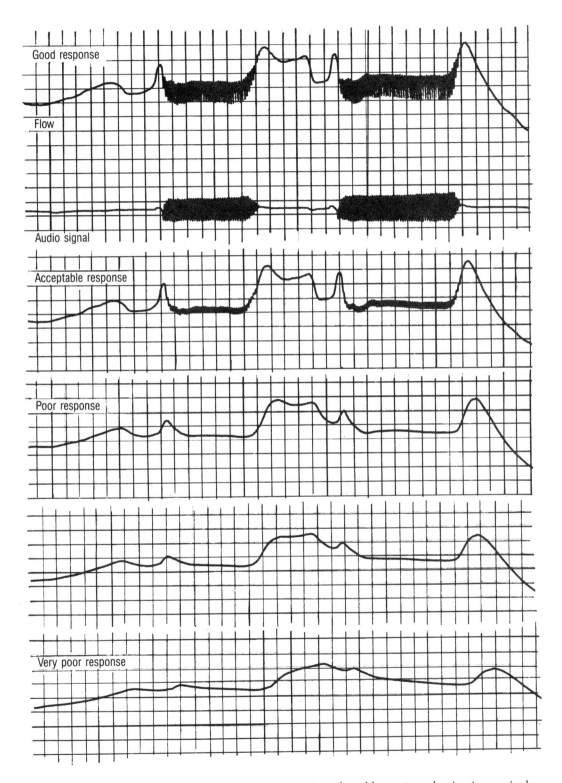

FIGURE 8–14. Flow records of the same utterance as transduced by systems having increasingly limited high-frequency response. (All of the traces are aligned in time.)

TABLE 8–4. Peak Airflow*

Phoneme	Flow (L/s) CV Syllables Mean	CV Syllables S.D.	VC Syllables Mean	VC Syllables S.D.
p —	0.933	0.065	1.019	0.057
— b	0.472	0.159	0.675	0.229
t —	0.968	0.136	0.821	0.157
— d	0.410	0.147	0.481	0.259
k —	0.940	0.159	0.882	0.226
— g	0.372	0.103	0.455	0.263
f —	0.352	0.073	0.525	0.113
— v	0.095	0.059	0.338	0.108
θ —	0.652	0.194	0.869	0.230
— ð	0.126	0.077	0.365	0.124
s —	0.466	0.053	0.455	0.254
— z	0.159	0.050	0.231	0.073
ʃ —	0.583	0.128	0.479	0.108
— ʒ	0.249	0.039	0.303	0.119
tʃ —	0.881	0.106	0.583	0.183
— dʒ	0.525	0.119	0.424	0.101
— m	0.168	0.080	0.287	0.145
— n	0.155	0.064	0.244	0.113
— l	0.133	0.072	0.213	0.108
— r	0.143	0.047	0.132	0.084

From Isshiki, N. and Ringel, R. Air flow during the production of selected consonants. *Journal of Speech and Hearing Research*, 7 (1964) 233–244. Table 1, p. 235. ©American Speech-Language-Hearing Association, Rockville, MD. Reprinted by permission.

*Four male and four female normal adults; "Normal vocal effort"; pitch and loudness uncontrolled. Single production of each syllable. Pneumotachograph system.

Expected results

Patient performance may be compared with the data in Table 8-8, which were compiled using a special computer program (Horii and Cooke, 1975).

If the flow associated with any particular phoneme in the passage is not of interest, the average flow during reading can be easily determined with a spirometer. A face mask is used to collect the expired air, but the connection to the spirometer is through a special valve (available from suppliers of pulmonary testing equipment). This device will pass expired air to the spirometer but will permit the patient to inhale room air, insuring that the spirometer volume is not reduced by inspiration. It is also possible to integrate the expiratory signals from a flow transduction system over the entire duration of the reading. In either case, the total expiratory volume divided by the expiratory time is the mean flow. Gross irregularities of flow will show as changes in the spirometer or integrator output record.

SUMMARY OF INFLUENCES ON CONSONANT AIRFLOW. Table 8-9 summarizes the ways in which airflow changes as a function of different speech phenomena.

Sustained Phonation

During production of a vowel the upper airway resistance is very small compared

TABLE 8–5. Peak Air Flow for Plosives: Effect of Position in Syllable*

Plosive	Mean Peak Oral Airflow (L/s)* Prevocalic Mean	Prevocalic S.D.	Intervocalic Mean	Intervocalic S.D.	Postvocalic Mean	Postvocalic S.D.
p	1.529	0.401	1.266	0.464	1.293	0.498
b	0.682	0.248	0.574	0.203	0.535	0.232
t	1.789	0.391	1.429	0.469	1.259	0.484
d	0.973	0.248	0.738	0.224	0.602	0.226
k	1.534	0.396	1.240	0.448	1.018	0.395
g	0.650	0.240	0.523	0.209	0.528	0.192

From Gilbert, H. R. Oral airflow during stop consonant production. *Folia Phoniatrica*, 25 (1973) 288–301. Table 1, p. 295. Reprinted by permission.

*Nine adult males; three repetitions each of /CʌC/ or /ʌCʌ/ syllables; pneumotachograph system.

**Converted from L/min. Significant differences were the following: voiced-voiceless; prevocalic-postvocalic (except /g/); prevocalic-intervocalic (except /g,b/); intervocalic-postvocalic (/t,d/ only).

TABLE 8-6. Relationship of Peak Oral Airflows of Voiced and Voiceless Plosives*

Syllable type	Plosives	Ratios of Mean Peak Airflows: Voiced/Voiceless			
		V = /i/		V = /a/	
		Male	Female	Male	Female
CV	d/t	.42	.41	.45	.30
	b/p	.40	.31	.38	.26
	g/k	.46	.38	.36	.28
VCV	d/t	.48	.37	.49	.26
	b/p	.37	.28	.41	.28
	g/k	.53	.45	.32	.26

From Emanuel, F. W. and Counihan, D. T. Some characteristics of oral and nasal air flow during plosive consonant production. *Cleft Palate Journal*, 7 (1970) 249-260. Tables 1 and 2, pp. 252-253. Reprinted by permission.

*Twenty-five male and twenty-five female adults, age 20-36 years; CV and VCV syllables, V = /i,a/; conversational loudness, comfortable pitch; split (oral and nasal) face mask, oral measures only; and warm-wire anemometer.

TABLE 8-7. Mean Peak Air Flow: Effect of Effort Level

Phoneme	Effort Level (L/s)*††		
	Conversational	Substantially Greater	Much Greater
ʃ	0.287	0.364	0.425
s	0.196	0.250	0.287

From Hixon, T. Turbulent noise sources for speech. *Folia Phoniatrica*, 18 (1966) 168-182. Reprinted by permission.

*Nine male adults; 10 repetitions each of /s/ and /ʃ/: (1 syllable/s— at each effort level. Split face mask (oral and nasal), oral measures only. Pneumotachograph system.

**Converted from L/min.

†All airflow differences for /ʃ/ are significant; for /s/ only the difference between the smallest and largest value is significant.

††The tendency for airflow rate to increase with effort level was consistent for all but one of the speakers.

to the resistance of the glottis. Since (other things being equal) airflow is a reflection of resistance, measuring it during sustained phonation of a vowel should provide insight into glottal function. In fact, a number of investigations have confirmed that this is indeed the case. There are even some data (Kelman et al., 1975) indicating that certain dysphonic patients will demonstrate abnormal airflow even during quiet nonspeech breathing.

The relationship among vocal fundamental frequency, intensity, and airflow rate is extremely complex. It would appear (Isshiki, 1964) that at low vocal pitches changes in the resistance of the glottis are used to regulate vocal intensity. Increases in subglottal pressure result in greater sound pressure but not necessarily in greater flow. At higher vocal frequency, however, flow does increase with increasing subglottal pressure and vocal intensity. It is important to note, however, that different speakers use different regulatory techniques (Isshiki, 1965). These findings are confirmed by the work of Yanagihara and Koike (1967) and Cavagna and Margaria (1965, 1968) whose reports also provide a lucid discussion of the complexities of the relationships involved.

Given the variability that characterizes the data, caution should be exercised in

TABLE 8-8. Average Airflow during Reading: Rainbow Passage (L/s)*

Sex	Expiratory			Inspiratory		
	Mean	S.D.	Range of Means	Mean	S.D.	Range of Means
Males	0.177	0.053	.142-.218	1.109	0.257	1.046-1.234
Female	01.59	0.020	.152-.170	1.105	0.175	0.963-1.194
Overall	0.168	0.023	.142-.218	1.107	0.086	0.963-1.234

*Four male and four female "young adults." Single reading of Rainbow Passage. Comfortable intensity. Face mask/pneumotachograph. Flow sampled and averaged by a special computer program.

Composite data derived from Horii and Cooke, 1978.

TABLE 8–9. Summary of Factors Affecting Consonant Airflow

Contract		
Greater Flow For	**Lesser Flow For**	**According to**
Stops	Fricatives	Isshiki & Ringel, 1964
Fricataves	"Vowel-like sounds"	Isshiki & Ringel, 1964
Voiceless phones	Voiced cognates	Isshiki & Ringel, 1964; Gilbert, 1973; Scully, 1971
Prevocalic*	Postvocalic	Gilbert, 1973
Prevocalic	Intervocalic	Gilbert, 1973
High effort level	Low effort level	Hixon, 1966
Adults	Children (under age 13)	Stathopoulos and Weismer, 1985
Adult males	Adult females	Stathopoulos and Weismer, 1985
No effect		
Word stress		Brown and
Syllable repetition rate		McGlone, 1974 Hixon, 1966

This summary presents general trends. See specific data tables.

*Postvocalic variability is higher than prevocalic variability.

drawing conclusions about normality of airflow across widely different vocal fundamental frequencies or intensities. A standard set of conditions for routine clinical assessment that meet the clinician's particular needs and clinical style should be consistently followed. (Dejonckere, Greindl, and Sneppe (1985) provide an example.) The data summarized below, however, can serve as basic guidelines for clinical interpretation of the results of controlled testing under comparable conditions.

Expected results

MODAL REGISTER. Koike and Hirano (1968) examined airflow rate in 21 male and 21 female adults as they sustained the vowel /ɑ/ for as long as possible at constant pitch and loudness. Three trials were done by each subject; all trials were used as data.

TABLE 8–10A. Mean Airflow During Sustained Phonation in Normal Adults

Group*	Mean Flow (mL/s)	
	Mean	**S.D.**
Male	112.4	36.2
Female	93.7	31.6

From Koike, Y. and Hirano, M. Significance of the vocal velocity index. *Folia Phoniatrica*, 20 (1968)285-296. Table I, p. 289. Reprinted by permission.

*Difference between groups is significant. For method, see text.

Mean airflow was derived by dividing the total air volume used by the duration of phonation. The results are summarized in Table 8-10A. A similar study by Yanagihara, Koike, and von Leden (1966) produced comparable results. Using similar methods Beckett, Thoelke, and Cowan (1971) derived the mean flow rates for children shown in Table 8-10B.

Relationship of Modal-Register Airflow to Vital Capacity: The Vocal Velocity Index. The difference between mean flow rates of men and women was hypothesized by Koike and Hirano (1968) to be related to the well-documented gender difference in vital capacity. They devised a measure to correct for this possible source of bias. Their *vocal velocity index* is defined as the "ratio of mean air flow [during sustained phonation of /ɑ/] to vital capacity in *pro mille*" (p. 287). That is, the measure is derived by dividing the mean flow in milliliters by the vital capacity expressed in liters. Values of the vocal velocity index (for the same experiment summarized in Table 8-10) are given in Table 8-11. The authors established a 95% confidence interval for these data. Vocal velocity index values greater than 44 or less than 14.3 should be considered abnormal.

Relationship to Frequency and Intensity. As pointed out above, airflow does not change in a consistent way as vocal fundamental frequency and intensity are altered. The

TABLE 8–10B. Mean Flow Rate During Sustained /ɑ/ in Seven-Year-Old Children*

Sex	Age (yr)	Height (cm)	Flow Rate (mL/s) Mean	Flow Rate (mL/s) Range
Boys				
Mean†	7.55	126.2	95.9	51.4–127.6
S.D.	0.23	4.4	23.8	
Girls				
Mean†	7.56	124.1	71.6	45.6–115.4
S.D.	0.25	4.4	20.7	

From Beckett, R. Thoelke, W., and Cowan, L. A normative study of airflow in children. *British Journal of Disorders of Communication*, 6 (1971) 13-16. Table I, p. 14. Reprinted by permission of the College of Speech Therapists, Harold Poster House, 6 Lechmere Rd., London NW25BU, England.

*Ten boys and ten girls; maximally sustained /ɑ/ spirometer measurement.

†Calculated from authors' data. Data differences between boys and girls are not significant.

TABLE 8–11. Vocal Velocity Index*

Group	Vocal Velocity Index Mean	Vocal Velocity Index SD
Male	23.5	7.45
Female	26.7	8.18
Combined	25.1	7.95

From Koike, Y. and Hirano, M. Significance of vocal velocity index. *Folia Phoniatrica*, 20 (1968) 285–296. Table III, p. 292. Reprinted by permission.

*Twenty-one male and 21 female adults; sustained phonation of /ɑ/ at comfortable pitch and loudness.

TABLE 8–12. Relationship of Airflow to Vocal Frequency and Intensity*

Intensity Level	Flow† (mL/s) Vocal Fundamental Frequency 98 Hz ("low")	Flow† (mL/s) Vocal Fundamental Frequency 196 Hz ("medium")	Flow† (mL/s) Vocal Fundamental Frequency 392 Hz ("high")
"Soft" (mean 70 dB)**	113	66	88
"Loud" (mean 82 dB)**	135	151	299

From Isshiki, N. Vocal intensity and air flow rate. *Folia Phoniatrica*, 17 (1965) 92–104. Table I, p. 95. Reprinted by permission.

*Eleven male and 11 female adults, *most with training in singing*. Phonation at 98, 196, and 392 Hz (musical G_3, G_4, and G_5); two trials each; pneumotachograph.

†Mean of the data for the two trials.

**Re: 0.0002 d/cm².

data in Tables 8-12 and 8-13 should be viewed as guidelines, not as norms. Brown and McGlone (1974) have also shown that airflow values and vocal intensity are strongly correlated.

PULSE REGISTER. Table 8-14 demonstrates the the significantly lower flow rates to be expected during pusle register phonation. In general, no consistent relationship between airflow and fundamental frequency has been observed. At comfortable intensity, airflow for males producing pulse-register vowels will range between 10 and approximately 72 mL/s, while females will use from 2 to about 63 mL/s (McGlone, 1967). Similar findings have been reported by Murry (1971).

LOFT REGISTER. McGlone (1970) has done a careful study of airflow during phonation in the "upper register," which he has defined as "that group of frequencies that occur above the modal register. This register may be falsetto,"—or loft (p.231). Eight college-age women sustained a vowel for 4 s at 10% intervals of their intensity range and at 10% intervals of their pitch range, within this register. Flow rate was derived by dividing the volume of air used by the duration of phonation. The resultant data are summarized in Table 8-15.

TABLE 8–13. Mean Rate of Increase in Airflow for a 10 dB Increase in Vocal Intensity*

| Frequency Level | Mean rate of Increase in Flow† | | | | | |
| | Males | | | Females | | |
	Mean	S.D.	Range	Mean	S.D.	Range
Low (98 Hz)	1.05	0.26	0.65–1.70	1.04	0.33	0.56–1.60
Medium (196 Hz)	1.30	0.32	0.91–2.10	1.88	0.46	1.05–2.70
High (392 Hz)	1.80	0.60	1.05–3.50	1.94	0.55	0.56–2.70

From Isshiki, N. Vocal intensity and air flow rate. *Folia Phoniatrica*, 17 (1965) 92–104. Table II, p. 98. Reprinted by permission.

*Conditions as for Table 8–12. *Reading the table:* The data entry represents the mean proportion of airflow at a given level to airflow during phonation at 10 dB lower intensity. Thus, at low pitch, if flow = 113 mLs, an increase of 10 dB would cause flow to increase to 113 × 1.05 = 118.7 mL/s. Brown and McGlone (1974) have also shown that airflow values and vocal intensity are strongly correlated.

†The difference in values between males and females is significant.

TABLE 8–14. Mean Airflow in Modal and Pulse Registers in Normal Males*

Register	F_0 (Hz) Mean	Range	Flow (mL/sec) Mean	Range
Modal	107.9	87–117	142.2	74.9–267.8
Pulse	34.4	18–65	40.4	0.†–145.3

From McGlone, R. E. and Shipp, T. Some physiologic correlates of vocal fry phonation. *Journal of Speech and Hearing Research*, 14 (1971) 769–775. Table 1, p. 772. © American Speech-Language-Hearing Association, Rockville, MD. Reprinted by permission.

*Nine young adult males; 2-s sustained phonations of a vowel at 10% pitch and 25% and 75% intensity levels in each subject's range; pneumotachograph measurement.

†Indicates a flow too small to be measured.

VOCAL PATHOLOGY. The expectation that the airflow rate should reflect the degree of laryngeal dysfunction is generally borne out by research reported in the literature. This is particularly true in those instances when adequate glottal closure is not achieved (Hirano, Koike, and von Leden, 1968; Hippel and Mrowinski, 1978). Airflow data, then, are useful in initial diagnosis or evaluation of the degree of dysfunction and also serve as an indicator of therapeutic progress.

The data presented in Table 8-16 are drawn from two comparable studies of patients with various laryngeal pathologies.

Measurements were made during sustained /ɑ/ at comfortable pitch and loudness. In some cases post-treatment measurements were also made; the resultant data are included in the table.

Note that the airflow values for any given group show very wide dispersion, and the standard deviations demonstrate that airflow measurements in these cases of pathology frequently overlap the normal range. Thus, an airflow value far beyond the normal is clearly indicative of disorder, but a value within the expected range is not presumptive evidence of normal laryngeal function. The results of measurement are always useful, however, in targeting therapeutic goals and choosing clinical courses of action.

VOLUME

Instrumentation

Spirometers

The classic instrument for evaluation of air volumes is the *wet spirometer*, an extremely simple device that has not changed much since its invention well over 100 years ago. It consists of an air-collecting "bell" inverted in a vessel of water. At the

TABLE 8–15.   Mean Airflow in the Loft Register: Females (mL/s)

Intensity Level (percentage intervals)	Pitch Level (percentage intervals)									Mean for Intensity Level
	10	20	30	40	50	60	70	80	90	
10	92.4	96.9	91.7	87.8	100.8	132.8	130.7	121.9	131.8	109.6
20	121.1	120.6	114.4	123.4	133.9	149.2	154.4	151.8	158.6	136.4
30	162.0	158.6	138.0	154.2	144.3	165.6	167.2	159.1	180.2	158.8
40	185.7	187.8	177.3	164.6	148.7	183.3	169.5	173.9	186.1	175.2
50	208.9	200.5	174.2	203.1	179.4	184.1	198.4	182.0	188.5	191.0
60	207.5	217.4	183.9	216.4	188.8	200.5	227.8	190.1	188.8	202.4
70	242.4	232.0	194.3	224.5	205.5	220.6	229.7	215.2	206.2	218.9
80	239.8	240.4	211.5	246.4	202.6	237.8	242.2	223.1	216.4	228.9
90	266.4	249.7	223.9	249.0	198.4	232.9	268.7	213.3	224.0	236.3
Mean for pitch level	191.8	189.8	167.7	185.5	166.9	189.6	198.7	181.2	186.7	

From McGlone, R. E. Air flow in the upper register. *Folia Phoniatrica*, 22 (1970) 231–238. Table II, p. 234. Reprinted by permission.

start of a test water fills the bell, but air from the patient is channelled into it, and the water is displaced. This causes the bell to float, so that its height is directly proportional to the amount of air in it. A pointer linked to the bell indicates the volume of air. Most spirometers also have a pen, moved by the bell via a pulley arrangement, that marks a moving chart paper to produce a permanent record of the volume events. Many spirometers are also equipped with a system to provide an electrical output proportional to the volume of air contained.

Although spirometers are widely available and are virtually unsurpassed for measurement of ventilatory volumes, their inherent characteristics limit their usefulness for observing small, rapid volume changes, such as those that may occur during speech (Hardy and Edmonds, 1968), Because they are mechanical devices, there is significant resistance to be overcome before bell displacement is achieved. Even when this is minimized, as it can be with careful design, the device still suffers from the effects of its inherently large inertia. That is, the spirometer is sluggish in its response. Therefore, rapid speech events are likely to be completely obscured by mechanical integration. The spirometer is not the instrument of choice for most evaluative tasks. Providing, however, that the

duration of phonatory or speech acts can be accurately marked on the spirometric record, it is quite acceptable in the determination of phonation volume or of total speech volume (Beckett, 1971). And, of course, the spirometer is the classic instrument for assessment of gross respiratory volumes.

Hand held, or *dry*, spirometers are compact and portable devices that do not depend on the displacement of water from a bell. Two types are in current use. One kind— exemplified by the Propper spirometer—is purely mechanical. A small turbine within its case is driven by the air blown into the mouthpiece. Its rotation moves a pointer around a dial on the outside of the case. Air volume is read from the position of the pointer at the end of the task. The instrument is rugged and reliable, but it may not be equally valid at all flow rates.

The other kind of portable spirometer is actually a flow transducer-and-integrator-circuit system. A digital readout shows volume. These electronic instruments are less rugged and more expensive than their purely mechanical counterparts, and they tend to be relatively insensitive to low flows, such as frequently occur during speech.

Compact spirometers are useful only for gross assessments of air volume, such as vital capacity (VC). Rau and Beckett (1984)

TABLE 8–16. Mean Airflow During Sutained Phonation in Laryngeal Pathology

Condition	Untreated N	Untreated Mean	Untreated S.D.	Treatment	posttreatment N	posttreatment Mean	posttreatment S.D.	Source
Uncompensated								
Unilateral	10	442.2	204.3	Teflon inj	4	200.5	34.7	a
Paralysis	11	312.8	154.9	Teflon inj	3	147.7	46.4	b
Unilateral								
Paralysis								
Medial or paramedial	?	346	105.8					c
Intermediate	?	845	106.7					c
Intermediate	19	353						d
Polyps	4	478.0	182.3					a
	10	218.5	91.9					b
Carcinoma	4	236.5	26.9					a
	5	224.0	171.5	Radiation and surgery	3	109.3	6.5	b
Large tumor	?	259	70.0					c
Chronic laryngitis	5	212.4	79.9					b
	M = 45	150						d
	F = 23	137						d
Vocal nodule	8	153.9	35.5					a
	8	160.9	66.4					b
Small tumor	?	189	94.3					c
Minor inflammation	11	133.8	29.2					a
Edema inflammation	?	173	93.8					c
Contact ulcer	?	144	42.4					c
Spasmodic dysphonia	8	110.4	49.7					b

*Means and standard deviations compiled from individual case data presented in sources a and b.

Sources: (a) Yanagihara and von Leden, 1967; (b) Hirano, Koike, and von Leden, 1968; (c) Isshiki and von Leden, 1964; (d) Iwata, von Leden, and Williams, 1972.

have determined that VC measures done with several hand-held units (including the Propper spirometer) compare quite well with VCs obtained with a standard water-displacement spirometer. For clinical purposes, then, compact spirometers may be confidently used in those situations where only a gross measure is needed and a paper record is not required.

Chest wall measurement

Lung volume changes can be determined from the changes in rib cage and abdominal size. Devices for transducing size chang-

es include magnetometers (Mead, Peterson, Grimby, and Mead, 1967), mercury strain gauges (Baken and Matz, 1973) and inductive plethysmographs (Sackner, 1980; Watson, 1979). The technology of these systems is discussed in Chapter 11.

The chest wall's two parts contribute independently to the total lung volume change, and the contributions need not be in the same direction. It is entirely possible, for example, for the rib cage to be enlarging (inspiring) while the abdominal wall is forcing the diaphragm upward (expiring). Therefore, derivation of a lung volume estimate requires that the separate motions of the rib cage and abdomen be added. Unfortunately the different geometric properties of the two chest-wall components cause them to make unequal contributions to the net lung volume change. That is, a 1 cm change in the diameter of the abdomen does not alter the lung volume as much as a similar change in rib cage size. Taking these factors into account (but ignoring changes due to air compression), estimating the lung volume change from movements of the chest wall entails solving an equation of the form

$$\Delta LV = k\,(\Delta RC + m\Delta Ab),$$

where ΔRC and ΔAb are the observed size changes of the rib cage and abdomen. The coefficient m expresses the relative effectiveness of abdominal to rib cage motion while k is a scaling constant to convert the sum of the terms to liters. Motion can be defined as the change in anteroposterior diameter (Mead, Peterson, Grimby, and Mead, 1967; Konno abd Mead, 1967), anterior hemicircumference (Baken, 1977), or body circumference (Sackner, Nixon, Davis, Atkins, and Sackner, 1980).

Because individuals differ in their anatomy, the rib-cage to abdominal equivalence ratio, m, varies greatly from one body to another. There is no practical way to predict it for a given person. Also, the scaling factor, k, changes as a function of system characteristics. This might seem to imply that application of this measurement method would require an inordinate amount of calibration for each subject. This is not the case, however. In practice, the equation can be solved electronically using very simple circuitry. It is not even necessary to determine the actual value of any of the unknowns. The method, which is built into instruments such as the Respi-Trace, is as follows.

The transduction system is attached to the subject, and its electrical outputs are connected to the inputs of a variable summing amplifier, as shown in Figure 8-15. This simple operational amplifier circuit (specific details are available in any ele-

mentary electronics text) produces an output representing the sum of the separate inputs. By using a variable resistance for the rib cage input, it is easy to adjust its contribution to the final output. The setting of the variable resistor, in short, represents m in the equation. Adjusting the feedback resistor changes the scaling factor, k. Thus, the simple circuit is an analog computer that, in voltage terms, solves for $k(\Delta RC + m\Delta Ab)$ when the m and k resistors are properly set.

To set the m resistor the subject performs a series of isovolume maneuvers: After inhaling a moderate quantity of air he closes his glottis ("hold your breath") and alternately contracts and relaxes his abdominal wall. Since, when the glottis is closed, no air can enter or leave the lungs the net volume change during the isovolume maneuver must be zero. Any contraction of the abdomen will cause an equivalent expansion of the rib cage. While the subject performs the isovolume maneuvers, the tester adjusts the m resistor until the summing amplifier's output shows minimal change. This indicates that the abdomen's voltage signal is cancelling the rib cage's, making the summing amplifier reflect no net lung volume change.

When the m resistor has been set, the output of the summing amplifier will be *proportional* to lung volume change, but it needs to be calibrated to actual volume values. This can be done in two ways. One is to match the output with that of an already calibrated volume transducer (spirometer, pneumotachograph and integrator, etc.). The two can be compared visually on an oscilloscope while the k (scaling) resistor is adjusted to make them match. More precise calibration can be obtained by subtracting one system output from the other (using a subtracting amplifier, also shown in Figure 8-15) while adjusting k until the two signals cancel each other completely. When k is properly adjusted the volume calibration of the chest wall system is the same as that of the volume instrumentation to which it has been compared, and the second system can be removed. The other

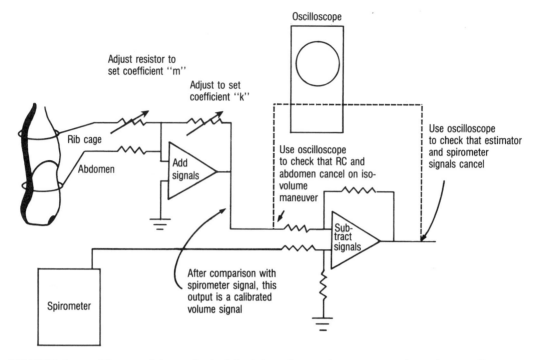

FIGURE 8–15. Diagram of the method of obtaining a lung-volume estimate from chest-wall signals. (See text. Chap. 11, Figure 11-19 shows the transducers in place on a subject.

method of calibration is easier, but less exact. The subject can simply be asked to inhale and exhale a known volume of air (to and from a spirometer, or into and out of a nonstretchable plastic bag of known capacity) while noting the change in the output voltage, from which the volts per liter calibration of the system is easily determined.

Articulatory and Phonatory Volumes

Instrumentation

In theory, all of the instrumentation used for measurement of ventilatory volumes can be made to serve for observation of the volumes associated with specific articulatory events or phonatory tasks. But the volumes involved may be very small and may be expended in very brief time intervals. This situation imposes special requirements with respect to resolution and frequency response. Any limitations along these lines must be considered in the light of the speech task to be evaluated so as to be certain that necessary compromises do not invalidate the data.

The shortcomings of the spirometer have been discussed above, but other volumetric instrumenation may have similar limitations, and several are also sensitive to compressional lung volume changes, which is undesirable if articulatory or phonatory volumes are to be examined. The method of choice for observing articulatory and phonatory volumes is integration of the output of a pneumotachograph. This instrumentation can show very small volume changes in time periods of only a fraction of a second. The improvement in resolution is clearly illustrated in Figure 8-16, in which the outputs of a spirometer and a pneumotachograph-integrator system are compared during production of the same utterance. Flow integrator modules are commercially available and Hardy and Edmonds (1968) have published a circuit that is easily constructed and can easily be

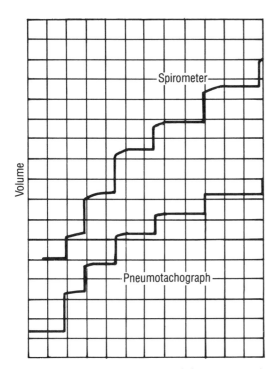

FIGURE 8–16. Comparison of the outputs of a spirometer (upper trace) and a pneumotachograph-integrator system (lower trace) for rapid incremental inputs of air. The greater squareness of the corners in the pneumotachograph record indicates better frequency response.

modified to take advantage of better, more modern circuit components.

Air volume measurements

Given the relationship between flow and volume (see "General Physical Principles" at the start of this chapter) it is clear that volume may always be calculated by multiplying the mean flow during an event by the event's duration. This indirect approach might not always be convenient, however, and it may not always be possible to determine the mean flow, particularly in the case of the flow pulses that characterize many articulatory gestures. Specific *volume* measures are, therefore, often useful.

ARTICULATORY VOLUMES. The volume of air used during a particular articulatory event depends on the subglottal pressure,

vocal tract impedance, and the event's duration. While generally a less useful measure than flow rate for understanding articulatory coordination, volumetric evaluation may provide special insights in particular cases.

Technique. Volume usage can be determined for whole syllables or for individual phonemes. In the former case a spirometer can be used to determine the *mean* volume per syllable by having the patient repeat the test utterance fairly rapidly on a single breath while the spirometer records the volume of air expired. The mean volume per syllable is the final spirometer volume divided by the number of syllables produced. This technique produces only approximate results. It obscures any significant variability among the syllables and may be very misleading if rapid, nonspeech inspirations are interspersed within the spoken text. (Itoh and Horii [1985] have shown this to be characteristic of some deaf speakers, for example.) Nonetheless, the method is often sufficiently discriminating for clinical purposes. Hardy (1961), for example, found that this method demonstrated differences in production of /bɑ/ by dysarthric and nondysarthric spastic children. More refined measures, however, will require better temporal and volumetric resolution than can be provided by a spirometer.

Instrumentation. Determining the air volume used during production of a phoneme will, ideally, involve three data signals: flow, volume, and audio. The flow and volume data are most commonly generated with a face mask-pneumotachograph-integrator system, while the audio signal is derived from a microphone mounted on or within the face mask. The three signals are read out on an oscilloscope or paper recorder. It is usually more convenient to record the data on an FM tape system (see Chap. 3) and perform the analysis after the test session.

Method. The phoneme of interest is placed in a syllable which is in turn embedded in a carrier phrase. For example, /t/ might be tested in the syllable /tɪp/ in the phrase "Say tip again." It is the usual practice to have the patient speak with comfortable loudness and pitch, although other conditions may be useful in special circumstances. Several repetitions are spoken; the mean and standard deviation of the trials are the data of interest.

The flow and audio channels are used to delineate the phoneme being tested. The carrier phrase should be constructed to provide a clear contrast between the event of interest and the surrounding phones.

Output Record. Figure 8-17 shows a typical output record. In this case air volume

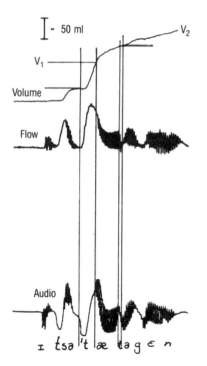

FIGURE 8–17. Volume usage during pre- and postvocalic /t/ in the phrase "It's a tat again." The flow and audio traces are used to delimit the onset (sudden increase in flow) and termination (initiation of voicing) of each /t/. The change in the volume trace between onset and termination is the volume used. Note that the (aspirated) prevocalic /t/ used somewhat over 50 mL of air, while the unaspirated postvocalic /t/ used a barely measurable volume.

for /t/ before a stressed and an unstressed vowel was of concern, so the test phrase was "Say tat again." The initial (prestressed vowel) and final (preunstressed vowel) /t/s of "tat" are measured. The flow signal and audio traces are used to mark the start of flow for /t/ and the beginning of postplosive voicing. The change in the integrator (volume) signal between these two points is the volume expended during /t/. Measurement of several repetitions of the phrase would be done in order to derive a mean value for these phones.

Typical Values. The data presented in Table 8-17A were derived by Warren and Wood (1969) according to the method described above. Thirteen male and seven female adults, speakers of "Southern dialect," spoke the carrier phrase "Say /Cæt/ again," where /C/ was each of the consonants shown.

Hardy and Arkebauer (1966) have used the respirometer to measure the mean air volume per syllable used by 32 normal children, aged 6 to 13 years. A face mask collected oral and nasal air. The mean volume per syllable was determined by division of the spirometer volume change during the task by the number of syllables produced. Resulting data are summarized in Table 8-17B.

SUSTAINED PHONATION. Determination of the volume of air used during a prolonged phonation is relatively easy, since the absence of sudden flow changes means that the dynamic response of the measurement system is not of great concern. Therefore, the volume can be accurately measured with a spirometer which is, in fact, the preferred instrument in this case. Unfortunately, phonatory volume is not, of itself, a very useful measure. It represents only the long-term integral of the flow (the mean flow times the phonatory duration), and thus it merges two variables of clinical interest. From a clinical point of view the flow rate and its stability during the task are much more important. (The former can be derived

TABLE 8–17A. Mean Air Volume for Selected Consonants (mL)

Sex*	/b,d/*		/p,t/*		/z,v/*		/s,f/*	
	Mean	S.D.	Mean	S.D.	Mean	S.D.	Mean	S.D.
Males	53	17	93	22	76	29	106	28
Females	40	13	84	21	50	17	75	14

From Warren, D. W. and Wood, M. T. Respiratory volumes in normal speech: A possible reason for intraoral pressure differences among voiced and voiceless consonants. *Journal of the Acoustical Society of America*, 45 (1969) 466–469. Table 1, p. 468. Reprinted by permission.

*Significant differences: male/female; voiced/voiceless.

TABLE 8–17B. Mean Volume per Syllable in Children*†

Speech Activity	Liters/syllable (BTPS)	
	Mean	S.D.
Counting 1–10	0.032	0.010
Repetition of /pʌ/	0.039	0.017
/tʌ/	0.035	0.017
/kʌ/	0.037	0.016
/sʌ/	0.056	0.018
/tʃʌ/	0.042	0.016
/fʌ/	0.052	0.018

From Hardy, J. C. and Arkebauer, H. J. Development of a test for velopharyngeal competence during speech. *Cleft Palate Journal*, 3 (1966) 6–21. Table 1, p. 11. Reprinted by permission.

†Also note that a modest ($r = -.40$) correlation exists between rate of repetition and air volume.

*Instructions: "Say _____ as fast as you can."

from the volume measure, while the latter is not easily observed in the spirometric record.)

Phonation Volume. A measure that is likely to be of great value to the speech pathologist is the *phonation volume*. It has been defined by Yanagihara and Koike (1967, p. 5) as "the maximum amount of air which is available for maximally sustained phonation." It is evaluated by requiring the patient to inhale maximally and then phonate for as long as possible, keeping vocal pitch and loudness constant. Volume is measured with a pneumotachograph-integrator or with a spirometer.

Expected Results. Phonation volume has been evaluated in 11 male and 11 female adults by Yanagihara and Koike (1967) and by Yanagihara, Koike and von Leden (1966). They had each subject phonate at three pitch levels: 1) "most comfortable and easiest"; 2) "highest pitch in chest register sustainable without special effort"; and 3) "lowest [modal] pitch sustainable without special effort." Comfortable loudness was used at all pitches, and three trials were performed at each level. Resulting data are summarized in Table 8-18A. Data for production at comfortable loudness by children are presented in Table 8-18B.

The same research established that there is, under all of the test conditions, a significant correlation ranging from $r = .59$ to $r = .90$) between a speaker's one-stage vital capacity (*VC*) and phonation volume (*PV*). The following regressions were computed to quantify this relationship:

1. at high pitch $PV = 0.85VC - 1133$
2. at comfortable pitch $PV = 0.86VC - 891$
3. at low pitch $PV = 0.94VC - 1186$

These equations may be used to generate a predicted phonation volume (for either men or women) that can be compared with the individual's measured phonation volume. In light of the modest correlations behind the equations, however, the predicted value should be liberally interpreted and not be construed as a rigid standard. No specific norms are available for children.

VOCAL ONSET. Different types of vocal *initiation* (*attack*) result in different flow rates during the vocal rise time. The nature

TABLE 8–18A. Mean Phonation Volume for Adults*†

Pitch	Mean F_o (Hz)	Phonation Volume in Liters		
		Mean	S.D.	Range
Males				
High	208	3.359	0.498	2.690–4.400
Comfortable	118	3.256	0.602	2.200–4.255
Low	95	2.946	0.408	2.540–3.550
Females				
High	390	2.161	0.451	1.480–2.980
Comfortable	230	2.146	0.345	1.520–2.723
Low	209	1.879	0.782	1.020–2.880

Compiled from Yanagihara, N. and Koike, Y. The regulation of sustained phonation. *Folia Phoniatrica*, 19 (1967) 1–18; and from Yanagihara, N. and von Leden, H. Respiration and phonation: the functional examination of laryngeal disease. *Folia Phoniatrica*, 19 (1967) 153–166. Reprinted by permission.

†Also note that volumes of males and females are significantly different.

*Eleven males, aged 30–43, and 11 females, aged 21–40; for method, see text.

TABLE 8-18B. Mean Phonation Volume for Children*†

	Age (yr)	Height (cm)	Phonation Volume (L)	
			Mean	Range
Boys				
Mean**	7.55	126.2	1.310	900–1650
S.D.	0.23	4.4	.242	
Girls				
Mean**	7.56	124.1	1.069	700–1500
S.D.	0.25	4.4	.239	

From Beckett, R., Thoelke, W., and Cowan, L. A normative study of airflow in children. *British Journal of Disorders of Communication*, 6 (1971) 13–16. Table II, p. 14. Reprinted by permission of the College of Speech Therapists, Harold Poster House, 6 Lechmere Rd., London NW25BU, England.

†Also note that differences in data for boys and girls are not significant.

*Ten boys and 10 girls; maximally sustained /ɑ/; spirometer measurement.

**Calculated from authors' data.

TABLE 8–19. Air Consumption During the First 200 ms of Phonation in Normal Men*†

Voice Initiation Type	Air Consumption (200 ms)		
	Mean	S.D.	Range
"Soft" (normal)	23	5.0	15–33
"Breathy"	97	52.1	23–215
"Hard"	46	16.4	29–77

From Koike, Y., Hirano, M., and von Leden, H. Vocal initiation: Acoustic and aerodynamic investigations of normal subjects. *Folia Phoniatrica*, 19 (1967) 173–182. Table II, p. 177. Reprinted by permission.

*Fourteen males; phonation of /a/ for several seconds ("over 200 samples"); pneumotachograph-integrator (other test details not given).

†Also note significant difference of voice initiation type.

TABLE 8–20. Air Consumption During the First 200 ms of Phonation in Laryngeal Pathology*

Disorder	Air Consumption (200 ms)		
	Number of Cases	Mean (mL)	Range
Cancer with glottal involvement	3	55.5	37–90
Unilateral paralysis	3	135.3	77–184
Papilloma	2	34.0	29–39

From Koike, Y. Experimental studies on vocal attack. *Practica Otologica Kyoto*, 60 (1967) 663–688. Table 5 p. 675. Reprinted by permission.

*Phonation of /a/; subjects using their best vocal attack; derived from author's data.

of these differences has been explored in men by Koike, Hirano, and von Leden (1967) and Koike 1967) who compared the amount of air consumed in the first 200 ms of phonations initiated with different attacks. The data (Table 8-19) may be useful in evaluation of voice onset characteristics and assessment of therapeutic progress. Note, however, that intrasubject variability tends to be high. Table 8-20 demonstrates how these data are elevated in at least some types of vocal pathologies.

TABLE 8–21. Mean Air Volume per Breath During Reading*

	Expiratory (in mL)			Inspiratory (in mL)		
	Mean	**S.D.**	**Range**	**Mean**	**S.D.**	**Range**
Males	650.5	99.4	541.8–782.5	640.3	101.4	422.8–770.1
Females	636.4	31.4	599.0–670.4	623.9	35.9	596.5–676.6
Overall	643.5	68.7	541.8–782.5	632.1	71.0	522.8–770.1

Data compiled from tables in Horii and Cooke, 1978.

*Four male and four female normal young adults; single reading of Rainbow Passage; comfortable intensity; pneumotachograph-integrator and special computer program.

CONTINUOUS SPEECH. The average expiratory and inspiratory volumes during ordinary speech may be of interest in certain cases. As was mentioned in the discussion of airflow during running speech, this is best assessed by having the patient read a standard passage. The "Rainbow Passage" is the almost-universal choice for this purpose. Horii and Cooke (1978) using a pneumotachograph-integrator system and special computer program (Horii and Cooke, 1975) have carefully generated relevant data (summarized in Table 8-21) that may be useful as broad guidelines in evaluation of clinical disorders. ∎

SELECT BIBLIOGRAPHY

Amerman, J. D. and Williams, D. K. Implications of respirometric evaluation for diagnosis and management of vocal fold pathologies. *British Journal of Disorders of Communication,* 14 (1979) 153-160.

Baken, R. J. Estimation of lung volume change from torso hemicircumferences. *Journal of Speech and Hearing Research,* 20 (1977) 808-812.

Baken, R. J. and Matz, B. J. A portable impedance pneumograph. *Human Communication,* 2 (1973) 28-35.

Bastian, H.-J., Unger, E., and Sasama, R. Pneumotachologische Objektivierung von Behandlungsverläufen und- ergibnissen. *Folia Phoniatrica,* 33 (1981) 216-226.

Beckett, R. L. The respirometer as a diagnostic and clinical tool in the speech clinic. *Journal of Speech and Hearing Disorders,* 36 (1971) 235-241.

Beckett, R. L., Thoelke, W., and Cowan, L. A normative study of airflow in children. *British Journal of Disorders of Communication,* 6 (1971) 13-16.

Brown, W. S., jr. and McGlone, R. E. Aerodynamic and acoustic study of stress in sentence productions. *Journal of the Acoustical Society of America,* 56 (1974) 971-974.

Brown, W. S., Murry, T., and Hughes, D. Comfortable effort level: an experimental variable. *Journal of the Acoustical Society of America,* 60 (1976) 696-699.

Catford, J. C. *Fundamental Problems in Phonetics.* Bloomington, Ind.: Indiana University, 1977.

Cavagna, G. A. and Margaria, R. An analysis of the mechanics of phonation. *Journal of Applied Physiology,* 20 (1965) 301

Cavagna, G. A. and Margaria, R. Airflow rates and efficiency changes during phonation. In Bouhuys, A. (Ed.). *Sound Production in Man (Annals of the new York Academy of Sciences* vol. 155). New York: New York Academy of Sciences, 1968. Pp. 152-163.

Collatina, S., Barone, E., Monini, S., and Bolasco, P. Realizzazione di un flussometro ad ultrasuoni e sua applicazione nella misura del flusso fonatorio: Primi risultati. *Acta Phoniatrica Latina,* 2 (1980) 61-68.

Comroe, J. H., jr., Forster, R. E. II, Dubois, A. B., Briscoe, W. A., and Carlsen, *The Lung.* Chicago: Year Book Medical Publishers, 1962.

Dejonckere, P. H., Greindl, M., and Sneppe, R. Débitmétrie aérienne à paramètres phonatoires standardisés. *Folia Phoniatrica,* 37 (1985) 58-65.

Diem, K. *Documenta Geigy: Scientific Tables.* Ardsley, NY: Geigy Pharmaceuticals, 1962.

Emanuel, F. W. and Counihan, D. T. Some characteristics of oral and nasal air flow during plosive consonant production. *Cleft Palate Journal,* 7 (1970) 249-260.

Fairbanks, G. *Voice and Articulation Drill Book* (second ed.). New York: Harper, 1960.

Fry, D. L., Hyatt, R. E., McCall, C. B., and Mallos, A. J. Evaluation of three types of respiratory flowmeters. *Journal of Applied Physiology,* 10 (1957) 210-214.

Gilbert, H. R. Oral airflow during stop consonant production. *Folia Phoniatrica,* 25 (1973) 288-301.

Gordon, M. T., Morton, M., and Simpson, I. C. Air flow measurements in diagnosisl assessment and treatment of mechanical dysphonia. *Folia Phoniatrica*, 30 (1978) 161-174.

Hardy, J. C. Intraoral breath pressure in cerebral palsy. *Journal of Speech and Hearing Disorders*, 26 (1961) 309-319.

Hardy, J. C. Air flow and air pressure studies. *ASHA Reports*, 1 (1965) 141-152.

Hardy, J. C. Techniques of measuring intraoral air pressure and rate of flow. *Journal of Speech and Hearing Research*, 10 (1967) 650-654.

Hardy, J. C. and Arkebauer, H. J. Development of a test for velopharyngeal competence during speech. *Cleft Palate Journal*, 3 (1966) 6-21.

Hardy, J. C. and Edmonds, T. D. Electronic integrator for measurement of partitions of the lung volume. *Journal of Speech and Hearing Research*, 11 (1968) 777-786.

Hippel, K. and Mrowinski, D. Untersuchung stimmgesunder und stimmkranker Personen nach der Methode deer Pneumotachographie. *Hals-, Nasen-, und Ohrenheilkeit*, 26 (1978) 421-423.

Hirano, M., Koike, Y. and von Leden, H. Maximum phonation time and air usage during phonation. *Folia Phoniatrica*, 20 (1968) 185-201.

Hixon, T. Turbulent noise sources for speech. *Folia Phoniatrica*, 18 (1966) 168-182.

Hixon, T. J. Some new techniques for measuring the biomechanical events of speech production: one laboratory's experiences. *ASHA Reports*, 7 (1972) 68-103.

Hixon, T. J., Saxman, J. H., and McQueen, H. D. A respirometric technique for evaluating velopharyngeal competence during speech. *Folia Phoniatrica*, 19 (1967) 203-219.

Horii, Y. and Cooke, P. A. Analysis of airflow and volume during continuous speech. *Behavior Research Methods and Instrumentation*, 7 (1975) 477.

Horii, Y. and Cooke, P. A. Some airflow, volume, and duration characteristics of oral reading. *Journal of Speech and Hearing Research*, 21 (1978) 470-481.

Isshiki, N. Respiratory mechanism of voice intensity variation. *Journal of Speech and Hearing Research*, 7 (1964) 17-29.

Isshiki, N. Vocal intensity and air flow rate. *Folia Phoniatrica*, 17 (1965) 92-104.

Isshiki, N. and Ringel, R. Air flow during the production of selected consonants. *Journal of Speech and Hearing Research*, 7 (1964) 233-244.

Isshiki, N. and von Leden, H. Hoarseness: aerodynamic studies. *Archives of Otolaryngology*, 80 (1964) 206-213.

Itoh, M. and Horii, Y. Airflow, volume, and durational characteristics of oral reading by the hearing-impaired. *Journal of Communication Disorders*, 18 (1985) 393-407.

Iwata S. von Leden H. and Williams, D. Air flow measurement during phonation. *Journal of Communication Disorders*, 5 (1972) 67-79.

Kelman, A. W., Gordon, M. T., Simpson, I. C., and Morton, F. M. Assessment of vocal function by air-flow measurements. *Folia Phoniatrica*, 27 (1975) 250-262.

Klatt, D. H., Stevens, K. N., and Mead, J. Studies of articulatory activity and airflow during speech. In Bouhuys, A. (Ed.) *Sound Production in Man (Annals of the New York Academy of Sciences, vol. 155)*. New York: New York Academy of Sciences, 1968. Pp. 42-55.

Koike, Y. Experimental studies on vocal attack. *Practica Otologica Kyoto*, 60 (1967) 663-688.

Koike, Y. and Hirano, M. Significance of vocal velocity index. *Folia Phoniatrica*, 20 (1968) 285-296.

Koike, Y., Hirano, M., and von Leden, H. Vocal initiation: acoustic and aerodynamic investigations of normal subjects. *Folia Phoniatrica*, 19 (1967) 173-182.

Konno, K. and Mead, J. Measurement of the separate volume changes of rib cage and abdomen during breathing. *Journal of Applied Physiology*, 22 (1967) 407-422.

Lubker, J. F. Aerodynamic and ultrasonic assessment techniques in speech-dentofacial research. *ASHA Reports*, 5 (1970) 207-223.

Lubker, J. F. and Moll, K. L. Simultaneous oral-nasal air flow measurements and cinefluorographic observations during speech production. *Cleft Palate Journal*, 2 (1965) 257-272.

McGlone, R. E. Air flow during vocal fry phonation. *Journal of Speech and Hearing Research*, 10 (1967) 299-304.

McGlone, R. E. Air flow in the upper register. *Folia Phoniatrica*, 22 (1970) 231-238.

McGlone, R. E. and Shipp, T. Some physiologic correlates of vocal fry phonation. *Journal of Speech and Hearing Research*, 14 (1971) 769-775.

Mead, J. Volume displacement body plethysmograph for respiratory measurements in human speech. *Journal of Applied Physiology*, 15 (1960) 736-740.

Mead, J., Peterson, N., Grimby, G., and Mead, J. Pulmonary ventilation measured from body surface movements. *Science*, 156 (1967) 1383-1384.

Micco, A. J. A sensitive flow direction sensor. *Journal of Applied Physiology*, 35 (1973) 420-422.

Murry, T. Subglottal pressure and airflow measures during vocal fry phonation. *Journal of Speech and Hearing Research*, 14 (1971) 544-551.

Peters, R. M. *The Mechanical Basis of Respira-*

tion. Boston: Little, Brown, 1969.

Quigley, L. F., jr., Shiere, F. R., Webster, R. C., and Cobb, C. M. Measuring palatopharyngeal competence with the nasal anemometer. *Cleft Palate Journal*, 1 (1964) 304-314.

Quigley, L. F., jr., Webster, R. C., Coffey, R. J., Kelleher, R. E., and Grant, H. P. Velocity and volume measurements of nasal and oral airflow in normal and cleft palate speech utilizing a warm-wire flowmeter and two-channel recorder. 2. *Journal of Dental Research*, 42 (1963)1520-1527.

Rau, D. and Beckett, R. L. Aerodynamic assessment of vocal function using hand-held spirometers. *Journal of Speech and Hearing Disorders*, 49 (1984) 183-188.

Rothenberg, M. A new inverse-filtering technique for deriving the glottal waveform during voicing. *Journal of the Acoustical Society of America*, 53 (1973) 1632-1645.

Rothenberg, M. Measurement of airflow in speech. *Journal of Speech and Hearing Research*, 20 (1977) 155-176.

Sackner, M. A. Monitoring of ventilation without a physical connection to the airway. In Sackner, M. A. (Ed.). *Diagnostic Techniques in Pulmonary Disease*, part I. New York: Dekker, 1980. Pp. 503-537.

Sackner, J. D., Nixon, A. J., Davis, B., Atkins, N., and Sackner, M. A. Non-invasive measurement of ventilation during exercise using a respiratory inductive plethysmograph. *American Review of Respiratory Disease*, 122 (1980) 867-871.

Scully, C. A comparison of /s/ and /z/ for an English speaker. *Language and Speech*, 14 (1971 187-200.

Smith, S. The electro aerometer. *Speech Pathology and Therapy*, 3 (1960) 27-33.

Stathopoulos, E. T. Effects of monitoring vocal intensity on oral air flow in children and adults. *Journal of Speech and Hearing Research*, 28 (1985) 589-593.

Stathopoulos, E. T. and Weismer, G. Oral airflow and air pressure during speech production: a comparative study of children, youths, and adults. *Folia Phoniatrica*, 37 (1985) 152-159.

Stevens, K. N. Airflow and turbulence noise for fricative and stop consonants: static considerations. *Journal of the Acoustical Society of America*, 50 (1971) 1180-1192.

Subtelny, J., Kho, G., McCormack, R. M., and Subtelny, J. D. Multidimensional analysis of bilabial stop and nasal consonants—cineradiographic and pressure-flow analysis. *Cleft Palate Journal*, 6 (1969) 263-289.

Subtelny, J. D., Worth, J. H., and Sakuda, M. Intraoral pressure and rate of flow during speech. *Journal of Speech and Hearing Research*, 9 (1966) 498-518.

Trullinger, R. W. and Emanuel, F. W. Airflow characteristics of stop-plosive consonant productions of normal-speaking children. *Journal of Speech and Hearing Research*, 26 (1983) 202-208.

van den Berg, Jw. Modern research in experimental phoniatrics. *Folia Phoniatrica*, 14 (1962) 81-149.

van Hattum, R., and Worth, J. H. Air flow rates in normal speakers. *Cleft Palate Journal*, 4 (1967) 137-147.

Warren, D. W. Aerodynamics of speech production. In Lass, N. (Ed.), *Contemporary Issues in Experimental Phonetics*. New York: Academic Press, 1976. Pp. 105-137.

Warren, D. W. and Wood, M. T. Respiratory volumes in normal speech: a possible reason for intraoral pressure differences among voiced and voiceless consonants. *Journal of the Acoustical Society of America*, 45 (1969) 466-469.

Watson, H. The technology of respiratory inductive plethysmography. *Proceedings of the Third International Symposium on Ambulatory Monitoring*, 1979.

Yanagihara, N. and Koike, Y. the regulation of sustained phonation. *Folia Phoniatrica*, 19 (1967) 1-18.

Yanagihara, N., Koike, Y. and von Leden, H. Phonation and respiration: function study in normal subjects. *Folia Phoniatrica*, 18 (1966) 323-340.

Yanagihara, N. and von Leden, H. Respiration and phonation: The functional examination of laryngeal disease. *Folia Phoniatrica*, 19 (1967) 153-166.

Yoshiya, I., Nakajima, T., Nagai, I., and Jitsukawa, S. A bidirectional respiratory flowmeter using the hot-wire principle. *Journal of Applied Physiology*, 38 (1975) 360-365.

CHAPTER **9**

Sound Spectrography

Stetson (1928) said that speech is "movements made audible." In some very real ways, he was correct. The sounds of speech are the product of actions of the complex acoustic system called the vocal tract. Any change in the acoustic characteristics of the speech signal must, of necessity, represent a change in the status of the organs of speech.

If the physiology and acoustics of speech production were completely understood, it might be possible to evaluate a speech signal and determine from its waveform exactly what the speaker's vocal tract was doing.* Our understanding is lamentably far from perfect, and so it is usually impos-

sible to draw unequivocal conclusions about specific motor events on the basis of acoustic analysis alone. Furthermore, there is no reason to believe in a strict one-to-one correspondence between individual motor acts and specific acoustic events. The entire speech system is characterized by many *degrees of freedom*. A given acoustic result can usually be produced by different combinations of vocal tract actions.

Still, acoustic analysis provides a very potent tool for assessing speech system functioning, especially when it is combined with appropriate physiological measures, such as air pressure or flow which increase certainty about the exact function of the speech organs. One of the most powerful acoustic analytic techniques, one for which the requisite instrumentation is widely available, is sound spectrography, the dissection of the acoustic wave into its most basic components.

The amount of information displayed in a spectrogram of even a simple utterance can be enormous. A great deal of research in spectrography has tried to determine which features are meaningful and which

---

*A large number of research studies have been devoted to exploring ways of plotting the shape of the vocal tract from an analysis of the speech signal or vice versa (Fant, 1962, 1980; Lindblom and Sundberg, 1971; Stevens and House, 1955, 1961; Ladefoged, Harshman, Goldstein and Rice, 1978; Atal, Chang, Mathews, and Tukey, 1978; Stevens, Kasowski, and Fant, 1953; Strube, 1977; Nakajima, 1977; Paige and Zue, 1970a, b; Schroeder, 1967; Mermelstein, 1967; Dunn, 1950). A truly practical, valid, and reliable means has yet to be found.

can be ignored in drawing conclusions about productive or perceptive behavior. Every aspect of speech motor behavior contributes to the final acoustic product and, therefore, the spectrogram is very likely to tell the clinician more than he or she wants to know about any given utterance. In consequence, the spectral features that are to be "read" and evaluated must be chosen according to the speech behaviors being examined.

The interpretation of spectrograms rests on a thorough knowledge of the acoustics and physiology of speech, on familiarity with the way in which spectrograms are generated, on experience, and on a trained eye. The richness of the technique has been explored in a vast and ever-expanding body of literature. Many excellent volumes have been written about its methodology and about the relationship of spectral features to various aspects of speech physiology, auditory perception, or basic acoustic processes. Hundreds and hundreds of research articles deal with spectrographic observations of just about every aspect of speech production and language. It is not possible, by any stretch of the imagination, to summarize even a fraction of this information here. Accordingly, the intent of this chapter is to introduce the newcomer to the principles underlying sound spectrography and to the methods by which it is accomplished.

Most sound spectrographs require that the user adjust the settings of the spectrographic instrument and choose among several options that determine precisely how a sample is analyzed. The adjustments made and the options selected can change the appearance of the resulting spectrogram a great deal, highlighting or obscuring various features. The choices made by the user will alter the ways in which the output must be interpreted. Because of this and because the user's decisions must be based on knowledge of how the spectrograph works, the functional details of the sound spectrograph will be considered in some detail in this chapter. The most basic features of the sound spectrogram will then be considered, with a very small sample of

some of the clinical measures that have been proposed. The intent is to provide only an introduction and overview of this very powerful analytical tool.

BASIC PHYSICAL PRINCIPLES

Understanding sound spectrography obviously requires a firm grounding in physical and psychological acoustics, at least at the elementary level. The physics of sound and the psychology of perception are both part of the required academic preparation of speech pathologists. It is assumed that the reader has mastered the relevant basic concepts in these areas. They will not be reviewed in detail here, but good summaries are provided by Lieberman (1977), Fry (1979), Pickett (1980) and Shoup, Lass, and Kuehn (1982) for those who may need to refresh their understanding. For the present purposes, an outline of the most salient and relevant points relating to the Fourier theorem, filtering, and the source-filter model of speech production will have to suffice.

Fourier Theorem

The physical rationale for spectrography lies in the Fourier theorem. Implementation of the technique depends on sophisticated use of electronic filtering or, in digital spectrographs, on the application of complex computational algorithms. Briefly, the Fourier theorem asserts that any periodic waveform can be analyzed into a series of sine waves, with different frequencies, amplitudes, and phase relationships. The frequencies of the component waves are all integral multiples of the repetition (*fundamental*) frequency (denoted F_0) of the wave and are known as *harmonics* (denoted f_1, $f_2, \ldots f_n$). Aperiodic waves have energy at many frequencies or over a continuous range of frequencies (at least within certain limits), although the amount of energy varies from place to place along the frequency continuum. To plot the amplitude of the components of a time waveform against their frequencies is to describe the *amplitude spectrum* of the wave.

Filters

The most common spectrographic method involves filtering of the speech signal with bandpass filters. A bandpass filter is one that transmits frequencies within a restricted range and attenuates higher or lower frequencies. The *bandwidth* of the filter specifies the extent of the range of frequencies that are passed. The upper and lower limits of the *pass band* are defined by those frequencies where attenuation is -3 dB compared to the center of the band. These are called the *cutoff frequencies* of the filter. Filters with a narrow passband can resolve closely spaced frequencies, but they are inherently sluggish in their response. Wide-band filters, on the other hand, are rapidly responding. Their time resolution is very good, but their frequency resolution is poor. There is always a tradeoff bbetween time and frequency: Resolution of one or the other, but not both, can be optimized. This is an important consideration in sound spectrography, since it means that the user must select filters to display *either* the fine points of temporal change (by using wide-band filters) *or* the precise frequencies of signal components (using narrow-band filters).

Fourier Analysis

The process of determining the components of a wave is called Fourier analysis. It is the dissection technique whereby a complex vibration is split into its component simple harmonic vibrations.

The application of the required mathematics is an incredibly formidable task, close to impossible to do by hand (see Steinberg, 1934, who managed to do it!). Even the early digital computer algorithms required impractically large amounts of time. However, the *Fast Fourier Transform* (Cooley and Tukey, 1965) simplified and speeded up the process enormously,

making it possible to implement a purely mathematical analysis even on fairly small computer systems. This has given rise to some of the instrumentation currently available. But it is also possible to sidestep the mathematical process altogether through the use of electronic filtering. Later portions of this chapter will concentrate on such analog electronic analysis systems, since they are by far the most commonly used.

Spectra

The spectrum of an acoustic wave is simply the result of a Fourier analysis of a sample of the waves under analysis. That is, it is a statement of what frequencies are present and what their amplitudes are. Because a list of numbers is not as easily assimilated as a graph of the same data, spectra are presented as a special kind of graph. For an amplitude spectrum (the kind with which the speech clinican will have to deal) the vertical axis is amplitude, and the horizontal is frequency.

Periodic waves: Line spectra

Figure 9-1 shows a square wave and its spectrum. Each frequency component (harmonic) of the wave is represented by a line appropriately positioned on the frequency axis. The height of each harmonic line shows its amplitude in dB. Note that the "graph" is discontinuous: There are no points between the harmonics. This is as expected, since the square wave was composed of discrete frequency components. The tops of the harmonic lines cannot be joined together to form a continuous, smooth curve. Doing so would imply that there are sine wave components that lie between the harmonics which have not been plotted. This is not the case: The blank spaces represent the absence of frequencies, not missing data. Because of its form, this kind of spectrum is usually called a *line spectrum*. All purely periodic signals can be analyzed into line spectra whose frequency components stand in integer realtionship.

Because each harmonic is a whole-num-

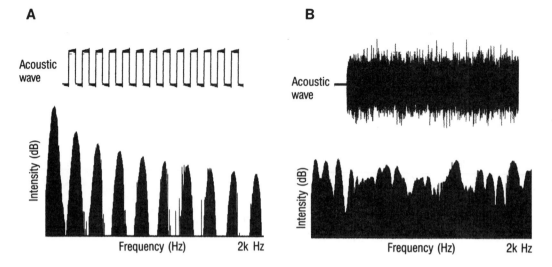

FIGURE 9–1. (A). The *line spectrum* of a *periodic* wave (in this case, a square wave. (B). *Continuous spectrum* of an *aperiodic* wave.

ber multiple of the fundamental frequency, the lines are regularly spaced across the spectrum. Assuming that all harmonics are present in the wave (the even harmonics are missing in the square wave), the spacing between the spectral lines will be equal to the fundamental frequency. Consider Figure 9-2, which shows the line spectra of the same waveform at two different frequencies—100 Hz and 300 Hz. The harmonic lines of the 100 Hz wave are much closer together than those of the 300 Hz wave, and the entire spectrum of the low-frequency version is "bunched up," but the *shape* of the two spectra are the same. The shape of the *spectrum envelope* represents the waveform, the line spacing represents the fundamental frequency.

Aperiodic waves: Continuous spectra

Aperiodic sounds are of two basic types. The first includes conntinuous signals of relatively long duration that are composed of random mixtures of frequencies within a given range or *bandwidth*. There is no discernible pattern to their sound pressure fluctuation over time, and there is no repetition of the waveform. A signal of this type (the /s/ in /su/) is shown

in Figure 9-3A, along with its spectrum.

The distinguishing characteristic of the spectrum of any aperiodic wave is that it is not composed of discrete lines. Within some portion of the frequency continuum there is energy at *all* frequencies within the signal's frequency band. Hence, these are called *continuous spectra*.

Daniloff, Schuckers, and Feth (1980 p. 89f) present an interesting way of viewing the continuous spectrum. Begin by considering a periodic wave with fundamental frequency F_0. The wave repeats F_0 times per second, and its harmonics are spaced F_0 Hz apart in its line spectrum. Now, àn aperiodic wave never repeats, which in a sense is the same as saying that its period, t, is infinite: t = ∞. Fundamental frequency is the reciprocal of the period, and therefore the "fundamental frequency" of an aperiodic wave is $F_0 = 1/∞$. That is, F_0 must be infinitesimally small. Since the separation of spectral lines is equal to the fundamental frequency, it follows that the spectral lines of an aperiodic signal must have only an infinitesimal space between them. In other words, for an aperiodic wave the spectral lines are right next to each other, and the "line spectrum," if drawn, would be a continuous blackened area. Rather than

100 Hz

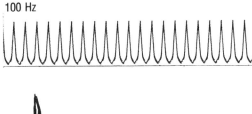

300 Hz

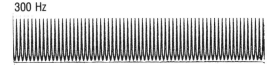

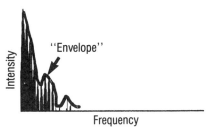

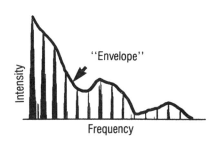

FIGURE 9–2. Line spectrum of two different waves, each at 100 Hz and 300 Hz. Note that the *shape* (more properly the *envelope*) of the spectrum does not change with fundamental frequency, but the space between the spectral lines is equal to F_0.

go through the mess and bother of blackening a graph, the convention is to draw an uninterrupted curve joining the tops of all the pressed-together spectral "lines," thereby defining the *spectrum envelope*. Doing so is perfectly valid in this case, since for an aperiodic signal there is in fact a component present at any point along the frequency scale.

The other type of aperiodic signal is a single event of very brief duration, such as the one shown in Fig. 9-3B. Such an impulse is often called a *transient*. While random noise spectra could extend over a very limited range of frequencies, the salient feature of the spectra of transients is that they always extend over a very wide bandwidth. They are therefore called *broad-band* signals.

SUMMARY Periodic waveforms will always be represented by line spectra. The spacing of the harmonic lines is equal to the fundamental frequency. The pattern of the harmonic amplitudes is independent of the fundamental frequency. Aperiodic waveforms generally have continuous spectra. Long-duration signals may have energy across a relatively restricted range of frequencies. Transients, however, are broadband signals.

It is very important that these principles be thoroughly understood. The interpreta-

tion of speech spectrograms depends on them.

Damped Waves

A damped wave is one whose amplitude decreases with time. Figure 9-4A shows a relatively simple damped wave, while Figure 9-4B is the repeated damped vocal waveform typically produced in pulse register (vocal fry) phonation (Coleman, 1963; Wendahl, Moore, and Hollien, 1963, Cavallo, Baken, and Shaiman, 1984).

A tuning fork provides an excellent example of damping. The amplitude of its vibrations, and hence of the tone it generates, diminishes exponentially after it is struck because it is continually losing energy (which is radiated out as an acoustic wave). The rate of energy loss can be increased by packing an energy-absorbing material, such as cotton, between the tines or dipping them in oil. The vibrations will then die out even more quickly. All sound sources lose energy, and unless it is replaced (from the power supply in an oscillator, the spring mechanism in the alarm clock, or what have you) the acoustic vibration ceases. If the energy loss is relatively rapid, the sound dies away quickly and the generator is said to be highly damped. Less damped systems conserve energy better and, like a

A **B**

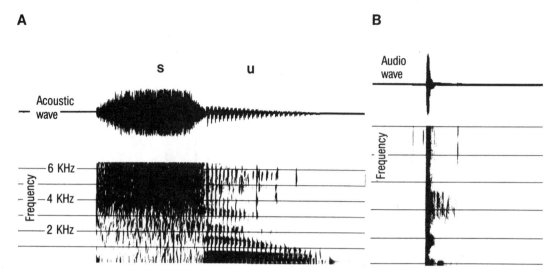

FIGURE 9–3. (A). Broad-band spectrogram of /su/. Note the spectral differences between the fricative and the vowel.(B). Broad-band spectrum of a single acoustic event of very brief duration. Note the distribution of energy through the frequency range.

church bell, continue to "ring" for a long time after initial excitation. The spectra of all damped oscillations have certain common characteristics. Because many speech sounds represent damped waves, and because the spectra of damped oscillations provide insight into the very important phenomenon called resonance, the subject merits some exploration at this point.

The bottom trace of Figure 9-5 shows a damped wave over a fairly short period of time. Clearly, taken as a whole, the segment shown is itself a complex wave whose period is the time it takes for the wave to decay to essentially zero amplitude. Since this is a complex wave, it must be composed of a set of sine waves. Some of these components are also shown in Figure 9-5. The frequencies of the constituent sine waves are *not* simple whole-number multiples of the fundamental frequency. They are, therefore, not harmonics. One of the components has a frequency of 90 Hz ($0.9 \times F_0$) and the other a frequency of 110 Hz ($1.1 \times F_0$). Close inspection of the diagram will show how these three components can add to produce the damped 100 Hz wave. At the start all the waves are pretty much synchronized—they are all rising together toward a maxi-

mum. But, given their frequency differences, they get out of synchrony with each other rather quickly, and pretty soon they are no longer adding constructively. The 110 Hz wave, for example, begins to go through its negative half cycle while the other two are still in their positive alternations. When this happens the amplitude of the 110 Hz wave begins to be subtracted from and to diminish the summed amplitude of the other two waves. The failure of synchrony increases with time until the net sum of the three waves is zero.

Figure 9-6 shows that the closer to the center frequency the component waves are (the narrower the band-width), the slower the decay (the less damping) of the waveform. That is, greater frequency spread of the components results in greater damping and, hence, faster decay. This should be intuitively appealing. A single, instantaneous pulse, or transient, can be considered to be infinitely damped. Recall that it was stated earlier that a pulse is a broad-band (very wide spectrum) signal.

In point of fact, the summations of Figure 9-5 only produce approximations of oscillations that decay to zero amplitude, and not very good approximations at that. A

A

B

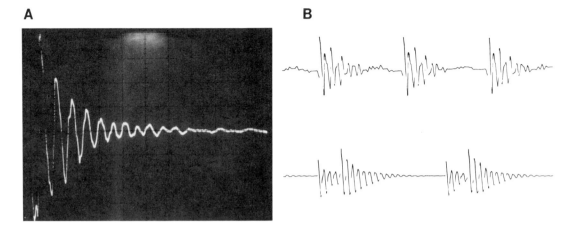

FIGURE 9–4. (A) A relatively simple damped wave—a lingualveolar "click." (B). Damped vocal wave-forms, typical of pulse-register phonation.

damped wave is really composed of a huge number of frequency components clustered about a cental value of maximal amplitude. In fact, since the damped wave is not a repeating (i.e., periodic) waveform, it is not surprising to find that it is composed of an *infinite number* of component frequencies. The amplitude of the envelope decreases exponentially with distance from the central value; therefore spectrum envelopes of all damped waves have a certain similarity. But for lightly damped waves the height drops rapidly to produce a sharply peaked narrow envelope, while highly damped waves have a broad spectrum envelope.

Resonance

The concept of impedance was introduced in Chapter 2. It was said that impedance has two components: resistive and reactive. The first represents energy dissipation, the second measures energy storage. When considering damping, in the section on "Damped Waves," these same factors were alluded to. That is, damping was said to be due to the dissipation of energy that had been stored in an oscillating body. In a mechanical system (such as a vibrating mass) energy is lost through friction, and it is stored in the momentum and compliance (the reciprocal of elasticity) of the

vibrating structure. (Momentum and compliance are the mechanical equivalents of electrical inductance and capacitance.) The degree to which energy can be stored as momentum is called the *mass reactance*; the capacity to store energy in the compliance is called *compliant reactance*.

In many ways, momentum and elasticity oppose each other. The magnitude of the energy that goes into momentum storage (mass reactance) increases as the frequency of the oscillation rises. The energy stored in elastic elements (compliant reactance)

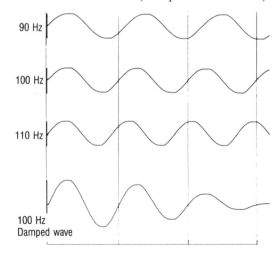

FIGURE 9–5. A damped 100 Hz wave (bottom) and three of its component frequencies (top: 90 Hz; second: 100 Hz; third: 110 Hz).

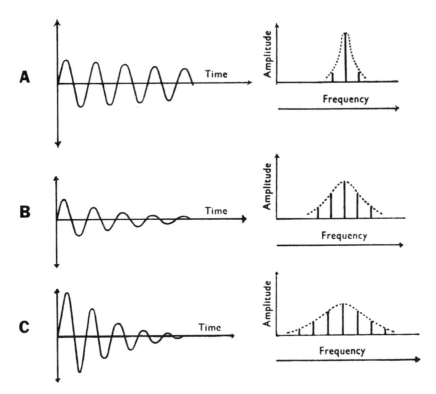

FIGURE 9–6. Relationship between the degree of damping and the width of the amplitude spectrum. Minimally damped waves (A) have very narrow spectra, while strongly damped waves (C) have wide spectra.

decreases as frequency increases. Furthermore, they are out of phase with each other. When one type of reactance is storing energy, the other tends to be losing it. In any given mechanical system the magnitude of the mass reactance is almost certain to be different from the magnitude of the compliant reactance. What this means is that they will not be well timed in terms of energy withdrawal from, and return to, the vibrating system. However, since the compliant reactance diminishes with increasing vibrational frequency, while the mass reactance grows as the vibration rate increases, for any given system there must be one particular frequency at which the two reactances are equal. At this special frequency, momentum and compliance are exactly out of phase with each other. As one is giving energy back to the system the other is absorbing it. In short, at one spe-

cial frequency in any system energy will be optimally transferred back and forth between the momentum and compliance storage capacities. The two reactances exactly cancel each other, and thus the net total reactance of the system at this particular frequency will be zero. Since impedance is the sum of resistive and reactive parts, it follows that at this particular frequency the total impedance must be minimal (and, in fact, is equal to the magnitude of the resistive component alone).

A system is said to be "resonant" at the frequency at which its impedance is thus minimized. Since impedance represents opposition to energy transfer, it is clear that a resonant system is at peak vibrational efficiency. At resonance, a system vibrates with maximum amplitude.

A basic law of physics says that power transfer is optimalized when the internal impedance of the power source exactly matches the impedance of the system it is feeding. At the resonant frequency, the impedance of a system is determined only by the resistive, or energy-dissipating, component. Recalling that energy dissipation is otherwise known as damping, it becomes clear that the impedance match between a source of power and a vibrational system at the resonant frequency is a function of the damping in the system. Consider the curves of Figure 9-7, which shows what earlier were referred to as the spectrum envelopes of damped waves. In this context we read the graph somewhat differently, however. It is taken to show how much attenuation of an input frequency occurs as that frequency deviates from the unique

frequency at which the system is exactly resonant. Figure 9-7A shows the spectrum of a vibrational system with very little damping. In other words, the frictional component is very small. Almost all of the impedance of the system is due to the reactive components. As the frequency of the system's vibration nears the resonant frequency, these reactive forces tend to cancel each other more and more, and at resonance they cancel each other completely, and thus play no role. Since the resistive component is very small, there is very little to prevent the response curve from growing very high and very rapidly as the reactive elements are cancelled out. Therefore, with very light damping a resonant system is very sharply tuned, which is to say that

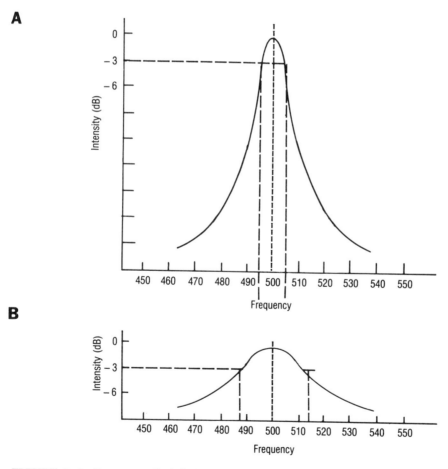

FIGURE 9–7. Response of lightly damped (A) and strongly damped (B) resonators. The dashed lines indicate the lower cutoff, resonant, and upper cutoff frequencies.

it responds with great efficiency in a very narrow band of frequencies. In the case of Figure 9-7B, however, the damping factor is great. There is a lot of frictional (resistive) loss in the system. As the reactive elements increasingly cancel each other, the total impedance of the system remains quite high because of the presence of its large resistive component. The response curve cannot grow as fast, nor can it grow as high. High damping is indicative of a broadly tuned resonant system, one that will respond with significant efficiency over a broad range of frequencies. Notice that all of this matches the statements made about the spectra of damped waveforms. In fact, we have arrived at the same conclusions from a different direction. Highly damped systems have broad frequency bands, and are, therefore, broadly-tuned resonators. Lightly damped systems are sharply tuned resonators with narrow bandwidth.

The bandwidth of the resonator is not sharply delimited, however. The response curve has no obvious cutoff, above or below which the system is utterly unresponsive. In fact, the spectrum envelope never actually reaches the zero line. Instead, it draws closer and closer to it, without ever actually touching it. It does get very close, however, and beyond some point we can say that for all intents and purposes a zero level has been reached. (In the language of mathematics, the curve is said to achieve an *asymptotic approximation* to zero.)

The lack of a clear frequency cutoff point for the system response leaves us with the problem of how we define the bandwidth. Like an old general, the system's response does not die, it just fades away. The question that has to be resolved is how much fading a general has to do before we no longer accord him military privileges? How much reduction in response must the system show before we call it effectively unresponsive. The answer must lie in some arbitrary value that everyone agrees to use in describing resonant systems. The agreement that has been reached is the following: The cutoff frequency is that point in the response curve where power transmis-sion is reduced by one-half. A power reduction of one-half is equivalent to a power loss of 3 dB. For a sine wave, a reduction of wave amplitude to 0.7071 times the peak amplitude represents a 3 dB power drop. Therefore, the cutoff frequencies are those frequencies whose amplitude is 0.7071 times the amplitude of the central frequency. We agree to say that the bandwidth of a system is the distance between the frequencies (one above and one below the central frequency on the curve) whose amplitudes are 0.7071 times the peak amplitude or, equivalently, whose power is 3 dB less than peak power. (The cutoff points of the response are sometimes called the "3 dB down" points or the "half-power" points.)

There is one other property of resonators that must be considered, because it greatly affects the methodology of spectrum analysis of speech sounds. The amount of damping in a system determines not only the sharpness of its tuning, but the amount of time required for vibrations at the resonant frequency to build up to their final amplitude. A lightly damped system (electrical or mechanical) responds to a very narrow range of frequencies, but it responds rather slowly. The amplitude of an applied vibration grows slowly until a final value is achieved. On the other hand, a strongly damped, broad-band resonator will respond very quickly to an applied vibration, but it will respond to vibrations over a broad range. The amount of time required for a system to respond is expressed in the *time constant*, which states the amount of time (in seconds) for the system to increase its vibration amplitude by a given percentage (the actual number need not concern us here).

The properties of resonators can therefore be summarized as follows:

- The bandwidth of a resonator is the distance between those frequencies at which the output is reduced to 0.7071 of the maximum ouput. These cutoff frequencies are also called the half-power points or the 3 dB down points.

- Highly damped resonators have wide bandwidths. That is, they respond relatively strongly to a broad range of frequencies.
- Lightly damped resonators have narrow bandwidths. Their response is limited to frequencies closely clustered about a central value.
- Highly damped resonators respond quickly, building up their vibrations to a maximal amplitude in a short time.
- Lightly damped resonators respond more sluggishly. Vibrational amplitude develops more slowly.
- The response time of a resonator is expressed in the time constant. Highly damped, broad bandwidth resonators have short time constants; lightly damped, narrow bandwidth resonators have long time constants. Therefore, the time constant is a somewhat indirect measure of bandwidth.

Air-space resonators

The discussion thus far has considered mechanical resonating systems. But air also has mechanical characteristics: It has mass and is compressible (implying that it has compliance). Therefore, if confined within a suitably constructed space, a quantity of air will behave as a resonator. Consider, for example, the simple bottle of air, shown in Figure 9-8, called a Helmholtz resonator. It has a narrow neck that is attached to a spherical bulb. When excited by brief acoustic pulse, the column of air in the neck is forced inward, acting as a cylindrical slug with inward momentum. The inward-moving air slug compresses the comparatively large air mass in the bulb, thereby transferring its kinetic energy to the air's compliance. The compressed air then begins to re-expand, and in doing so tranfers energy back to the slug of air in the neck, which regains momentum in an outward direction. The rate at which this sequence of events occurs is determined by the volume of the bulb and the width of the neck. Therefore, the system is resonant at a certain frequency. If a periodic pulse wave ex-

cites this system at its resonant frequency, the air in the neck will oscillate back and forth with maximal amplitude. At other pulse frequencies the response will be very weak.

The Helmholtz resonator is a very simple system, but it is easy to imagine much more complex ones. For instance, the neck of the resonator could open into another bulb, which is connected via another neck to yet another bulb, and so on. Not surprisingly, such a complex system will have more than one resonance peak in its response. Furthermore, the various chambers will interact with each other so that the resonance peaks of the whole system are not

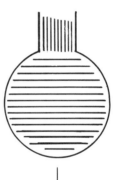

A Helmholtz resonator can be considered to contain two air masses.
A slug of air in the neck,

and a larger pillow of air in the body.

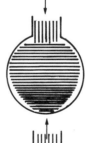

When a momentary pulse of high pressure arrives, it pushes the slug of air inward,

forcing it to compress the pillow of air in the body.

When the high pressure disappears, the slug of air is pushed back out by the decompression recoil of the compressed air pillow.

The size of the air masses determines the speed of the air-pillow's response. If the high-pressure pulses arrive at an interval that matches the air mass's response time, the system will resonate. Any other pulse repetition rate elicits a much weaker response.

FIGURE 9-8. The Helmholtz resonator.

at the frequencies of the isolated chambers.

The complex resonator just described very much resembles the vocal tract, which is also an air-filled cavity of complex shape.

SOURCE-FILTER THEORY OF THE VOCAL TRACT

A powerful model that explains how the vocal tract produces different vowels is called the *source-filter theory* of vowel production (Stevens, Kasowski, and Fant, 1953; Stevens and House, 1961). The model describes the glottis as the source of a harmonic-rich signal that is applied to the complex filter of the vocal tract resonances. Some of the harmonics in the glottal signal fall at or near the resonance peaks in the vocal tract transfer function, and are therefore enhanced. Other harmonics are attenuated because they lie beyond the cut-off points of the resonance peaks. Therefore, they contibute very little to the shape of the final waveform at the mouth opening. As the vocal tract changes shape its resonance frequencies change, and different vowels are perceived by a listener.

Glottal Source Characteristics

Figure 9-9A shows the waveform of the airflow signal (*glottal volume velocity*) actually produced at the glottis. Note that it is very different from the waveshape of any of the vowels shown elsewhere in this text. Since the glottal waveform is not a sine wave (but is periodic), it must have a line spectrum, as shown in Figure 9-9B. The F_0 in this illustration is 100 Hz, and the spectrum's lines are spaced 100 Hz apart. Note that the harmonics grow weaker as their frequency increases. The roll-off is about 6 dB per octave.* This is characteristic of the glottal signal.

----

*At the level of the larynx itself the roll-off is actually steeper. The radiation properties of the mouth opening, however, change this to produce an *effective* slope of -6 dB/octave.

Vocal Tract Filter

The supralaryngeal vocal tract behaves as a tube resonator, in many ways similar to an organ pipe. (The acoustics of such a system are complex and will not be discussed in detail here.) Figure 9-10, however, shows some configurations of the vocal tract and the transfer functions associated with them. At the top is the relaxed shape of the tract, asssumed for the neutral vowel. This is the simplest shape of the tract, and it results in a simple transfer function. In fact, this transfer function is very similar to that of a straight tube. The peaks show the frequencies at which the vocal tract is resonant. The resonance peaks of the vocal tract are called *formants*. There is a popular misconception that the formants are the emphasized frequencies in the final speech output. This is NOT the case. The formants represent vocal tract resonances. It will be seen shortly that the distinction between vocal tract formants (resonances) and the amplitude of the spectral lines (emphasized frequencies) of the speech signal is an important one.

For a neutral vowel the formants are spaced regularly across the frequency scale and have comparable, if not equal, amplitudes. Movements of the articulators, especially the tongue and lips, produce more complex configurations of the vocal tract and hence much more complicated formant patterns. As the vocal tract assumes the postures required for different vowels, the formant peaks in the transfer function shift around and assume unequal heights. The transfer function may come to have an overall slope to it, either positive or negative (as shown in Figure 9-10 for /u/ and /i/). A large body of literature has shown that the perception of vocalic sounds (vowels, liquids, glides, and nsasls) depends heavily on the formant characteristics as reflected in the final acoustic signal radiated from the lips. These characteristics in turn depend on the location of constrictions in the vocal tract (Chiba and Kajiyama, 1941; Stevens and House, 1955, 1961; Fant, 1960; Dunn, 1950). A good technical review of

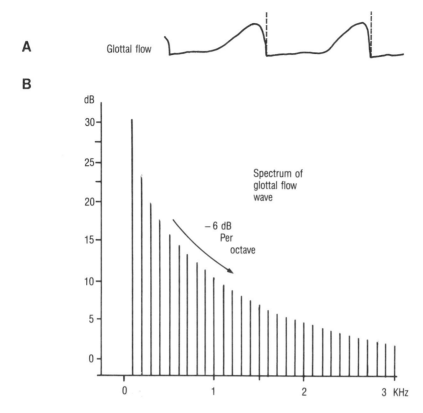

FIGURE 9–9. (A).Typical glottal waveform. (B). Line spectrum of the glottal wave as it would be measured at the lips. Note the *roll-off* of about 6 dB/octave.

the relationships between vocal tract shape and the resultant acoustic signals has been published by Fant (1980).

Source-Filter Interaction:
The Spectra of Vowels

What we have for vowel production, then, is a glottal signal, whose component harmonics progressively diminish in amplitude, and a vocal tract transfer function that has irregularly spaced resonant peaks of differing heights. The spectrum of the vowel that is ultimately produced is a function of the characteristics of both contributions, glottal and tract. (The contribution of the glottal source does not vary significantly with changes in the vocal tract shape.) As shown in Figure 9-11, the two *interact*. Therefore, any acoustic analysis of the final product simultaneously evaluates both

the glottal source and the supralaryngeal filter characteristics. One of the tasks of spectrographic analysis is to separate the two functions.

In passing, it should be noted that the source-filter model assumes that the vocal tract acoustic characteristics do not significantly affect vocal-fold function. In other words, the source is considered to be independent of the filter. This is not really the case. For instance, constriction of the vocal tract results in higher supraglottal air pressure. This alters the magnitude of the transglottal pressure drop, and thereby modifies the vocal signal. Furthermore, the vocal tract characteristics affect vocal fold function. Low-frequency first formants tend to raise vocal F_0, while higher-frequency first formants lower it (Flanagan, Coker, Rabiner, Schafer, and Umeda, 1970). From a clinical point of view, these effects are

Vocal tract shape

Acoustic transfer function

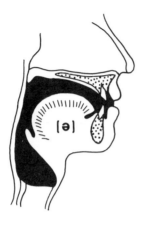

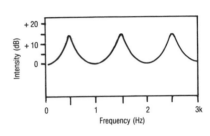

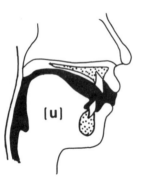

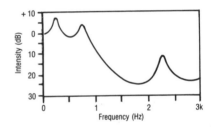

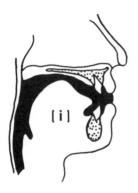

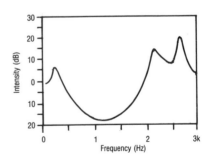

FIGURE 9–10. Configurations of the vocal tract and the acoustic transfer functions associated with them.

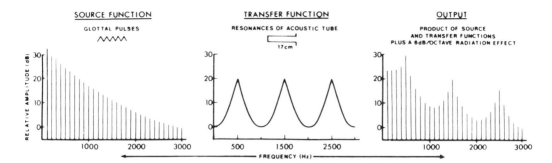

FIGURE 9–11. The spectral characteristics of the glottal source (left) interact with the resonant properties (or *transfer function*) of the vocal tract (center) to produce the spectral characteristics of the radiated sound wave. (Reprinted from Borden and Harris: *Speech Science Primer*. Baltimore: Williams and Wilkins, 1984. ©1984, The Williams and Wilkins Co., Baltimore, MD. Reprinted by permission.)

likely to be negligible. Nonetheless, the clinician will want to bear in mind that significant interactions are possible and, if they occur, they can alter the interpretation of a spectrum analysis.

Nonvowel Sounds

Airstream turbulence within the vocal tract produces aperiodic noises, and sudden release of impounded air pressure generates acoustic transients. These phenomena are associated with fricative and plosive production. In these cases the vocal tract serves as its own excitation source, but it retains its filter function. Sounds generated in the vocal tract itself are still radiated from the mouth only after being subjected to the resonant properties of the vocal tract.

Nasalization

Opening of the velopharyngeal port couples the nasal resonating cavities to the rest of the vocal tract, creating an entirely different vocal-tract transfer function. The spectral features of nasalization are considered in greater detail in Chapter 10.

SPECTROGRAPHIC INSTRUMENTATION

Although the physical and mathematical principles of spectrum analysis are well understood, their application for speech

spectrography nonetheless presents a number of problems. The speech signal constantly changes, so any practical method must be capable of continuous analysis. At the same time, it is often useful to determine the exact spectral characteristics of a single sound at a single time point selected from a flow of speech, and therefore a practical method should also be able to do "spot analysis." The display of the spectrum as it changes during an utterance must be in a form that is easily interpreted. (Imagine trying to make sense of a very large succession of transfer-function graphs!) Finally, practical spectrography should be relatively simple to do. If the instrumentation requires an elaborate setup procedure or critical adjustments, the results will not usually be worth the time and trouble invested.

Sound spectrograms can be generated by two different methods. Analog techniques use electronic filtering of the speech signal, while digital methods involve direct numeric implementation of Fourier analysis.

Analog Methods

A conceptually simple means of visualizing the ever-changing spectrum of a speech signal is exemplified by the *visible speech translator* of Dudley and Gruenz (1946), shown in Figure 9-12. The speech input from a microphone is fed to a bank of bandpass filters. When there is a harmon-

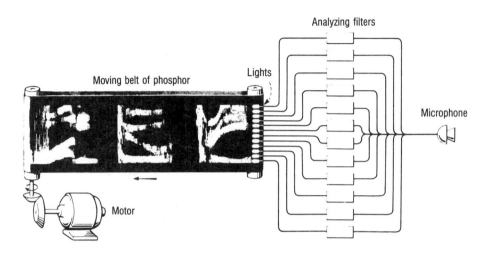

FIGURE 9–12. The *Visible Speech Translator* of Dudley and Gruenz, 1946. (From Potter, R. K., Kopp, G. A. and Kopp, H. G. *Visible Speech.* New York: van Nostrand, 1947. Figure 1, p. 17. Reprinted by permission.)

ic whose frequency falls within the band of one of the filters, it is passed to the output of that filter with an amplitude that is proportional to its strength. This output is used to light a miniature lamp associated with each filter. The lamp shines on a moving belt of phosphorescent material, which then glows with a brightness related to the brightness of the bulb. As the belt moves it displays the recent history of the brightness of each of the lamps. The result is a three-dimensional record that shows the changes in frequency components and their amplitudes (shown as brightness variations) over time. The phosphorescent screen thus displays a spectrogram of the type that is still most prevalent.

A major advantage of this system is that it generates a "real-time" display. The spectrogram appears with almost no delay at all. But even when the complications of the phosphor belt are eliminated by substitution of a cathode-ray (oscilloscope) tube as the display device (Riesz and Schott, 1946), this instrument has significant limitations imposed by the large number of filters, each of which (although not shown in the diagram) has an amplifier and other support circuitry associated with it. Increasing

frequency resolution requires narrower filter bandwidths, which in turn implies that a larger number of filters is needed to cover the frequency range of the speech signal. Despite special techniques that reduce the number of filters involved (Wood and Hewitt, 1963), the amount of circuitry is likely to grow quickly as increased frequency precision is called for. Reducing the *frequency* resolution in order to improve *time* resolution (so as to be able to see transient speech events) also involves changing all of the filters. In short, the system is inflexible and therefore limited in the types of analyses it can achieve without major modification. For these reasons, the visible speech translator was superceded by another instrument developed at about the same time: the sound spectrograph. It is this instrument, with surprisingly little modification, that is still the most popular for sound spectrum analysis. Developed by Koenig, Dunn, and Lacy (1946), the sound spectrograph is by far the most widely used device for spectrum analysis of speech. It is a very versatile instrument that can operate in a number of different analytic modes. It is also flexible, allowing important parameters such as filter bandwidth to be selected by the user. The versatility and flexibility come at a price, however. The analysis method is different from, and somewhat more complex than, the relatively simple approaches considered thus far. A moderately large number of parameters need to be adjusted by the user (see Figure 9-13). Therefore, the user needs to understand the workings of this instrument somewhat better than is usual for other instrumentation in order to obtain even minimally acceptable results. This section will dissect a typical sound spectrograph and explore in some detail how its functional elements work interact. The specific unit to be considered is the Sonagraph® of Kay Elemetrics, which is the most popular sound spectrograph. It is very similar to the other widely used analog spectrograph, the Voice Identification Laboratories series 700.

Overview of Sonagraph function

The Sonagraph stores the signal to be analyzed on a built-in magnetic recording surface. During analysis this recording is played back over and over again, hundreds of times. With each repetition the center frequency of a band pass filter system is increased. Each scan, then, serves to detect the presence of vibrational energy at a somewhat higher frequency than was detected during the previous scan. When a frequency within the bandwidth of the filter is present, a voltage is generated that causes a stylus to blacken a sensitive sheet of paper.

The paper on which the spectrogram is printed (actually, etched) is wrapped around a drum mounted on top of the unit. The drum rotates once for each playback of the recorded signal. Each point on the circumference of the rotating drum is thus associated with a single point in time in the recording. When the paper is unwrapped, each location along its horizontal dimension will similarly be associated with a single point in the recording that was analyzed. As the center frequency of the analyzing filter moves higher, so does the position of the marking stylus. Therefore, when the stylus marks the paper (indicating detection of a certain frequency) the height of the stylus (and thus the mark) on the paper will show what the center frequency of the filter was, while the location along the papers length represents the point in time at which this frequency component was present. After many repetitions, a spectrogram is built up.

Recording, playback, and writing systems

Under the top cover of the Sonagraph is a large, heavy metal disc whose edge is coated with a magnetic medium (Fig. 9-14). An electromagnetic record and reproduce head (see Chap. 4) is held against the surface by a spring-lever system. In essence, this assembly constitutes a tape recorder in which the tape is fused to the edge of the disc. The disc is turned by a motor system at a speed of 25 rpm, moving the entire recording surface past the heads in 2.4 s, which, therefore, represents the longest segment that can be recorded. Input can be from a microphone or an external tape recorder. If analysis of a sample longer than 2.4 s is to be done, the tape recording can be advanced and analyzed in sequential 2.4 second increments. Circuits have been designed that automate the tape advance (Carmeci and Jorgensen, 1960).

(The Voice Identification spectrographs use a design by Prestigiacomo [1957] that circumvents the need to re-record contiguous short samples. The prerecorded tape to be analyzed is wrapped around the base of the drum, and it serves as the magnetic surface that is repeatedly scanned by a revolving playback head. At the end of the analysis the tape is automatically advanced the proper distance for the next sample.)

Firmly bolted atop the large metal disc is a tall drum on which the recording paper is mounted. Drum and disc are a single mechanical unit and rotate together. This linkage assures the exact correspondence of points on the paper with points in the magnetic recording. The disc-drum assembly is also linked by a drive belt (Figure 9-14C) to a vertical screw that moves

A

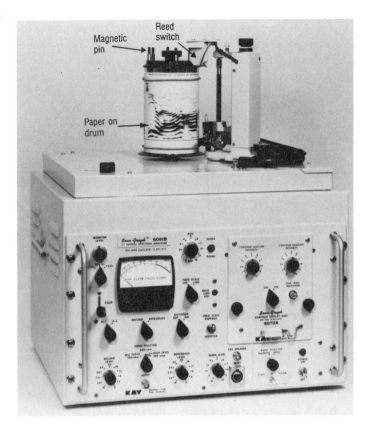

B

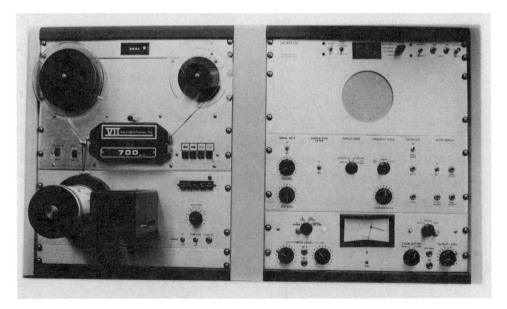

FIGURE 9–13. Sound spectrographs. (A). The Kay Elemetrics model 6061. (B). Voice Identification Laboratories' series 700.

the marking stylus. Rotation of the disc causes the screw to turn, carrying the stylus upward along the vertical axis of the drum and the paper mounted on it. The vertical stylus movement, in turn, tunes the analyzing filter system to ever higher frequencies (by a system described below).

In the Sonagraph, then, the record and reproduce surface (disc edge), paper carrier (drum), display marker. positioner (drive screw), and analyzing-filter center-frequency control are all linked to each other to form a single mechanical system.

Analysis and display systems

Figure 9-15 illustrates the general scheme of signal processing in the Sonagraph. The discussion of how the Sonagraph performs a spectrum analysis will be organized to follow the signal path as shown in this diagram.

After a speech sample has been captured on the magnetic surface, the recording process is stopped by switching to the *reproduce mode*. The reproduce amplifiers now receive signals *from* the record head, allowing the user to verify that the recording is adequate. As mentioned ear1ier, the Sonagraph analyzes the sample by doing many scans of it, each time detecting a higher frequency than during the previous scan. The analysis range is normally from 80 to 8000 Hz. For recording, the disc turns at a rate of 25 rpm to provide a 2.4 s recording time. At this speed the multiple scans needed for analysis would take an inordinately long time—on the order of 15 min—to complete. Therefore, when set for analysis, the playback is done at 12 times recording speed, or 300 rpm. A single scan thus requires only 0.2 s, and the analysis takes only about 1.3 min.

Playback at 12 times the recording speed also means that all waveforms will be reproduced at 12 times their real-time frequency. So, instead of detecting frequency components up to 8000 Hz the Sonagraph will really scan from 0 to 96 kHz. The functional block diagram shows the output of the reproduce amplifier as lying in this range, and all the circuitry of the analyzer is designed to work with these frequencies.

The output of the reproduce section is connected to one input of a mixer circuit called a *balanced modulator*.* The modulator also receives an input from a *carrier oscillator*, whose output frequency is varied from 200 kHz to 296 kHz during the course of the analysis. The output of the demodulator is fed to a band pass filter whose center frequency is fixed at 200 kHz. When two sine waves are mixed together the resulting signal includes components at frequencies equal to the sum of the mixed frequencies and to the difference between the mixed frequencies. To understand how this can be used in the analysis, suppose that the signal recorded on the Sonagraph is a 1000 Hz sine wave. When played back at high speed for analysis, the recorded signal becomes a 12000 Hz wave applied to the modulator. With each scan, the output frequency of the variabile oscillator increases, from a low of 200 kHz to a high of 296 kHz. At some point during the frequency sweep the oscillator's output will be 212 kHz. When it is, the difference between it and the input signal of 12 kHz will equal exactly 200 kHz. Since this corresponds to the center frequency of the filter, an output will get through to the marking circuit, and the recording paper will be blackened. When, in this sample, the variable oscillator is feeding any frequency other than 212 kHz to the modulator, its output will be simply the oscillator frequency. Because the sample being analyzed contains only a 12 kHz (originally 1 kHz) component, the difference between any other oscillator frequency, F_{Osc}, and the sample frequency is $F_{Osc} - 0$ Hz $= F_{Osc}$. If the recorded sample contained only two frequencies, say 1 kHz and 4 kHz, then there would be an output from the 200 kHz filter only when the oscillator was producing 212 kHz and 248 kHz.

In the case of a complex signal, such as

---

*The entire method of frequency detection and recording is an extension of a plan originally developed by Ballantine (1933).

A

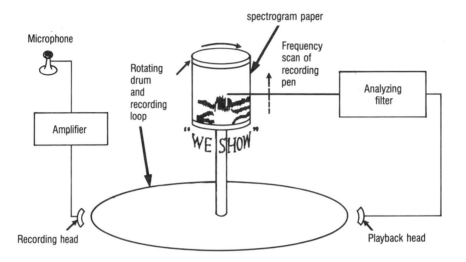

Microphone

Amplifier

Rotating drum and recording loop

spectrogram paper

Frequency scan of recording pen

"WE SHOW"

Analyzing filter

Recording head

Playback head

B

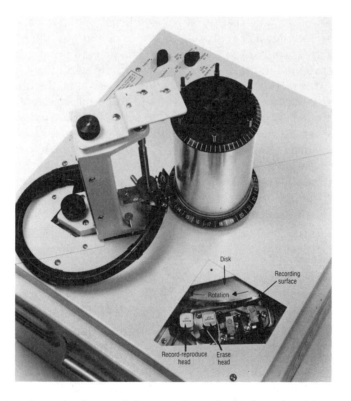

Disk

Recording surface

Rotation

Record-reproduce head

Erase head

FIGURE 9–14. (A). General schema of the recording, playback, and writing system of the Kay Sonagraph. (From Pickett, *The Sounds of Speech Communication*. Baltimore: University Park Press, 1980, Figure 15, p. 36. ©1980 by University Park Press. Reprinted by permission.) (B).Recording surface (disc edge) and record and playback head of the Sonagraph. (C). A drive belt transfers rotation of the recording surface (disc) to a vertically mounted screw on which the stylus travels. As the

C

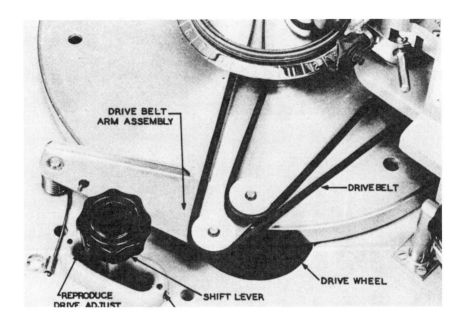

DRIVE BELT
ARM ASSEMBLY

DRIVE BELT

DRIVE WHEEL

REPRODUCE
DRIVE ADJUST

SHIFT LEVER

D

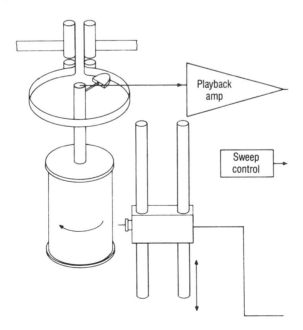

Playback
amp

Sweep
control

recording is repeatedly played, the turning of the screw carries the stylus upward along the drum on which the sensitive paper is mounted. The stylus assembly is attached to a variable resistor that controls the Sonagraph's oscillator. (D). Recording and playback system of the Voice Identification series 700 spectrograph.

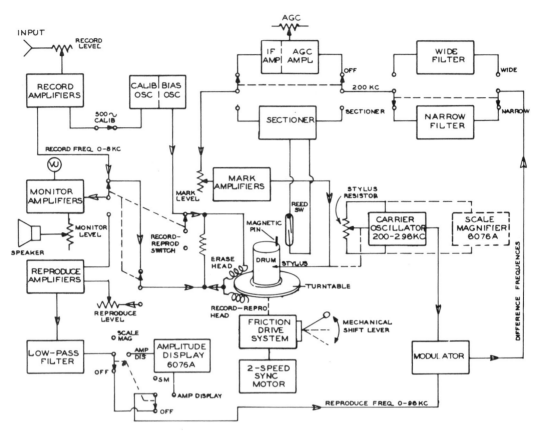

FIGURE 9-15. Functional block diagram of the Kay Elemetrics Sonagraph.

speech, mixing the oscillator frequency with the frequencies of the sample produces a great number of difference frequencies. But there will be an output from the 200 kHz filter if and only if one of those difference frequencies is 200 kHz. This can only happen if there is a frequency component in the sample signal (in its speeded-up form) that is 200 kHz lower than the oscillator frequency at any given moment. Therefore, sweeping the oscillator from 200 kHZ to 296 kHz will cause analysis for frequencies from 0 to 96 kHz, which is equivalent to 0 to 8000 Hz at the original recording speed. (A much simpler "Visual Speech Spectrum Analyzer" that uses this principle to produce a display on an oscilloscope screen has been described by Potvin, Foreit, Lam, Trued, and Potvin, 1980).

The frequency of the oscillator in the sound spectrograph is controlled by a potentiometer that is physically linked to the marking stylus. We have already seen that the stylus is mounted on a screw that moves it vertically on the paper as the drum system turns. Height of the stylus, therefore, corresponds to the carrier oscillator frequency, which in turn determines what component frequencies (if any) will be different by exactly 200 kHz and will, therefore, cause an output through the filter to the marking stylus.

FILTERS. Up to this point it has been assumed that the filter passes only signals that exactly correspond to its center frequency of 200 kHz. This cannot actually be the case, of course: every bandpass filter has a bandwidth that includes a range of frequencies. What this means in the Sonagraph is that the filter causes the paper to be marked not only when the modulator output contains a 200 kHz output, but whenever the output frequency is near 200 kHz and within the bandwidth of the filter.

This has significant consequences for the appearance of the spectrogram and for the kind of information that is displayed. Consider again the case in which the signal recorded on the magnetic surface is a pure 1000 Hz sine wave. As the carrier oscillator increases its frequency from 200 to 296kHz, the difference frequencies out of the modulator will go from 188 to 284 kHz. (Remember that a recorded signal of 1000 Hz becomes a signal of 12,000 Hz on playback.) Suppose now that the output filter has a bandwidth of 45 Hz. In that case, the filter will pass any difference signal that is less than 22.5 Hz away from the center frequency, that is lying between 199,977.5 Hz and 200,022.5 Hz. Since the carrier oscillator frequency depends on the height of the stylus on the page, it is clear that a 1000 Hz signal will produce a bar on the paper rather than a single line falling exactly at

the height that corresponds to precisely 1000 Hz. The bar will have a thickness equivalent to 45 Hz-worth of height on the paper, and it will be centered on the height equivalent to 1000 Hz. Such a spectrogram is shown in Figure 9-16A.

Imagine that the filter is changed. Its center frequency is still 200 kHz, but its bandwidth is increased to 300 Hz. Now the difference frequencies that are passed lie within 150 Hz on either side of the center frequency—from 199,850 Hz to 200,150 Hz. The stylus will, therefore, mark a broader band centered on a height equivalent to 1000 Hz; the marked area will have a width equivalent to 300 Hz on the vertical scale, as shown in Figure 9-16B.

Clearly, the bandwidth of the analyzing filter determines the *frequency resolution* of the system. That is, with a 300 Hz filter two frequencies must lie at least 300 Hz apart in order to be seen as two separate lines in the spectrogram. The narrow-band 45 Hz filter can resolve two frequencies separated by only 45 Hz. It might seem that one would be better off always using a

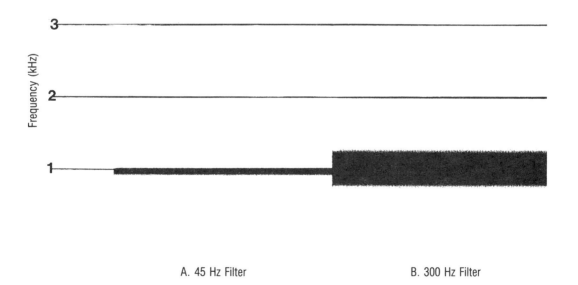

A. 45 Hz Filter

B. 300 Hz Filter

FIGURE 9–16. Effect of filter bandwidth on the spectrographic representation of a 1 kHz sine wave.

narrow-band filter. But this overlooks an important characteristic of filters that was discussed earlier: There is a trade-off between frequency resolution and time resolution. The narrow-band filter does, in fact, depict frequencies more precisely, but it is more sluggish in its response and, therefore, cannot show very rapid events. The wide-band filter does not permit as much accuracy in frequency determination, but it responds quickly, providing better resolution in time.

Speech signals often contain components less than 300 Hz apart that the speech pathologist might wish to resolve. However, speech is also characterized by rapid events (such as the opening and closing of the vocal folds) that the speech clinician may wish to see too. A single filter cannot serve both purposes, and therefore spectrographs usually provide a way to change the filter bandwidth. Typically, 45 Hz and 300 Hz filters are used, but other bandwidths may be selected for particular cases.

MARKING SYSTEM AND AUTOMATIC GAIN CONTROL. The final element in the analysis system is the mark amplifier. It produces a high-frequency, high-voltage signal that energizes the stylus for marking the paper. Each difference frequency from the modulator has an amplitude that is proportional to the amplitude of the signal component producing it. Therefore the signal passed by the analyzing filter system represents not only a given frequency in the recorded signal but the intensity of that frequency as well. The mark amplifer causes the stylus to darken the paper in proportion to the intensity of the frequency component being passed. This gives the spectrogram a third dimension—grayness—that represents component intensity.

Unfortunately, the paper on which the spectrogram is produced has a limited gray range. The difference between the lightest and darkest shades that can be produced is about 10 dB on an optical (reflectivity) scale. The components of the speech signal, on the other hand, can easily encompass a 30 dB intensity range. Without some

modification of the signal it is very likely that the marking system would be easily saturated. All components more than 10 dB stronger than minimal intensity would be marked maximally black, eliminating a great deal of useful information from the spectrogram. To avoid this, and to permit the full range of speech-component intensities to be displayed in the limited gray range of the paper, the spectrograph has a circuit that compresses the analyzing-filter output into a limited voltage range. The *automatic gain control* (AGC) makes intense signals weaker (attenuates them) and weak signals stronger (amplifies them) so that they all lie within a 10 dB intensity range. Figure 9-17 illustrates this process. The amount of compression required depends on the range of intensities in the signal being analyzed. If a very "flat" signal is being processed, very little compression need be used. If, on the other hand, the signal has very large intensity variations, a lot of compression will be required to fit it into the available 10 dB gray range. The AGC is adjustable by the user by means of a front panel control.

Sectioning

The system just described produces three-dimensional (time x frequency x intensity) spectrograms. But a classic amplitude-over-frequency spectrum display of a given instant in the sample is often quite useful, since it quanitifies the harmonic intensities much more precisely than the gray scale can. The spectrograph uses a system devised by Kersta (1948) for generating such a display. In the jargon of spectrography it is called a *section* (because it represents a slice through the continuous time display of the standard spectrogram).

On top of the drum that carries the display paper is a circular plate with equally spaced holes around its circumference. The point in the recording at which a section is to be done is selected by screwing a small, rod-shaped magnet into the hole that is located just above it. A special reed switch, which closes in the presence of a

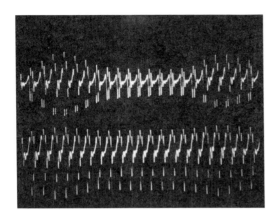

FIGURE 9–17. Function of an automatic gain control (AGC). The top trace, the input to the AGC circuit, shows considerable amplitude variability. The AGC works to minimize the amplitude changes and produces a more stable output, as shown in the bottom trace.

magnetic field, is swung into position over the plate. With each revolution of the drum, the magnet comes very close to the switch, causing it to close for just a brief moment. The switch closure causes a capacitor to be charged to a voltage proportional to the amplitude of the signal during the duration of the switch closure. As the drum rotates and the magnet is carried past the switch, it opens again, leaving the charged capacitor attached to a 100 kHz oscillator. The capacitor begins to lose charge, but the oscillator will produce an output just as long as any charge remains. The amount of time required for the capacitor to discharge will be determined by the amount of charge it originally acquired from the signal being analyzed. Therefore, the duration of the oscillator burst is proportional to the amplitude of the signal that was present at the time the reed switch closed. The oscillator output drives the mark amplifier, which produces a mark on the rotating paper for the duration of the burst. In this way, the magnitude of the signal being analyzed is converted to a horizontal line on the display paper.

When the reed switch closes the signal applied to the capacitor is not the signal in the recording but rather the 200 kHz signal out of the modulator. That is, the signal that charged the capacitor is one that represents the magnitude of a given frequency in the original recording. As was the case with the standard (frequency vs. time) spectrogram, the stylus moves across the paper, changing the frequency being analyzed. What the sectioner produces, however, is a series of lines that show the amplitude (on a dB scale) at successive frequencies. Figure 9-18 shows sections through a vowel and a fricative, using a 45 Hz and a 300 Hz bandpass analyzing filter.

Auxiliary functions

CALIBRATION AND TIMING MARKERS. Older spectrographs include a provision for generating a special tone that has strong harmonics, say every 500 Hz, that can be printed on the spectrogram together with the analysis of the signal. Newer models produce a line across the display at selected frequencies. Either way, the resultant marks (shown in Figure 9-18 along with the sections) serve as a scale for the vertical (frequency) dimension of the display. Similarly, timing marks can be made along the horizontal dimension of the spectrograph to facilitate evaluating the time course of events.

RECORDING PRE-EMPHASIS. By means of a front-panel switch, the characteristics of the record amplifier can be altered to permit two types of signal recordings. When the switch is set to "FL" the system has a flat frequency response: The recorded components will have amplitudes that are within a couple of dB of their original values. In the "HS" (High Shaping) position, however, the switch causes the recording to be made with a 13 dB "pre-emphasis." In other words, the amplitude of the recorded components increases with frequency so that 8 kHz components are recorded with 13 dB more gain than 100 Hz signals. This shaping of the recorded signal offsets (approximately) the roll-off in the spectrum of the glottal source, and thereby componen-

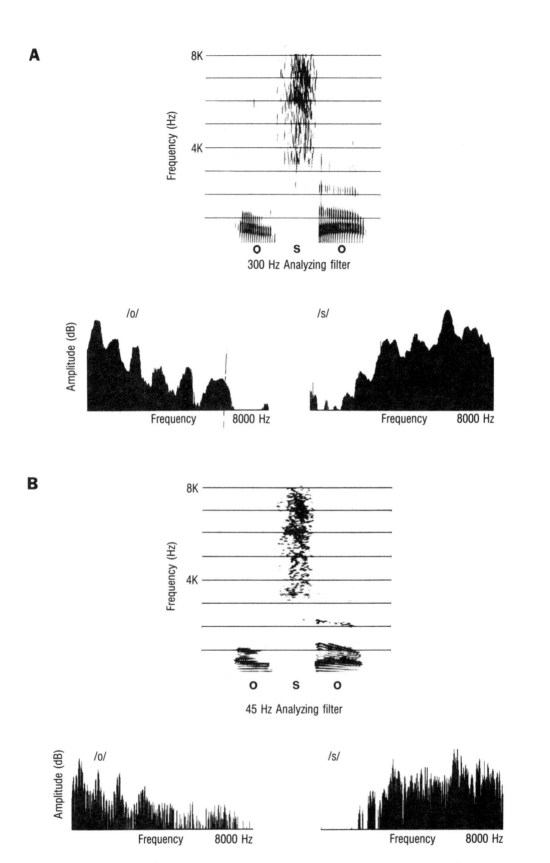

FIGURE 9–18. Spectral analysis of /oso/ using (A) 300 Hz and (B) 45 Hz filters. Below each spectrogram is a "section" (amplitude spectrum) through /o/ and /s/.

sates for it. Generally, speech spectrographic work is done with the HS function.

CONTOUR DISPLAY. Normally, intensity information is coded in the spectrogram as continuous gray shading. Grayness is the third dimension of the spectrogram, and it can be conceptualized as showing the height of the trace off the surface of the paper. The intensity scale can be more conveniently quantified by drawing what amounts to a contour map of intensities. A special *contour display* module provides this function. The output of the analyzing filter is connected to this module, whose output amplitude increases in discrete steps, rather than continuously, as the amplitude of the analyzing-filter output increases. Each step is equivalent to a 6 dB increase, and each step causes the page to be marked with a distinctly darker gray. Provision is also made for a very dark mark to be produced each time the contour display unit switches from one level to another. This produces clear contour lines separating the gray levels. Typically, a 42 dB range can be accomodated. Figure 9-19 shows a standard spectrogram and a contoured display of the same speech utterance.

ANCILLARY DATA DISPLAYS. Relating other (especially physiological) data to events shown in the spectrogram often helps in evaluating the nature of a clinical problem. Since the spectrograph is a frequency analyzer, it is possible to display other data along with the spectrum if those data can be put into frequency-modulated form. Horii (1980), for example, describes a means of displaying his HONC index (see Chapter 10) on a spectrogram of the speech sample during which it was generated. Suppose, as another example, that a pressure probe (see Chapter 7) is used to sense intraoral pressure during production of an utterance to be analyzed with the spectrograph. The output of the pressure transduction system need only be applied to a frequency modulator (see Chapter 3) to produce a variable-frequency signal that is recorded along with the speech signal. The spectrogram of the combined signals will show a standard spectrum analysis, together with an analysis of the frequency of the pressure signal. Typically, as in Figure 9-20, the speech signal is filtered before recording to eliminate any frequencies above about 4 kHz, leaving the upper half of the spectrogram vacant. The center frequency of the modulated signal is then set for 6 kHz, with a maximum deviation of 2 kHz, so that the ancillary signal occupies the otherwise-empty top part of the spectrogram.

Commercial spectrographs may include an *amplitude display* capability (first described by Carmeci and Jorgensen, 1960) that takes advantage of this process to show the (relative) amplitude of each point in the signal being evaluated. Kay Elemetrics also manufactures a plug-in unit that allows a pressure transducer to be connected directly to their Sonagraph to produce a pressure trace in the top half of the spectrogram. With just a little circuit design, however, the clinician will find it fairly easy to add any physiological signal to the spectrogram.

Digital Spectrography

Advances in integrated circuitry in the last several years opened the way for the creation of spectrographs that perform purely digital analysis of the sample. Analysis can be done by implementing the Fast Fourier Transform (Cooley and Tukey, 1965), cepstrum analysis (Noll, 1964, 1967; Schafer and Rabiner, 1970) or digital inverse filtering (Wakita, 1976) or more complex schemes (Paul, House, and Stevens, 1964).

Very recently, special circuits have been fitted to microprocessor (personal computer) systems to perform "on line" spectrum analysis. Companies such as Eventide Clockworks in New York, or IQS Inc. of Long Beach, CA have marketed models specifically for Pet and Apple computers. As yet, however, these units do not have sufficient resolution or flexibility for clinical use in speech pathology. The rapid evolution of faster, 16-bit microcomputers, however, may change this in the not-too-distant future.

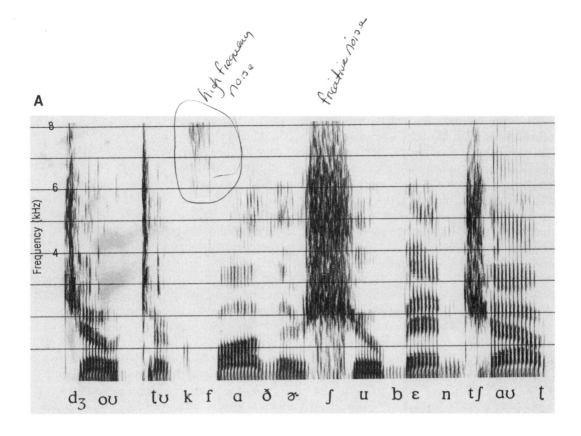

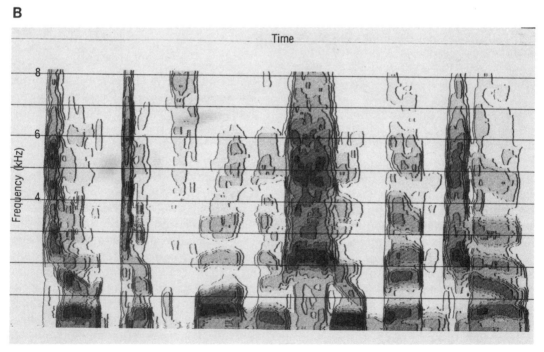

FIGURE 9–19. Standard (A) and contoured (B) spectrograms of the utterance "Joe took father's shoe bench out."

A

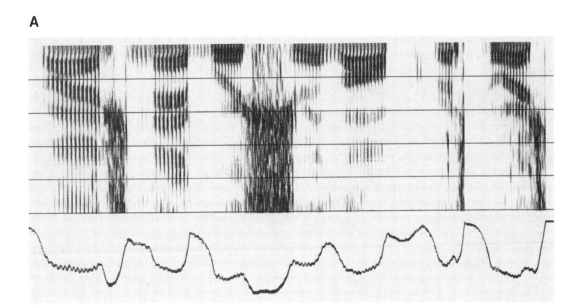

B

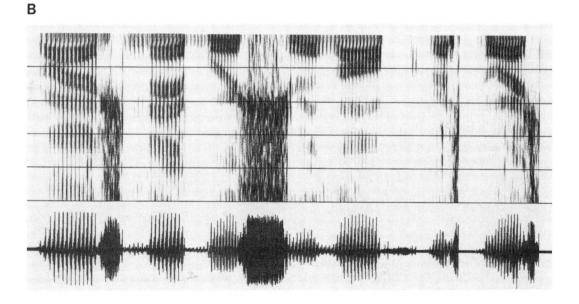

FIGURE 9–20. Ancillary displays on the spectrogram: 300 Hz-filter analyses of the sentence "Joe took father's shoe bench out." (A). Audio wave shown above spectrogram. (B). Audio amplitude shown above spectrogram.

The prime advantage of a purely digital system lies in the fact that the analysis is close to instantaneous, allowing the spectrogram to be generated as the sample is being spoken. Paper copies of the spectrogram, however, can only be produced by a special, add-on device. Changing characteristics of the system to meet special needs (shaping, filter bandwidth, frequency range, etc.) may be difficult. Amplitude-over-frequency sections often cannot be produced. To some extent, versatility has been sacrificed to convenience.

On the other hand, digital control techniques (implemented by incorporating a microprocessor into a spectrograph) can be applied to spectrograph function to facilitate much of the work that the speech clinician needs to do. Voice Identification, Inc. has produced a "real time digital spectrograph" that, in addition to producing video displays of spectrograms in color, can determine the duration of speech segments, calculate fundamental frequency, formant ranges, and the like. As with everything else in the digital electronics field, progress is rapid and the very term "status-quo" has little meaning.

Hybrid Analog and Digital Spectrography

Quite recently, Kay Elemetrics introduced a new spectrograph, the model 7800 (Figure 9-21). Although they call it a "digital Sonagraph," it is really a hybrid system. The input is digitized and stored in numeric form, but the analysis of the signal is accomplished with analog circuitry similar in most ways to the older models'.

The improvement over earlier, all-analog spectrographs is significant. Digital storage of the signal results in considerably less noise than magnetic recording. But more important, converting the input signal to a series of sequential numerical values and assigning an "address" to each value in memory sets the stage for precisely controlled access to any part of the signal. Also, it is possible to sample the input at one rate and read it out of memory at a different rate.

(This is equivalent to recording at on speed and playing back at another with a standard tape recorder.) Doing so changes the frequency range of the analysis.

The advantages of the hybrid technique are throroughly exploited in this instrument, which is extremely flexible and easy to tailor to the needs of a particular situation. Furthermore, many of the features that were add-on options in earlier Sonagraphs and other company's spectrographs have been included as standard capabilities in this model. Precise scale magnification, variable frequency range, three different filter bandwidths, amplitude display, and time-wave display are all built in the standard, unmodified instrument. (Examples of these functions are shown in Figure 9-20). The mechanical system for driving the display printer is also changed, making it considerably easier to use. The new "digital" Sonagraph really does not perform many functions that cannot be done by other units on the market. But it requires less in the way of add-on circuitry and "tinkering" to achieve what might otherwise require several different instruments. It is, in short, a convenient, highly flexible, extremely precise spectrographic system that can do almost anything that any other spectrograph can do. It is very rapidly gaining in popularity among both researchers and clinicians, and it will probably be the standard spectrograph for the next several years.

Another combined analog and digital spectrograph is the Speech Spectrographic Display (SSD) of Spectraphonics, Inc., illustrated in Figure 9-22. The analysis system is housed in the small case, and the display appears on a television monitor. The input signal is sampled by an analog-to-digital converter and stored in memory as a series of amplitude values. Analysis is by analog filtering. The analyzing filter bandwidths are 450 Hz and 600 Hz (a 300 Hz bandwidth is available as an option). Maximal sample duration is either 0.75 or 1.5 s, and input can be "live"or prerecorded. An unusual feature of the SSD is the fact that two separate inputs can be displayed simultaneously on the screen, greatly facil-

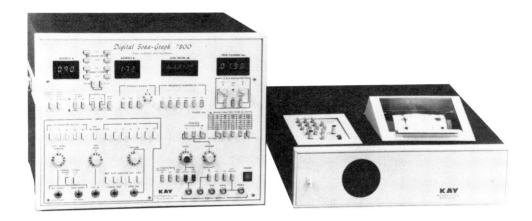

FIGURE 9–21. The Kay Elemetrics model 7800 spectrogaph, a hybrid (analog and digital) spectrum analyzer.

itating comparison of different samples.

There is no doubt that the SSD is convenient and easy to use, and its "real time" output may, as the manufacturers claim, make it ideal for use in therapy, especially since it has been shown that patients can differentiate "correct" from "incorrect" productions on the basis of the SSD display (Maki, Gustafson, Conklin, and Humphrey-Whitehead, 1981).* But it is somewhat limited (compared to the more traditional spectrographs) in what it can perform. It is probably for this reason that it has not yet made significant inroads against Kay Elemetrics and Voice Identification units. It is likely that, for the near future, serious users will prefer more traditional spectrographic methods.

THE SPECTROGRAM

Before moving to a discussion of specific details, a general consideration of spectral features as they are demonstrated by various analysis techniques is in order.* This information forms the basis for deciding on the type of display that will be most useful for demonstrating features of interest in particular cases. Furthermore, it will give the reader some preliminary practice in reading and interpreting simple sound spectrograms.

Source and Filter: Harmonics and Formants

Earlier in the chapter, reference was made to the source-filter model of vowel production. The speech signal, it was said, represents the interaction of the acoustic components of the glottal wave with the complex filtering properties of the vocal tract. Figure 9-23 demonstrates how the vocal and resonant components appear in spectrograms. A number of spectral analyses have been done on two utterances: (1) the vowel /ɛ/, sustained with alternation between two fundamental frequencies, and (2) alternation between /ɛ/ and /ɑ/.

The left side of Figure 9-23A shows the alternation of /ɑ/ and /ɛ/ as analyzed with

---

*When using the dual-channel SSD in the "comparative" (therapist vs. patient) mode, it is important that the therapist not expect a patient to match his or her spectral features exactly. Many acoustic characteristics are fixed by the specific structure of the vocal tract and are not amenable to modification.

*An excellent concise summary of the effect of the spectrograph's physical characteristics on the spectrogram has been published by Peterson (1952).

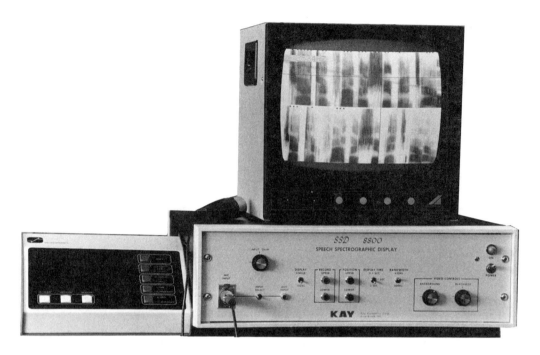

FIGURE 9–22. The Speech Spectrographic Display.

a filter having a bandwidth of 300 Hz. The dark horizontal bars represent the frequency components emphasized by the vocal tract formants. They have been labelled F_1, F_2, and so on. The movement of the several formant bars is a consequence of the change in shape (and therefore the change in resonant properties) of the vocal tract as it moves from one vowel to the other. The vowels were spoken with a fundamental frequency of about 100 Hz. The harmonics of the glottal (source) signal itself, then, are about 100 Hz apart. Since the analyzing filter used for this analysis had a bandwidth of 300 Hz, the individual vocal harmonics are too close to each other to be resolved. The position of the formant bars, then, does not tell us anything about the vocal signal itself, only about the vocal tract resonances. This is made clear by Figure 9-23C, in which the vowel /ɛ/ was sustained at two quite distinct vocal pitches. The analysis on the left was also done with a 300 Hz filter. Note that the position of the formant bands remains remarkably constant despite

shifts of vocal fundamental frequency. (There is *some* movement of the formant bands, however. It results from the speaker's inability to maintain an absolutely stable vocal tract posture in the face of laryngeal adjustments.) To the right of each of these two "broad-band" analyses are spectrograms of precisely the same utterances done with a 45 Hz filter. This bandwidth is narrow enough to resolve the individual harmonics in the vocal signal. Therefore, the horizontal bands ruunning across these two spectrograms show vocal signal components. The harmonics are more intense (darker) in the region of the formants than elsewhere, showing that they are the ones emphasized by the resonant characteristics of the vocal tract. In fact, outside of the formant regions the harmonics are often so weak as to disappear from the printout. In the narrow-band spectrograms the horizontal lines represent, from bottom to top, harmonic 1 (f_1), harmonic 2 (f_2), and so forth, rather than formants. If one of the harmonic lines in the /ɛ/-/ɑ/ alternation is traced across the printout, it will be found to be interrupted (because of severe weakening) but straight. The formant bars are not formed by movement of the harmonics, but rather by emphasis of different harmonics as the vocal tract resonances change. The invariance of harmonics shows that the two vowels were produced at a stable fundamental frequency. On the other hand, Figure 9-23C, the 45 Hz bandwidth analysis of /ɛ/ at alternating pitches, demonstrates just the reverse phenomenon. The horizontal lines again show the harmonics, and they move up and down with the pitch changes. The formants, however, are demonstrated by darkening of harmonic lines, and the vertical position of the darkened zones remains essentially constant across the paper, showing that the formants have not changed with the pitch. In summary, Figure 9-23A shows formant emphases moving across harmonic levels, while Figure 9-23C shows harmonics moving in and out of formant resonances. Narrow bandwidth, by providing fine resolution of frequency, allows us to see the characteristics of the source (vocal) signal; wide bandwidth demonstrates vocal tract resonances (formants). Formants are largely indpedendent of glottal harmonics.

The same demonstration can be done using amplitude versus frequency spectra, as in Figures 9-23B and D, which are *sections* of the vowels taken at the points indicated. The horizontal scale for each is frequency, increasing from left to right; the vertical scale is relative intensity. Because vowels represent periodic waves, they have line spectra. The narrow-band sections show the individual harmonic lines fairly well. Note that the line spectra of /ɛ/ and /ɑ/ (9-23B) are quite different: The peaks showing maximal harmonic intensity (due to formants) have very different locations on the frequency scale. However, the change of fundamental frequency during /ɛ/ (9-23D) produces only slight displacement of the resonance peaks (indicating that the same vowel was produced), while the spacing of the harmonic lines in the narrow-band analysis shows how the vocal fundamen-

tal frequency varied. Obviously the same conclusions apply to the sections: Broad band analysis shows vocal tract resonances, while narrow-band demonstrates vocal (source) characteristics.

The spectrograms also show another important difference between broad and narrow filter bandwidth. In both of the analyses done with the 300 Hz filter, the spectrogram is actually made up of a series of closely spaced vertical stripes. These striations represent the acoustic result of individual glottal closures. Every time the vocal folds snap together the sudden cessation of airflow generates an acoustic excitation of the vocal tract resonators. The vocal tract is then acoustically quiet until the next closure. Hence, a series of vertical dark stripes (response to excitation) separated by blank spaces (quiet between pulses). Since the rate of glottal closure is the fundamental frequency, and because there is a single striation for each closure, the vocal fundamental frequency is indicated by the spacing of the vertical striations (see Chap. 5).

The narrowband (45 Hz) analysis does not have glottal striations. This is a consequence of the poor time-resolution that results because a narrow bandwidth filter must be lightly damped , and lightly damped filters are "sluggish" in their response. In other words, the output of the narrow-band filter system cannot change fast enough to show the very rapid sound-silence alternations. The striations are blurred together into a continuous line. The loss of vertical striations is another example of the trade-off between time and frequency resolution imposed by the laws of physics. To improve one is to worsen the other.

Frication

The aerodynamic feature that characterizes fricatives is airstream turbulence generated by airflow through a tight constriction in the vocal tract (Catford, 1977). The turbulence, of course, is random fluctuation of local air pressure, the acoustic correlate of which is aperiodic noise. The vocal tract in which the noise is gen-

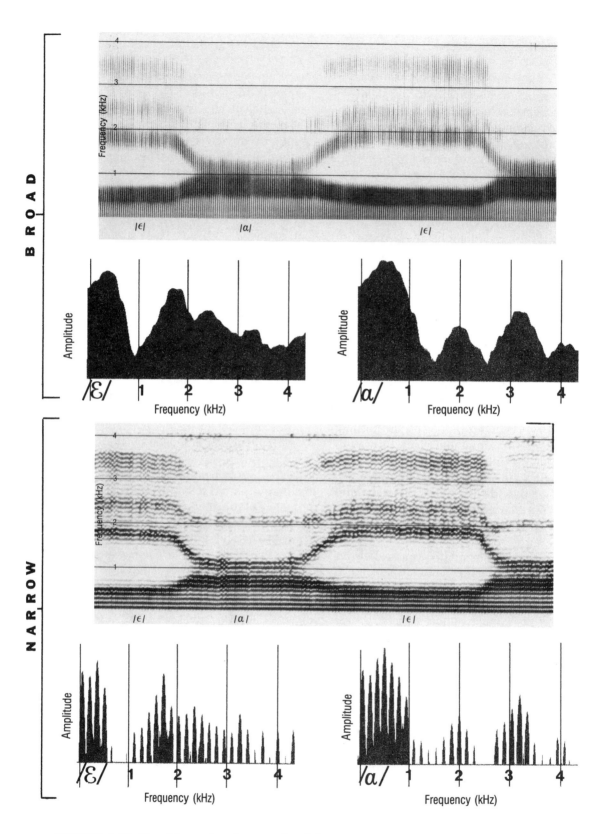

FIGURE 9-23. Broad (upper) and narrow-band (lower) spectrograms of the utterance /ε-ɑ-ε/ with sections through both vowels. The narrow-band analysis shows that the harmonics are stable but different harmonics are emphasized as the formants change.

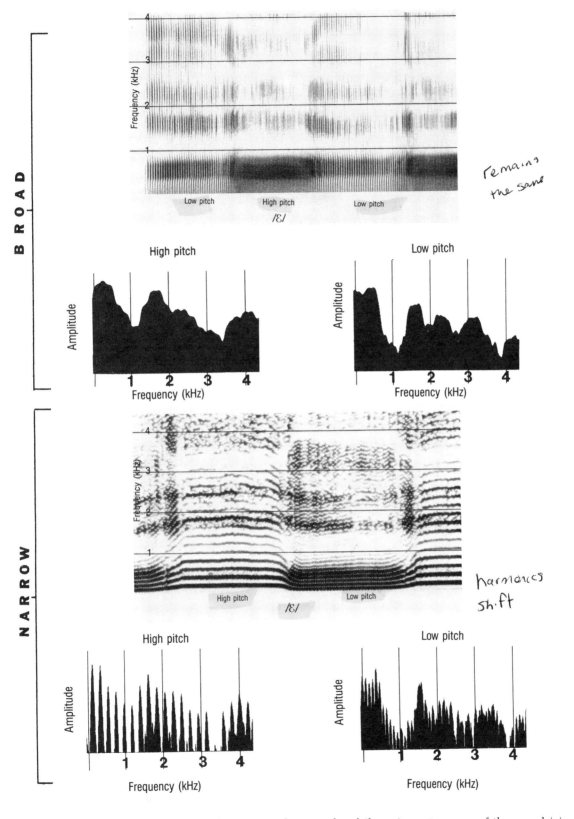

FIGURE 9-23 *(continued).* Broad (upper) and narrow-band (lower) spectrograms of the vowel /ɛ/ produced at two fundamental frequencies, with sections through the vowel at both frequencies. The narrow-band analysis shows how the harmonics rise and fall with the frequency change, while the formants are (relatively) stable.

erated, however, is an active resonant space with a real transfer function that influences the radiated noise signal, limiting its bandwidth. Therefore, the spectra of fricatives contain a strong continous-spectrum component extending over a frequency range that is broad, but limited. This is shown clearly in Figure 9-24A. Note the ways in which /s/ differs from /i/: absence of glottal pulses (voiceless), continuous spectrum (noise) and noise energy concentrated in the higher frequencies due to the

influence of the vocal tract transfer function . When a voiced fricative is analyzed, as in Figure 9 24B, the spectrum shows the combined contributions of glottal pulsing and frication turbulence. Glottal pulsing continues throughout the fricative although there is also a distinct high-frequency noise component. The amplitude versus frequency spectrum (section) shows the same evidence: During /z/ the harmonics in the line spectrum are interspersed with random noise.

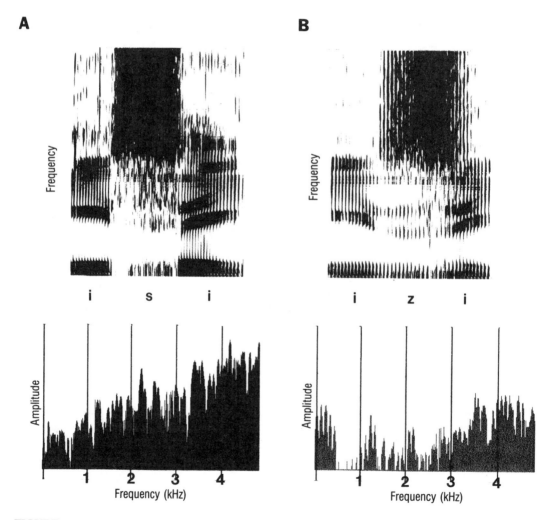

FIGURE 9–24. Time (top) and amplitude (bottom) spectra of (A) /isi/, and (B) /izi/. Note the presence of regular glottal pulses during /z/. The amplitude spectrum of /z/ shows harmonics, which are particularly evident in the low-frequency region.

Effect of Shaping

The spectrograph has a "high shape" circuit that modifies the input signal by emphasizing high-frequency components. This compensates for the normal roll-off of the glottal signal, boosting high-frequency vocal harmonics sufficiently so that they can be seen in the final spectrogram. Figure 9-25 shows the effect of this circuit. This signal processing results in distortion of the true speech signal. But it is only the representation of the source spectrum that is affected, and frequently this component of the speech signal is of secondary interest. The boosting of high-frequency components makes it much easier to evaluate vocal tract characteristics, and therein lies the val-

ue of the shaping circuits. If necessary, the measured amplitude of the vocal harmonics can be arithmetically adjusted to compensate for the extra emphasis in the higher frequencies since the spectrograph manual specifies the exact amount of boosting done by the shaping circuitry.

Influence of Fundamental Frequency

The fundamental frequency of the speech sample affects the spectrogram in two important ways. Unfortunately, both ways make it increasingly difficult to interpret the spectrogram as the fundamental frequency rises. One of these problems will be considered more fully in the section dealing with formant evaluation. The other, however, so alters the general appearance of the spectrogram as to mislead the unwary and so will be considered here.

In the preceding discussion filters were described as "wide" or "narrow." While these descriptive terms have obvious value as a way of comparing filters to each other, they also have meaning in terms of a more important comparison. A filter is said to have a wide or narrow bandwidth in relation to the spacing of the harmonics of the signal being analyzed. Figure 9-26 illustrates what this means and shows its significance for applied spectrography. In each case a sustained /i/ is analyzed using a filter with a bandwidth of 300 Hz. In Figure 9-26A the fundamental frequency of the vowel is about 100 Hz. The spectrogram has the same general appearance as the previous figures of wide-band spectra. Individual harmonics are blurred into formant bands. However, when the fundamental frequency is raised to around 300 Hz, as in Figure 9-26B, the appearance of a spectrogram done with the same 300 Hz filter is very different. The individual harmonics are separately resolved, and they come to look like closely spaced formants.

The reason for this is not difficult to understand. When the fundamental frequency and harmonic spacing is only 100 Hz, a filter with a 300 Hz bandwidth "sees" more

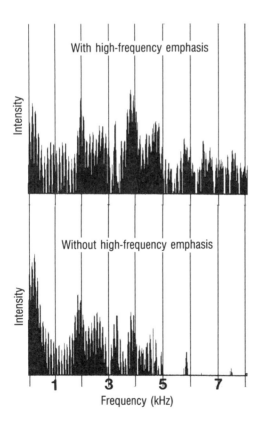

FIGURE 9–25. The effect of high-frequency "shaping" of a signal. Note the increased amplitude of the high-frequency components in the shaped (top) line spectrum, compared to the obvious high-frequency roll-off in the natural (unshaped) version (bottom) of the same vowel.

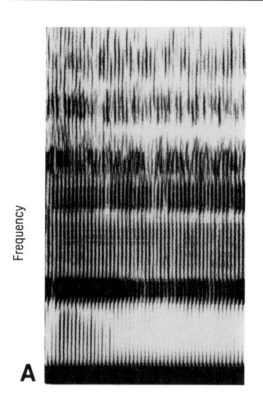
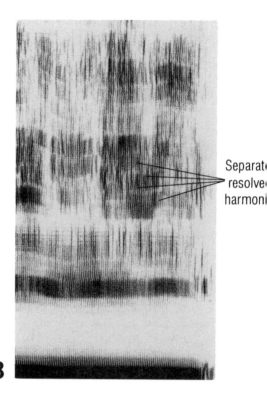

Separat‹
resolve‹
harmoni‹

FIGURE 9–26. When the filter bandwidth is wide compared to the fundamental frequency (as in A), individual harmonics are not resolved, making it easier to see the formants. But when the fundamental frequency and the filter bandwidth are comparable (as in B) the harmonic lines may be separately resolved, and they may, in some cases, actually be mistaken for formant bands.

than one harmonic at a time. Therefore, adjacent harmonics are blended together by the filter system. There is always a filter output, of greater or lesser amplitude according to how much the harmonics included in the filter band have been emphasized by the vocal tract resonances. Hence, the spectrogram shows the formant locations. When, however, the harmonics are over 300 Hz apart the pass-band of the filter never includes more than a single harmonic. As it sweeps across the frequency range of its analysis, the filter resolves each harmonic individually, as is typical of a narrow-band filter. The bars representing the harmonics are wide, because the filter keeps "seeing" a given harmonic until its center frequency has moved 300 Hz away from it. Since it keeps producing an output until it no longer detects the harmonic, the line that

it causes to be made on the paper is 300 Hz wide. This might fool the user into believing that the wide line represents a formant, but examining the spectrogram shows that formants are actually indicated by darkening of several adjacent harmonic lines—as in any narrow-band printout.

The same 300 Hz filter is wide-band with respect to 100 Hz spacing, but narrow-band for harmonics that are over 300 Hz apart. The same principle holds true for any filter bandwidth. A 150 Hz filter bandwidth is narrow with respect to a fundamental frequency of 600 Hz, but wide in comparison to a fundamental frequency of 80 Hz. The practical problem is obvious. High fundamental frequency makes it difficult to blur harmonics together to emphasize formant peaks, and so interpreting the spectrogram is something of a problem.

SPECTRAL FEATURES

The information displayed in the spectrogram is considered here under several broad headings. They have been assigned somewhat arbitrarily, but are likely to represent the spectrographic features of most interest to the practicing speech pathologist.

Vowels

Vowels are the nuclei around which syllables are built. They are charcterized by pulsed glottal airflow that remains laminar as it traverses the open vocal tract. Aside from the spectral characteristics of vowel sounds, considerable attention has been focussed on their duration, which varies in a language-specific way as a function of tense-lax distinction, consonant environment, position in the breath group, stress or prominence, speech rate, and even the information content of the word of which they are a part. All of these factors interact in very complex ways (House and Fairbanks, 1953; Fry, 1955; Fonagy and Magdics, 1960; Peterson and Lehiste, 1960; Lehiste and Peterson, 1961; Lehiste, 1972; Klatt, 1973, 1975b, 1976; DiSimoni, 1974b; Umeda 1975; Allen, 1978; Kent, Netsell, and Abbs, 1979; Pickett, 1980; Prosek and Runyan, 1982). The discussion to follow, however, will be limited to a basic consideration of vowel spectral features.

The vowel resonances are probably the most immediately obvious feature in the spectrogram of a speech utterance. While interest in them dates from the 19th century, the sound spectrograph, by making them readily observable, unleashed a flood of research into their characteristics and significance. As a result, formant patterns are understood better than most other spectral characteristics of speech. As in so many areas of scientific inquiry, the understanding achieved often points more to unresolved questions and the inability to formulate inviolable rules than to a complete and settled model. A number of significant caveats must therefore be kept in mind.

The formant pattern of a vocalic sound (and in particular the relationship of its first two formants) is crucial to its perceptual categorization by a listener (Potter and Peterson, 1948; Potter and Steinberg, 1950; Delattre, Liberman, Cooper, and Gerstman, 1952; Potter, Kopp, and Green, 1947). However formant frequencies do not necessarily uniquely specify the vowel that is perceived. Some vowels share a common formant pattern yet are perceptually distinct (Peterson and Barney, 1952; Fairbanks and Grubb, 1961). Identification is influenced by the listener's linguistic experience, speaker fundamental frequency, the vowel's phonetic context, stress or prominence, and formant amplitude (Peterson, 1961; Tiffany, 1959; Ladefoged and Broadbent, 1957).

Since formants reflect the size and shape of the vocal tract, there is no reason to expect that absolute formant frequencies should remain constant in the face of anatomical variation among speakers. What are important are the *relative* frequencies of the formant peaks, their positions with respect to each other and to the formants of other vowels produced by the same speaker (Ladefoged and Broadbent, 1957). However, even the relativity of formant frequencies may not be perfectly preserved across speakers. If it were, one would expect that, for a given vowel, the ratio of the frequencies of the first and second formants would remain stable across men and women, and across older and younger children, whose vocal tracts are all different in size and shape. There are indeed linear trends in interpersonal formant scaling, but the exact relationships are neither simple nor perfectly understood (Broadbent, Ladefoged, and Lawrence 1956; Fant, 1966; Gerstman, 1968; Eguchi and Hirsh, 1969; Kent, 1976, 1978, 1979; Kent and Forner, 1978; 1979).

It is clear, then, that clinical use of formant data must be approached with due regard for constraints on their applicability and interpretation. For example, attempts to have a child exactly match the therapist's formant patterns would probably be futile and almost certainly be pointless. Still, formant measures can have value in assessing developmental normality (Buhr, 1980) and a range of speech disorders, including dysfluency, dyslalia, and dysarthria (Kent, 1979; Adams, 1978; Gilbert, 1970).

Formant quantification

Formants can be described in terms of three parameters: frequency, amplitude, and bandwidth. The latter two are of limited interest to the speech clinician, and therefore will not be considered here. Good reviews of the problems of assessing them are provided by Fant, Fintoft, Liljencrants, Lindblom and Martony (1963) and Dunn (1961).

Formant frequencies

A formant is a local maximum in the vocal tract transfer function. It is a single frequency at which vocal tract transmission is more efficient than at nearby frequencies. The emphasis on transmission characteristics is important here: The vocal tract system has formants even if no sound is being produced. The fact is, however, that a formant frequency can be detected only when there is acoustic energy being transmitted. Therefore, a formant can be operationally defined as a peak in the displayed amplitude spectrum that is not due to source-spectrum properties.

This pragmatic definition raises a significant problem in that the vocal signal, which is the wave usually being transmitted, has a line spectrum. That is, it has significant energy only at discrete (harmonic) frequencies. So the formant becomes that point on the frequency scale where a harmonic has greater amplitude than its neighbors. It would be a fortunate coincidence if the frequency of a harmonic fell at exactly the true frequency of formant peak: One could then be certain that the formant frequency had been precisely indicated. It is not surprising, given the essential independence of the glottal source and

vocal-tract filter, that such a happy correspondence is likely to be rare and certainly not to be assumed.

Individual harmonics serve as "samples" of the vocal tract's resonant responses. We must assume that the amplitude of a harmonic represents (other factors being equal) transmission characteristics that the vocal tract would have for nearby frequencies that are not actually present. The greater the space between harmonics, the larger the gaps between samples and the less certain the formant determination can be. Harmonic spacing is a direct correlate of fundamental frequency, and so formant frequency determination becomes less precise as vocal pitch rises. Figure 9-27 shows how serious the situation can become. At the top is the true spectrum envelope of a vowel by a hypothetical speaker. Figure 9-27B shows the line spectrum that results when the vowel is actually spoken at a fundamental frequency of 100 Hz. The tops of the spectral lines are joined by a dashed line to generate an estimate of true spectral envelope. That estimate is reasonably accurate because the harmonic are close enough to sample all of the envelope's peaks. However, when the fundamental frequency is raised to 400 Hz (Fig. 9-27C) the widely spaced spectral lines sample only a few points of the vocal tract response. In fact, the spacing is so wide that a reconstruction of the spectral envelope from the available harmonic amplitudes fails to show the second formant. It is not that the formant is not there, it is just not detected. A gross error of formant assessment has resulted.

Obviously, the voices of women and especially of children are most likely to suffer this kind of estimation inaccuracy. Peterson (1959), after a lucid and concise review of the difficulty, found it to be essentially irresolvable. Even more recently developed mathematical analytic methods do not seem to hold the promise of a solution (Monsen and Engebretson, 1983). There are, however, a few tricks that circumvent the problem. One is to analyze whispered speech, since the broad-band noise signal

A

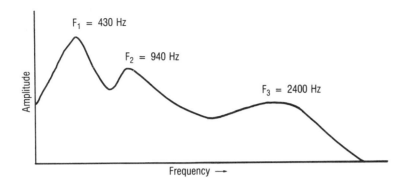

B

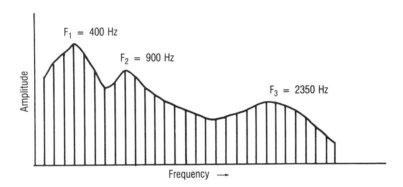

C

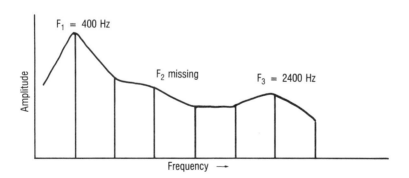

FIGURE 9–27. (A). True spectral envelope of a vowel-like sound. (B). A line spectrum of the vowel spoken with a fundamental frequency of 100 Hz provides lines that are close enough to give good estimates of where the formants are. (C). When the fundamental frequency is 400 Hz, however, the harmonics are so far apart that it is possible for none of them to lie in a given formant region. In this case, a formant peak might be missed when reconstructing the spectral envelope.

of whispering will excite all the formants (Watterson and Emanuel, 1981). Another is to substitute an external noise source or low-frequency signal for the patient's voice. A clever way of doing this is to have the speaker mouth the utterance while using an electrolarynx (Huggins, 1980).* The tricks do have their problems, however (Weiss, Yeni-Komshian, and Heinz, 1979). There is sound leakage from the electrolarynx directly to the microphone; the spectrum of the electrolaryngeal excitation is different from the natural vocal spectrum, and may result in spurious peaks in the speech amplitude spectrum (Sáfrán, 1971); and speech rate tends to be slower both when using the electrolarynx and when whispering (Parnell, Amerman, and Wells, 1977). But, as shown in Figure 9-28, there is enormous improvement in formant resolution.

Still another approach to the problem of high-pitched voices is to increase the bandwidth of the analyzing filter beyond the 300 Hz generally designated "wide band." Filters with bandwidths of 450 or 600 Hz are available for the more popular spectrographs. In their absence, one more "trick" can be used. Playback at half of the recording speed reduces the frequency of all recorded signals by half. A 300 Hz filter analyzing a half-speed playback, therefore, has its effective "real-time" bandwidth doubled to twice its nominal rating, or 600 Hz. At the same time, of course, the spectrograph's vertical frequency scale is also doubled: Instead of extending from 0 to 8 kHz, for example, the analysis range will really be 0 to 16 kHz. (If the spectrograph has scale expansion this is easily dealt with.) Also, the true frequency of any calibration lines will be twice their apparent value. It might seem that this method is ideal, solving all

of the problems of formant specification in the face of high F_0. But increasing the bandwidth of the analyzing filter proportionally broadens the formant bars making it harder to pinpoint the exact formant frequency, which presumably lies at the center of the band marked on the paper. There is a moral in this: The laws of physics cannot really be circumvented. If there is uncertainty in the signal, there is uncertainty no matter what is done to the signal. It's all summed up in a common expression of working scientists: "There is no free lunch."

EXPECTED VALUES. If there is one thing that early spectrographic investigations of speech made clear, it is that there are no static signals. This holds true for vowels. The voluminous examples presented in the classic work of Potter, Kopp, and Green (1947) show that vowel formants change as they "grow" out of the preceding phoneme and merge into the following one. Not only do the formant transitions change as a function of the acoustic surroundings, but the formants of the vowel's *hub*, or mid-portion, show accommodative shifting as well. Therefore, studies designed to assess formant characteristics have usually used either a standard phonetic context or a simple prolongation of an isolated vowel. (Some investigation of diphthongs has also been done. See Holbrook and Fairbanks [1962], for example.) Measurements are commonly made at the midportion of the vowel production. Assessment of a patient's speech should do the same if comparability with published data is to be preserved.

Table 9-1 summarizes formant frequency data from three research studies:

1. Peterson and Barney (1952) evaluated a population of 33 men, 28 women, and 15 children (ages unspecified) that had been studied earlier by Potter and Steinberg (1950). Each speaker did two readings of a list of 10 words: heed, hid, head, had, hod, hawed, who'd, hud, and heard. Formant frequencies were located

---

*An externally applied sine wave signal, rapidly swept through a wide frequency range, can provide an excellent delineation of formants (Fujimura and Lindqvist, 1971). However, it requires the speaker to maintain a static articulatory posture and entails more complexity than the clinical situation is likely to warrant.

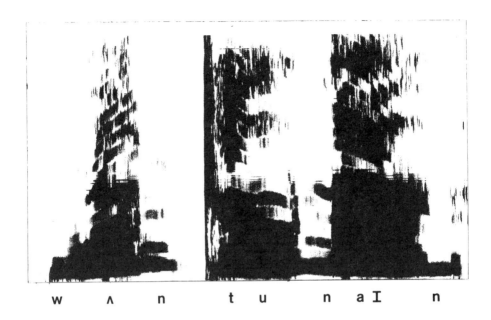

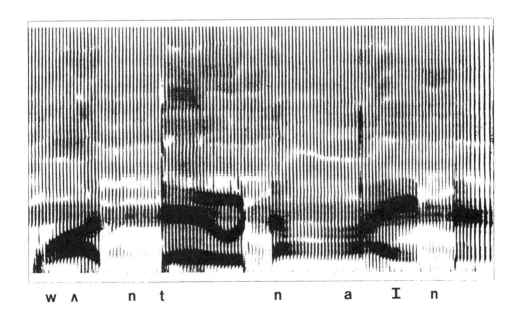

FIGURE 9–28. Two analyses (300 Hz bandwidth of the utterance "one-two-nine" spoken by the same individual. (A) Using normal phonation, fundamental frequency about 400 Hz. (B) Using a Western Electric electrolarynx instead of phonation as the "source" signal.

TABLE 9–1. Mean Formant Frequencies in Hz

F_n	i	I	ɛ	æ	ɑ	ɔ	ʊ	u	ʌ	ɝ	Source
					VOWEL						
					MEN						
F_0*	136	135	130	127	124	129	137	141	130	133	a
F_1	270	390	530	660	730	570	440	300	640	490	a
F_2	2290	1990	1840	1720	1090	840	1020	870	1190	1350	a
F_3	3010	2550	2480	2410	2440	2410	2240	2240	2390	1690	a
F_1	288		555	616		653		344			c
F_2	2217		1726	1723		1048		1256			c
					BOYS						
F_0*	199	191	189	187	188	189	194	204	195	194	b
F_1	262	410	606	588	917	762	500	363	671	396	b
F_2	2776	2300	2079	2231	1376	1067	1216	1061	1427	1459	b
F_3	3251	2974	2908	2961	2705	2750	2791	2757	2813	1909	b
F_1	370		652	645		724		427			c
F_2	2794		2047	1987		1193		1347			c
					WOMEN						
F_0*	235	232	223	210	212	216	232	231	221	218	a
F_1	310	430	610	860	850	590	470	370	760	500	a
F_2	2790	2480	2330	2050	1220	920	1160	950	1400	1640	a
F_3	3310	3070	2990	2850	2810	2710	2680	2670	2780	1960	a
F_1	338		589	761		666		356			c
F_2	2810		2111	2054		1135		1460			c
					GIRLS						
F_1	386		635	703		812		433			c
F_2	2994		2244	2188		1503		1443			c
					CHILDREN						
F_0*	272	269	260	251	256	263	276	274	261	261	a
F_1	370	530	690	1010	1030	680	560	430	850	560	a
F_2	3200	2730	2610	2320	1370	1060	1410	1170	1590	1820	a
F_3	3730	3600	3570	3320	3170	3180	3310	3260	3360	2160	a

*Fundamental frequency.

Sources: (a)Peterson and Barney., 1952; (b) Angelocci, Kopp, and Holbrook, 1964 (comparison to a group of deaf boys); and (c) Eguchi and Hirsh, 1969. Data for boys and girls averaged over tabled values for 11-14 year olds.

in narrow-band sections taken at the midpoint of each vowel.

2. Angelocci, Kopp, and Holbrook (1964) studied two groups (normal and deaf) of 18 boys each, age 11-14. (Only data for the normal boys are included in Table 9-1.) The same vowels as in the Peterson and Barney study (in a different phonetic context) were analyzed in very much the same way.

3. Eguchi and Hirsh (1969) explored developmental changes of a number of speech variables, including formant frequencies. The subject population included 5 children at each age from 3 to 10 years, 5 boys and 5 girls at each age from 11 to 13, five adult men and five adult women. Each subject spoke two sentences: "He has a blue pen" and "I am tall." Narrow-band sections were used to locate the first two formants of each of the italicized vowels (and of the first vowel in /aI/).

There is an orderly progression of formant frequencies in the table, a regularity which is made clearer in actual spectrograms of the same vowels (produced in the same /h--d/ contexts), as in Figure 9-29. There is a definite pattern of formant change across vowels. The pattern is most easily explored by preparing a graph, in which the second formant is plotted against the first formant. Figure 9-30A shows just such a plot, prepared by Peterson and Barney (1952) to demonstrate the formant positions of vowels spoken by all their subjects. Note that there is considerable dispersion of the data points; the same vowel can have a very different F_1/F_2 relationship when produced by different speakers. Outlining the zone within which each vowel lies shows that the dispersion is great enough to produce overllap of vowel areas (for example, /ɝ/ and /ɛ/). What this indicates is that the formant pattern of, say, /ɔ/ for one speaker might be the same as a different speaker's pattern for /ɑ/. The formant similarity of two different vowels by two different speakers is a demonstration of the fact that formants do not uniquely specify the vowel category.

Isovowel Lines and Formant Scaling

The F_2/F_1 graph can be simplified by plotting the mean formant values for each vowel. This has been done separately for the men, women, and children in Figure 9-30B. It now becomes even clearer that the orderly progression of formant changes across vowels is related in some way to the vocal tract configuration assumed for each one. Note how the mean relationships of the formants outline the classic vowel diagram. More important for the present purposes is the fact that there seems to be a regular relationship among the formant locations of men, women, and children. In Figure 9-30C the F_2/F_1 loci of vowels as produced by the three groups are connected together to demonstrate this. The "isovowel lines" (Broad, 1976) show that the progression is not fully regular, but there is a strong sense that the loci are "fleeing" from the origin of the graph.

What significance, validity, and applicability does this have? It helps, in answering these questions, to begin by considering

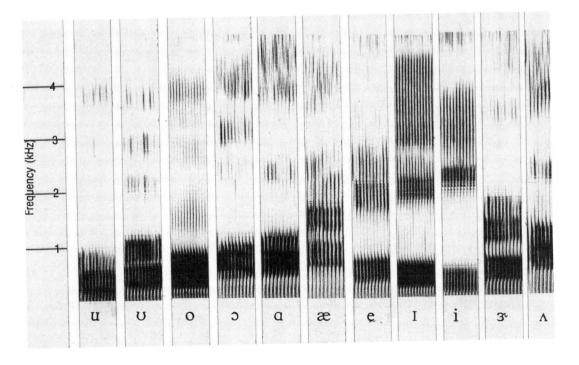

FIGURE 9-29. Formant patterns of the English vowels.

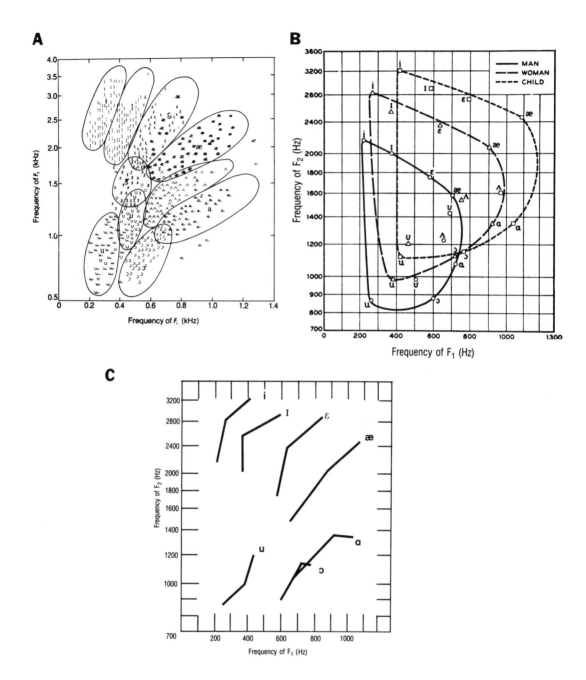

FIGURE 9–30. (A). Frequency of the second formant plotted against the frequency of the first formant for vowels spoken by 76 speakers. (Adapted from Peterson and Barney, *Journal of the Acoustical Society of America*, 24 (1954) p. 182. Reprinted by permission from Lieberman, P., *Speech Physiology and Acoustic Phonetics*, New York: Macmillan, 1977, p. 68.) (B). F_2/F_1 relationships for vowels spoken by men, women, and children. (Reprinted by permission from Bogert and Peterson, "The Acoustics of Speech" in Travis, L. E. (Ed.), *Handbook of Speech Pathology*. New York: Appleton-Century-Crofts,. 1957. p. 152.) (C). *Isovowel lines* created by connecting the "man", "woman" and "child" loci of Figure 9-30B. Although the relationship is not completely regular, there is a strong sense that the formant ratios are moving away from the graph's origin. (The "child" end of each line has been labelled by the IPA symbol for each vowel.)

how isovowel lines can be generated. Suppose a group of speakers all produce several vowels. The formant frequences of each production are determined and plotted, as in Figure 9-31A, forming "clouds" on the graph. Using a mathematical technique called regression analysis two very important characteristics about each group of data points can be determined. One is the equation of a *best fit* line (also called a *least squares* line) that can be drawn through each aggregation of points. (It is called "best fit" because the average distance of the data points from the line is minimized.) The equation of the line has the general form $F_2 = bF_1 + a$. The coefficient b is the slope of the line on the graph. It is the average F_2/F_1 ratio for the data points included in the analysis. Conceptually, the best-fit line represents the locus of points along which all F_2/F_1 relationships would lie if the data were "pure," uninfluenced by any external factor and not contaminated by any error.

The extent to which this last concept holds is quantified in the *correlation coefficient,* which is the second important parameter determined by regression analysis. It specifies how spread out the data are, that is, how far on the average the data points lie from the idealization represented by the best-fit line. Obviously, the closer the points are to the line, the more likely it is that it does, in fact, represent some real underlying relationship and not just the meaningless product of a mathematical manipulation. Even better, the square of the correlation coefficient (called the coefficient of determination) is the proportion of F_2/F_1 position change that is attributable to the relationship represented by the best fit line. (The rest of the data-point variability is attributable to other unknown influences and to error.) If, for example, the coefficient of determination is 0.5 or higher, we may conclude that there is a significant linear relationship among the points because at least 50% of the change in the F_2/F_1 position is accounted for by the equation of the best-fit line.

This kind of scaling has been explored by a number of acoustic phoneticians (e.g., Mol, 1963; Fant, 1973), but most relevantly by Kent (1978, 1979) and Kent and Forner (1979) who studied the formants of /i,æ, ɑ,u,ɝ/ as produced by 4-, 5-, and 6-year-old boys and girls and by adult men and women. Regression analysis of the sort just described resulted in F_2/F_1 isovowel lines as shown in Figure 9-31B. As the coefficients of determination show, linear relationships are quite strong, except in the case of /æ/. If the "a" term is dropped from the best-fit equation, leaving only the "b" (slope) coefficient, extensions of the best fit lines will all pass through the graph's origin, forming a set of radiating isovowel "rays."

Each of the rays represents the change in the F_2/F_1 ratio as the vocal tract increases in size. Data for the small vocal tracts of children lie more distant from the origin than those for men whose large vocal tracts have lower formant frequencies. Also, in many ways the rays of the diagram represent the life history of the vocal tract. As an individual's vocal tract grows and changes, his vowel formants travel down the rays toward the graph's origin. Most of the movement will occur during childhood but, as Kent (1979) points out, both anatomic (Israel, 1968, 1973) and acoustic (Endres, Bombach, and Flösser, 1971) studies provide reason to believe that vocal tract development extends across the life span.

Kent (1979) describes how the "universal" isovowel lines can be of use to the clinician. It is simply a matter of measuring a patient's formant frequencies and plotting them onto a graph with the appropriate isovowel lines (Figure 9-31C). The distance of the plotted data points from their respective isovowel lines is at least an approximate measure of deviance. Kent shows, for instance, how plotting the data of Angelocci, Koopp, and Holbrook (1964) for deaf boys on the isovowel lines results in a vowel triangle that is much smaller than normal (that is, its vertices do not extend to the isovowel lines), demonstrating severe vowel centralization in this population. (Similar data from Monsen [1976] also

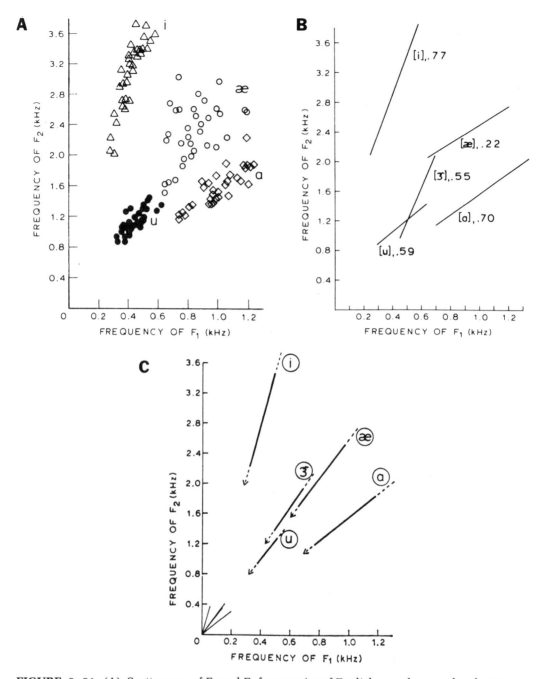

FIGURE 9–31. (A). Scattergram of F_2 and F_1 frequencies of English vowels as spoken by 33 men, women, and children. (Reprinted by permission from Kent and Forner, Developmental study of vowel formant frequencies in an imitation task. *Journal of the Acoustical Society of America*, 65 (1979) p. 210.) (B). Isovowel lines (least-squares regression) for the data points of Figure 9-31A. The number associated with each line is its coefficient of determination, which indicates the proportion of variability accounted for by the F_2/F_1 relationship. (Same reference as Fig. 9-31A, p. 211.) (C). Isovowel lines as determined by Kent, 1979. The solid midportion of each line represents the region for which normative data are available; dashed segments are extrapolated. Each line can be described by an equation of the form $F_2 = b \cdot F_1$ where b is the slope of the lines. The coefficients for the lines shown are: /i/ = 7.11; /u/ = 2.48; /ɑ/ = 1.545; /æ/ = 2.65; /ɝ/= 2.79. (Reprinted with permission from Kent, Isovowel lines for the evaluation of vowel formant structure in speech disorders. *Journal of Speech and Hearing Disorders*, 44 (1979) 513-521, Figure 1, p. 515. ©American-Speech-Language-Hearing Association, Rockville, MD.)

show this effect.) Using the same evaluation procedure Kent, Netsell, and Abbs (1979) demonstrated that formant structure was largely undisturbed in cerebellar dysarthria, while Kent and Rosenbek (1983) have explored vowel errors in apraxics.

Kent (1979) suggests that F_3/F_2 plots can also be used to improve vowel-formant assessment. He also adds an important caution to the effect that the position of a patient's F_2/F_1 locus in relationship to an isovowel line is not as important as its position with respect to the *age appropriate segment* of the line. For example, an F_2/F_1 point for an adult male might fall directly on the isovowel line, but quite far from the origin. The distant (upper right) reaches of the line are normally the province of young children. As noted earlier, advancing age should move the F_2/F_1 points toward the lower left. Therefore, the hypothetical adult male in question has a highly abnormal set of formants, despite their exact coincidence with the isovowel norm.

While no exact age-division of the line can be done, Table 9-2 may help the clinician locate regions broadly associated with different ages. The data are taken from the Eguchi and Hirsh (1969) study described earlier. There are five children in each of the age or age-sex groups. In using these data, remember that the phonetic context of the vowels was very different from that of Kent's studies.

Specific Influences on Vowel Spectra

VOCAL TRACT SHAPING. From the studies cited at the opening of this chapter and others, it is possible to formulate a set of "rules" that relate specific changes in formant patterns to actions or shapes of the vocal tract. Caution is required in drawing inferences from them, since many were derived by changing a vocal tract analog (often an electrical circuit or digital model) and noting the effect on the resulting vowel formants. Reasoning in the other direction, from formant frequencies to vocal

TABLE 9–2. Mean Formant Frequencies of Vowels at Different Ages*

Age	/i/ F_1	/i/ F_2	/ɛ/ F_1	/ɛ/ F_2	/æ/ F_1	/æ/ F_2	/ɔ/ F_1	/ɔ/ F_2	/u/ F_1	/u/ F_2
	BOYS AND GIRLS									
3	484	3318	673	2683	786	2599	802	1485	578	1664
4	444	3050	566	2397	567	2281	762	1390	472	1528
5	408	3235	642	2418	643	2423	901	1513	452	1477
6	397	3108	512	2281	611	2238	689	1308	431	1385
7	411	3204	664	2280	736	2299	817	1398	481	1525
8	397	3104	585	2195	685	2222	743	1359	450	1437
9	403	3106	308	2296	647	2295	836	1352	469	1392
10	403	3028	645	2193	735	2255	814	1336	469	1351
	BOYS									
11	397	2778	671	2109	620	2063	724	1284	448	1388
12	359	2877	618	2059	658	2012	705	1175	404	1253
13	355	2727	668	1974	658	1885	744	1120	428	1347
	GIRLS									
11	423	3134	628	2359	736	2266	799	1325	478	1474
12	358	2940	687	2169	700	2136	830	1382	422	1436
13	377	2907	590	2205	672	2161	806	1802	399	1420

From Eguchi, S. and Hirsh, I. J. Development of speech sounds in children. *Acta Otolaryngologica*, suppl. 257 (1969) 5-43. Table 1, pp. 9-13. Reprinted by permission.
*Method: Five children in each group. Analysis of the italicized vowels in, "He *has* a *blue* pen" and "I am *tall*."

tract shape, is not necessarily valid, since there are many degrees of freedom. In theory, there are an infinite number of vocal tract shapes that could produce a given formant frequency. However, as a rough guide, the following relationships may prove useful. They are schematized in Figure 9-32.

1. *Length.* The frequency of all formants lowers as the length of the vocal tract increases.
2. *Lip rounding.* Increasing constriction of the labial port lowers all formant frequencies.
3. *Anterior oral constriction.* Elevation of the front of the tongue lowers the first formant and raises the second formant.
4. *Posterior oral constriction.* Raising the posterior part of the tongue tends to lower the second formant.
5. *Pharyngeal constriction.* Narrowing the pharynx raises the frequency of the first formant.
6. *Nasalization.* The effects of coupling the nasal resonant space to the vocal tract are very complex. Not only are resonant frequencies altered, but anti-

resonances are introduced. The overall result is highly variable. Specific nasalization characteristics are summarized in Chap. 10.

VOCAL EFFORT OR INTENSITY. A number of studies (e.g., Flanagan, 1958; Fant, 1973; Rothenberg, 1973) have shown that the glottal (source) wave changes with increasing vocal effort or intensity: Its rise and decay become steeper and its turning points sharper and more abrupt. Spectrally, these changes indicate more energy at high frequencies. In fact, the extended bandwidth of the vocal signal is one of the acoustical correlates of increased loudness (Brandt, Ruder, and Shipp, 1969; Zwicker, Flottorp, and Stevens, 1957). Therefore, as vocal intensity increases the vocal source spectrum shows increased amplitude of high frequency harmonics, which results in elevation of the amplitude of formants 2 and 3.

SPEECH RATE. The effect of the rate of syllable production on the formant frequencies is still a matter of some dispute. Lindblom (1963) found that formants (and espe-

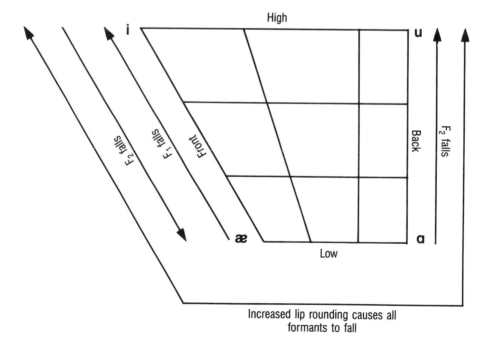

Increased lip rounding causes all formants to fall

FIGURE 9–32. Relationship between vowel position and formant values.

cially the second formant) did change as speech rate increased (vowel duration decreased). In essence this was considered to represent an "undershoot" in the approximation of a target vocal-tract posture as increasing speed demands were placed on the system. On the other hand, a study by Gay (1978) failed to detect a change in the formants of the vowel midpoint when speakers changed from a slow to a fast syllabic rate.

Consonants

Öhman (1967) has proposed that it is useful to view consonants as articulatory gestures superimposed on an underlying continuous variation of vowel productions. The consonants have several important characteristics that cause their spectra to differ in fundamental ways from those of the background vowels. Aside from the fact that consonants may include silent intervals, nasalizations, and aspirations, consonantal spectra are profoundly influenced by two critical facts:

1. While the sound source for normal English vowels is always the periodic and harmonic-rich glottal pulse, consonants can be formed from periodic glottal tone, aperiodic turbulence noise, or a combination of the two. The effects of this latitude on the spectrogram are obvious.
2. Consonants (even the relatively-open /j/ and /w/) are produced with significantly more constriction of the vocal tract than vowels. (Constriction reaches an extreme in the case of the plosives, for which there is a brief period of airway closure.) The tighter constriction of the consonants results in less radiated sound energy than vowels (See Chap. 4).

In discussing vowels, the point was made that formant frequencies change during the transitions from the preceding, and to the following, sounds. Furthermore, it was said that even in its stable midsection the formant frequencies of a given vowel could be expected to be different as a function of the phonetic surroundings. This same effect is seen in consonants. Each begins with an onset transition period during which its acoustic characteristics are built up on the foundation of the preceding sound, and each terminates as an offset transition as its acoustic signal modifies toward that of the following sound. And, as was the case for the vowels, the acoustic midportion of the consonant can be expected to show accomodation to its neighbors.

These effects, of coursse, are the acoustic manifestation of the constant motion of the articulators. Speech is not a sequence of static postures, each representing a discrete phoneme. Rather, the higher neurological control calls for, and the vocal tract biomechanics impose, an overlapping of sounds on the motor and acoustic level. In saying "spot" lip closure for /p/ is occurring during /s/ production. The resonances of /s/ will reflect the ever-diminishing labial opening: Part of the /p/ resides in the /s/. In short, coarticulatory effects are significant.

Just as elementary courses in phonetics present a picture of rather idealized speech sounds so, for the same reasons, the following sections on the English consonants will deal with idealized spectral features. The physiological classification of speech sounds according to articulatory *manner* has its counterpart in spectral features and, thus, will be used to organize the discussion.

Temporal aspects of consonants are important to their perceptual differentiation but, with a few exceptions, durational aspects of consonant features will not be dealt with here. (More information on this subject is available in Denes, 1955; Liberman, 1957; Liberman, Delattre, and Cooper, 1952; Liberman, Delattre, Gerstman, and Cooper, 1956; Liberman, Harris, Hoffman, and Griffith, 1957; DiSimoni, 1974b,c; Umeda, 1975, 1977; Klatt, 1974; Prosek and Runyan, 1982; Parnell, Amerman, and Wells, 1977).

Sonorants: Semivowels

Phoneticians use the term *sonorant* in various ways. For the present discussion it is considered to mean a voiced speech sound produced with airflow that is neither fully laminar (as for vowels) nor totally turbulent (as is the case with fricatives). There are three generally recognized subclasses in the sonorant group: semivowels, laterals, and retroflexes.

It has become clear that all of the sonorants share an important spectral feature—rapid formant transitions. Not unreasonably, Pickett (1980) therefore chose to classify them all as glides. While such a classificatory decision makes sense, in that it highlights a unifying similarity, traditional phonetics generally restricts the term glide to /j/ and /w/. It seems best to honor that convention.

The *semivowels*, /j/ and /w/, are aptly named. Although more constricted, they are physiologically and acousticallyy similar to /i/ and /u/. When combined with a vowel, these consonants produce a pattern of formant change that very much resembles a diphthong (Figure 9-33). The greater constriction of the consonants, however, results in lower F_1 and F_2 frequencies than is typical of these vowels. The third formant of /w/ is commonly weak or missing (weaker sound radiation for consonants), and the third formant of /j/ is often at a higher frequency than that of /i/.

An important difference between diphthongs and semivowel glides is the much briefer duration of the consonants, meaning that formant transitions are faster. Furthermore, the duration of these phonemes may be too short for the formants to stabilize at all. In that case, of course, /w/ and /j/ reduce to little more than a formant transition between two other sounds. This is not a problem, since perceptual discrimination of different sonorants depends heavily on the transitional patterns of F_2 and F_3 (Lisker, 1957a; O'Connor, Gerstman, Liberman, Delattre, and Cooper, 1957).

Sonorants—lateral and retroflex: /l/ and /r/

/l/ is characterized by great formant variability, particularly of F_2, whose frequency is strongly influenced by the surrounding vowels. Syllabic /l/ is somewhat more stable (Tarnóczy, 1948; Lehiste, 1964). The syllable-final /ł/, however, tends to show a higher first and lower second formant than the more common /l/.

Despite the very great variety of articulator postures used for the retroflex /r/ (Delattre, 1965), the acoustic product is almost always characterized by extreme lowering of F_3, bringing it close to F_2. This phenomenon is the signature of /r/ in English (Lehiste, 1964). /ɟ/, on the other hand, has a higher F_3. Acoustically, /r/ is influenced by its position in the utterance (initial, medial, etc.) more than by the physiological differences in production style. Initial /r/, for instance, has generally lower formants than other /r/s and, in general, is relatively immune to the influence of the following vowel. The formants of final /r/ are strongly influenced by the preceding vowel, however.

Dalston (1975) has studied word-initial /l, r, w/ as produced by normal children and adults. His data are comparable to those of the other investigators cited above, and he confirmed that the formant transitions of the sonorants are important to their discrimination. Tables 9-3 and 9-4 summarize his findings of formant frequencies of the steady-state portions of the sonorants and their formant transition characteristics.

Fricatives

Spectrograms of fricatives are easily recognized by the quasi-random turbulence noise that is their distinguishing characteristic. Voiced fricatives, of course, have an additional periodic component generated at the glottis. It is easily distinguished from the broad-band noise, especially in the lower frequencies. Voiced and unvoiced fricative cognates are otherwise essentially identical.

Although spectrally distinct as a group from other classes of speech sounds, the specific acoustic characteristics underlying perceptual discrimination of individual fricative phones remain largely unknown. A number of listener identification criter-

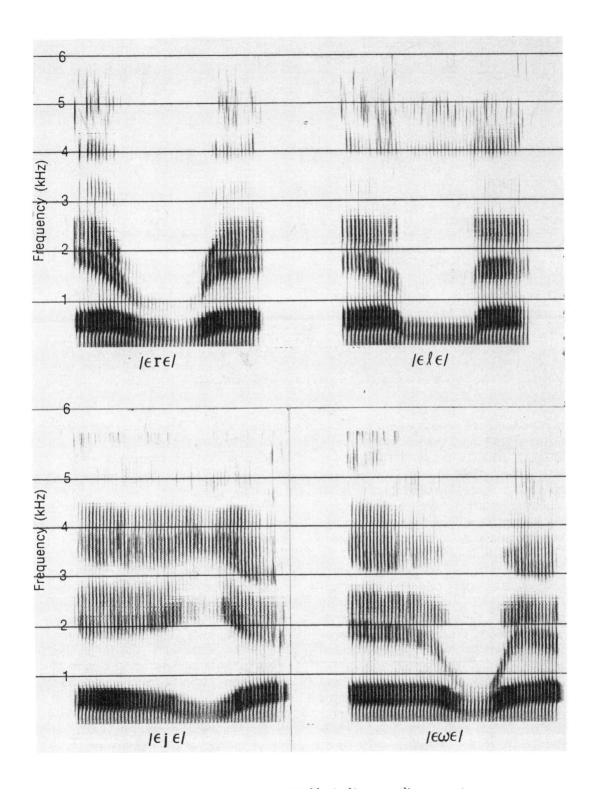

FIGURE 9–33. Spectra (300 Hz filter) of intervocalic sonorants.

TABLE 9–3. Steady-State Formant Frequencies (Hz) of /w, r, l/ in Normal Speakers*

	Men		Women		Children	
	Mean	**S.D.**	**Mean**	**S.D.**	**Mean**	**S.D.**
/r/						
F_1	348	45.9	350	38.3	431	49.8
F_2	1061	92.5	1065	85.4	1503	191.8
F_3	1546	94.8	2078	346.1	2491	369.8
/w/						
F_1	336	39.2	337	30.4	402	59.7
F_2	732	87.6	799	87.8	1020	148.8
F_3	2290	335.8	2768	141.7	3547	223.7
/l/						
F_1	344	55.2	365	11.6	412	38.4
F_2	1179	141.2	1340	96.8	1384	175.3
F_3	2523	197.8	2935	174.4	3541	293.0

From Dalston, R. M. Acoustic characteristics of /w, r, l/ spoken correctly by young children and adults. *Journal of the Acoustical Society of America*, 57 (1975) 462-469. Table II, p. 464. Reprinted by permission.

*Subjects: 6 boys, age 3 years 3 months to 4 years 3 months (mean 4 years 0 months); 4 girls, age 3 years 5 months to 4 years 3 months (mean 3 years 11 months); 3 men, age 19 years 9 months to 27 years 8 months (mean 25 years 4 months); 2 women, age 18 years 6 months to 18 years 9 months (mean 18 years 8 months). Word-initial /r, l, w/ combined with /i, a, u/ in simple words; 5 repetitions of each word.

ia have been proposed but none seems to completely separate a given fricative from all others (Hughes and Halle, 1956; Heinz and Stevens, 1961; Jassem, 1965). In fact, Harris (1954, 1958) has shown that discrimination of fricatives may depend heavily on the formant transitions of the post-fricative vowel rather than on the spectral properties of the consonant itself.

Most attempts at characterizing the spectra of fricatives have centered on determination of the frequency limits of the noise band and on the location of any energy peaks within it. Differences in these parameters should, in theory, reflect changes in the length of the portion of the vocal tract anterior to the turbulence-producing constriction, since that is the effective resonating space. Several studies support that hypothesis (Heinz and Stevens, 1961; Pentz, Gilbert, and Zawadzki, 1979, Daniloff, Wilcox, and Stephens, 1980). Peak energy for /f/, which has an exceptionally short length of vocal tract in front of the labiodental constriction, is at higher frequencies than peak energy of /ʃ/, whose constriction opens into a much longer res-

onating tube. The pattern of airflow and obstructions in the airstream also create acoustic differences by generating "spoiler" or "edge" noise that is added to the turbulence.

The formant peaks of the fricatives are not very strong, and they seem to show significant variation as a function of the following vowel. Further complicating any attempt at a clear specification of their spectral properties is the fact that fricatives are prone to a great deal of allophonic modification and intersubject variability (Hughes and Halle 1956). All things considered, only a broad and general description of any given fricative can be offerred. Figure 9-34 and Table 9-5 summarize their most salient features.

Given the fact that fricatives, and in particular /s/, are so often misarticulated in the school-age population, it is unfortunate that a firm grasp of the exact basis of their acoustic characteristics has been elusive. Daniloff, Wilcox, and Stephens (1980), for example, studied the spectral features of children's /s/ misarticulations. They concluded that listener's auditory impressions of ab-

TABLE 9–4. Mean Formant Durations of Word-Initial /w,r,l/ in Milliseconds for Normal Speakers*

		Adults		Children	
		Mean	SD	Mean	SD
/r/					
Steady-state portion	F_1	39.2	23.2	40.3	15.3
	F_2	35.5	14.8	41.2	15.0
Transition duration	F_1	33.7	20.4	32.7	19.2
	F_2	50.4	17.3	52.3	21.5
Transition rate (Hz/ms)	F_1	3.9	2.2	8.0	7.7
	F_2	10.5	6.6	11.7	6.9
/w/					
Steady-state portion	F_1	39.6	16.1	39.0	23.1
	F_2	44.4	20.2	39.5	21.9
Transition duration	F_1	32.7	18.7	36.9	18.2
	F_2	58.3	26.8	55.0	24.7
Transition rate (Hz/ms)	F_1	3.5	3.5	7.7	7.5
	F_2	11.8	6.9	7.4	9.5
/l/					
Steady-state portion	F_1	67.0	19.0	56.7	14.6
	F_2	57.0	19.9	55.4	15.9
Transition duration	F_1	21.3	15.7	21.8	14.1
	F_2	41.3	26.7	41.1	28.1
Transition rate (Hz/ms)	F_1	8.5	6.6	11.2	9.5
	F_2	11.4	4.5	19.0	7.0

From Dalston, R. M. Acoustic characteristics of /w, r, l/ spoken correctly by young children and adults. *Journal of the Acoustical Society of America*, 57 (1975) 462-469. Table III and IV, pp. 466 and 467. Reprinted by permission.

*For method, see Table 9-3.

normality had a basis in the acoustic signal, but intersubject variability was so high as to preclude a classification of the more subtle /s/ distortions.

Stops

The stops are unique among the sounds of speech in that they include a variable period of total blockage of airflow during which sound output may cease. During this interval air pressure rises behind the point of closure to be released as a burst of acoustic energy. (The dynamics of airflow during stop consonants has been examined in detail by Rothenberg, 1968.) Stop consonants are discriminated on the basis of three major parameters: (1) the characteristics of the burst (or impulse); (2) the nature of formant transitions before and after the silent (closure) period; and (3) the time required

for reestablishment of glottal pulsing (voice onset time) following release of the closure. The appearance of these features in the spectrogram is illustrated in Figure 9-35.

BURST (IMPULSE) CHARACTERISTICS. Release of the high pressure associated with "voiceless" stops gives rise to a more intense burst and often to significant aspiration. These are important cues to the voicing distinction in English. Intensity and aspiration aside, a number of studies have shown that place of plosive articulation can be discriminated on the basis of the spectral characteristics of the first 20 ms or so of the release burst (Halle, Hughes, and Radley, 1957; Liberman, 1957; Stevens and Blumstein, 1978; Blumstein and Stevens, 1979; Winitz, Scheib, and Reeds, 1972).

The important features seem to be that

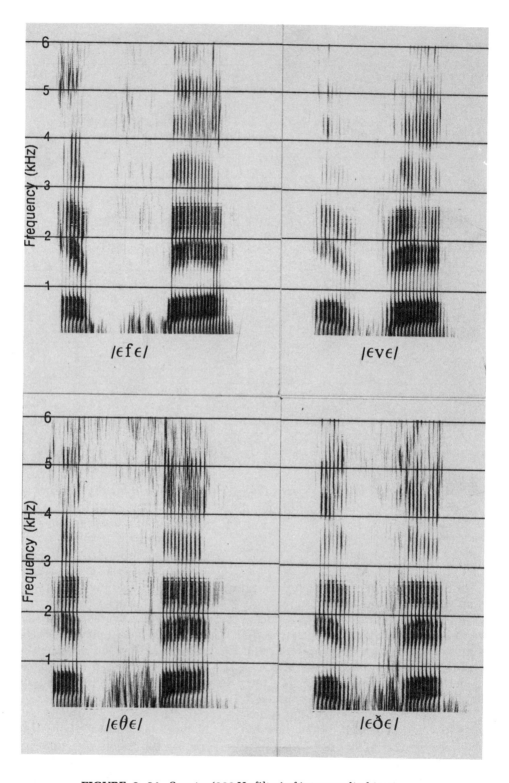

FIGURE 9–34. Spectra (300 Hz filter) of intervocalic fricatives.

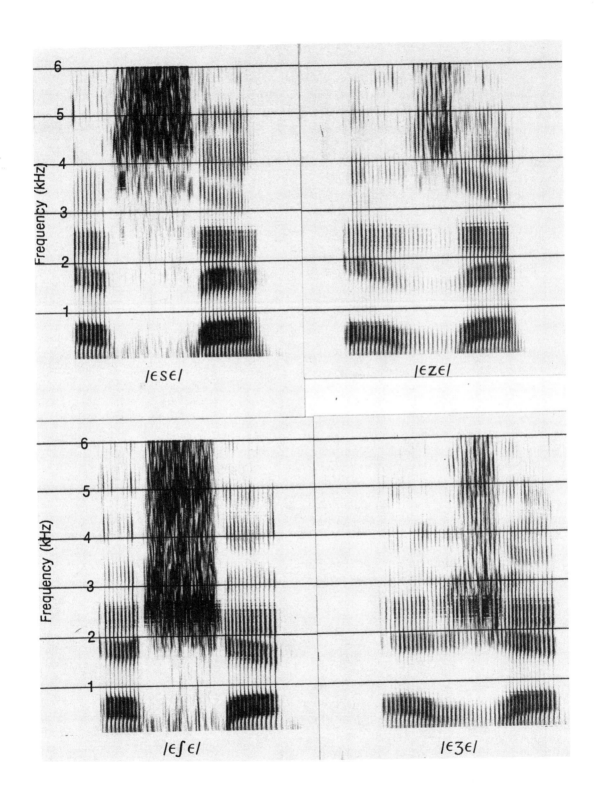

/ɛsɛ/

/ɛzɛ/

/ɛʃɛ/

/ɛʒɛ/

TABLE 9–5. Spectral Characteristics of Fricatives: Normal Speakers

Phone		Noise Band Limits (Hz)	Energy Peak Locations (Hz)	Intensity	Source
f/v	Adult	1500–7000+	1900, 4000, 6800–8400,	Low	a
			8200–12,000+		b
	Child		11,200–11,400		c
o/ð		1400–7200+	2000	Low	a
s/z	Adult	>3500–8000+	Variable:	Moderate	a
			3500–6400, 8000–8400		b
	Child		8300–8400		c
			6500–10,000		d
ʃ/ʒ	Adult	1600–7000	Near Lower end:	Moderate	a
			2200–2700, 4300–5400		b
	child		5300		c

(a) Strevens, 1960; (b) Heinz and Stevens, 1961; (c) Pentz, Gilbert, and Zawadzki, 1979; (d) Daniloff, Wilcox, and Stephens, 1980.

1. the *labials* /p,b/ have a primary energy concentration at low frequency (500 to 1500 Hz);
2. the *alveolars* /t,d/ show either a flat burst spectrum or one in which energy is concentrated above 4000 Hz. There is also an energy peak at about 500 Hz;
3. the *velar* stops /k,g/ have their burst energy concentrated in the intermediate 1500 to 4000 Hz region.

These characteristics are by no means invariant and, in general, are subject to the following modifications:

1. Voiced plosives are likely to have continuous glottal pulsing that shows as a major concentration of energy below 300 Hz or so. (The burst interval will also have faint glottal striations in its spectrogram.)
2. The lower pressure of voiced plosives (see Chap. 7) results in less high-frequency energy in the burst. Hence, for example, /d/ would be expected to have less spectral amplitude above 4000 Hz than /t/.
3. The burst characteristics are modified by coarticulation of the following vowel (Fischer-Jørgensen, 1954). The velar stops seem particularly susceptible to this effect. Their spectral peaks tend to

shift toward the second formant of the vowel in which they are released.

FORMANT TRANSITIONS. A number of studies (most of them done at Haskins Laboratories) have demonstrated the extreme importance of the formant transitions of the following vowel to identification of a stop's

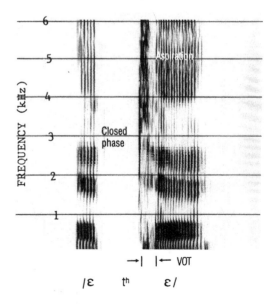

FIGURE 9–35. Spectrographic appearance of an intervocalic stop.

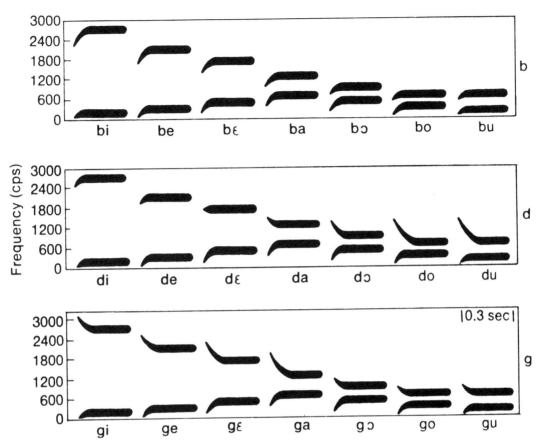

FIGURE 9–36. Formant transitions associated with perception of specific stop-vowel syllables. (Adapted from Delattre, P. C., Liberman, A. M., and Cooper, F. S. Acoustic loci and transitional cues for consonants. *Journal of the Acoustical Society of America*, 27 (1955), 769-773. Reprinted by permission from Lieberman, P. *Speech Physiology and Acoustic Phonetics.* New York: Macmillan, 1977, Figure 7-3, p. 119.)

place of articulation (Cooper, Delattre, Liberman, Borst, and Gerstman, 1952; Delattre, Liberman, and Cooper, 1955; Malmberg, 1955; Liberman, 1957; Harris, Hoffman, Liberman, Delattre, and Cooper, 1958; Hoffman, 1958). While third-formant transitions contribute to the discrimination, most of the necessary information is carried by the second formant.

The patterns of the formant transitions associated with different stops do not show a strict one-to-one correspondence with perceived phonemic categories. Figure 9-36 illustrates the formant-transitions pattern of synthetic stimuli that listeners identified as the syllables indicated. The first-formant

movements are always the same and, therefore, can be presumed to play little if any role in discrimination of specific stops. For a given stop, the second formant can be assumed to originate at some frequency locus that does not appear in the pattern but that iis "pointed at" by the onset transition. Clearly, for /b/ the indicated second formant frequency-of-origin is very low, and the second formant of /b/ always "rises" from it. Hence, /b/ always has a rising F_2 transition. By the same reasoning, it can be assumed that the origin of F_2 of /g/ must be quite high, since all of /g/'s F_2 transitions are falling. /d/ must originate at a locus of intermediate frequency. The transitions into the high second formants of /i, e, and ɛ/ rise, while the transitions into the lower second formants of the other vowels fall. That the formant transitions should signal the place of stop production is not surprising, since they reflect movement of the articulators on release of the plosive.

Final stops are often unreleased in English, so there are no burst and postrelease formant transitions to identify them. It is clear in these cases that formant transitions of the pre-stop sound provide the basis for perceptual categorization. Wang (1959) showed that the greater these formant transitions were, the more certain a listener was of the stop's identity. However, the reduction of information caused by the loss of the release phenomena was reflected in greater listener confusion than would be the case were the stop release available. English partially compensates for the reduced acoustic cues of unreleased final stops by requiring that the vowel preceding a voiced stop have longer duration than a vowel preceding its voiceless cognate (Denes, 1955; House and Fairbanks, 1953; Peterson and Lehiste, 1960; Raphael, 1972).

Nasal consonants

The primary resonator for the nasal consonants is the pharynx-nasal cavity tube. The oral cavity serves as a dead-end (occluded) resonator that is coupled to the rest of the vocal tract approximately at its midpoint. The length of this side branch is longest for /m/ (labial occlusion) and shortest for /ŋ/ (linguavelar closure). Pharyngeal shape is essentially the same for all three nasal consonants, and the geometry of the nasal cavity itself cannot be voluntarily altered. It is, therefore, not surprising that the nasal consonants have similar formant peaks.

The addition of a side branch to the resonating system creates *antiresonances* in its transfer function. These are the opposite of formants: valleys in the spectral envelope that represent spectral minima (in contrast to the formant peaks that represent spectral maxima). Like formants, however, antiresonances are located at specific frequencies. It has been shown by Fant (1960, 1973) that each antiresonance produced by coupling in a side-branch resonator is associated with an added resonance in the transfer function. Thus, the oral side branch produces resonance-antiresonance *pairs*. The frequency-separation between the added resonance peak and its associated antiresonance is a function of the amount of coupling between the side branch (oral cavity and the main resonator pharynx-nasal cavity). Strong coupling (that is, a large connecting orifice) results in wide separation of the resonance and antiresonance on the frequency scale. Weak coupling causes the two to be closer together. In fact, with a very narrow communicating orifice between the two resonating chambers the resonance and antiresonance may fall at essentially the same frequency. In this case, of course, they will cancel each other and produce no net change of the vocal tract transfer function. Specific spectral features of nasalization are considered in Chapter 10, to which the reader should refer for a more detailed listing of the effects of side-branch coupling on the speech signal.

The three nasal consonants of English (whose spectrograms are shown in Figure 9-37) are distinguished from each other by the frequency location of the resonances-antiresonances and by the formant transitions between the consonant and its surrounding sounds.

Resonances and Antiresonances

The nasalization resonances and antiresonances are added to (or subtracted from) the transfer function of the major resonating tube. The antiresonance may be most easily detected in the spectral envelope. Its position depends on the length of the side branch: The longer it is, the lower the antiresonance frequency (Hattori, Yamamoto, and Fujimura, 1958; House, 1957). Typically, the major antiresonances are at about 1000 Hz for /m/, 3500 Hz for /n/, and above 5000 Hz for /ŋ/.

Second-formant frequencies also play an important role in perception of place of

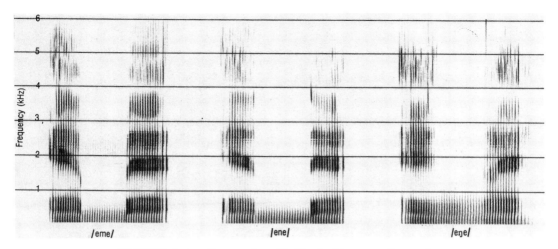

FIGURE 9–37. Spectra (300 Hz filter) of intervocalic nasals.

articulation. Nakata (1959) and Hecker (1962) have explored this parameter using synthetic speech signals. Their results indicate that second-formant frequencies in the range of 1200 Hz, 1800 Hz, and 2100 Hz are strong cues to /m/, /n/, and /ŋ/, respectively.

It is clear that the formant transitions associated with oral occlusion and opening also play an important role in nasal-consonant discrimination (Fujimura, 1962; Malécot, 1956). The transition patterns are very complex and not yet completely characterized.

Voice Onset Time

Voice onset time (VOT), an essential characteristtic of plosive phones, is easily read from a broad-band spectrogram. It can be viewed as a variable that, in a sense, summarizes a very complex and extremely important aspect of articulator-laryngeal coordination. It can be measured from simple, easily elicited utterances that can be produced even by very young children. (Bond and Korte [1983] have found that the VOT of spontaneous and imitative productions of 2- and 3-year-olds are not significantly different.) The pattern of VOT change during the period of speech acquisition is clear and relatively well docu-

mented, and there is the possiblity that it is sensitive to senescent involution as well. All of these facts point to VOT as a measure that is likely to be of use in describing or categorizing a range of developmental, neuromotor, or linguistic disorders. This potential utility to the speech pathologist may be one of the reasons for the heavy emphasis VOT has received in the research literature. It seems worthwhile, then, to consider it in some detail here.

The voice onset time is defined as the interval between the release of an oral constriction and the start of glottal pulsing (Lisker and Abramson, 1964). Although it is a temporal value that can be determined directly from the speech signal using relatively simple circuitry (Till and Stivers, 1981) it is more common to measure it from a wide-band spectrogram. In this context VOT is defined as the time equivalent of the space from the onset of the stop release-burst to the first vertical striation representing glottal pulsing (Liberman, Delattre, and Cooper, 1952; Lisker and Abramson, 1964, 1967). An example of VOT measurement is shown in Figure 9-38.

Viewed solely from the perspective of physiological capability of glottal and supraglottal coordination, the VOT is free to vary over a wide and continuous range. However, most languages limit VOT to two

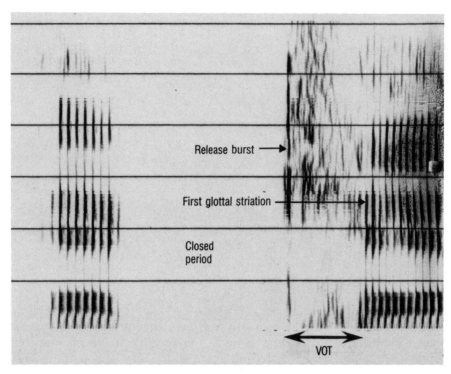

Release burst

First glottal striation

Closed
period

VOT

FIGURE 9–38. Measurement of voice onset time (VOT) in the utterance /ɛkɛ/. The VOT is defined as the interval from release of intraoral pressure to the onset of glottal pulsing.

or three relatively narrow and non-overlapping ranges. For prevocalic stops the range into which a given VOT falls serves the listener as an important cue to the voicing category of the phone (Lisker and Abramson, 1964; Abramson and Lisker, 1965; 1968). The traditional distinction of phoneticians, based on a dichotomous presence or absence of voicing during stop production, has been found inadequate to explain categorization along the voiced-voiceless dimension (Malécot, 1970; Ladefoged, 1971).

Interruption of glottal pulsing during stops can be either passive or active. Passive unvoicing results when the air pressure behind an oral closure rises near the level of the subglottal pressure. With the effective elimination of a transglottal pressure drop, voicing must halt. On the other hand, voicing can be actively stopped by the simple expedient of abducting the vocal folds. Numerous studies have shown that the larynx commonly behaves as an active articulator in controlling unvoicing, although its function in this regard is complex and only dimly understood (Kim, 1970; Hirose and Gay, 1972; Hirose and Ushijima, 1978; Sawashima, 1970; Warren and Hall, 1973; Löfqvist and Yoshioka, 1979, 1980). It is not yet clear whether variation of VOT is achieved by manipulation of glottal width during abduction for a stop or by direct timing control by higher CNS centers (Kim, 1970; Benguerel, Hirose, Sawashima, and Ushijima, 1978; Benguerel and Bhatia, 1980). No matter what the control mechanism, it is widely recognized that the VOT is a reliable and easily measured correlate of an important and precisely regulated aspect of speech motor coordination. Furthermore, a moderately large body of work has confirmed a clear developmental pattern of VOT change that provides a basis for evaluation of one aspect of a patient's early developmental status.

VOT in English

By convention, a VOT of 0 signals simultaneous onset of release-burst noise and glottal pulsing. Negative VOT values denote the time *before* burst noise that voice began (prevoicing, voice lead), while positive VOT values show the time of vocal striations *after* burst onset (voice lag).

In their early studies of isolated words with initial stops, Lisker and Abramson (1964, 1967) determined that VOT fell into three distinct ranges. Voiceless stops had a long VOT, ranging from +60 to +100 ms. On the other hand, VOTs associated with voiced stops fell into two ranges: -75 to -25 ms voicing lead) and 0 to +25 ms (short voicing lag). It has been demonstrated that perceptual categorization of English stops along the voicing dimension requires only two categories (Lisker, 1957b; Abramson and Lisker, 1965; Lisker and Abramson, 1964; Zlatin, 1974). Listeners classify stops with prevoicing or short voicing lags as voiced, while a long voicing lag underlies the perception of voiceless.* Therefore, the two "voiced" VOT ranges are generally collapsed into one category when discussing the English language.

The data in Table 9-6 are taken from a study by Zlatin (1974) in which normal English-speaking adults each produced 35 tokens of each of eight test words. There is very little overlap of the voiced and voiceless ranges. By and large the categories are quite distinct. The data also reveal that VOT tends to increase as the place of articulation is retracted. Labial plosives have the shortest VOTs, velars the longest. This effect was also noted by Lisker and Abramson (1964, 1967) and possible explanations for it, in terms of articulatory dynamics, have been proposed by Klatt (1975a). Thus, in stressed single-word utterances a VOT less than 25 ms or so can be said to signal an English voiced plosive. Longer VOTs

indicate a voiceless phoneme. Within the two ranges there are obviously overlapping subdivisions that offer some cue to place of articulation.

Contextual variability

The VOT of a given stop also varies as a function of the phonetic and suprasegmental characteristics of its environment. On the segmental level, the VOT of both voiced and voiceless stops is significantly longer before sonorants. VOTs of voiceless stops are lengthened by about 15% before the high vowels /i, u/ as compared to the low vowels /a, æ/ (Klatt, 1975a; Port and Rotunno, 1979; Weismer, 1979). A similar effect can be seen in the data for "bees" and "bear" in Table 9-6. Addition of a second syllable to a plosive-initial word shortens VOT only by about 8% (Klatt, 1975a).

The larger context, beyond the one or two syllables directly associated with the stop, also influences its VOT. In particular, there is demonstrable sensitivity to such suprasegmental characteristics as speech rate, word stress, semantic importance, and utterance length (Umeda, 1977; Lisker and Abramson, 1967). Based on his own research findings, Klatt (1975a) has generated a series of rules for predicting VOT in sentence contexts. They are summarized in Table 9-7, along with his data for average VOT values for word-initial stops and consonant clusters.

It is also important to realize that "citational" utterances of a single word for testing purposes may have VOTs that are significantly different from, and less variable than, the VOTs occurring in more realistic speech samples (Baran, Laufer, and Daniloff, 1977).

Developmental changes in VOT

Life-span changes in the VOT voicing contrast have been explored from the point of view of both perception and production. Most of the research has examined childhood development, but there are also indications that certain involutional changes

---

*Other acoustic phenomena, including formant transition characteristics, burst intensity, and the like, play a role in real-life categorization (Slis and Cohen, 1969a, b; Stevens, 1971; Stevens and Klatt, 1972, 1974; Klatt, 1975a; Summerfield and Haggard, 1977).

TABLE 9-6. Voice Onset Time in Milliseconds for Word-Initial Plosives
in Single-Word Utterances*†

Word	Mean	S.D.	Mode	Median	Minimum	Maximum
bees	−23.17	(50.74)	10	5.79	−170	+30
bear	−12.02	(43.02)	10	7.54	−210	+50
dime	−5.20	(42.50)	10	10.30	−200	+50
goat	−0.08	(49.67)	20	19.75	−210	+50
Voiced	−10.12		10		−210	+50
peas	+78.99	(23.67)	70	74.05	+40	+220
pear	+83.77	(25.06)	70	80.26	+10	+170
time	+87.12	(25.66)	70	82.52	+30	+180
coat	+90.73	(23.66)	70	86.93	+40	+170
Voiceless	+85.15		70		+10	+220

From Zlatin, M. A. Voicing contrast: Perceptual and productive voice onset time characteristics of adults. *Journal of the Acoustical Society of America*, 56 (1974) 981-994. Table 5, p. 989.

*Ten males, 10 females; age 23–40 years, mean 29 years; general American dialect; 35 repetitions of each stimulus word, measured from broad-band spectrograms.

†The large differences among the mean, median, and mode in each class are indicative of the marked skewing of the distributions.

might be associated with advanced age (Preston and Yeni-Komshian, 1967; Preston and Port, 1969; Eguchi and Hirsh, 1969; Kewley-Port and Preston, 1974; Menyuk and Klatt, 1975; Gilbert, 1975; Zlatin and Koenigsknecht, 1975, 1976; Sweeting and Baken, 1982; Neiman, Klich, and Shuey, 1983).

The picture of childhood development of VOT control that emerges indicates that very young children (age <1 year) produce stops whose VOTs fall rather uniformly along the VOT continuum. With further development the VOTs of *all* stops tend to cluster around the short-lead/short-lag (equivalent to the adult's "voiced") part of the range. As the child matures the voiceless stops are increasingly associated with greater voicing lag (that is, with longer VOT).

Just around the time of speech onset, then, children's stops have a unimodal distribution of VOTs: They all tend to fall on what an adult would categorize as the "voiced" side of the perceptual dichotomy. Put another way, the VOT ranges used by very young children to indicate the voiced-voiceless distinction tend to overlap almost completely, so that they are collapsed into a single productive category. This situation is readily apparent in the data of Kewley-Port and Preston (1974) and Zlatin and Koenigsknecht, (1976). By the age of 6 or so the categories overlap very much less, thanks to the increased mean voicing lag that has come to the voiceless cognates. Somewhere past the age of 6, movement of voiceless stops further into the lag range results in complete separation of the two categories, with no overlap in the VOT ranges for isolated words. The skill that is acquired by children in controlling VOT is that of *delaying* voice onset a precise amount of time in order to mark a voiceless phoneme.*

---

*It should be noted that acquisition of the voicing contrast does not seem to depend on learning to perceive the difference between long and short VOT. Zlatin and Koenigsknecht (1975) have shown that 2 year olds are capable of perceiving the VOT distinction, even though they may not be able to reproduce it. There is reason to believe that the perceptual ability is a function of inborn auditory feature detectors (Eimas, Siqueland, Jusczyk, and Vigorito, 1971; Kuhl, 1979) that are not unique to humans (Kuhl and Miller, 1975, 1978).

TABLE 9–7A. Voice Onset Time in Milli-seconds: Average Values for Word-Intial Consonant Clusters*

Voiced		Voiceless		/s-/ initial	
/b/	11	/p/	47	/sp/	12
/d/	17	/t/	65	/st/	23
/g/	27	/k/	70	/sk/	30
/br/	14	/pr/	59	/spr/	18
/dr/	2	/tr/	93	/str/	37
/gr/	35	/kr/	84	/skr/	35
/bl/	13	/pl/	61	/spl/	16
/gl/	26	/kl/	77	/skw/	39
		/tw/	102		
		/kw/	94		

From Klatt, D. H. Voice onset time, frication, and aspiration in word-initial consonant clusters. *Journal of Speech and Hearing Research*, 18 (1975) 686-706. Table 1, p. 689. © American Speech-Language-Hearing Association, Rockville, MD. Reprinted by permission.

*Three normal adult males. Five words for each cluster, embedded in the carrier "Say _____ again." Measured from broad-band spectrograms.

An important index of a child's speech-motor development may be the restriction of VOTs for a given stop to an acceptably narrow range that lies wholly to one side of the voiced-voiceless boundary.* In the terminology of statistics, the mean VOTs of voiced and voiceless stops should be widely separated, and the standard deviation associated with each should be small enough to prevent significant overlap of the distributions. On the motor-control level, what is implied is that a speaker should be able to attain a desired VOT target with minimal variation from trial to trial.

Eguchi and Hirsh (1969) provide mean intrasubject standard deviations that provide a useful gauge of the attainment of the required precision. Data for each of the age groups they studied are summarized in Table 9-8.

*There is some evidence that VOT control may be slightly poorer in "language delayed" children compared to their normal peers (Bond and Wilson, 1980). The differences between the two groups are not dramatic, however.

TABLE 9–7B. Rules for Predicting VOT in Sentence Productions*

Condition	Multiply Tabled Average Value by:
Voiced stops /b, d, g/	
Not in blend	1
Preceded by voiceless consonant	1.3
Preceded by nasal consonant	0.8
Voiceless stops /p, t, k/	
In prestressed cluster	1
Not stressed, word-initial:	
not in blend	0.7
preceded by voiceless consonant or silence	0.9
Not stressed, word medial or final	
not in blend	0.4
preceded by voiceless consonant	0.7

From Klatt, D. H. Voice onset time, frication, and aspiration in word-initial consonant clusters. *Journal of Speech and Hearing Research*, 18 (1975) 686-706. Appendix, p. 706. C American Speech-Language-Hearing Association, Rockville, MD. Reprinted by permission.

*Caution: :"Individual VOT values may differ from the predictions due to unaccounted-for variability, especially in unstressed environments" (p. 706)

VOICE QUALITY: EVALUATION OF THE SOURCE SPECTRUM

Because the acoustic spectrum of speech is the product of the vocal source signal as well as the filter characteristics of the vocal tract, spectrum analysis provides a window on laryngeal function as well as on articulatory movements. Evaluative methods rely primarily on spectrograms of the types already discussed. Another form of analysis—the long-term average spectra (LTAS)—uses the mean of all spectra of sounds during a relatively long sample. Recent research shows that it holds promise as an index of vocal quality (Carr and Trill, 1964; Frøkjaer-Jensen and Prytz, 1976; Wedin, Leanderson, and Wedin, 1978; Hammarberg, Fritzell, Gauffin,

TABLE 9–8.   Average Intra-Subject Standard Deviations Associated with Word-Initials /p/ and /t/*

Age (yr)	/p/		/t/	
	ms	Relative (Adult = 100)	ms	Relative (Adult = 100)
3	26.1	253	27.8	281
4	19.8	192	24.2	244
5	17.4	169	22.2	224
6	17.1	166	18.7	189
7	11.8	115	11.3	114
8	11.2	109	10.5	106
9	10.8	105	11.4	115
10	10.6	103	9.9	100
11	10.4	101	9.8	99
12	9.9	96	11.0	111
13	10.0	97	10.6	107
Adult	10.3	100	9.9	100

Eguchi, S. and Hirsh, I. J. Development of speech sounds in children. *Acta Otolaryngologica*, suppl. 257 (1969) 5-43. Table 3, p. 28. Reprinted by permission.
*Five or six subjects, each age group (separate male and female groups over age 10). Utterances: "He has a blue pen"; "I am tall."

Sundberg, and Wedin, 1980; Izdebski, 1980; Weinberg, Horii, and Smith, 1980; Wedin and Ögren, 1982). Because the hardware and computer support needed for LTAS are not widely available in speech clinics, the method remains somewhat esoteric. While it will not be considered here, the references just cited can provide a moderately comprehensive introduction to the technique. The several techniques discussed in this section have been found to be useful in the evaluation of vocal fold pathology (Rontal, Rontal, and Rolnick, 1975a,b; Wolfe and Ratusnik, 1981), esophageal voice (Tato, Mariani, de Piccoli, and Mirasov, 1954), spasmodic dysphonia (Frint, 1974), metabolic disorder (Rontal, Rontal, Leuchter, and Rolnick, 1978), and vocal abnormalities associated with severe hearing impairment (Monsen, 1979; Wirz, Subtelny, and Whitehead, 1981).

The search for spectrographic methods of analyzing vocal quality has concentrated on characterizing or quantifying the acoustic energy that lies between the harmonic frequencies. The harmonic content of the vocal signal results from quasi-periodic interruption of airflow by the vocal folds. The interharmonic (noise) energy, however, is the acoustic correlate of an uninterrupted turbulent transglottal flow. By analogy with electrical signals, the "chopped" airflow is described as AC; the turbulent but continuous flow represents a DC component (Isshiki, Yanaghihara, and Morimoto, 1966; Yanagihara, 1967a). As laryngeal function deteriorates and glottal efficiency declines, vocal-fold modulation of the airstream becomes less complete: The AC component weakens as the DC component grows. The spectral manifestation of this shift is progressive replacement of harmonic lines by aperiodic noise.*

Different aspects of glottal-source noise can be observed in wide- and narrow-band spectrograms (Cornut, 1971) such as those shown in Figure 9-39, in which normal and hoarse vowel productions are compared. Abnormality can be seen in the irregular spacing of the glottal striations and in the obvious high-noise background of the wide-band analyses. But the differences between the normal and hoarse voices are even more apparent in the narrow-band spectrograms because of the clear delineation of the vocal harmonics. It is obvious why narrow-band analyses form the basis of spectrographic evaluation.

Spectrographic Categories of Hoarse Voice

Yanagihara (1967a,b) evaluated male and female speakers with varying degrees of hoarseness. Narrow band-spectrograms of their sustained /u, ɔ, ɑ, ɛ, and i/ at "moderate loudness and medium pitch" could be categorized into 4 types that correlated well with hoarseness severity. Narrow-band spectrograms are assigned to the various classes according to the following criteria (Yanagihara, 1967b).

*Another major source of noise—cycle-to-cycle period variability—is discussed in the section on "Jitter" in Chap. 5.

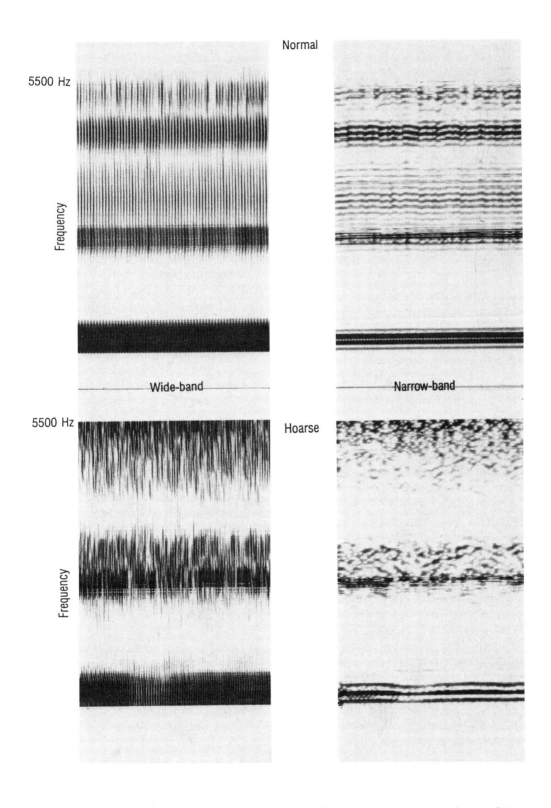

FIGURE 9–39. Wide- (300 Hz, left) and narrow-band (45 Hz, right) spectrograms of normal (top) and hoarse (bottom) productions of /i/.

Type I. "The regular harmonic components are mixed with the noise component chiefly in the formant region of the vowels."

Type II. "The noise components in the second formants of /ɛ/ and /i/ dominate over the harmonic components, and slight additional noise components appear in the high-frequency region above 3000 Hz in the vowels /ɛ/ and /i/."

Type III. "The second formants of /ɛ/ and /i/ are totally replaced by noise components, and the additional noise components above 3000 Hz further intensify their energy and expand their range."

Type IV. "The second formants of /ɑ, ɛ/ and /i/ are replaced by noise components, and even the first formants of all vowels often lose their periodic components which are [supplanted] by noise components. In addition, more intensified high frequency additional noise components are seen."

Spectral Noise Level

Spectral noise and its relationship to vowel *roughness* (a term specially used to avoid the confusion associated with the term *hoarseness*) has been a particular interest of Emanuel and his coworkers (Emanuel and Sansone, 1969; Sansone and Emanuel, 1970; Lively and Emanuel, 1970; Emanuel, Lively, and McCoy 1973; Whitehead and Emanuel, 1974; Emanuel and Whitehead, 1979; Arnold and Emanuel, 1979; Whitehead and Lieberth, 1979; Emanuel and Scarinzi, 1979, 1980; Emanuel and Austin, 1981).

Their method of analysis is best exemplified by the first of their reports (Emanuel and Sansone, 1969; Sansone and Emanuel, 1970). Speakers sustained each of several vowels for 7 s at a monitored intensity of 75 dB SPL. A two-second tape segment of the vowel recording was formed into a loop and repeatedly scanned by a spectrum analyzer operated with a very narrow (3 Hz) bandwidth. The strip-chart output was an amplitude-by-frequency spectrum, equivalent to a section produced by a standard spectrograph (but with much finer frequency resolution, of course). From this record

the minimum noise value (in dB SPL) was measured for each 100 Hz segment of the spectrum from 200 to 8000 Hz. In this first study, normal men produced the vowels using their habitual voice and then using a "rough" voice. Findings were not always fully consistent across speakers, but several conclusions were justified:

1. All vowels—both normal and rough—have noise components over a broad spectral range, but rough vowels have much more noise. This finding is consistent with the earlier work of Isshiki, Yanagihara, and Morimoto (1966), Yanagihara (1967a,b), and Nessel (1960).

2. The noise level is related to the amount of frequency perturbation.

3. Spectral noise level varies with tongue height of the vowel. For both normal and rough productions, the high /u/ and /i/ had the least, /æ/ the most, and /ɑ/ /ʌ/ intermediate noise levels.

4. The correlation coefficients for overall spectral noise level and perceived vowel roughness were all significant ($p < .05$), ranging from 0.74 to 0.92. The correlations were even higher (0.97-0.98) when noise levels only in the range of 100 to 2600 Hz were considered. (Correlation coefficients resulting from several studies are summarized in Whitehead and Emanuel, 1974.)

Similar, and hence confirmatory, results have been obtained in studies of simulated rough vowels produced by women (Lively and Emanuel, 1970; Emanuel, Lively, and McCoy, 1973). Phonatory register also influences spectral noise levels. In normal speakers, pulse register is associated with more spectral noise, and loft register with less, than modal register (Emanuel and Scarinzi, 1979, 1980).

The validity of spectral noise levels as a measure of roughness of genuinely (as opposed to simulated) dysphonic vowels has been assessed by Arnold and Emanuel (1979). They studied 10 normal boys and 10 with confirmed laryngeal lesions and rough voices. The analytic methods were the same as in the simulation studies, but two pitch levels were examined. Spectral noise was found to be higher in the voices of the dysphonic children. For all children, vowels differed in median noise level, generally following the order observed in adults. Among the normal children, high vocal pitch was associated with lower noise levels, but this effect did not hold for the dysphonic children. It has also been determined that spectral noise levels correlate moderately well with ratings of the "tension/harshness" of the voices of deaf speakers (Whitehead and Lieberth, 1979; Wirz, Subtelny, and Whitehead, 1981). Unfortunately, spectral noise alone has been found to be only a fair differentiator of rough and abnormal voices (Emanuel and Austin, 1981).

The other side of the spectral-noise coin, so to speak, is the harmonic amplitude level. As (interharmonic) spectral noise increases, it might be supposed that the energy at the harmonic frequencies would decrease. Emanuel and Whitehead (1979) found that this is indeed the case—up to a point. They reanalyzed the taped samples used by Sansone and Emanuel (1970) using the same spectrum analyzer. This time, however, the variable of interest was the amplitude of each of the first five harmonics and its relationship to perceived vowel roughness.

Unfortunately, their results were not unequivocal. With a single exception (the third harmonic of /i/), the amplitude of the first three harmonics decreased as judged roughness increased. The correlation coefficients for the median of the judges' roughness ratings and harmonic amplitude level ranged from -0.32 to -0.74 (excluding the correlation for the third harmonic of /i/). Interestingly, the correlation coefficients for the second harmonic were considerably higher than those for the first and third, ranging from -0.70 to -0.74. These correlations are statistically significant ($p < .05$), but on the whole they are not impressive. A coefficient of -0.32 indicates that the harmonic amplitude change accounts for a scant 10% of the change in perceived roughness. Even a coefficient of -0.74 means that

only 55% of the roughness variability is accounted for.

Confounding the harmonic-level interpretation even more is the fact that the fourth and fifth harmonics sometimes showed a significant *increase* in amplitude as roughness grew more severe. The authors hypothesized that this was due to high-frequency noise additively contributing to the energy of the upper formants. The supposition could not be tested, however.

Harmonic-to-Noise Ratio

The major problem with Emanuel's approaches is that either the noise or the harmonic level is considered in isolation. However, work of Isshiki, Yanagihara, and Morimoto (1966), Yanagihara (1967a,b) and Kim, Kakita, and Hirano (1982) has shown that a characteristic feature of hoarseness is the replacement of harmonics by noise energy. That is, aperiodic sound intensifies at the expense of periodic signal. It is reasonable to conclude that the best measure of hoarseness might be the ratio of one to the other. This was the approach taken by Kojima, Gould, and Lambiase (1979), Kojima, Gould, Lambiase, and Isshiki (1980) and Kitajima (1981). Their computational procedure, however, was complex and inconvenient. It was soon improved upon by Yumoto, Gould, and Baer (1982) and Yumoto, Sasaki, and Okamura (1984), whose purpose was to objectify and quantify the features that appear in the spectrogram of the hoarse voice.

While the actual mathematical method is beyond the scope of the present discussion, the conceptual basis of Yumoto et al.'s measure is fairly simple and worth some consideration. The voice is considered to have two components: perfectly periodic waves and random noise. Because the noise component represents random sound pressure variation about a zero value, summing the instantaneous noise amplitudes over a moderately long time interval will result in a net noise amplitude of zero. On the other hand, similarly adding the consecutive waves of the purely periodic component results in an ever-larger net-sum wave. Therefore, if the average amplitude of every point in a real vowel waveform is taken for a moderately large number of periods, the noise component should cancel out, leaving a pure periodic signal.

Now, it can be assumed that the pure (average) periodic wave is increasingly contaminated by random noise as hoarseness worsens. The degree of contamination can best be expressed as a periodic-to-noise amplitude ratio. It has just been shown that the periodic amplitude can be determined fairly easily by averaging waveforms. How can the noise level associated with each vocal period be determined?

It turns out that the answer is relatively simple. Since the averaged waveform represents a pure, noise-free vocal period, it suffices to subtract its value at every point in time from a real (noise contaminated) vocal period. The remainder is the isolated noise content of the real waveform. The *harmonic-to-noise (H/N) ratio* is then just the mean amplitude of the average wave divided by the mean amplitude of the isolated noise components for the train of waves. For convenience, the H/N ratio is expressed in dB.

To test the utility of their index, Yumoto and his coworkers assessed the sustained /ɑ/ of 22 men and 20 women with no demonstrable vocal disorder. They were compared to the pre- and post-operative phonations of a roughly comparable group of 12 men and 8 women with various laryngeal pathologies and widely different degrees of hoarseness. The mean H/N ratio for the normal subjects was 11.9 dB (S.D. = 2.32; range 7.0 to 17.0). Men and women were not significantly different. The 95% confidence limit was 7.4 dB. In contrast, the mean H/N ratio of the preoperative dysphonics was only 1.6 dB (range -15.2 to 9.6). Three of the 20 preoperative subjects had H/N ratios greater than the 7.4 dB lower limit of normality, but they were the ones with very slight clinical hoarseness. Postoperatively, the patients' mean H/N ratio rose to 11.3 dB (S.D. = 3.13; range 5.9 to 17.6) with about 95% achieving a ratio in the expected normal range. Equally interesting was the fact that the correlation between the H/N ratios and the spectrogram type (as determined by an experienced clinician) was an impressive 0.849. The pre- to postoperative change in H/N ratio was correlated with change in spectrogram type to the extent of a near-perfect coefficient of 0.944. In a later study (Yumoto, Sasaki, and Okamura, 1984) it was found that the correlation of the H/N ratio and psychophysical scaling of hoarseness was 0.809.

Yumoto et al. did their assessment by computer processing of the vocal signal after analog-to-digital conversion at a rate of 20 thousand samples per second. In fact, computer processing is the only practical way to perform this analysis. This is not likely to keep H/N ratio determination beyond the reach of the voice clinician for long. The analysis algorithm is not overly complex, and the digitizing is not likely to remain outside the range of what fairly inexpensive microcomputers will be able to achieve in the easily forseeable future. In consequence, a modest amount of development and refinement could turn this evaluative method into valuable clinical diagnostic procedure. ■

SELECT BIBLIOGRAPHY

Abramson, A. S. and Lisker, L. Voice onset time in stop consonants: acoustic analysis and synthesis. *Fifth International Conference on Acoustics* (Liège, Belgium), 1965.

Abramson, A. S. and Lisker, L. Voice timing: Cross-language experiments in identification and discrimination. *Haskins Laboratories Status Report of Speech Research*, SR13/14 (1968) 49-63.

Adams, M. R. Further analysis of stuttering as a phonetic transition defect. *Journal of Fluency Disorders*, 3 (1978) 265-271.

Allen, G. D. Vowel duration measurement: A reliability study. *Journal of the Acoustical Society of America*, 63 (1978) 1176-1185.

Angelocci, A. A., Kopp, G. A., and Holbrook, A. The vowel formants of deaf and normal-hearing eleven- to fourteen-year-old boys. *Journal of Speech and Hearing Disorders*, 29 (1964) 156-170.

Arnold, K. S. and Emanuel, F. W. Spectral noise levels and roughness severity ratings for vowels produced by male children. *Journal of Speech and Hearing Research*, 22 (1979) 613-626.

Atal, B. S., Chang, J. J., Mathews, M. V., and Tukey, J. W. Inversion of articulatory-to-acoustic transformation in the vocal tract by a computer-sorting technique. *Journal of the Acoustical Society of America*, 63 (1978) 1535-1555.

Ballantine, S. A logarithmic recorder for frequency response measurements at audiofrequencies. *Journal of the Acoustical Society of America*, 5 (1933) 10-24.

Baran, J. A., Laufer, M. Z., and Daniloff, R. Phonological contrastivity in conversation: a comparative study of voice onset time. *Journal of Phonetics*, 5 (1977) 339-350.

Benguerel, A.-P. and Bhatia, T. K. Hindi stop consonants: An acoustic and fiberscopic study. *Phonetica*, 37 (1980) 134-148.

Benguerel, A.-P., Hirose, H., Sawashima, M., and Ushijima, T. Laryngeal control in French stop production: A fiberscopic, acoustic, and electromyographic study. *Folia Phoniatrica*, 30 (1978) 175-198.

Blumstein, S. E. and Stevens, K. N. Acoustic invariance in speech production: evidence from measurements of the spectral characteristics of stop consonants. *Journal of the Acoustical Society of America*, 66 (1979) 1001-1017.

Bogert, B. P. and Peterson, G. E. The Acoustics of Speech. In Travis, L. E. (Ed.). *Handbook of Speech Pathology*. New York: Appleton-Century-Crofts, 1957. Chap. 5 pp. 109-173.

Bond, Z. S. and Korte, S. S. Children's spontaneous and imitative speech: an acoustic-phonetic analysis. *Journal of Speech and Hearing Research*, 26 ((1983) 464-467.

Bond, Z. S. and Wilson, H. F. Acquisition of the voicing contrast by language-delayed and normally speaking children. *Journal of Speech and Hearing Research*, 23 (1980) 152-161.

Borden, G. J. and Harris K. S. *Speech Science Primer: Physiology, Acoustics, and Perception of Speech* (2nd ed.). Baltimore: Williams and Wilkins, 1984.

Brandt, J. F., Ruder, K. F., and Shipp, T., jr. Vocal loudness and effort in continuous speech. *Journal of the Acoustical Society of America*, 46 (1969) 1543-1548.

Broad, D. J. Toward defining acoustic phonetic equivalence for vowels. *Phonetics*, 33 (1976) 401-424.

Broadbent, D. E., Ladefoged, P., and Lawrence, W. Vowel sounds and perceptual constancy. *Nature*, 178 (1956) 815-816.

Buhr, R. D. The emergence of vowels in an infant. *Journal of Speech and Hearing Research*, 23 (1980) 73-94.

Carmeci, P. and Jorgensen, R. Sonagraph recording techniques. *Journal of the Acoustical Society of America*, 32 (1960) 1959-1961.

Carr, P. B. and Trill, D. Long-term larynx-excitation spectra. *Journal of the Acoustical Society of America*, 36 (1964) 2033-2040.

Catford, J. C. *Fundamental Problems in Phonetics*. Bloomington, IN: University of Indiana, 1977.

Cavallo, S. A., Baken, R. J., and Shaiman, S. Frequency perturbation characteristics of pulse register phonation. *Journal of Communication Disorders*, 17 (1984) 231-243.

Chiba, T. and Kajiyama, M. *The Vowel: Its Nature and Structure*. Tokyo: Kaiseikan, 1941.

Coleman, R. F. Decay characteristics of vocal fry. *Folia Phoniatrica*, 15 (1963) 256-263.

Cooley, J. W. and Tukey, J. W. An algorithm for the machine calculation of the complex Fourier series. *Mathematics of Computation*, 19 (1965) 297-301.

Cooper, F. S., Delattre, P. C., Liberman, A. M, Borst, J. M., and Gerstman, L. J. Some experiments on the perception of synthetic speech sounds. *Journal of the Acoustical Society of America*, 24 (1952) 597-606.

Cornut, G. Vibrations normales et pathologiques des cordes vocales étudiées à l'aide du Sonagraph. *Folia Phoniatrica*, 23 (1971) 234-238.

Dalston, R. M. Acoustic characteristics of /w, r, l/ spoken correctly by young children and adults. *Journal of the Acoustical Society of America*, 57 (1975) 462-469.

Daniloff, R., Schuckers, G., and Feth, L. *The Physiology of Speech and Hearing: An Introduction*. Englewood Cliffs, NJ: Prentice-Hall, 1980.

Daniloff, R. G., Wilcox, K., and Stephens, M. I. An acoustic-articulatory description of children's defective /s/ productions. *Journal of Communication Disorders*, 13 (1980) 347-363.

Delattre, P. *Comparing the Phonetic Features of English, German, Spanish, and French: An Interim Report*. Heidelberg: Julius Groos Verlag, 1965.

Delattre, P. C., Liberman, A. M., Cooper, F. S. Acoustic loci and transitional cues for consonants. *Journal of the Acoustical Society of America*, 27 (1955) 769-773.

Delattre, P., Liberman, A. M., Cooper, F. S., and Gerstman, L. J. An experimental study of the acoustic determinants of vowel color. *Word*, 8 (1952) 195-210.

Denes, P. Effect of duration on the perception of voicing. *Journal of the Acoustical Society of America*, 27 (1955) 761-764.

DiSimoni, F. G. Effect of vowel environment on the duration of consonants in the speech of three-, six-, and nine-year-old children. *Journal of the Acoustical Society of America*, 55 (1974a) 360-361.

DiSimoni, F. G. Influence of consonant environment on duration of vowels in the speech of three-, six-, and nine-year-old children. *Journal of the Acoustical Society of America*, 55 (1974b) 362-363.

DiSimoni, F. G. Influence of utterance length upon bilabial closure duration of /p/ in three-, six-, and nine-year-old children. *Journal of the Acoustical Society of America*, 55 (1974c) 1353-1354.

Dudley, H. and Gruenz, 0. jr. Visible speech translators with external phosphors. *Journal of the Acoustical Society of America*, 18 (1946) 62-73.

Dunn, H. K. The calculation of vowel resonances, and an electrical vocal tract. *Journal of the Acoustical Society of America*, 22 (1950) 740-753.

Dunn, H. K. Methods of measuring formant bandwidths. *Journal of the Acoustical Society of America*, 33 (1961) 1737-1746.

Eguchi, S. and Hirsh, I. J. Development of speech sounds in children. *Acta Oto-laryngologica*, suppl. 257 (1969) 5-43.

Eimas, P. D., Siqueland, E. R., Jusczyk, P., and Vigorito, J. Speech perception in infants. *Science*, 171 (1971) 303-306.

Emanuel, F. W. and Austin, D. Identification of normal and abnormally rough vowels by spectral noise level measurements. *Journal of Communication Disorders*, 14 (1981) 75-85.

Emanuel, F. W., Lively, M. A., and McCoy, J. F. Spectral noise level and roughness rating for vowels produced by males and females. *Folia Phoniatrica*, 25 (1973) 110-120.

Emanuel, F. W. and Sansone, F. E., jr. Some spectral features of "normal" and simulated "rough" vowels. *Folia Phoniatrica*, 21 (1969) 401-415.

Emanuel, F. and Scarinzi, A. Vocal register effects on vowel spectral noise and roughness: Findings for adult females. *Journal of Communication Disorders*, 12 (1979) 263-272.

Emanuel, F. and Scarinzi, A. Vocal register effects on vowel spectral noise and roughness: Findings for adult males. *Journal of Communication Disorders*, 13 (1980) 121-131.

Emanuel, F. W. and Whitehead, R. L. Harmonic levels and vowel roughness. *Journal of Speech and Hearing Research*, 22 (1979) 829-840.

Endres, W., Bombach, W. and Flösser, G. Voice spectrograms as a function of age, voice disguise, and voice imitation. *Journal of the Acoustical Society of America*, 49 (1971) 1842-1848.

Fairbanks, G. and Grubb, P. A psychophysical investigation of vowel formants. *Journal of Speech and Hearing Research*, 4 (1961) 203-219.

Fant, G. *Acoustic Theory of Speech Production*. The Hague: Mouton, 1960.

Fant, G. M. Descriptive analysis of the acoustic aspects of speech. *Logos*, 5 (1962) 3-17.

Fant, G. A note on vocal tract size and nonuniform F-pattern scalings. *Quarterly Progress and Status Report, Speech Transmission Laboratory*, 4 (1966) 22-30.

Fant, G. *Speech Sounds and Features*. Cambridge, MA: MIT Press, 1973.

Fant, G. The relations between area functions and the acoustic signal. *Phonetica*, 37 (1980) 55-86.

Fant, G., Fintoft, K., Liljencrants, J., Lindblom, B., and Martony, J. Formant-amplitude measurements. *Journal of the Acoustical Society of America*, 35 (1963) 1753-1761.

Fischer-Jørgensen, E. Acoustic analysis of stop consonants. *Miscellanea Phonetica*, 2 (1954) 42-59.

Flanagan, J. L. Some properties of the glottal sound source. *Journal of Speech and Hearing Research*, 1 (1958) 99-116.

Flanagan, J. L., Coker, C. H., Rabiner, L. R., Schafer, R. W., and Umeda, N. Synthetic voices for computers. *IEEE Spectrum*, 7 (1970) 22-45.

Fönagy, I. and Magdics, K. Speed of utterance in phrases of different lengths. *Language and Speech*, 3 (1960) 179-192.

Frint, T. Experimentelle Untersuchungen Seltner Stimmphänomene bei einem Fall von spastischer Dysphonie. *Folia Phoniatrica*, 26 (1974) 422-427.

Frøkjaer-Jensen, B. and Prytz, S. Registration of voice quality. *B & K Technical Review*, 3-1976, 3-17.

Fry, D. B. Duration and intensity as physical correlates of linguistic stress. *Journal of the Acoustical Society of America*, 27 (1955) 765-768.

Fry, D. B. *The Physics of Speech*. New York: Cambridge University, 1979.

Fujimura, O. Analysis of nasal consonants. *Journal of the Acoustical Society of America*, 34 (1962) 1865-1875.

Fujimura, O. Analysis of nasal consonants. Joursurements of vocal-tract characteristics. *Journal of the Acoustical Society of America*, 49 (1971) 541-558.

Gay, T. Effect of speaking rate on vowel formant movements. *Journal of the Acoustical Society of America*, 63 (1978) 223-230.

Gerstman, L. J. Classification of self-normalized vowels. *IEEE Transactions: Audio-Electroacoustics*, AV-16 (1968) 78-80.

Gilbert, J. H. Formant concentration positions in the speech of children at two levels of linguistic development. *Journal of the Acoustical Society of America*, 48 (1970) 1404-1406.

Gilbert, J. H. V. A voice onset time analysis of apical stop production in 3-year olds. *Journal of Child Language*, 4 (1975) 103-110.

Halle, M., Hughes, G. W., and Radley, P. A. Acoustic properties of stop consonants. *Journal of the Acoustical Society of America*, 29 (1957) 107-116.

Hammarberg, B., Fritzell, G., Gauffin, J., Sundberg, J. and Wedin, L. Perceptual and acoustic correlates of abnormal voice qualities. *Acta Oto-laryngologica*, 90 (1980) 441-451.

Harris, K. S. Cues for the identification of the fricatives of American English. *Journal of the Acoustical Society of America*, 26 (1954) 952A.

Harris, K. S. Cues for the discrimination of American English fricatives in spoken syllables. *Language and Speech*, 1 (1958) 1-7.

Harris, K. S., Hoffman, H. S., Liberman, A. M., Delattre, P. C., and Cooper, F. S. Effect of third-formant transitions on the perception of the voiced stop consonants. *Journal of the Acoustical Society of America*, 30 (1958) 122-126.

Hattori, S., Yamamoto, K., and Fujimura, 0. Nasalization of vowels in relation to nasals. *Journal of the Acoustical Society of America*, 30 (1958) 267-274.

Healey, E. C. and Gutkin, B. Analysis of stutterers' voice onset times and fundamental frequency contours during fluency. *Journal of Speech and Hearing Research*, 27 (1984) 219-225.

Hecker, M. H. L. Studies of nasal consonants with an articulatory speech synthesizer. *Journal of the Acoustical Society of America*, 34 (1962) 179-188.

Heinz, J. M. and Stevens, K. N. On the properties of voiceless fricative consonants. *Journal of the Acoustical Society of America*, 33 (1961) 589-596.

Hirose, H. and Gay, T. The activity of the intrinsic laryngeal muscles in voicing control. *Phonetica*, 25 (1972) 140-164.

Hirose, H. and Ushijima, T. Laryngeal control for voicing distinction in Japanese consonant production. *Phonetica*, 35 (1978) 1-10.

Hoffman, H. S. Study of some cues in the perception of the voiced stop consonants. *Journal of the Acoustical Society of America*, 30 (1958) 1035-1041.

Holbrook, A. and Fairbanks, G. Diphthong formants and their movements. *Journal of Speech and Hearing Research*, 5 (1962) 38-58.

Horii, Y. An accelerometric approach to nasality measurement: a preliminary report. *Cleft Palate Journal*, 17 (1980) 254-261.

House, A. S. Analog studies of nasal consonants. *Journal of Speech and Hearing Disorders*, 22 (1957) 190-204.

House, A. S. and Fairbanks, G. The influence of consonant environment upon the secondary acoustical characteristics of vowels. *Journal of the Acoustical Society of America*, 25 (1953) 105-113.

Huggins, A. W. F. Better spectrograms from children's speech: a research note. *Journal of Speech and Hearing Research*, 23 (1980) 19-27.

Hughes, G. W. and Halle, M. Spectral properties of fricative consonants. *Journal of the Acoustical Society of America*, 28 (1956) 303-310.

Israel, H. Continuing growth in the human cranial skeleton. *Archives of Oral Biology*, 13 (1968) 133-137.

Israel, H. Age factor and the pattern of change in craniofacial structures. *American Journal of Physical Anthropology*, 39 (1973) 111-128.

Isshiki, N., Yanagihara, N., and Morimoto, M. Approach to the objective diagnosis of hoarseness. *Folia Phoniatrica*, 18 (1966) 393-400.

Izdebski, K. Long-time-average spectra (LTAS) applied to analysis of spastic dysphonia. In Lawrence, V. and Weinberg, B (Eds.). *Transcripts of the Ninth Symposium: Care of the Professional Voice*, part I. New York: The Voice Foundation, 1980. Pp. 89-94.

Jassem, W. The formants of fricative consonants. *Language and Speech*, 8 (1965) 1-16.

Kent, R. D. Anatomical and neuromuscular maturation of the speech mechanism: evidence from acoustic studies. *Journal of Speech and Hearing Reserach*, 18 (1976) 421-447.

Kent, R. D. Imitation of synthesized vowels by preschool children. *Journal of the Acoustical Society of America*, 63 (1978) 1193-1198.

Kent, R. D. Isovowel lines for the evaluation of vowel formant structure in speech disorders. *Journal of Speech and Hearing Disorders*, 44 (1979) 513-521.

Kent, R. D. and Forner, L. L. Age-sex differences in vowel formant frequencies: Normalization criteria. Presentation at the 1978 Convention of the American Speech and Hearing Association.

Kent, R. D. and Forner, L. L. Developmental study of vowel formant frequencies in an imitation task. *Journal of the Acoustical Society of America*, 65 (1979) 208-217.

Kent, R. D. and Forner, L. L. Speech segment durations in sentence recitations by children and adults. *Journal of Phonetics*, 8 (1980) 157-168.

Kent, R. D., Netsell, R., and Abbs, J. H. Acoustic characteristics of dysarthria associated with cerebellar disease. *Journal of Speech and Hearing Research*, 22 (1979) 627-648.

Kent, R. D. and Rosenbek, J. C. Acoustic patterns of apraxia of speech. *Journal of Speech and Hearing Research*, 26 (1983) 231-249.

Kersta, L. G. Amplitude cross-section representation with the sound spectrograph. *Journal of the Acoustical Society of America*, 20 (1948) 796-801.

Kewley-Port, D. and Preston, M. S. Early apical stop production: a voice onset time analysis. *Journal of Phonetics*, 2 (1974) 195-210.

Kim, C. W. A theory of aspiration. *Phonetica*, 21 (1970) 107-119.

Kim, K. M., Kakita, Y., and Hirano, M. Sound spectrographic analysis of the voice of patients with recurrent laryngeal nerve paralysis. *Folia Phoniatrica*, 34 (1982) 124-133.

Kitajima, K. Quantitative evaluation of the noise level in the pathologic voice. *Folia Phoniatrica*, 33 (1981) 115-124.

Klatt, D. H. Interaction between two factors that influence vowel duration. *Journal of the Acoustical Society of America*, 54 (1973) 1102-1104.

Klatt, D. The duration of /s/ in English words. *Journal of Speech and Hearing Research*, 17 (1974) 51-63.

Klatt, D. H. Voice onset time, frication, and aspiration in word-initial consonant clusters. *Journal of Speech and Hearing Research*, 18 (1975a) 686-706.

Klatt, D. H. Vowel lengthening is syntactically determined in a connected discourse. *Journal of Phonetics*, 3 (1975b) 129-140.

Klatt, D. H. Linguistic uses of segmental duration in English: acoustic and perceptual evidence. *Journal of the Acoustical Society of America*, 59 (1976) 1208-1221.

Koenig, W., Dunn, H. K., and Lacy, L. Y. The sound spectrograph. *Journal of the Acoustical Society of America*, 18 (1946) 19-49.

Kojima, H., Gould, W. J., and Lambiase, A. Computer analysis of hoarseness. *Journal of the Acoustical Society of America*, 65 suppl. 1 (1979) S67.

Kojima, H., Gould, W. J., Lambiase, A., and Isshiki, N. Computer analysis of hoarseness. *Acta Oto-laryngologica*, 89 (1980) 547-554.

Kuhl, P. K. The perception of speech in early infancy. In Lass, N. J. (Ed.). *Speech and Language* vol. I. New York: Academic Press, 1979. Pp. 1-47.

Kuhl, P. K. and Miller, J. Speech perception by the chinchilla: Voiced-voiceless distinction in alveolar plosive consonants. *Science*, 190 (1975) 69-72.

Kuhl, P. K. and Miller, J. M. Speech perception by the chinchilla: Identification for synthetic VOT stimuli. *Journal of the Acoustical Society of America*, 63 (1978) 905-917.

Ladefoged, P. *Preliminaries to Linguistic Phonetics*. Chicago: University of Chicago, 1971.

Ladefoged, P. and Broadbent, D. E. Information conveyed by vowels. *Journal of the Acoustical Society of America*, 29 (1957) 98-104.

Ladefoged, P., Harshman, R., Goldstein, L., and Rice, L. Generating vocal tract shapes from formant frequencies. *Journal of the Acoustical Society of America*, 64 (1978) 1027-1035.

Lehiste, I. Acoustical characteristics of selected English consonants. *International Journal of American Linguistics*, 30 (1964) 1-197.

Lehiste, I. The timing of utterances and linguistic boundaries. *Journal of the Acoustical Society of America*, 51 (1972) 2018-2024.

Lehiste, I. and Peterson, G. E. Transitions, glides, and diphthongs. *Journal of the Acoustical Society of America*, 33 (1961) 268-277.

Liberman, A. M. Some results of research on speech perception. *Journal of the Acoustical Society of America*, 29 (1957) 117-123.

Liberman, A. M., Delattre, P., and Cooper, F. S. The role of selected stimulus variables in the perception of the unvoiced stop consonants. *American Journal of Psychology*, 65 (1952) 497-516.

Liberman, A. M., Delattre, P. C., Gerstman, L. J., and Cooper, F. S. Tempo of frequency change as a cue for distinguishing classes of speech sounds. *Journal of Experimental Psychology*, 52 (1956) 127-137.

Liberman, A. M., Harris, K. S., Hoffman, H. S., and Griffith, B. C. The discrimination of speech sounds within and across phoneme boundaries. *Journal of Experimental Psychology*, 54 (1957) 358-368.

Lieberman, P. *Speech Physiology and Acoustic Phonetics: An Introduction*. New York: Macmillan, 1977.

Lindblom, B. Spectrographic study of vowel reduction. *Journal of the Acoustical Society of America*, 35 (1963) 1773-1781.

Lindblom, B. E. F. and Sundberg, J. E. F. Acoustical consequences of lip, tongue, jaw, and larynx movement. *Journal of the Acoustical Society of America*, 50 (1971) 1166-1179.

Lisker, L. Minimal cues for separating /w, r, l, j/ in intervocalic position. *Word*, 13 (1957a) 256-267.

Lisker, L. Closure duration and the intervocalic voiced-voiceless distinction in English. *Language*, 33 (1957b) 42-49.

Lisker, L. and Abramson, A. S. A cross-language study of voicing in initial stops: acoustical measurements. *Word*, 20 (1964) 384-422

Lisker, L. and Abramson, A. S. Some effects of context on voice onset time in English stops. *Language and Speech*, 10 (1967) 1-28.

Lively, M. A. and Emanuel, F. W. Spectral noise levels and roughness severity ratings for normal and simulated rough vowels produced by adult females. *Journal of Speech and Hearing Research*, 13 (1970) 503-517.

Löfqvist, A. and Yoshioka, H. Laryngeal activity in Swedish voiceless obstruent clusters.

Haskins Laboratories Status Report on Speech Research, SR59/60 (1979) 103-125.

Löfqvist, A. and Yoshioka, H. Laryngeal activity in Icelandic obstruent production. *Haskins Laboratories Status Report on Speech Research*, SR63/64 (1980) 275-292.

Maki, J. E., Gustafson, M. S., Conklin, J. M., Humphrey-Whitehead, B. K. The Speech Spectrographic Display: interpretation of visual patterns by hearing-impaired adults. *Journal of Speech and Hearing Disorders*, 46 (1981) 379-387.

Malécot, A. Acoustic cues for nasal consonants: an experimental study involving a tape-splicing technique. *Language*, 32 (1956) 274-284.

Malécot, A. The lenis-fortis opposition: its physiological parameters. *Journal of the Acoustical Society of America*, 47 (1970) 1588-1592.

Malmberg, B. The phonetic basis for syllable division. *Studia Linguistica*, 9 (1955) 80-87.

Menyuk, P. and Klatt, M. Voice onset time in consonant cluster production by children and adults. *Journal of Child Language*, 2 (1975) 223-231.

Mermelstein, P. Determination of the vocal tract shape from measured formant frequencies. *Journal of the Acoustical Society of America*, 41 (1967) 1283-1294.

Mol, H. *Fundamentals of Phonetics (Janua Linguarum no. 26)* The Hague: Mouton, 1963.

Monsen, R. B. Normal and reduced phonological space: The production of English vowels by deaf adolescents. *Journal of Phonetics*, 4 (1976) 189-198.

Monsen, R. B. Acoustic qualities of phonation in young hearing-impaired childen. *Journal of Speech and Hearing Research*, 22 (1979) 270-288.

Monsen, R. B. and Engebretson, A. M. The accuracy of formant frequency measurements: a comparison of spectrographic analysis and linear prediction. *Hearing Research*, 26 (1983) 89-97.

Nakajima, T. Identification of a dynamic articulatory model by acoustic analysis. In Sawashima, M. and Cooper, F. S. (Eds.) *Dynamic Aspects of Speech Production*. Tokyo: University of Tokyo, 1977. Pp. 251-275.

Nakata, K. Synthesis and perception of nasal consonants. *Journal of the Acoustical Society of America*, 31 (1959) 661-666.

Neiman, G. S., Klich, R. J., and Shuey, E. M. Voice onset time in young and 70-year-old women. *Journal of Speech and Hearing Research*, 26 (1983) 118-123.

Nessel, E. Uber das tonfrequenz spektrum der pathologisch verandertenstimme. *Acta Otolaryngologica*, suppl. 157 (1960) 3-45.

Noll, A. M. Short-term spectrum and "cepstrum" techniques for vocal pitch detection. *Journal of the Acoustical Society of America*, 36 (1964) 296-302.

Noll, A. M. Cepstrum pitch determination. *Journal of the Acoustical Society of America*, 41 (1967) 293-309.

O'Connor, J. D., Gerstman, L. J., Liberman, A. M., Delattre, P. C., and Cooper, F. S. Acoustic cues for the perception of initial /w, j, r, l/ in English. *Word*, 13 (1957) 24-43.

Öhman, S. E. G. Numerical model of coarticulation. *Journal of the Acoustical Society of America*, 41 (1967) 310-320.

Paige, A. and Zue, V. W. Computation of vocal tract area functions. *IEEE Transaction: Audio and Electroacoustics*, AU18 (1970a) 7-18.

Paige, A. and Zue, V. W. Calculation of vocal tract length. *IEEE Transactions: Audio and Electroacoustics*, AU18 (1970b) 268-270.

Parnell, M., Amerman, J. D., and Wells, G. B. Closure and constriction duration for alveolar consonants during voiced and whispered speaking conditions. *Journal of the Acoustical Society of America*, 61 (1977) 612-613.

Paul, A. P., House, A. S., and Stevens, K. N. Automatic reduction of vowel spectra: an analysis-by-synthesis method and its evaluation. *Journal of the Acoustical Society of America*, 36 (1964) 303-308.

Pentz, A. Gilbert, H. R., and Zawadzki, P. Spectral properties of fricative consonants in children. *Journal of the Acoustical Society of America*, 66 (1979) 1891-1893.

Peterson, G. E. Parameter relationships in the portrayal of signals with sound spectrography techniques. *Journal of Speech and Hearing Disorders*, 17 (1952) 427-432.

Peterson, G. E. Vowel formant measurements. *Journal of Speech and Hearing Research*, 2 (1959) 173-183.

Peterson, G. E. Paramters of vowel quality. *Journal of Speech and Hearing Research*, 4 (1961) 10-29.

Peterson, G. E. and Barney, H. L. Control methods used in a study of the vowels. *Journal of the Acoustical Society of america*, 24 (1952) 175-184.

Peterson, G.. E. and Lehiste, I. Duration of syllable nuclei in English. *Journal of the Acoustical Society of America*, 32 (1960) 693-703.

Pickett, J. M. *The Sounds of Speech Communication*. Baltimore: University Park Press, 1980.

Port, R. F. and Rotunno, R. Relation between voice-onset time and vowel duration. *Journal of the Acoustical Society of America*, 66 (1979) 654-662.

Potter, R. K., Kopp, G. A., and Green, H. *Visible Speech*. New York: Van Nostrand, 1947. Reprinted as: Potter, R. K., Kopp, G. A., and Green, H. G. *Visible Speech*. New York: Dover, 1966.

Potter, R. K. and Peterson, G. E. The representation of vowels and their movements. *Journal of the Acoustical Society of America*, 20 (1948) 528-535.

Potter, R. K. and Steinberg, J. C. Toward the specification of speech. *Journal of the Acoustical Society of America*, 22 (1950) 807-820.

Potvin, A. R., Foreit, K. G., Lam, K., Trued, S., and Potvin, J. H. *Archives of Physical Medicine and Rehabilitation*, 61 (1980) 542-546.

Prestigiacomo, A. J. Plastic-tape sound spectrograph. *Journal of Speech and Hearing Disorders*, 22 (1957) 321-327.

Preston, M. S. and Port, D. K. Further results of voicing in stop consonants in young children. *Haskins Laboratories Status Report on Speech Research*, SR13/14 (1969) 181-184.

Preston, M. S. and Yeni-Komshian, G. Studies on the development of stop consonants in children. *Haskins Laboratories Status Report on Speech Research*, SR-11 (1967) 49-53.

Prosek, R. A. and Runyan, C. M. Temporal characteristics related to the deiscrimination of stutterers' and nonstutterers' speech samples. *Journal of Speech and Hearing Research*, 25 (1982) 29-33.

Raphael, L. J. Preceding vowel duration as a cue to the perception of the voicing characteristic of word-final consonants in American English. *Journal of the Acoustical Society of America*, 51 (1972) 1296-1303.

Riesz, R. R. and Schott, L. Visible speech cathode-ray translator. *Journal of the Acoustical Society of America*, 18 (1946) 50-61.

Rontal, E., Rontal, M., and Rolnick, M. I. Objective evaluation of vocal pathology using voice spectrography. *Annals of Otology, Rhinology, and Laryngology*, 84 (1975a) 662-671.

Rontal, E., Rontal, M., and Rolnick, M. I. The use of spectrograms in the evaluation of vocal cord injection. *Laryngoscope*, 85 (1975b) 47-56.

Rontal, M., Rontal, E., Leuchter, W. and Rolnick, M. Voice spectrography in the evaluation of myasthenia gravis of the larynx. *Annals of Otology, Rhinology, and Laryngology*, 87 (1978) 722-728.

Rothenberg, M. The breath-stream dynamics of simple released plosive production. *Bibliotheca Phonetica*, 6 (1968) 1-117.

Rothenberg, M. A new inverse-filtering technique for deriving the glottal air flow waveform during voicing. *Journal of the Acoustical Society of America*, 53 (1973) 1632-1645.

Sáfrán, A. Vergleichende Untersuchungen der Leistung der normal-, Flüster- und Ösophagussprache sowie der Stimmprothese mit dem Sona-Graph. *Folia Phoniatrica*, 23 (19971) 323-332.

Sansone, F. E., jr. and Emanuel, F. Spectral noise levels and roughness severity ratings for normal and simulated rough vowels produced by adult males. *Journal of Speech and Hearing Research*, 13 (1970) 489-502.

Sawashima, M. Glottal adjustments for English obstruents. *Haskins Laboratories Status Report on Speech Research*, SR21/22 (1970) 180-200.

Schafer, R. W. and Rabiner, L. R. System for the automatic analysis of voiced speech. *Journal of the Acoustical Society of America*, 47 (1970) 634-648.

Schroeder, M. R. Determination of the geometry of the human vocal tract by acoustic measurements. *Journal of the Acoustical Society of America*, 41 (1967) 1002-1010.

Shoup, J. E., Lass, N. J., and Kuehn, D. P. Acoustics of speech. In Lass, N. J., Northern, J. L., and Yoder, D. E. (Eds.). *Speech, Language, and Hearing*, vol. I. Philadelphia: Saunders, 1982. Pp. 193-218.

Slis, I. H. and Cohen, A. On the complex regulating the voiced-voiceless distinction I. *Language and Speech*, 12 (1969a) 80-102.

Slis, I. H. and Cohen, A. On the complex regulating the voiced-voiceless distinction II. *Language and Speech*, 12 (1969b) 137-155.

Steinberg, J. C. Application of sound measuring instruments to the study of phonetic problems. *Journal of the Acoustical Society of America*, 6 (1934) 16-24.

Stetson, R. H. Motor phonetics. *Archives Néerlandaises de Phonétique Expérimentale*, 3 (1928) 1-216.

Stevens, K. N. Airflow and turbulence noise for fricative and stop consonants: static considerations. *Journal of the Acoustical Society of America*, 50 (1971) 1180-1192.

Stevens, K. N. and Blumstein, S. E. Invariant cues for place of articulation in stop consonants. *Journal of the Acoustical Society of America*, 64 (1978) 1358-1368.

Stevens, K. N. and House, A. S. Development of a quantitative description of vowel articulation. *Journal of the Acoustical Society of America*, 27 (1955) 484-493.

Stevens, K. N. and House, A. S. Studies of formant transitions using a vocal tract analog. *Journal of the Acoustical Society of America*, 28 (1956) 578-585.

Stevens, K. N. and House, A. S. An acoustical theory of vowel production and some of its implications. *Journal of Speech and Hearing Research*, 4 (1961) 303-320.

Stevens, K. N., Kasowski, S., and Fant, C. G. M. An electrical analog of the vocal tract. *Journal of the Acoustical Society of America*, 25 (1953) 734-742.

Stevens, K. N. and Klatt, D. H. Current models of sound sources for speech. In Wyke, B. D.

(Ed.). *Ventilatory and Phonatory Control Systems.* New York: Oxford, 1972.

Stevens, K. N. and Klatt, D. H. The role of formant transitions in the voiced-voiceless distinction for stops. *Journal of the Acoustical Society of America,* 55 (1974) 653-659.

Strevens, P. Spectra of fricative noise in human speech. *Language and Speech,* 3 (1960) 32-49.

Strube, H. W. Can the area function of the human vocal tract be determined from the speech wave? In Sawashima, M. and Cooper, F. S. (Eds.). *Dynamic Aspects of Speech Production.* Tokyo: University of Tokyo, 1977. Pp. 233-248.

Stuart, R. D. *An Introduction to Fourier Analysis.* London: Chapman and Hall, 1966.

Summerfield, Q. and Haggard, M. On the dissociation of spectral and temporal cues to the voicing distinction in initial stop consonants. *Journal of the Acoustical Society of America,* 62 (1977) 435-448.

Sweeting, P. M. and Baken, R. J. Voice onset time in a normal aged population. *Journal of Speech and Hearing Research,* 25 (1982) 129-134.

Tarnóczy, T. Resonance data concerning nasals, laterals, and trills. *Word,* 4 (1948) 71-77.

Tato, J. M., Mariani, N., DePiccoli, E. M. W., and Mirasov, P. Study of the sonospectrographic characteristics of the voice in laryngectomized patients. *Acta Oto-laryngologica,* 44 (1954) 431-438.

Tiffany, W. R. Nonrandom sources of variation in vowel quality. *Journal of Speech and Hearing Research,* 2 (1959) 305-317.

Till, J. A. and Stivers, D. K. Instrumentation and validity for direct-readout voice onset time measurement. *Journal of Communication Disorders,* 14 (1981) 507-512.

Umeda, N. Vowel duration in American English. *Journal of the Acoustical Society of America,* 58 (1975) 434-445.

Umeda, N. Consonant duration in American English. *Journal of the Acoustical Society of America,* 61 (1977) 846-858.

Wakita, H. Instrumentation for the study of speech acoustics. In Lass, N. J. (Ed.). *Contemporary Issues in Experimental Phonetics.* New York: Academic Press, 1976. Pp. 3-40.

Wang, W. S.-Y. Transition and release as perceptual cues for final plosives. *Journal of Speech and Hearing Research,* 2 (1959) 66-73.

Warren, D. W. and Hall, D. J. Glottal activity and intraoral pressure during stop consonant productions. *Folia Phoniatrica,* 25 (1973) 121-129.

Watterson, T. and Emanuel, F. Effects of oral-nasal coupling on whispered vowel spectra. *Cleft Palate Journal,* 18 (1981) 24-38.

Wedin, S., Leanderson, R., and Wedin, L. Evaluation of voice training. *Folia Phoniatrica,* 30

(1978) 103-112.

Wedin, S. and Ögren, J.-E. Analysis of the fundamental frequency of the human voice and its frequency distribution before and after a voice training program. *Folia Phoniatrica,* 34 (1982) 143-149.

Weinberg, B., Horii, Y., and Smith, B. E. Long-time spectral and intensity characteristics of esophageal speech. *Journal of the Acoustical Society of America,* 67 (1980) 1781-1784.

Weismer, G. Sensitivity of VOT measures to certain segmental features in speech production. *Journal of Phonetics,* 7 (1979) 197-204.

Weiss, M. S., Yeni-Komshian, G. H., and Heinz, J. M. Acoustical and perceptual characteristics of speech produced with an electronic artificial larynx. *Journal of the Acoustical Society of America,* 65 (1979) 1298-1308.

Wendahl, R. W., Moore, P., and Hollien, H. Comments on vocal fry. *Folia Phoniatrica,* 15 (1963) 251-255.

Whitehead, R. L. and Emanuel, F. W. Some spectrographic and perceptual features of vocal fry, abnormally rough, and modal register phonations. *Journal of Communication Disorders,* 7 (1974) 305-319.

Whitehead, R. L. and Lieberth, A. K. Spectrographic and perceptual features of vocal tension/harshness in hearing-impaired adults. *Journal of Communication Disorders,* 12 (1979) 83-92.

Winitz, H. E., Scheib, M. E., and Reeds, J. A. Identification of stops and vowels from the burst portion of /p, t, k/ isolated from conversational speech. *Journal of the Acoustical Society of America,* 51 (1972) 1309-1317.

Wirz, S. L., Subtelny, J., and Whitehead, R. L. Perceptual and spectrographic study of tense voice in normal hearing and deaf subjects. *Folia Phoniatrica,* 33 (1981) 23-36.

Wolfe, V. I. and Ratusnik, D. L. Vocal symptomatology of postoperative dysphonia. *Laryngoscope,* 91 (1981) 635-643.

Wood, D. E. and Hewitt, T. L. New instrumentation for making spectrographic pictures of speech. *Journal of the Acoustical Society of America,* 35 (1963) 1274-1278.

Yanagihara, N. Hoarseness: investigation of the physiological mechanisms. *Annals of Otorhinolaryngology,* 76 (1967a) 472-488.

Yanagihara, N. Significance of harmonic changes and noise components in hoarseness. *Journal of Speech and Hearing Research,* 10 (1967) 531-541.

Yumoto, E., Gould, W. J., and Baer, T. Harmonics-to-noise ratio as an index of the degree of hoarseness. *Journal of the Acoustical Society of America,* 71 (1982) 1544-1550.

Yumoto, E., Sasaki, Y., and Okamura, H. Harmonics-to-noise ratio and psychophysical measurement of the degree of hoarseness. *Journal of Speech and Hearing Research, 27* (1984) 2-6.

Zlatin, M. A. Voicing contrast: perceptual and productive voice onset time characteristics of adults. *Journal of the Acoustical Society of America,* 56 (1974) 981-994.

Zlatin, M. A. and Koenigsknecht, R. A. Development of the voicing contrast: perception of stop consonants. *Journal of Speech and Hear-* *ing Research,* 18 (1975) 541-553.

Zlatin, M. A. and Koenigsknecht, R. A. Development of the voicing contrast: a comparison of voice onset time in stop perception and production. *Journal of Speech and Hearing Research,* 19 (1976) 93-111.

Zwicker, E., Flottrop, G., and Stevens, S. S. Critical bandwidth in loudness summation. *Journal of the Acoustical Society of America,* 29 (1957) 548-557.

CHAPTER 10

Velopharyngeal Function

Nasality and nasal emission of air are symptoms of many different kinds of speech disorders. Not only are they the central concern in cases of cleft palate and similar maxillofacial defects (Spriestersbach, 1965), but they may be concommittants of dysarthria and dyspraxia as well. Nasality also figures prominently in the speech of the hearing impaired. Nasality and nasal emission clearly are problems that the speech pathologist encounters often. Because of the complexity of these symptoms and the many different approaches to their evaluation, they are considered in this separate chapter.

Nasalization may be defined as the existence of significant communication between the nasal cavity and the rest of the vocal tract. When inappropriate in degree or timing, such communication can result in two related, but clinically different, problems. *Nasal emission* refers to the abnormal escape of air via the nasal route. The abnormal "shunt" may reduce intraoral pressure, causing distortion of consonants. When the nasal air escape results in an audible "snort," the nasal emission becomes

even more obtrusive and the speech is more seriously impaired. *Nasality* (more properly *hypernasality*) refers to the unacceptable voice quality that results from inappropriate addition of the nasal resonance system to the vocal tract. In contrast to nasal emission, nasality does not involve large nasal airflows, nor does it significantly change intraoral air pressure. Obviously, nasality and nasal emission are often associated, and they may represent two facets of the same problem. It is possible for a patient to show one symptom and not the other. Both disorders of nasalization will be considered in this chapter.

Nasal emission is a fairly straightforward concept, not subject to much debate. On the other hand, while reliably perceived, nasality is an ill-defined phenomenon. Its basis lies in nasalization, and it is useful to consider nasality as nasalization that is inappropriate in degree or in timing. Such an operational definition places the full burden on the velopharyngeal port and would seem to point the way to fairly easy assessment methods. This, alas, is not the case.

Nasality is a *perceptual attribute* whose

detection requires the judgment of a listener (Moll, 1964). The degree of nasality reflects the complex interaction of a number of factors. There is general agreement that, as expected, the most important of these is the size of the velopharyngeal opening. But the degree of nasality is not by any means a direct function of this alone (Subtelny, Koepp-Baker, and Subtelny, 1961). For example, Massengill and Bryson (1967) found that, in normal speakers, the amount of velopharyngeal opening was significantly correlated to the perceived nasality of /i/, /u/ and /æ/, but not of /ɑ/. Spriestersbach and Powers (1959a) have provided complementary findings in cleft palate children to the effect that isolated productions of high vowels are perceived as more nasal than similar productions of low vowels. The explanation for this seems to lie in the fact that, in normal speakers, the tongue posture of the high vowels facilitates velopharyngeal closure, while the low vowels' tongue position reduces closure effectiveness (Moll, 1962; Harrington, 1944, 1946; Hardy and Arkebauer, 1966). Schwartz (1968a) has presented sound pressure level data that support this contention. Listeners have learned to be expectant of, and tolerant toward, greater nasalization of low vowels, but are surprised by it in high vowels and are more attentive to it. If an isolated vowel is used to judge nasality, the choice of vowel may influence the severity rating.

Defectiveness of a speaker's articulation also affects listeners' perceptions of nasality (Sherman, 1954; McWilliams, 1954; Spriestersbach, 1955; van Hattum, 1958; Spriestersbach and Powers, 1959b). So does his vocal intensity (Lintz and Sherman, 1961) and rate of speech (Bzoch, 1968). In short, while nasality is fundamentally a matter of velopharyngeal function, the judgment of the severity of velopharyngeal malfunction is confounded by many other aspects of speech.

Lest all of this leave the impression that nasality results from incomplete velopharyngeal closure alone, let it be added

immediately that *timing* is also a critical variable. A perfectly competent velopharyngeal port is of little value if it is closed at the wrong times during an utterance; perceived nasality can result from nasal coupling that is too early or too late. Since velar movement shows very extensive coarticulation (Moll and Daniloff, 1971; Ali, Gallagher, Goldstein, and Daniloff, 1971; Thompson and Hixon, 1979) the opening and closure timing patterns in running speech can be very complex. It would be surprising if this complicated coordination were not disrupted in the dysarthric or dyspraxic speaker (Itoh, Sasanuma, and Ushijima, 1979), and it would be a rare clinician who could reliably discriminate nasality due to mistiming from nasality due to velopharyngeal incompetence simply by listening to running speech.

It is likely that "the perception of nasality, while dependent upon listener judgment, is a complex phenomenon, and that attempts to explain nasal speech through perceptual measures alone may be limited" (Counihan, 1972). Since the goal of speech therapy is to *modify* perceived nasality, the first task of the speech pathologist is to isolate its basic causes. To achieve this the contributing factors need to be sorted out. Because they are more or less inextricably confounded in the perceptual judgment, objective tests will be needed. They are particularly important when data are required for informing decisions about surgical or prosthetic management. Instrumental measures of nasality can also be used to track the progress of therapy (Moser, 1942) and to provide feedback (Garber, Burzynski, Vale, and Nelson, 1979; Netsell and Daniel, 1979) especially to patients who, like the hearing-impaired, cannot use auditory cues (Stevens, Nickerson, Boothroyd, and Rollins, 1976).

The field of speech pathology has been greatly concerned with the problem of nasality for a long time, and a great many observational methods have been devised. Some of these, for example, the rheadeik of Vealey, Bailey, and Belknap (1965), are perhaps useful for patient motivation, but they do not greatly enhance the therapist's insight into the precise nature of the patient's problem. These methods will not be discussed here. Rather, this chapter will focus on techniques that facilitate evaluation of the mechanisms of nasality or allow quantification of its severity. The prime emphasis will be on the measurement of the effectiveness and timing of velopharyngeal closure.

BACKGROUND CONSIDERATIONS

Decisions concerning testing procedures to be used must be made carefully and with full consideration of the peculiar circumstances of any given case. The velopharyngeal port is a very complex structure whose specific functional modalities are not well understood. It is known that activity patterns differ from task to task and from subject to subject. The following points should be kept in mind when planning the evaluation procedure:

1. The principle of motor equivalence is fully applicable to velar and pharyngeal function. At our present level of understanding, ordinary testing procedures cannot clearly indicate the specific contributions of the several muscles of the system (Bell-Berti, 1976, 1980; Seaver and Kuehn, 1980).

2. The relationship between the size of the velopharyngeal port and perceived nasality is not, by any stretch of the imagination, a direct or linear one. Furthermore, openings of less than approximately 20 mm^2 do not seem to cause perceptible nasality (Warren, 1964b, 1967) or articulatory defectiveness (Shelton, Brooks, and Youngstrom, 1964; Isshiki, Honjow, and Morimoto, 1968; Shelton and Blank, 1984). Also, the effects of larger port openings can be masked by variations of oral port size, nasal airway resistance, and respiratory effort (Warren and Ryon, 1967).

3. Circumspection is required in generalizing from data gathered on normal speakers to those with maxillofacial defects. Closure mechanisms may be very different in the two groups (Moll, 1965b; Hagerty, Hill, Pettit, and Kane, 1958a; Buck, 1954). Nor can the nature of the maxillofacial deformity be considered a predictor of the closure pattern that will be used (Shelton, Brooks, and Youngstrom, 1964).

4. Nonspeech tasks are generally poor indicators of velopharyngeal behavior during speech. Impounding of intraoral air and sucking can be accomplished by linguapalatal valving. Cleft palate patients who cannot achieve velopharyngeal closure during speech routinely do so on swallowing (Moll, 1965b). Blowing and sucking tasks (Chase, 1960) are particularly suspect. Several studies (Moll, 1965b; McWilliams and Bradly, 1965; Calnan and Renfrew,, 1961) have indicated that velar elevation, and hence velopharyngeal closure, is significantly greater during blowing tasks than during speech, perhaps because the high intraoral pressure forces the velum more tightly against the pharyngeal wall.

5. Measurement of static productions (for example, of a sustained vowel) may yield results that differ from those obtained during speaking tasks (Powers, 1962) since crucial timing elements are not being tested.

Not all of the techniques available for assessment of velopharyngeal function are suitable for routine clinical use. Electromyography, for example, has been of great value to the researcher (Fritzell, 1963, 1969, 1979; Broadbent and Swinyard, 1959; Basmajian and Dutta, 1961; Cooper, 1965; Shelton, Harris, Sholes, et al., 1970; Bell-Berti, 1976; Fritzell and Kotby, 1976; Hering, Hoppe, and Kraft, 1965; Ushijima, Sawashima, Hirose, et al., 1976; Li and Lundervold, 1958). But it is highly invasive, generally painful, and often disruptive of normal speech movements (see Chap. 11). Likewise, a number of special X-ray techniques have been devised for visualizing palatal activity (Powers, 1962; Carrell, 1952; Hagerty, Hill, Pettit, and Kane, 1958b; Massengill, 1966, 1972; Massengill and Brooks, 1973; Massengill, Quinn, Barry, and Pickrell, 1966; Moll, 1960, 1965a, 1965b; Shelton, Brooks, and Youngstrom, 1964; Skolnick, 1970; Williams, 1972; Zwitman, Gyepes, and Sample, 1973; Croatto, Cinotti, et al., 1980; Williams and Eisenbach, 1981). It is also possible to combine X-ray observation with electromyography (Fritzell, 1963; Lubker and Curtis, 1966; Lubker, 1968; Subtelny, McCormack, Subtelney et al., 1968), with sound spectroscopy (Björk and Nylen, 1961) and with airflow measurement (Lubker and Moll, 1965).

These applications of special technology have been of enormous value in the exploration of velopharyngeal functioning. Most practicing clinicians, however, will vastly prefer less invasive or dangerous means of clinical assessment. Horii (1980) has pointed out that an ideal technique for evaluating physical correlates of nasality would meet the following criteria:

1. psychological and physical noninvasiveness;
2. capability of assessing velopharyngeal function during speech;
3. nondisruptive of articulatory, phonatory, or ventilatory processes;
4. noninterference with sensory feedback of speech activity;
5. excellent correlation with perceived nasality;
6. low cost, ease of operation, and portability;
7. ease of interpretation.

From the early flame tests and stretched-diaphragm systems (Moser, 1942) to the present sophisticated integrated circuitry, no method meets all of these requirements. Compromise is always necessary: The criteria must be prioritized for each case and setting. The rest of this chapter will explore those techniques that are most likely to meet the priorities of speech clinicians.

VISUALIZATION OF PALATAL STRUCTURES

Intuitively, it would seem that the easiest method of evaluating velopharyngeal function might be to watch the velum during speech or to take motion pictures of it for fine analysis. Unfortunately, such simple methods are very problematic. One study (Eisenback and Williams, 1984), for example, has found that adequacy judgments made from simple visual observations showed relatively poor agreement with judgments based on cinefluorographic examination.

Part of the problem is due to the fact that the working velopharyngeal port is inaccessible to direct visual inspection by an observer.* It is therefore necessary to insert some sort of telescopic device into the pharyngeal area, a technique referred to as endoscopy. A typical instrument for this purpose has been the Taub oral panendoscope, shown in Figure 10-1. The long shaft of the instrument is inserted into the subject's mouth until its distal end lies in the oropharynx. The telescope within its plastic shield is rotated to view the velopharynx above, while a small light bulb next to the viewing lens provides illumination. The examiner can observe directly, or the panendoscope can be mounted on a camera (Taub, 1966a, b). More recently, clinicians have also used the panendoscope with video recording or monitoring systems, thereby providing for simultaneous audio and visual recording (Willis and Stutz, 1972) and immediate visual feedback to the patient of his own velar activity (Shelton, Paesoni, McClelland, and Bradfield, 1975).

The disadvantages of the panendoscope

---

*Except in those rare cases in which a maxillofacial defect (usually created surgically) provides an opening through which the posterior oral cavity can be seen. Several of the early investigations of velopharyngeal valving (e.g., Harrington, 1944 and Bloomer, 1953) took advantage of such situations. While some insights into palatal function were gained, conclusions based on grossly abnormal oropharyngeal structures may have little applicability to more anatomically normal speakers.

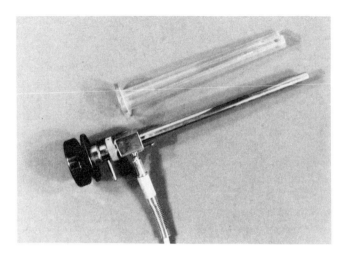

FIGURE 10-1. An oral endoscope.

are readily apparent. Many subjects gag if the tongue base, faucial region, velum, or pharyngeal wall is touched by the instrument, as is almost inevitable. Less disturbing to the patient, but much more important to the therapist, is the fact that a fairly large instrument must traverse the length of the oral cavity pretty much in the midline. Articulation is thus limited to low or neutral vowels and labial phones. The development of much thinner fiber-optic endoscopes has diminished problems of speech interference only a little (Zwitman, Sonderman, and Ward, 1974) although moving the light source out of the working end of the instrument has placed a source of considerable heat far away from oral tissues. A thin fiber-optic nasendoscope can be passed via the naris into the nasopharynx, allowing the velopharngeal region to be viewed from above (Pigott, 1969; Pigott, Bensen, and White, 1969; Sawashima and Ushijima, 1971, 1972; Itoh, Sasanuma, and Ushijima, 1979; Niimi, Bell-Berti, and Harris, 1982). This leaves the articulators unencumbered, but it is at the price of more invasiveness than is likely to be tolerated by many patients, especially children.

While visual observations of velopharyngeal structures accord well with radiographic findings (Zwitman, Gyepes, and Ward, 1976), endoscopy leaves much to be desired, except when simple photograph-ic documentation of structural abnormality is wanted. Most optical instruments so encumber the oral cavity that it is not possible to observe a wide range of activity during speech. While the pernasal approach solves that problem, it is apt to provoke considerable patient anxiety. Furthermore, careful evaluation of velopharyngeal activity will require relatively minute analysis of sound-synchronized motion pictures, a procedure that is time-consuming, laborious, and often expensive.

INDIRECT ASSESSMENT METHODS

The limited utility of photographic techniques and the drawbacks of electromyography and radiography encourage the use of indirect assessment techniques. That is, the correlates of velopharyngeal function are measured so that inferences about malfunction may be drawn.

Articulation Tests

Obviously, one could use articulatory performance as an indirect index of velopharyngeal function. This has the appeal of a certain straight-forwardness. Leakage of air through an incompetent port would be expected to interfere with high-pressure consonants and produce perceptible nasality. Conversely, inadequate opening should severely distort /m/, /n/, and /ŋ/. Different phonemes might be expected to suffer in varying degrees according to the nature and magnitude of the malfunction. Differential diagnosis and severity scaling might, therefore, be possible.

Interest in the articulation profiles of cleft palate children is hardly recent (see, for example, Spriestersbach, Darley, and Rouse, 1956). Some attempts have been made to devise articulation tests that will, in fact, provide a firm basis for drawing conclusions about actual or potential velopharyngeal valving function (van Demark, 1979). Morris, Spriesterbach, and Darley (1961) created the Iowa Pressure Articulation Test (IPAT), a subset of items from the popular Templin-Darley test, in an attempt to do just this. While its correlation with other tests of velopharyngeal valving is only fair (Barnes and Morris, 1967), it does seem to have promise as an indicator of the need for secondary management (van Demark and Morris, 1977). Van Demark and Swickard (1980) have reported preliminary results of a screening articulation test for detection of velopharyngeal inadequacy that can be used with 3 1/2 year olds. Validity is yet to be assessed.

Appealing as such methods may be, they are fraught with problems. Velopharyngeal malfunction may cause speech changes other than outright distortion of phonemes, and misarticulations may be due, in whole or in part, to abnormalities other than those involving the velopharyngeal port (Pitzner and Morris, 1966). In general, one cannot accurately measure and describe the specific movements of the velopharyngeal system that are defective on the basis of articulatory deficits. Instead, the clinician must have recourse to corrrelates of velopharyngeal action whose relationships to system functioning are stronger or better understood.

Acoustic Measures

Quantification of nasality by means of acoustic measures would be very conve-

nient. Because no invasive instrumentation is required, speech performance would not be changed by the evaluation procedure and patient anxiety would be minimized. In principle, measurement could even be done from tape recordings. It is, therefore, not surprising that considerable effort has been devoted to the search for valid and reliable acoustic measures of velopharyngeal function. While a definitive method has yet to be established, considerable progress has been made and several options are now available for (carefully interpreted) use by clinical practitioners.

Vocal tract damping

If, during phonation, the supraglottal airway is suddenly blocked, the air pressure above the vocal folds will quickly rise to a level close to the subglottal pressure. Since this eliminates the transglottal pressure drop, vocal fold vibration must stop. The time required for the supraglottal pressure to reach a value sufficient to inhibit phonation depends on a number of inherent physical characteristics, including the volume of the vocal tract and its compliance. Equally important, however, is the fact that air leakage around the blockage (that is, a shunt or "bleed" airflow) will significantly slow down the rise in supraglottal pressure and, therefore, delay phonatory shut-down. The greater the shunt airflow, the longer the delay should be.

Zemlin and Fant (1972) applied this reasoning to the development of a simple and completely noninvasive measure of velopharyngeal closure. Called the *Zemlin Index of Palatopharyngeal Opening* (ZIPPO), the measurement can be done with relatively simply apparatus (Figure 10-2). A mouthpiece, fitted with a special valve, is connected to a rotameter-type flow meter (see Chap. 8). The valve is kept open by an electromagnet that holds a stopper away from its seat. When current to the electromagnet is interrupted the stopper drops and prevents egressive air flow. A microphone mounted on the outside of the valve system picks up the "clunk" of the valve clo-

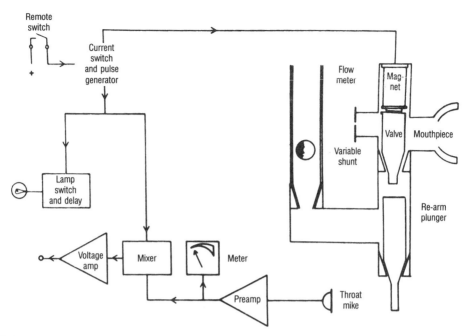

FIGURE 10-2. Instrumentation for "ZIPPO." (From Zemlin, W. R. and Fant, G. The effect of a velopharyngeal shunt upon vocal tract damping times: An analog study. *Speech Transmission Laboratory Quarterly Progress and Status Report*, 4 (1972) 6-10. Figure 1, p. 7. Reprinted by permission.)

sure that signals airflow interruption. A contact microphone placed on the thyroid cartilage detects laryngeal vibrations. The amplified microphone signals are displayed on separate channels of a dual-trace oscilloscope.

The test requires that the subject phonate /i/ into the mouthpiece while maintaining an airtight lip seal around it. Consistency of test conditions across trials is maintained by providing the subject with feedback of phonatory airflow and vocal intensity by having him watch the rotameter and a VU meter. When the tester presses a button the valve closes; its pickup microphone produces a deflection on the oscilloscope screen. Supraglottal pressure builds rapidly and layrngeal vibration (also shown on the oscilloscope) soon stops.

The relevant measure is the damping time, the interval between the valve-microphone deflection and the disappearance of laryngeal waves. Zemlin and Fant (1972) tested this system with normal speakers

and found that the average damping time was about 100 ms. When shunts were added to the valve, the damping time increased as predicted.

Plattner, Weinberg, and Horii (1980) have tested ZIPPO on a group of 15 normal young adult women. Damping times were determined (using an online computer) for 100 trials each (requiring about 30 min of testing). The times ranged from 5 to 900 ms (mean: 108 ms; SD: 68 ms). Ninety-five percent of the measured times were less than 300 ms. Unfortunately, the subjects vaired widely in performance. Most had a narrow range of damping times, but some were highly variable. Both improvement and deterioration of performance over trials were noted.

ZIPPO is clearly not ready for diagnostic application at this time. But its "sound theoretical basis and ease of . . . administration provide sufficient grounds to prompt needed additional research into its clinical application" (Plattner et al., 1980, p.

215). ZIPPO may be on the relatively near clinical horizon.

Spectral features of nasalization

Abnormal nasalization can be reliably perceived. Therefore, the acoustic content of nasalized speech must be different from that of normal speech. When the velopharyngeal valve is opened, the nasal cavity is coupled to the rest of the vocal tract. One would, therefore, expect that nasalization might be the perception of the simple addition of a *nasal resonance* to the other resonance characteristics of the vocal tract.

This reasoning led to a search for relatively simple and invariant changes in the acoustic spectrum attributable to a nasal resonance that would signal nasalization. So, for example, Hattori, Yamamoto, and Fujimura (1958) found that the spectra of nasalized vowels showed "selective attenuation at 500 cps . . . due to the antiresonance of the nasal cavity acting as a side branch connected to the major vocal tract at its midpoint" (p. 269). Other "nasalization phenomena" were also identified, but they varied from one speaker to another (Bloomer and Peterson, 1955; Dickson, 1962), were different for different vowels (Stevens, Nickerson, Boothroyd, and Rollins, 1976), and failed to correlate well with the degree of perceived nasality. Using synthetic speech stimuli, investigators (House and Stevens, 1956; Farnetani, 1979b) have confirmed that the perception of nasality depends on highly complex and very variable acoustic cues. It is now clear that the discovery of "precise acoustic correlates of nasalization appears to be a far more formidable and perhaps questionable task than [had been] suspected" (Schwartz, 1972, p. 198).

In fact, the search for invariant acoustic features of nasalization is almost certain to be fruitless. The reasoning behind this conclusion was excellently presented by Curtis (1968, 1970), and is summarized here. The basic flaw in earlier research is the assumption that the nasal space represents one more fixed resonantor that adds its own particular contribution to the combined acoustic properties of the other relatively independent resonators making up the vocal tract. In other words, the difficulty lies in the assumption of a separate "nasal resonance" added to other separate resonances. Dunn (1950) has presented a model of the vocal tract that has been shown to be more explanatory of speech acoustics. According to his construct, the vocal tract can be said to consist of a set of cylinders arranged in series. Each of these, in some sense, has acoustic properties but, because the cylinders are connected in a string, they are enormously interdependent. None makes an identifiable isolated contribution to the final acoustic product. Quite the contrary: the contribution of any given region of the vocal tract is very much a function of all of the other regions. The final result is very different from the simple sum of a set of independent parts. Consequently, coupling of the nasal cavity to the rest of the system does not add an invariant resonator, but rather it just changes the overall nature of a complex acoustic system. The resonance characteristics of the nasal cavity *interact with* the variations in vocal tract shaping required for different vowels. Therefore, different vowels have different acoustic "nasalization" characteristics. Similarly, individual variations in vocal tract anatomy lead to differences in the acoustic correlates of nasality from one speaker to another. "The conclusion," Curtis (1970, p. 71) says,

> seems self-evident. An adequate theoretical model for vocal resonance gives little reason to predict that nasalization will lead to invariant changes in the acoustic spectra of speech. On the contrary, the spectral changes which are to be expected will depend very considerably on what is happening in other portions of the vocal cavity system. If one accepts this conclusion the apparent inconsistency and lack of invariance in the data concerning the acoustic effects of nasalization are not mystifying. This lack of invariance is in fact consistent with theory and should have been expected.

Despite inconsistency among speakers and

among the phonemes produced by a single individual, certain spectral features are generally agreed to be associated with nasalization. While not useful for differential diagnosis (Dickson, 1962; Accordi, Croatto-Accordi, and Cassin, 1981), change in any such feature in a standard speech context produced by a given speaker may serve as a useful, although perhaps tentative, means for observing the effect of therapy. It is entirely conceivable that the speech spectrum will show changes that are real but too subtle for reliable perceptual detection. The more-or-less "established" features of nasalization are summarized in Table 10-1. Figure 10-3 shows how nasalization of a vowel might appear in a standard wideband spectrogram (see Chap. 9). More extensive discussions of the acoustics of nasalization are available in Schwartz (1968b, 1972) and in Curtis (1970).

Oral and nasal sound pressure

Lowering the velum increases the coupling of the nasal cavity and the rest of the vocal tract. More of the vocal signal is then propagated through the nose. In somewhat simpler terms, velopharyngeal opening increases the intensity of nasal sound emission. Increased nasal sound pressure at the nares provides a rather direct indication of a lowered velum, and the audio signal from a nasal microphone can be used to provide a patient with instantaneous feedback of nasalization (Hultzen, 1942).

Nasal sound pressure level can be measured fairly easily by inserting a probe microphone just inside the naris (Hirano, Takeuchi, and Hiroto, 1966) or by erecting a barrier that will separate oral and nasal signals (Hyde, 1968). The microphone output can be amplified, rectified, and filtered

TABLE 10-1. Spectral Features of Nasalization

Effect	Reference
Increased formant bandwidth	Bloomer & Peterson, 1955
	Dickson, 1962
(first formant)	House & Stevens, 1956
Formant frequency shift	Dickson, 1962
	Stevens, et al., 1976
	Watterson & Emanuel, 1981
	Gonay, 1972
(third formant higher)	Hanson, 1964
	Bloomer & Peterson, 1955
(first formant higher)	House & Stevens, 1956
	Fujimura, 1960
Extra resonances	Watterson & Emanuel, 1981
	Dickson, 1962
	Bloomer & Peterson, 1955
	House & Stevens, 1956
(at about 250 Hz)	Hattori et al., 1958
Diminished or anti-resonances	Dickson, 1962
(reduced first formant)	House & Stevens, 1956
(about 500 Hz)	Hattori et al., 1958
(about third formant)	House & Stevens, 1956
	Bloomer & Peterson, 1955
Noise between formants	Hattori et al., 1958
(friction noise)	Bloomer & Peterson, 1955
Decreased overall intensity	Dickson, 1962
	House & Stevens, 1956
	Bernthal & Beukelman, 1977

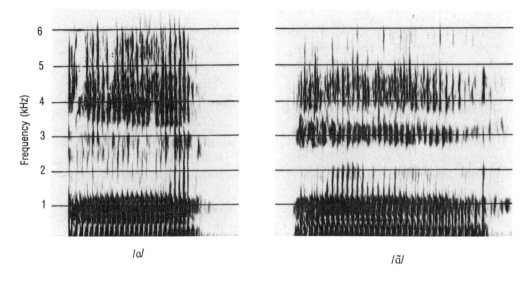

/ɑ/   /ɑ̄/

FIGURE 10-3. Broad-band spectrograms of /ɑ/ and /ɑ̄/ spoken by the same normal male. Note the formant at about 3 kHz in the nasalized vowel.

(Figure 10-4) to produce a signal prepresenting the nasal sound amplitude. This can be displayed on an oscilloscope (in which case it can be used for feedback to the patient) or recorded on paper. While simple, this method has a number of problems that limit its use as an evaluative tool. Even in normal speakers, supposedly nonnasal vowels are routinely produced with measurable nasal sound emission, the intensity of which varies, but not very predictably, with the vowel being produced (Schwartz, 1968a). Also, the sensitivity of the probe microphone to airflow through the nose can confound the measurement. Finally, the nasal sound pressure is not simply a function of the degree of nasal coupling: It obviously also reflects the vocal intensity. Thus, an increase of intra-nasal sound intensity might represent nothing more than increased phonatory effort.

Something of a solution to the last problem can be achieved by separately and simultaneously measuring intranasal and oral sound pressure levels and comparing them.* As vocal intensity changes, the oral

*A brief review of the rationale, advantages, and difficulties of this method has been prepared by Counihan (1972). Note also that the HONC index, described later, can be implemented with microphone pickups.

and nasal signals would, presumably, change together, maintaining a constant relationship. Most commonly the difference (in dB) between the oral and nasal sound pressures has been used, but the ratio of one to the other (nasal/oral) has also been tried (Shelton, Knox, Arndt, and Elbert, 1967; Fletcher, 1970). For patient feedback purposes, rectified oral and nasal signals can both be applied to a stereo balance meter (available at many audio equipment shops) to provide a real-time visual indication of oral to nasal balance (Yules, Josephson, and Chase, 1969).

Appealing though its theoretical basis may be, the results of nasal to oral sound pressure comparisons do not correspond very closely to listener judgments of nasality. Shelton, Knox, Arndt, and Elbert (1967) found that the correlation between listener ratings of nasality and nasal sound pressure level was 0.47; between listener ratings and the difference of oral and nasal sound pressures, 0.41; and between listener ratings and the ratio of the two pressures, 0.37. These coefficients are significant ($p < .01$) from the point of view of inferential statistics, but the relationship is clearly too weak to permit the use of such measures as indices of the severity of perceived nasality.

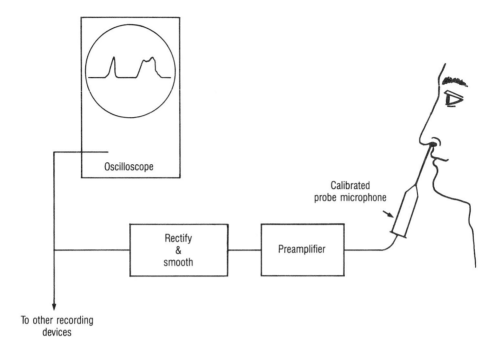

FIGURE 10-4. Measuring nasal sound pressure.

(They may, however, reflect nasalization itself fairly well.) It should also be noted that the nasal to oral sound pressure ratio may show sex differences (Clarke, 1975, 1978).

TONAR and the Nasometer

Automatic derivation of the ratio of nasal to oral sound pressure at different frequencies was achievved by an electronic system, named *The Oral Nasal Acoustic Ratio (TONAR)* by its developer (Fletcher, 1970). While TONAR itself is no longer available commercially, Kay Elemetrics Corp. has recently marketed the Nasometer, a computer-based system that uses the TONAR method. Performing a somewhat more complex function than its name might at first imply, the basic organization of the TONAR system is diagrammed in Figure 10-5.

Inputs from nasal and oral microphones (or from a dual-channel recording) are individually amplified and conditioned by identical bandpass filters. Rectification and smoothing of the filtered signals results in DC voltages proportional to the amplitude of the portion of each input within the filters' passband. A special circuit performs an analog division function. Its output is the ratio of the (filtered) nasal amplitude to the (identically filtered) oral amplitude. The ratio signal is read out on a multichannel strip chart, together with the signals representing the oral and nasal sound pressures. The variable filters may be electronically controlled by the user to provide for different bandwidths in the frequency range of 10 to 65 kHz. Alternatively, the filters can be automatically swept across several frequency ranges at various rates.

The instrument may be used with the filtering inactivated, in which case the output is a simple nasal/oral ratio. But the filtering results in a more complex output product: the ratio of the amplitude in a limited range of the speech frequency spectrum. The term *nasalance* has been coined to describe this measure, and it has been found to correlate moderately with perceived nasality (Fletcher and Bishop,

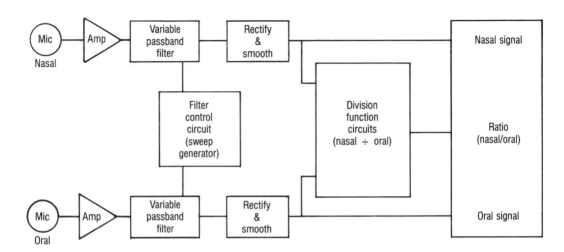

FIGURE 10-5. Functional block diagram of TONAR.

1973).* Although the developer obviously attaches importance to the frequency-limitation capability of the instrument and has found it to be useful (Fletcher, 1970), the specific advantages conferred have not been clearly demonstrated. A special version of the device, TONAR II, has been developed for biofeedback and contingency-management therapies (Fletcher, 1972). It has also been used in nasalance studies of esophageal (Colyar and Christensen, 1980) and hearing impaired (Fletcher and Daly, 1976) speakers.

Hutchinson, Robinson, and Nerbonne (1978) have provided typical nasalance values for normal speakers of various ages. Measures were made for readings of the Rainbow Passage and for sustained /ɑ/. Nasalance was also assessed using two special passages: one containing no nasal phonemes, the other heavily loaded with them (Fletcher, 1973). The TONAR II filters were centered at 500 Hz, with a bandwidth of 300 Hz. The resultant data (Table 10-2) are not normative (too few subjects were tested) but may serve as clinical approximations of normal values.

----

*When set to automatic passband sweep TONAR is useful only for steady-state prolongations of a sound. This is a result of the fact that the frequency range being analyzed constantly changes during the sweep; if the input also changes, the results are likely to be uninterpretable.

Accelerometry

Nasal sounds induce vibration of the soft tissue of the nose that is easily detectable. Using accelerometers (see Chap. 3) to pick up the nasal vibration has two major advantages over the use of microphones to monitor the airborne nasal sound. First, the accelerometer is in no way affected by normal nasal airflow that can confound microphone signals. Second, because the accelerometer is insensitive to airborne waves it is minimally influenced by simultaneous oral sound emission. This means that better separation of the nasal signal from the total speech output can be achieved. To be sure, accelerometers are not without problems. Detection obviously varies with different tissue transmission characteristics and may also be affected by the angle of attachment to the nose and the degree of contact intimacy achieved. Therefore, it is not possible to compare absolute values of outputs between subjects nor, in fact, from one test session to another with the same subject. The drawbacks, however, can be circumvented by careful design of the evaluation procedure.

Stevens, Kalikow, and Willemain (1975) have successfully used a very small accelerometer attached to the nose to provide feedback (via an oscilloscope) for management of nasality in deaf children. Stevens, Nickerson, Boothroyd, and Rollins (1976)

TABLE 10-2. Mean Nasalance Values for Normal Speakers*†

Age	N	Rainbow Passage		Sustained /a/		Non-nasal Passage		Highly nasal Passage	
		Mean	SD	Mean	SD	Mean	SD	Mean	SD
MEN									
18–38	11*	16.8	5.8	8.0	10.6	8.7	1.9	32.9	13.0
50–55	5	24.6	3.7	14.4	5.1	16.0	4.3	40.8	5.4
56–60	5	25.0	2.4	14.2	6.8	18.0	3.4	39.0	5.5
61–65	5	22.2	4.1	16.8	6.2	18.8	4.3	37.4	7.8
66–70	5	24.0	6.4	18.4	8.3	14.4	2.4	36.0	11.0
71–75	5	20.2	2.6	15.4	5.6	16.6	5.0	34.2	3.1
76–80	5	25.5	7.5	18.0	7.5	16.4	4.4	42.0	10.8
All men over age 50	50	23.5	5.1	16.2	6.8	14.7	4.2	38.2	8.4
WOMEN									
18–38	11*	18.8	7.0	6.5	9.4	8.3	2.5	38.9	14.5
50–55	5	31.2	13.0	25.0	15.1	22.2	9.9	45.4	15.2
56–60	5	38.2	10.2	30.4	8.1	25.4	7.6	55.2	9.8
61–65	5	27.0	8.4	13.2	7.0	17.6	6.6	42.2	5.3
66–70	5	25.4	10.1	15.0	3.0	20.2	5.6	37.2	14.8
71–65	5	32.6	4.4	25.6	9.4	23.2	9.0	50.0	8.3
76–80	5	37.8	12.7	32.2	12.0	25.4	7.7	56.0	17.4
All women over age 50	50	32.0	10.7	23.6	4.4	27.3	8.4	47.5	14.5

From Hutchinson, J. M., Robinson, K. L., and Nerbonne, M. A. Patterns of nasalance in a sample of normal gerontologic subjects. *Journal of Communication Disorders*, 11 (1978) 469-481. Table 1, p. 474. © 1978 by Elsevier Science Publishing Co., Inc. Reprinted by permission.

*Six of the subjects in each of these groups were tested in a study by Fletcher, 1976 (unpublished).

†Male-female differences are significant (p < .01). Age differences are not significant.

also used this method.* Although they noted that the accelerometer signal reflected changes in vocal intensity as well as varying nasalization, it was felt that the problem was not serious. Changes in vocal effort, they noted, were not likely to amount to more than about ± 2 dB, whereas nasalization increased accelerometer output by 10 to 20 dB. The problem of changing vocal intensity has been addressed by Horii and Monroe (1983). They describe a very simple system that displays the ratio of the nasal accelerometer and oral microphone signals on an oscilloscope screen in a form that can easily be used for visual feedback during therapy.

*Lippman (1981) has shown that an ultraminiature accelerometer available from Knowles Electronics performs just as well for detecting nasalization as the much more expensive devices previously used.

HONC

Horii (1980) has devised an electronic system for producing the ratio of nasal to oral accelerometer output (similar in principle to the sound pressure ratios discussed earlier) during running speech. The *Horii Oral Nasal Coupling (HONC)* index is a relative scale, with a value of 1 representing maximal nasalization. HONC ratios can be compared across speakers. The scaling procedure also compensates for changes in accelerometer mounting characteristics and tissue attenuation properties, thereby providing comparability of one test session with another for the same patient. Preliminary evidence (Horii, 1983; Redenbaugh and Reich, 1985) indicates a high correlation between HONC and perceived nasality/ denasality.

The HONC index can be defined mathematically as

$$\text{HONC} = A_{\text{rms}(n)}/(k \times A_{\text{rms}(v)}).$$

$A_{\text{rms}(n)}$ is the root mean square amplitude (see Chap. 2) of the output of a nasal accelerometer; $A_{\text{rms}(v)}$ is a similar value for a vocal (neck-mounted) accelerometer. The constant k is a number (determined for each test condition) that causes the ratio to equal 1 when maximal nasalization occurs. Although the HONC index can be continuously derived by a computer, Redenbaugh and Reich (1985) describe a relatively uncomplicated analog system that provides a strip-chart record without digital processing. Implementation is, therefore, quite simple and direct.

The block diagram of Horii's instrumentation (Figure 10-6) illustrates its operating principles. A master amplifier is provided for separately boosting the output of both accelerometers, but the signal from the neck transducer is first amplified by a variable preamplifier. This additional gain represents k in the mathematical equation. After amplification, the signals from the two channels are independently rectified and smoothed to provide DC voltages representing the amplitude, A_{rms}, of each. An analog divider circuit then generates the ratio, $A_{\text{rms}(n)}/(k \times A_{\text{rms}(v)})$, of the two voltages. A special circuit acts as a voice detector and produces an output only when the neck accelerometer is active. This output is used to control an electronic switch that cuts off the divider output if a voiceless sound is being produced. The display system (an oscilloscope or pen recorder) therefore shows the ratio only during phonated speech segments.

TEST METHOD. The nasal accelerometer is attached with adhesive tape to the external surface of the nose, somewhat above the ala. Redenbaugh and Reich (1985) point out that the accelerometer site should be chosen with some care. Septal deviation is common in many patients with velopharyngeal insufficiency. The nasal accelerometer should be located on the more patent side. The vocal accelerometer is located between the thyroid cartilage and the sternal notch or at any location where tactile evaluation shows strong vibration during phonation. The patient then sustains /m/ or /n/ at a loud, but still comfortable, vocal level while the variable (voice) amplifier, whose gain represents k, is adjusted until the display shows a maximal output. This represents a ratio of 1, indicating maximal nasalization. It is important that a moder-

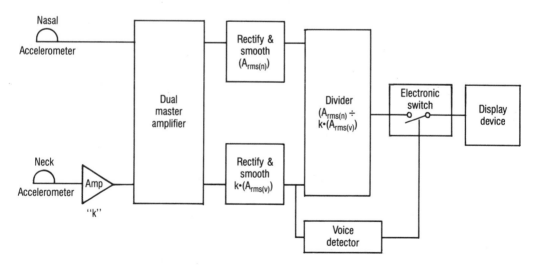

FIGURE 10-6. Functional block diagram of HONC.

ately loud /m/ or /n/ be used for this adjustment to insure that the system will not later be overdriven by greater degrees of vocal effort. If necessary the master amplifier may be adjusted to change the scale width on the display device without altering the relationship of nasal and vocal signals. Full scale deflection on the display represents complete nasalizationn (HONC = 1); no deflection indicates total denasalization (HONC = 0). Using /m/ or /n/ as the basis for calibration allows the system to be used with normaal subjects and with those who have velopharyngeal incompetence. The fully nasalized reference condition also provides a basis for comparison of results over time and across subjects. (If evaluating denasality, a fully oralized sound can be used as the baseline reference.)

OUTPUT. Because some vocal energy is always transmitted to the nasal tissues (even during normally non-nasal speech) the HONC value only rarely reaches 0 in actu-

al practice. Also, since tissue transmission characteristics and the orientation of the transducer can change with patient movement and muscle tension adjustments, it is possible for HONC to slightly exceed a value of 1. A sample of a HONC output is shown in Figure 10-7. Horii (1980) also provides instructions for displaying the HONC trace on a sound spectrogram, facilitating phonetic segmentation. While still experimental, the HONC index holds significant promise.

Airflow and Air Pressure Tests

Lowering the velum not only results in the propagation of the phonatory acoustic wave through the nasal cavity, it also diverts at least part of the airstream through the nose. Nasal escape of air, and the attendant rise of the intranasal air pressure can, therefore, serve as indicators of nasalization. (This, of course, is the rationale for the classic, but very crude, "mirror test"

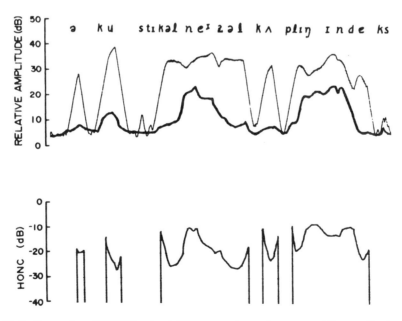

FIGURE 10-7. Examples of HONC output. The upper trace shows nasal (heavy line) and oral (light line) sound pressure levels. The lower trace is the corresponding HONC index in dB. Discontinuities are produced by the electronic switch that disables the instrument during voiceless sounds. (From Horii, Y. An accelerometric approach to nasality measurement: A preliminary report. *Cleft Palate Journal*, 17 (1980) 254-261. Figure 6, p. 259. Reprinted by permission.)

that has seen service for so many years.)
The physics of air pressure and flow is reviewed in Chapters 7 and 8, as are the principles of their measurement. This section
will deal primarily with the special application of those methods to evaluation of
velopharyngeal activity.

Nasal airflow

Nasal airflow measurement is done in order to detect and quantify "nasal emission"
(alternatively called "nasal escape"). Mc-
Donald and Koepp-Baker (1951, p. 12) have
suggested that this term "be restrictively
employed to describe the escape of air
through the nasal passages when the speaker attempts to produce any sound requiring intra-oral breath pressure such as
plosives or fricatives." Nasal emission may
be monitored with a pneumotachograph
(Warren, 1967; Warren, Duany, and Fischer,
1969; Lubker, Schweiger, and Morris, 1970;
Dickson, Barron, and McGlone, 1978;
Thompson and Hixon, 1979) or with a
warm-wire anemometer (Kelleher, Webster,
Coffey, and Quigley, 1960; Quigley, Webster, Coffey, Kelleher, and Grant, 1963;
Quigley, Shiere, Webster, and Cobb, 1964)
fitted to nasal masks. A special version of
the electro-aerometer (Smith, 1960; van den
Berg, 1962) is also available commercially. Some literature ((Subtelny, McCormack,
Subtelny, Worth, Cramer, Runyon, and
Rosenblum, 1968; Worth, Runyon, and
Subtelny, 1968; Subtelny, Kho, McCormack, and Subtelny, 1969) reports the use
of warm-wire systems arranged in front of
the nostrils without the rather cumbersome
nose mask, but the validity of such instrumentation is highly questionable
(Hardy, 1967).

At first glance it might seem that the
amount of nasal emission might be very directly related to the degree of velopharyngeal opening and would, therefore, serve
by itself as an excellent index of the degree
of nasalization. More careful consideration
of the relationship of oral and nasal pathway aerodynamics, schematized in Figure
10-8, shows why such an expectation is un-

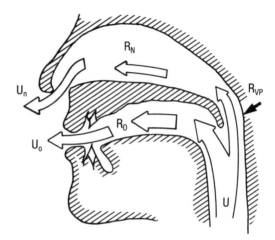

FIGURE 10-8. Airflows (U) and resistances (R)
in the upper vocal tract.

likely to be realized. Assume that the vocal tract posture is fixed, as indicated in
the figure. There is a small velopharyngeal
opening between essentially wide-open nasal airways. Air under pressure streams up
from the lower pharynx. Because the oral
airway is unobstructed it presents very little resistance to this flow. But some small
fraction of the airstream will be pushed by
the pressure through the slightly open
velopharyngeal port. (The resistance
through the opening is high, but it is not
infinite; some small amount of air gets
through.) The flow-pressure relationship
(discussed in Chap. 8) indicates that the
flow through the velopharyngeal port will be

$$U_n = P/R_{vp}.$$

That is, the airflow through the nose, U_n,
is equal to the pressure in the oropharynx,
P, divided by the resistance of the velopharyngeal port, R_{vp}. (It is assumed for the
moment that the nasal passage, being totally unobstructed, has no resistance of its
own to complicate the situation.) The nasal airflow, then, does not change only with
change in velopharyngeal resistance (which
in turn reflects the amount of port opening) but with the intraoral pressure as well.
Since a given speaker's intraoral pressure
varies from phoneme to phoneme and also
changes with the amount of vocal effort, it

is clear that these variables also significantly affect the rate of nasal airflow. There is also reason to believe that velopharyngeal insufficiency causes greater respiratory effort (Warren, Wood, and Bradley, 1969).

The problems do not end there, however. Even if the intraoral air pressure were to remain constant, the amount of air being forced through the velopharyngeal port would vary according to the degree of oral constriction—including, for example, the amount of lip rounding. This is because increasing oral constriction implies higher oral pathway resistance. As the oral resistance rises, more and more of the air finds it less "inconvenient" to squeeze through the velopharyngeal resistance. Hence, nasal airflow also reflects oral port constriction, which changes not only for different phonemes but also from one production to another of the same phoneme. Furthermore, oral port constriction can be abnormal in cleft palate cases (Claypoole, Warren, and Bradley, 1974; Warren and Mackler, 1968). A way out of the tangle—simultaneous measurement of oral and nasal airstream characteristics—will be discussed later.

There remains yet another difficulty. It was assumed earlier that the nasal passages were wide open and presented no resistance of their own to the flow of nasal air. In the anatomically normal individual this is a useful approximation of the truth. But patients with structural anomalies of the velopharynx (who are, after all, very likely to be the subjects of evaluation) are also likely to have such nasal defects as deviated septum, bony spurs, mucous membrane thickening, and the like (Powers, 1962; Morris, 1968). They are, in short, the very individuals for whom the assumption of a wide open nasal airway is least likely to be valid. The amount of nasal flow will decrease as nasal airway resistance increases, even if the velopharyngeal port is wide open. Nasal airflow measures reflect many aspects of vocal tract function, all confounded in a very complex way (Warren and Ryon, 1967).

Of the several problems mentioned, the nasal resistance factor is the most difficult to control for in testing. It can, however, be measured. Clinicians might wish to do so to determine the extent to which the nasal cavity resistance is facilitating non-nasal speech. Nasal resistance is also of obvious importance in cases of clinical denasality, where the therapist must determine if the problem is due to velopharyngeal malfunction or to nasal obstruction.

A fairly simple screening test for nasal patency can be performed with a spirometer (Davies, 1978). The maximal volume that can be inhaled in 0.5 s ($FIV_{0.5}$) is measured, first through the nose alone (N - $FIV_{0.5}$) *and then through the mouth alone* (M - $FIV_{0.5}$). The *Nasal Patency Index* is defined as the ratio of nasal to oral volume:

$$NPI = (N - FIV_{0.5}) / (M - FIV_{0.5}).$$

Because the resistance of the nasal passage is normally greater than that of the oral airway, the NPI is much less than unity in normal subjects. Davies (1978) found the NPI to range from 0.19 to 0.74 (mean = 0.47, S.D. = 0.15) in eleven healthy men. Values below this range may signal nasal obstruction.

Warren, Duany, and Fischer (1969) evaluated airway resistance with the instrumentation diagrammed in Figure 10-9. One catheter is used to sense intraoral pressure, and another catheter is attached to a tightly fitting nose mask. The two are connected to a differential pressure transducer that senses the pressure difference (ΔP_n) from one end of the nasal cavity to the other. (Subjects produce nasal phonemes so that the velopharyngeal resistance approximates zero.) A pneumotachograph at the outlet of the nose mask measures the nasal airflow (U_n). The resistance of the nasal cavity is, therefore,

$$R_n = \Delta P_n / U_n.$$

In their study of the nasal resistance of 29 normal men and women and of 27 men and women with different types of repaired and untreated palatal clefts, resistance was determined at a point during a prolonged nasal phoneme when nasal flow, $U_n = 0.5$ L/s. The resultant data, summarized in Ta-

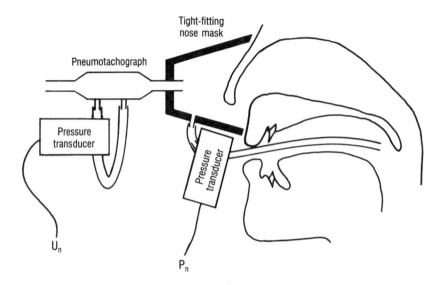

FIGURE 10-9. Determination of nasal airway resistance.

ble 10-3, may be useful in evaluation of other clinical cases.

Lotz, Shaugnessy, and Netsell (1981) used a nose mask, pneumotachograph, and oral pressure probe to assess nasal airway resistance in 15 male and 15 female normal adult speakers. Their finding of a mean resistance of 3.1 cm $H_2O/L/s$ (S.D. = 0.3) during sustained /m/ and 3.9 cm $H_2O/L/s$ (S.D. = 0.4) during quiet breathing confirms the assumption that velopharyngeal resistance can be considered negligible during production of a nasal phone. It is, as these researchers put it, a "happy finding" in that it demonstrates that an accurate measure of minimal nasal cavity resistance can be obtained during a few seconds of sustained /m/. This is much easier to achieve than trying to get subjects to breathe quietly while maintaining an open velopharynx without disturbing the oral pressure sensing tube with their tongue.

Despite all the caveats and limitations, nasal airflow measures are likely to be useful if interpreted conservatively. They are particularly suited for assessment of the effects of speech therapy or medicosurgical management in a given case.

Emanuel and Counihan (1970) have studied peak oral and nasal airflows using a two-chambered face mask and calibrated warm-wire anemometers. Normal adult subjects produced the six English plosives in combination with /i/ or /ɑ/; measurement was at the point of maximal oral flow. Their data are summarized in Table 10-4.

Thompson and Hixon (1979) also evaluated nasal airflow. Their subjects were 92 normal boys and girls aged 3 to 18 and 20 men and women aged 18 to 37. They sustained /i, s, z, n/, repeated /ti, di, si, zi, ni/ and produced repetitions of /iti, idi, isi, izi, ini/ in a carrier phrase. Flow was measured with a nasal mask and pneumotachograph. No nasal flow at all was detected except during utterances with a nasal phoneme. Therefore, they concluded, "the anticipated clinical observation in normal velopharyngeal closure on oral sounds would be no flow. However, a small amount of flow should not be interpreted to mean velopharyngeal incompetence" (p. 419). The latter point is underscored by the findings of Emanuel and Counihan. Lotz, Shaughnessy, and Netsell (1981, p. 6) also warn that "most normal adults close completely for oral productions, but small and inconsistent leaks can be expected."

Warren (1967) has explored the relationship of nasal emission to the area of the

TABLE 10-3. Nasal Resistance in cm $H_2O/L/s$*

Age range	Normal		Cleft Palate	
	Mean	SD	Mean	SD
9–11	3.0	0.4	4.9	2.1†
12–13	2.4	0.6	3.6	1.1
Over 15	2.0	1.1	3.5	1.8†

Compiled from raw data in Warren, Duany, and Fischer, 1969.

*Males and females. Measured when nasal flow = 0.5 liter/sec.

†Difference between normal and cleft palate group significant (p < .05). No significant sex differences. Note that there is a clear tendency for nasal resistance to diminish with age.

velopharyngeal port. He studied 28 subjects, aged 8 to 47, with surgically repaired or prosthetically closed palatal clefts. They produced the word /pɑpɑ/ while peak nasal airflow of the initial /p/ was measured with a pneumotachograph. Simultaneous estimates of the velopharyngeal orifice area (by a method discussed later) were derived. His results indicate that the degree of nasal emission is strongly correlated to velopharyngeal port size only when the area of the latter is less than 20 mm². When the area of the opening is greater, the nasal airflow is a poor indicator. The same situation seems to prevail in cases of oronasal fistulas (Shelton and Blank, 1984).

Even if nasal airflow is not highly valid as a discriminator of the degree of velopharyngeal opening, there is little reason to doubt that it can distinguish normal from abnormal velopharyngeal closure. Lubker, Schweiger, and Morris (1970), whose data are summarized in Table 10-5, illustrated the magnitude of the differences that may be observed. The peak airflow during the several utterances was obtained by a nose mask and pneumotachograph. Normal subjects were free of speech defect or distortion; cleft palate subjects were all prosthetically managed and their speech quality was perceptually categorized as "good, fair, or poor." For all but one of the tasks the cleft palate subjects had significantly higher nasal flow rates (p < .01) than

the normal speakers. The exception, surprisingly, occurred for /m/, during which the prosthetically managed cleft palate speakers had significantly lower (p < .05) nasal flow rates than normals. This probably reflects the restriction of velopharyngeal port size by the prosthesis.

In summary, nasal airflow rate, like any solitary measure, is only a fair predictor of how a listener will judge the severity of nasality. It is nonetheless an important contributor to that judgment. It can also serve grossly to differentiate good, fair, and poor velopharyngeal function in cleft palate speakers, and it can clearly distinguish such speakers from normals.

Volume measures

Since air volume is the product of airflow and time, determination of the volume of nasal escape represents an alternative approach to velopharyngeal assessment that is sometimes simpler. Spirometers, the most common instruments for respiratory volume measurement, tend to be more widely available and easier to use than airflow transduction systems.

Kantner (1947) seems to have been the first to suggest using a set of vital capacity tasks to assess nasal leakage. He recommended that the patient first do several vital capacity trials (to stabilize the reading). The patient's nares are then occluded with a clip, and the vital capacity again determined. The nasal clip is removed, and the vital capacity is measured one last time. It is assumed that inadequacy of the velopharyngeal seal will result in nasal escape when the nares are open, and so the variable of interest is the ratio of the two vital capacity measures: with nares open and with nares occluded. A unity ratio would indicate no difference between the two conditions and hence (presumably) no nasal escape of air. As the ratio diminishes air escape is assumed to be increasing. The test shares the advantages of the oral breath pressure ratio (discussed subsequently) to which it is logically related. It is quick and easy and poses no threat to a patient who

TABLE 10-4. Peak Oral and Nasal Airflow in Normal Speakers*

Syllable Type	C	V	Mean Peak Flow (mL/s)†			
			Male		Female	
			Oral	Nasal	Oral	Nasal
CV	t		1045	5	798	16
	p		936	17	690	26
	k		644	2	576	8
		i				
	d		437	6	324	10
	b		370	14	215	15
	g		293	6	216	4
	t		1324	6	1162	16
	p		1103	26	880	18
	k		1144	7	904	5
		a				
	d		598	8	346	7
	b		425	23	232	17
	g		415	9	258	5
VCV	t		342	4	276	7
	p		304	10	237	20
	k		221	3	189	4
		i				
	d		166	8	103	5
	b		112	12	66	10
	g		116	10	85	7
	t		441	7	420	5
	p		357	17	270	14
	k		363	8	310	6
		a				
	d		218	12	110	6
	b		148	18	77	11
	g		118	9	82	4

Modified from Emanuel and Counihan, 1970.

*Twenty-five men, 25 women; age 20–36 years: Split face mask, warm-wire anemometers; conversational loudness, comfortable pitch; measured at point of maximal oral airflow.

†Data originally in liters/min.

may have experienced countless failures when confronted with speech tasks. At least in terms of group comparisons, the test seems to have validity. Spriestersbach and Powers (1959b) tested 103 cleft palate children, aged 5 to 15, and found that those who could achieve velopharyngeal closure (as determined by X-ray studies) had a mean ratio of 0.99, while those could not achieve such closure had a mean ratio of only 0.68. (The difference is significant at $p < .01$.)

Unfortunately, the test also has all the limitations of the breath pressure ratio. Velar function is evaluated under conditions of higher-than-normal intraoral pressure which, as noted earlier, may promote a degree of closure not achieved in speech. It also evaluates a static velar posture, thereby ignoring the fact that it is the adequacy of rapid velar movements that is of prime concern in speech. Other methodological problems reside, for instance, in the assumption that equal effort underlies both

TABLE 10-5. Mean Peak Nasal Airflow*

Utterance	Peak flow in mL/s†	
	Normal	Prosthetically Managed
/ipi/	3	206
/isi/	3	188
/æpæ/	8	177
/s/	<<1	164
/izi/	7	163
/æsæ/	8	154
/z/	6	138
/æzæ/	5	124
/ibi/	5	122
/æbæ/	7	118
/i/	<<1	66
/u/	2	48
/æ/	1	8
/ɑ/	2	5
/m/	212	168
"connected speech"**	3	189

From Lubker, J. F., Schweiger, J. W., Morris, H. L. Nasal airflow characteristics during speech in prosthetically managed cleft palate speakers. *Journal of Speech and Hearing Research*, 13 (1970) 326-338. Table 2, 331. © American Speech-Language-Hearing Association, Rockville, MD. Reprinted by permission.

*Thirty-six subjects (18 male, 18 female) each group; age 8–44, mean 19 years. Nose mask and pneumotachograph.

†Originally in liters/min.

**Simulated by six rapid repetitions of /isi/.

vital capacity trials and that there is no active middle-ear disorder (Morris, 1966).

Hardy and Arkebauer (1966) proposed a different method of respirometric testing that obviates some of these limitations. To the extent that the velopharyngeal port leaks air, they reasoned, the volume of oral emission should be less than that total (oral + nasal) air volume used during a speech task having no nasal phonemes. The test they proposed requires that the patient produce at least 25 repetitions of each of the following CV syllables: /pʌ, tʌ, kʌ, sʌ, tʃʌ, fʌ/. A mouth mask is used to collect the orally emitted air in a recording spirometer. The spirometer chart is hand-marked to indicate the beginning and the end of each task. The volume of air expired is divided by the number of syllables produced to derive the mean oral air per syllable. The en-

tire process is then repeated, but this time a full face mask is used, allowing the spirometer to record total air volume. The oral volume per syllable is divided by the total volume per syllable, generating a ratio that serves as an index of velopharyngeal closure.

Hardy and Arkebauer assessed their technique with 32 normal children, aged 6 to 13 years, using a 9 L spirometer and kymograph. In addition to performing the task described, the children counted from 1 to 10. The presence of five /n/s in the eleven syllables of the count allowed a test of the sensitivity of the method to the presence of nasalization. The data they obtained are summarized in Table 10-6. It is clear from the lower ratio for counting that the method is a moderately good detector of relatively small amounts of nasalization. The comparatively low standard deviations attest to acceptable intersubject reliability. In addition, it was determined that simple hand marking of the spirometer record was adequate and that trial to trial reliability was acceptable. There was some relationship (r = -.40) of syllable rate to mean syllable volume. The ratios that are greater than 1, however, imply that the volume of orally expired air exceeds the total air usage, a logical impossibility. The fault, no doubt, lies in the fact that two separate trials are measured. Different respiratory effort on each trial could account for the error.

Despite this obvious (and relatively minor) flaw, Hardy and Arkebauer felt that the method had promise as an assessment technique. It requires only simple instrumentation, and is non-invasive. Children do not have to meet any difficult performance criteria; they need only be instructed to "say _____ as fast as you can." Each task is done three times and the results averaged.

At the expense of considerably more elaborate instrumentation, Hixon, Saxman, and McQueen (1967) have modified the Hardy and Arkebauer test to eliminate the possibility of ratios greater than unity. At the same time they achieved lower ratio variability. The task to be performed by the patient remains essentially unchanged:

TABLE 10-6. Mean Ratios of Spirometric Volumes (Oral ÷ Total Volume)

| Task | Single Spirometer[a] | | Dual Spirometers | | | |
| | | | Adults[b] | | Children[c] | |
	Mean	SD	Mean	SD	Mean	SD
/pʌ/	0.997	0.258			0.963	0.010
/tʌ/	1.147	0.409	0.9941	0.042	0.962	0.019
/kʌ/	1.145	0.282	0.936	0.047	0.963	0.023
/sʌ/	1.062	0.200	0.913	0.051	0.953	0.013
/ʃʌ/			0.924	0.031	0.958	0.016
/tʃʌ/	1.094	0.325			0.947	0.013
/fʌ/	1.045	0.263	0.938	0.057	0.963	0.016
Count 1–10	0.939	0.259	0.797	0.061	0.841	0.061

From (a) Hardy and Arkebauer, 1966; (b) Hixon, Saxman, and McQueen, 1967; (c) Shaw and Gilbert, 1982.

three sets of 25 repetitions of /tʌ, kʌ, sʌ, ʃʌ, fʌ/. Air usage variation due to rate of utterance is controlled by pacing the repetitions with a metronome set for four beats per second. The patient is instructed to inspire maximally before each task and to produce all repetitions on a single breath. A split face mask channels oral air to one spirometer and nasal air to another, while a dual electromechanical marker system, controlled by the tester, puts reference marks on both spirometer charts to provide common time references. The ultimate ratio is the oral spirometer volume divided by the sum of the two volume records. In order to control for voice onset and offset phenomena, only repetitions 4 through 23 of each utterance (20 syllables) are used in the measurement. Shaw and Gilbert (1982) have tested this evaluation method on 5 boys and 5 girls (age 6 years 7 months to 10 years 5 months) using a comparable methodology: 3 sets of 15 repetitions each of several CV syllables at a rate of 3 syllables per second and counting from 1 to 10.

The results of the several validation studies, summarized in Table 10-6, show the improvement achieved by the test modifications. None of the ratios exceeds 1, and the difference between the syllable repetition and counting ratios is more pronounced, indicating greater sensitivity to the presence of nasalization. The much smaller standard deviations imply greater intersubject reliability. Children do not gen-

erate ratios different from those of adults. Although neither of the two spirometric tests has been validated on subjects with demonstrated velopharyngeal deficits, both clearly hold promise and should find wider use in clinical evaluation.

Air pressure

ORAL BREATH PRESSURE RATIO. The oral breath pressure ratio has enjoyed considerable popularity among speech pathologists. It is defined as the ratio of intraoral pressure with the nares open to the pressure with the nares occluded (P_{open}/P_{sealed}). A ratio of 1 is assumed to demonstrate that occlusion of the nares has no effect, an indication that the velopharyngeal seal is effective. Ratios less than one (lower oral air pressure with the nares open) are considered demonstrative of nasal air leakage and hence are presumptive evidence of poor velopharyngeal closure.

Instrumentation. The U-tube manometer or Boudon-type manometer are traditionally employed. Any standard pressure transducer will serve, however.

Method. The maximum intraoral breath pressure is measured by having the patient blow as forcefully as possible into the sensing tube. Two trials are run—one with a nose clip in place and the other without it.

It is important that a bleed valve be used during both trials. It is possible to do these measurements on negative pressure by having the subject generate a maximal inspiratory effort on both trials. But the task is difficult to describe, and most subjects will find it more difficult to perform than blowing. One is, therefore, best advised to restrict testing to positive (expiratory) pressure.

Advantages and Limitations. Morris and Smith (1962) point out that, by avoiding a speech activity, this does not arouse feelings of frustration and defeatism in handicapped individuals. Furthermore, the task lends itself to easy quantification and comparison of evaluations done at different times in the therapeutic course. On the other hand, the nonspeech nature of the task severely constrains interpretation of the results. The static measure is not necessarily reflective of a patient's ability to achieve the rapid velopharyngeal closure needed for speech, a fact demonstrated by McWilliams and Bradley (1965).

The air pressures involved in testing the breath pressure ratio are very different from those needed for speech production. This point is related to a more subtle problem discussed by Hardy (1965), who points out that the test rests on the assumption that the patient is producing a maximum (or at least equal) expiratory effort during the nares-open and nares-occluded conditions. The examiner cannot be certain that this is so when the ratio is significantly less than 1. Furthermore, maximal lung pressure is strongly influenced by lung volume, and a difference in maximal oral pressure may, therefore, reflect differences in lung inflation. It is probably wise, therefore, to measure maximal oral pressure under standardized ventilatory conditions—at the end of a maximal inspiration or at the rest expiratory level, for instance.

Lastly, the oral breath pressure ratio may be adversely affected by active disorders of the middle ear. When an individual with eustachian tube malfunction blows into the manometer with the nares occluded, pain or discomfort may be felt in the ear, causing him to blow less forcefully. The result is that the nares-occluded pressure is spuriously lowered, raising the open to closed ratio. If velopharyngeal closure is indeed normal, the ratio may exceed 1. More serious, however, is the fact that the ratio may benefit from this artifact and approach unity in cases where there actually is a degree of velopharyngeal incompetence that would have been detected if the tympanic problem did not exist. Morris (1966) discusses this particular problem of "false negatives" more fully.

The limitations of this test, then, are very real and have been evaluated by Shelton et al. (1965, p. 42) who conclude that the clinician "dealing with an individual . . . patient must continue to base . . . treatment decisions on a variety of observations. Clinical testing with simple manometers should be included with caution pending further study."

Expected Results. Spriestersbach and Powers (1959b) used a Bourdon-type manometer to determine oral breath pressure ratios in two groups of cleft palate boys and girls, ages 5 to 15. Those who chould achieve adequate velopharyngeal closure (demonstrated by lateral X-rays) achieved a mean ratio of 0.98, while those with deficient velopharyngeal function had a mean ratio of 0.70. Note, however, that test results should only be interpreted on the basis of an "adequate/inadequate dichotomy." At present, there is no justification for interpreting a ratio of 0.80 as necessarily indicating better function than a ratio of 0.75.

Pitzner and Morris (1966 p. 39) have found that cleft palate children who have breath pressure ratios less than 0.89 "display poorer articulation [as measured by the Templin-Darley Diagnostic Test] not only on plosives, fricatives, and affricates, but also on vocalic /r/ and /l/." Cleft palate children with higher ratios had articulation abilities similar to those of normal children. One might, therefore, wish to take a ratio of 0.90 as the dividing point between adequate and inadequate.

INTRANASAL PRESSURE. Airflow through the nose necessarily implies elevated intranasal pressure. Logically, then, nasal air pressure reflects velopharyngeal opening. Simple nasal pressure detection methods—a nasally connected water manometer (Hess and McDonald, 1960) or strain-gauge transducer (Condax, Howard, et al., 1974)—can be used to signal nasalization. While their simplicity suggests possible use in biofeedback-based therapies, these techniques provide no information about the size of the velopharyngeal port. Although provision of a variable "bleed" in the pressure measurement system might improve resolution, the results of such a method have been disappointing (Hess, 1976).

Warren (1979) has recommended using the difference between intraoral and intranasal pressures during production of /p/ as an index of *palatal efficiency*. After studying 75 normal and cleft palate subjects, he concluded that an oral-nasal pressure difference of 3 cm H_2O or more indicates adquate closure, while a difference less than 1 cm H_2O clearly demonstrates inadequacy. Pressure differences between these cutoff points are presumed to signal "borderline" closure. Not only is the borderline region problematic, but is must also be understood that the method does not evaluate actual speech performance. Further, valid measures are not possible in the presence of incomplete lip closure, such as might be seen in cases of severe open bite or labial flaccid paralysis. The simplicity of the test, however, might recommend it to some practitioners. A special instrument, dubbed the *Palatal Efficiency Rating Computed Instantaneously* (PERCI) has been designed to provide an instantaneous digital readout of the oronasal pressure difference.

Oral Pressure and Nasal Flow

Observing nasal airflow and oral pressure at the same time greatly enhances the potential for drawing inferences about the function of the velopharyngeal valve. The intraoral air pressure is the force tending to drive air through the port, while the nasal flow represents the failure of the velopharyngeal system to withstand that pressure. The presence of both measures on a strip-chart record provides an excellent illustration of the effectiveness of velar closure during all the combinations of oral and velopharyngeal status needed for speaking. Furthermore, the timing characteristics of velar function are readily apparent.

Implementation of this observation method is straightforward and simple. Intraoral air pressure is sensed with an oral probe tube and pressure transducer while a nose mask and pneumotachograph monitor nasal airflow (Figure 10-10). The speech signal, picked up by a microphone in front of the speaker's mouth, is also displayed in the output. Typical records for a normal speaker might look like those of Figure 10-11. Rapid and well-timed movements of the velum are apparent in the brief bursts of appropriate nasal expiration. No nasal emission occurs, even during the high-pressure fricatives and plosives.

Warren (1964a,b) has used a slightly different measurement system, diagrammed in Figure 10-12. One pressure probe is placed in the posterior area of the mouth, while another is secured in the subject's nostril by means of a cork. Both are connected to a differential pressure transducer, whose output is, therefore, the transvelar pressure difference. A flow transducer is connected to the other nostril, again by means of a tube secured by a cork. (Note that the assumption of equal patency of the two nasal passages must be valid.) Warren has used this system to evaluate velopharyngeal adequacy of cleft palate individuals during running speech. He points out that incomplete velopharyngeal closure is frequently signalled by a reversal of the flow and pressure patterns. Normally, stop consonants are characterized by a relatively high transvelar pressure and very little, if any, nasal air flow. An incompetent velopharyngeal valve, however, often causes a severe reduction of the pessure and a great increase in the nasal flow (Warren and Devereux, 1966).

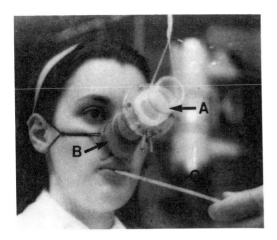

FIGURE 10-10. Simultaneous measurement of nasal flow and intraoral pressure. (A) pneumotachograph; (B) nose mask; (C) pressure sensing probe. (Courtesy of Dr. R. Netsell.)

This situation is dramatically illustrated in Figure 10-13, taken from Warren (1964b, p. 19). The left side shows the pressure and flow outputs when a cleft palate speaker said "Bessie stayed all summer." Nasal flow is very high during plosives and fricatives, higher, in fact, than for /m/. The transvelar pressure difference, however, is virtually nil. When the same speaker used a palatal appliance (right side of Figure 10-13) the pressure trace shows appropriate peaks, while nasal flow drops to zero except during /m/. (In fact, Warren reports that the speaker's voice quality was denasal.) This method, then, provides a valuable means of assessing nasality and the results of its management.

Dysarthric speakers, of course, may have poor velopharyngeal closure only during some phonemes, and some show dysfunction only when the rate of syllable production is changed. Netsell (1969) has, therefore, proposed a special paradigm for evaluation of velopharyngeal function in such speakers. Intraoral pressure and nasal airflow are observed while the patient produces utterances as shown in Table 10-7. The consonants /t/, /d/, and /n/ provide a contrast of voiceless, voiced, and nasal productions at a single place of articulation that is not disturbed by a post-molar sensing tube. The neutral vowel also prevents probe disruption that might result from the need to achieve more extreme lip or tongue postures. Conversational pitch and loudness are used.

The sensitivity of Netsell's test method as a detector of several different types of problem is illustrated in the output records shown in Figure 10-14, which are taken from Netsell (1969).

Difficulty with velar timing is particularly well documented by this technique. Hardy, Netsell, Schweiger, and Morris (1969) have presented a series of case histories that demonstrated the applicability of Netsell's test to children with neuromuscular disorders. Interestingly, the pessure-flow record showed that persistent nasality was associated with residual incompetence of the prosthetically-aided velopharyngeal port in cases where lateral X-rays had indicated adequate anteroposterior closure.

Area of the velopharyngeal opening

If the pressure difference between the oropharynx and the nasal cavity (ΔP) and the airflow through the nose (U_n) are both known, then the resistance of the velopharyngeal-nasal system (R) is given by $R = \Delta P / U_n$. The laws of hydrodynamics specify the way in which the resistance of an opening is related to its area. Specifically,

$$Area = \frac{U}{\sqrt{2 \times \dfrac{P}{density}}}$$

By implication, if the transvelar pressure difference and the nasal airflow are known, it should be possible to calculate the actual area of the velopharyngeal opening.

The equation, however, is valid only for the special case in which there is no turbulence or nonuniformity of flow. To be applicable to estimation of velopharyngeal port size, a correction factor must be introduced to compensate for very real deviations from the ideal case. Warren and DuBois (1964) have used a physical model of the oral and nasal pathways to determine

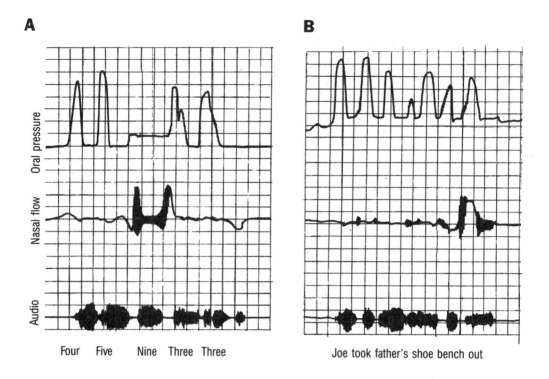

FIGURE 10-11. Typical records of nasal flow and oral pressure. (A) Normal speaker saying "4, 5, 9, 3, 3." There is significant nasal flow only during "nine." (B) Same speaker saying "Joe took father's shoe bench out."

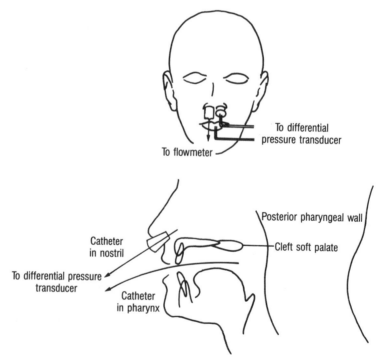

FIGURE 10-12. Connection of sensing tubes for simultaneous trans-velar pressure and nasal flow measurement. (From Warren, D. W. Velopharyngeal orifice size and upper pharyngeal pressure-flow patterns in normal speech. *Plastic and Reconstructive Surgery,* 33 (1964) 148-161. Figure 2, p. 150. Reprinted by permission.)

A **B**

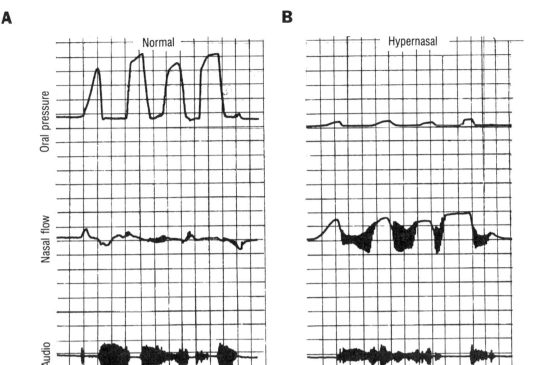

FIGURE 10-13. Intraoral pressure and nasal airflow patterns during speech. Note that the pressure and flow patterns are "reversed" during hypernasal speech.

the required value of such a correction factor.* They found that under different conditions of flow, pressure, and orifice size, the value varied from 0.59 to 0.72. Using a mean value of 0.65, they felt, would provide an estimate sufficiently accurate for most purposes. The area of the velopharyngeal opening, then, is estimated by a hydrokinetic equation[†] of the form:

$$\text{Area} = \cfrac{U_n}{0.65 \sqrt{2 \times \cfrac{P_o - P_n}{D}}}$$

where U_n = nasal flow in mL/s
$\quad P_o$ = oral pressure in dynes/cm^2
$\quad P_n$ = nasal pressure in dynes/cm^2
$\quad D$ = density of air = 0.001g/cm^3

Computation of the estimate can be done in real-time by an on-line analog computer, making it possible to derive a continuous curve on a paper readout that shows velopharyngeal port area along with other relevant variables. Such a computer is not overly difficult to construct from integrated circuits that are widely available.

When tested on the physical model, the hydrokinetic equation was found to produce an error of about 9% when orifice size was about 120 mm^2, and of about 8% with an orifice size of 2.4 mm^2. Further testing on models has since been done by Lubker (1969) and by Smith and Weinberg (1980), both of whom found it to be a valid estimator. The latter study reported a mean accuracy of about 5% for airflows of 50 to more than 400 mL/s, but the error reached as much as 20% with some flow-orifice size combinations. It is difficult to achieve a

---

*Müller and Brown (1980, p. 328) argue strongly (and correctly) for great caution in the choice of a correction factor. They point out its dependence on the user's assumptions about the geometry of the velopharyngeal port—assumptions which might not be valid.

[†]Derivation of the equation and validation methods are presented in Warren and DuBois (1964). Further aerodynamic implications are explored in Warren and Devereux (1966).

TABLE 10-7.   Test Utterances or Evaluation
of Velopharyngeal Competence
in Dysarthria

Utterance	Testing Condition
tʌ	Repetition at rates of 1, 2,
dʌ	4, and 5 per second
nʌ	
ʌtʌd	Five repetitions of each
ʌdʌt	at conversational rate
ʌndʌntʌn	
ʌntʌndʌn	
ʌtʌnʌ	
ʌdʌnʌ	
ʌnʌtʌ	
ʌnʌdʌ	

From Netsell, R. Evaluation of velopharyngeal function in dysarthria. *Journal of Speech and Hearing Disorders*, 34 (1969) 113-122. Table 1, p. 115. © American
Speech-Language-Hearing Association, Rockville,
MD. Reprinted by permission.

good estimate of a large velopharyngeal area
if airflow is low, since ΔP then becomes too
small to measure accurately. Estimation reliability appears to be adequate (Warren
and DuBois, 1964).

As described, the measurement procedure does not take account of nasal resistance. It, therefore, misestimates the
velopharyngeal orifice area. What it really
provides is a measure of the *equivalent*
nasal-velopharyngeal area. Where necessary, a better estimate can be achieved by
correcting for the contribution of the nasal
cavity according to the (somewhat tedious)
method that Warren and DuBois (1964)
describe.*

The originators of the "hydrokinetic equation method" have pointed out its clear advantages. It is less complex, less dangerous,
and perhaps more accurate than X-ray techniques, and is the only means currently
available for tracking velopharyngeal port
area during running speech. It, therefore,
seems very useful, especially for assessing

*Note that the Warren-DuBois method can also be
used to estimate the equivalent area of oral articulatory constrictions. See Hixon (1966), Claypoole, Warren, and Bradley (1974), and Smith, Allen, Warren,
and Hall (1978).

the success of therapeutic intervention (Hogan, 1973). Still, one is confronted yet again
with the difference between the *perception*
of nasality and the physiological correlates
of nasalization. While Warren (1964b) and
Warren and Mackler (1968) suggest that
velopharyngeal orifice areas greater than 20
mm^2 are associated with perceived nasality, and areas over 100 mm^2 with extreme
nasality, no clear and direct corres-
pondance between the two has been demonstrated.

Aerodynamic bridge

For cases in which no invasiveness can
be tolerated, the rather novel method proposed by Hixon, Bless, and Netsell (1976)
can be used. Employing the special equipment diagrammed in Figure 10-15, the
procedure is based on the aerodynamic
equivalent of bridge-balancing (see Chap.
2). A special three-tube glass model that
simulates the oral, nasal, and pharyngeal
airways is needed. Continuously variable
shutter valves are installed at the model's
equivalent of the nasal, oral, laryngeal, and
velopharyngeal openings to permit the size
of these ports to be adjusted. A nose mask
couples the patient's airway to a hard-
walled tube, the other end of which is connected to the nasal port of the model. A
sidearm at the tube's midpoint connects it
to a generator of oscillatory airflow (made
of a series of loudspeakers driven by a sine-
wave power generator). Identical pneumotachograph and pressure transducer
systems are attached to the patient's mouth
and to the oral port of the model. When the
oscillatory airflow generator is turned on,
equal signals are applied to both halves of
an aerodynamic bridge, schematized in Figure 10-15B. The shutter valves at the model's oral, nasal, and laryngeal ports are
preadjusted to resistances typical of these
structures (the authors suggest 0.5, 2.0, and
75 cm H$_2$O/L/s, respectively). Any difference in the magnitude of the sine-wave outputs of the two oral pneumotachographs (as
observed on an oscilloscope or balance meter) should then be due to an inequality of
the model's and patient's velopharyngeal

port area. The two outputs can be equated by adjusting the velopharyngeal shutter valve of the model and, thereby, balancing the bridge, until the balance meter is centered or nulled.*

Actual measurement is done by impressing the forced oscillatory flow on the airway while the patient sustains a voiced continuant sound. The size of the model's velopharyngeal opening is adjusted until there is no difference in the flow signal from the two pneumotachographs. When this balance condition is achieved the patient stops phonating and the area of the velopharyngeal shutter-valve is measured. This area is an estimate of the patient's velopharyngeal port area.

A number of conditions must be satisfied if a valid area estimate is to result. Clearly, the patient's nasal pathway resistance must be very low compared to the resistance of his velopharyngeal port. Like the Warren and DuBois method, this procedure really generates an estimate of the equivalent area of the nasal-pharyngeal combination. Low nasal resistance means that the estimate more nearly reflects the state of the velopharyngeal resistance alone. The oral resistance must also be much less than that of the velopharyngeal port, while the laryngeal resistance must be relatively high. All of these must also be approximated by the glass-tube model. There are obvious restrictions on patient performance: A single phoneme has to be sustained long enough for the tester to achieve a balance condition, and the prolongation must be stable.

This method hass several apparent drawbacks, the most serious of which is that it does not permit tracking of running speech. Further development work, however, may lead to easier implementation and greater utility under a wider variety of conditions.

VELAR MOVEMENT

Although velopharyngeal closure involves more than a simple velar movement,

this particular aspect is often important to the clinician, especially in cases of paralysis or higher CNS dysfunction. A number of means are available for transduction of structural displacement in general (see Chap. 11) and several have been tried on the soft palate. None has found widespread acceptance for this purpose, nor is any complete system available commercially. Further work might lead to an instrument of everyday practicality. Several velar-motion transduction schemes are described here as examples of what might be on the horizon.*

Strain Gauges

Bonded strain gauges can be mounted on special supports and anchored in the oral cavity in such a way as to transduce movements of the soft palate. Moller, Martin, and Christiansen (1971) and Christiansen and Moller (1971) report on the use of such a system, one that they found to be accurate and reliable. It consisted of a thin (0.01 inch thick) steel beam on which the gauges were mounted. A fine spring wire extended from the beam and rested on the center line of the velum, whose movement thus deformed the strain gauges. The entire unit was anchored in place by an orthodontic band that fit around the maxillary second molar.

When correctly fitted, this kind of transducer does not interfere significantly with articulation, and its frequency response is at least adequate for tracking the velar movements of speech. While such a device is clearly useful for real-time biofeedback in managing the "sluggish" velum (Moller, Path, Werth, and Christiansen, 1973), the difficulty in achieving identical placements of the sensing wire at different test sessions seriously limits its usefulness for documenting long-term changes of velar function.

Photoelectric Detectors

The intensity of light transmitted through the velopharyngeal port or reflected from

---

*The electronic circuitry of the instrument contains a bandpass filter that eliminates the phonatory signal and any relatively slow intensity changes.

*While possible, capacitative transduction seems to hold less promise than other methods. Therefore, it has been omitted from this discussion. It is, however, considered by Cole (1972).

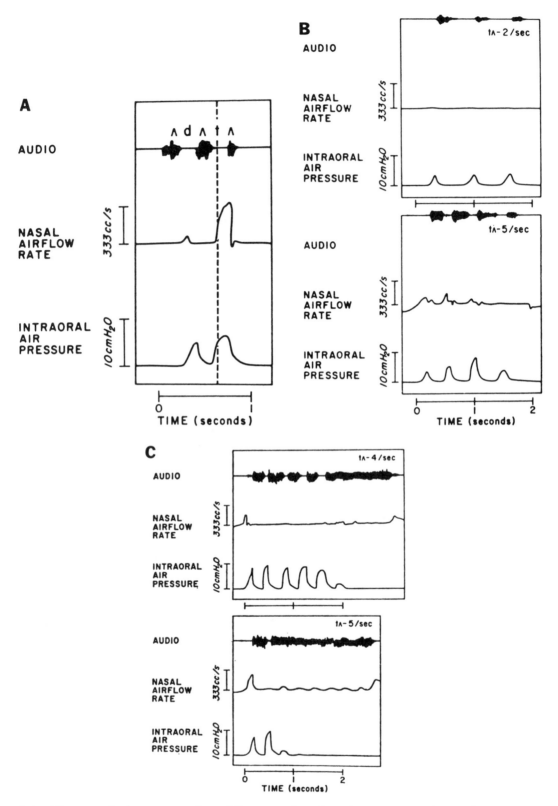

FIGURE 10-14. Oral pressure and nasal flow records in dysarthria. (A) Dysarthric male repeating /ʌdʌtʌ/, showing premature velopharyngeal opening. (B) Dysarthric male repeating /tʌ/ at rates of 2 (upper) and 5 (lower) per second. The lower record shows gradual closure of the velopharyngeal port. (C) Dysarthric female repeating /tʌ/ at rates of 4 (upper) and 5 (lower) per second. The records

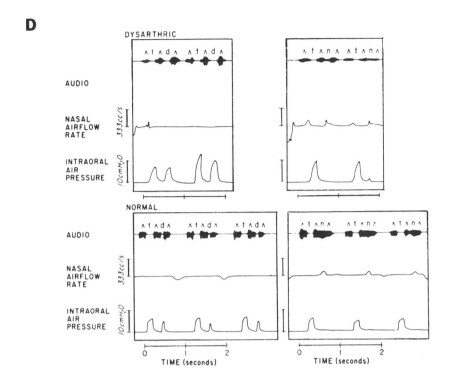

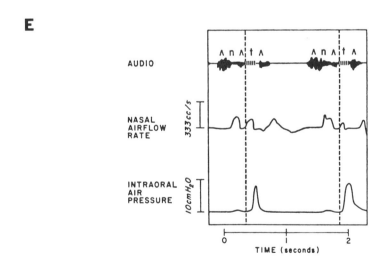

illustrate gradual opening of the velopharyngeal port. (D) Repetitions of /ʌtʌdʌ/ and /ʌtʌnʌ/ by a dysarthric (upper) and a normal (lower) female. The dysarthric speaker uses an inappropriate anticipatory velopharyngeal opening. (E) Repetition of /ʌnʌtʌ/ by a dysarthric male showing inappropriate maintenance of velopharyngeal opening. (All illustrations from Netsell, R. Evaluation of velopharyngeal function in dysarthria. *Journal of Speech and Hearing Disorders*, 34 (1969) 113-122. Figures 3 through 7, pp. 116-120. © American Speech-Language-Hearing Association, Rockville, MD. Reprinted by permission.)

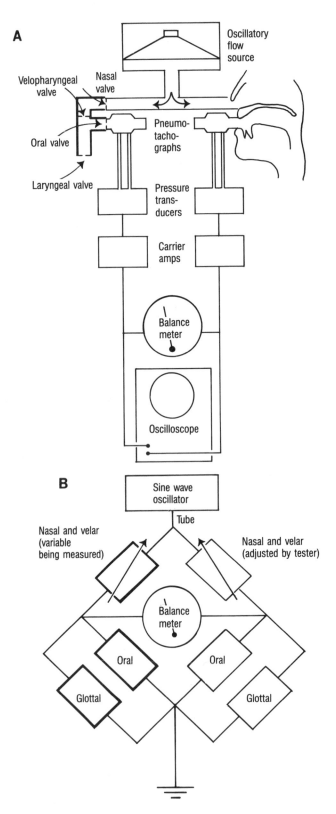

FIGURE 10-15. (A) A non-invasive measurement of velopharyngeal port area. (Modified after Hixon, Bless, and Netsell, 1976). (B) Electrical bridge equivalent of the Hixon, Bless, and Netsell method. Elements of the physical model are in heavy lines on the left. Subject impedances are on the right.

the velar surface can also serve as an indicator of velar motion. Ohala (1971) has constructed a photodetector system consisting of a highly compressible polyethylene tube that contains a miniature lamp and a more proximal photodetector. (The device is also described in Abbs and Watkin, 1976.) The tube is inserted pernasally far enough to place the light source below and the detector above the velopharyngeal port. As the velopharyngeal port narrows, the amount of light transmitted to the detector diminishes, and its output falls accordingly. Unfortunately there appears to be no easy way to calibrate this system and, therefore, it can provide only a relative measure of oronasal coupling.

Condax, Acson, Miki, and Sakoda (1976) have used a reflective system for their phonetic research. A probe containing two fiber-optic bundles is inserted into the nasal cavity. One bundle shines a beam of light posteriorly, while the other conveys reflected light back to an external detector. Elevation of the velum from its rest (open) position results in increased reflection from its superior surface and hence a greater output from the phototransducer. This system does not seem amenable to accurate calibration either, and its use is thereby limited. However, a similar device, the *velograph* of Künzel (1977, 1978, 1979a,b) has been successfully used to provide feedback of velar motion in therapy (Künzel, 1982). ■

Select Bibliography

Abbs, J. H. and Watkin, K. L. Instrumentation for the study of speech physiology. In Lass, N. J. (Ed.), *Contemporary Issues in Experimental Phonetics.* New York: Academic Press, 1976. Pp. 41–75.

Accordi, M., Croatto-Accordi, D., and Cassin, F. Possibilità e limiti dell'indagine spettrografica nella valutazione della rinolalia aperta. *Acta Phoniatrica Latina*, 3 (1981) 25–31.

Ali, L., Gallagher, T., Goldstein, J., and Daniloff, R. Perception of coarticulated nasality. *Journal of the Acoustical Society of America*, 49 (1971) 538–540.

Barnes, I. J. and Morris, H. L. Interrelationships among oral breath pressure ratios and articulation skills for individuals with cleft palate. *Journal of Speech and Hearing Research*, 10 (1967) 506–514.

Basmajian, J. V. and Dutta, C. R. Electromyography of the pharyngeal constrictors and levator palati in man. *Anatomical Record*, 139 (1961) 561–563.

Bell-Berti, F. An electromyographic study of velopharyngeal function in speech. *Journal of Speech and Hearing Research*, 19 (1976) 225–240.

Bell-Berti, F. Velopharyngeal function: A spatial-temporal model. In Lass, N. J. (Ed.) *Speech and Language: Advances in Basic Research and Practice* vol. 4. New York: Academic Press, 1980. Pp. 291–316.

Bernthal, J. E. and Beukelman, D. R. The effect of changes in velopharyngeal orifice area on vowel intensity. *Cleft Palate Journal*, 14 (1977) 63–77.

Björk, L. and Nylen, B. 0. Cineradiography with synchronized sound spectrum analysis. *Plastic and Reconstructive Surgery*, 27 (1961) 397–412.

Bloomer, H. Observation of palatopharyngeal movements in speech and deglutition. *Journal of Speech and Hearing Disorders*, 18 (1953) 230–246.

Bloomer, H. and Peterson, G. A spectrographic study of hypernasality. *Cleft Palate Bulletin*, 5 (1955) 5–6.

Broadbent, T. R. and Swinyard, C. A. The dynamic pharyngeal flap: Its selective use and electromyographic evaluation. *Plastic and Reconstructive Surgery*, 23 (1959) 301–312.

Buck, M. Post-operative velo-pharyngeal movements in cleft palate cases. *Journal of Speech and Hearing Disorders*, 19 (1954) 288–294.

Bzoch, K. Variations in velopharyngeal valving: The factor of vowel changes. *Cleft Palate Journal*, 5 (1968) 211–218.

Calnan, J. and Renfrew, C. E. Blowing tests and speech. *British Journal of Plastic Surgery*, 13 (1961) 340–346.

Carrell, J. A. A cinefluorographic technique for the study of velopharyngeal closure. *Journal of Speech and Hearing Disorders*, 17 (1952) 224–228.

Chase, R. A. An objective evaluation of palatopharyngeal competence. *Plastic and Reconstructive Surgery*, 26 (1960) 23–29.

Christiansen, R. L. and Moller, K. T. Instrumentation for recording velar movement. *American Journal of Orthodontia*, 59 (1971) 448–455.

Clarke, W. M. The measurement of the oral and nasal sound pressure levels of speech. *Journal of Phonetics*, 3 (1975) 257–262.

Clarke, W. M. The relationship between subjective measures of nasality and measures of the oral and nasal sound pressure ratio. *Language and Speech*, 21 (1978) 69–75.

Claypoole, W. H., Warren, D. W., and Bradley, D. P. The effect of cleft palate on oral port constriction during fricative productions. *Cleft Palate Journal*, 11 (1974) 95–104.

Cole, R. M. Electrical capacitance measures of oropharyngeal functions. In Bzoch, K. R. (Ed.), *Communicative Disorders Related to Cleft Lip and Palate*. Boston: Little, Brown, 1972. Pp. 172–177.

Colyar, T. C. and Christensen, J. M. Nasalance patterns in esophageal speech. *Journal of Communication Disorders*, 13 (1980) 43–48.

Condax, I. D., Acson, V., Miki, C. C. and Sakoda, K. K. A technique for monitoring velic action by means of a photoelectric nasal probe: Application to French. *Journal of Phonetics*, 4 (1976) 173–181.

Condax, I. D., Howard, I., Ikranagara, K., Lin, Y. C., Crosetti, J, and Yount, D. E. A new technique for demonstrating velic opening: Application to Sundanese. *Journal of Phonetics*, 2 (1974) 297–301.

Cooper, F. S. Research techniques and instrumentation: EMG. *ASHA Reports* 1 (1965) 153–168.

Counihan, D. T. Oral and nasal sound pressure measures. In Bzoch, K. R. (Ed.). *Communicative Disorders Related to Cleft Lip and Palate*. Boston: Little, Brown, 1972. Pp. 186–193.

Croatto, L., Cinotti, A., Moschi, P., and Toti-Zattoni, A. Il contributo xeroradiografico nello studio dell'insufficienza velo-faringea. *Acta Phoniatrica Latina*, 2 (1980) 31–50.

Curtis, J. F. Acoustics of speech production and nasalization. In Spriestersbach, D. C. and Sherman, D. (Eds.). *Cleft Palate and Communication*. New York: Academic Press, 1968. Pp. 27–60.

Curtis, J. F. The acoustics of nasalized speech. *Cleft Palate Journal*, 7 (1970) 380–396.

Daly, D. A. Bioelectronic measurement of nasality in trainable mentally retarded children. *Journal of Speech and Hearing Disorders*, 42 (1977) 436–439.

Daly, D. A. and Johnson, H. P. Instrumental modification of hypernasal voice quality in retarded children: Case reports.

Davies, H. J. Measurement of nasal patency using a Vitalograph. *Clinical Allergy*, 8 (1978) 517–523.

Dickson, D. R. An acoustic study of nasality. *Journal of Speech and Hearing Research*, 5 (1962) 103–111.

Dickson, S., Barron, S., and McGlone, R. E. Aerodynamic studies of cleft-palate speech. *Journal of Speech and Hearing Disorders*, 43 (1978) 160–167.

Dunn, H. K. The calculation of vowel resonances, and an electrical vocal tract. *Journal of the Acoustical Society of America*, 22 (1950) 740–753.

Eisenback, C. R. II and Williams, W. N. Comparing the unaided visual exam to lateral cinefluorography in estimating several parameters of velopharyngeal function. *Journal of Speech and Hearing Disorders*, 49 (1984) 136–139.

Emanuel, F. W. and Counihan, D. T. Some characteristics of oral and nasal air flow during plosive consonant production. *Cleft Palate Journal*, 7 (1970) 249–260.

Farnetani, E. Aerodinamica della nasalizzazione. *Rivista Italiana di Acustica*, 3 (1979a) 5–21.

Farnetani, E. Foni nasali e nasalizzazione. *Acta Phoniatrica Latina*, 1 (1979b) 30–57.

Fletcher, S. G. Theory and instrumentation for quantitative measurement of nasality. *Cleft Palate Journal*, 7 (1970) 601–609.

Fletcher, S. G. Contingencies for bioelectronic modification of nasality. *Journal of Speech and Hearing Disorders* 37 (1972) 329–346.

Fletcher, S. G. *Manual for Measurement and Modification of Nasality with TONAR II*. Birmingham, Ala.: University of Alabama, 1973.

Fletcher, S. G. and Bishop, M. E. Measurement of nasality with TONAR. *Cleft Palate Journal*, 10 (1973) 610–621.

Fletcher, S. G. and Daly, D. A. Nasalance in utterances of hearing-impaired speakers. *Journal of Communication Disorders*, 9 (1976) 63–73.

Fritzell, B. An electromyographic study of the movements of the soft palate in speech. *Folia Phoniatrica*, 15 (1963) 307–311.

Fritzell, B. A combined electromyographic and cineradiographic study: Activity of the levator and palatoglossus muscles in relation to velar movements. *Acta Otolaryngologica*, Suppl. 250 (1969) 1–81.

Fritzell, B. Electromyography in the study of the velopharyngeal function—a review. *Folia Phoniatrica*, 31 (1979) 93–102.

Fritzell, B. and Kotby, N. M. Observations on thyroarytenoid and palatal levator activation for speech. *Folia Phoniatrica*, 28 (1976) 1–7.

Fujimura, 0. Spectra of nasalized vowels. *Quarterly Progress Report of the Research Laboratory of Electronics* (MIT), 15 (1960) 214–218.

Garber, S. R., Burzynski, C. M., Vale, C., and Nelson, R. The use of visual feedback to control vocal intensity and nasalization. *Journal of Communication Disorders*, 12 (1979) 399–410.

Gonay, P. Effet du nasonnement sur les formants vocaliques. *Acta Oto-Rhino-Laryngologica Belgica*, 26 (1972) 757–770.

Hagerty, R. F., Hill, M. J., Pettit, H. S., and Kane, J. J. Posterior pharyngeal wall movement in normals. *Journal of Speech and Hearing Research*, 1 (1958a) 203–210.

Hagerty, R. F., Hill, M. J., Pettit, H. S., and Kane, J. J. Soft palate movements in normals. *Journal of Speech and Hearing Research*, 1 (1958b) 325–330.

Hanson, M. L. A study of velopharyngeal competence in children with repaired cleft palates. *Cleft Palate Journal*, 1 (1964) 217–231.

Hardy, J. C. Air flow and air pressure studies. *ASHA Reports*, 1 (1965) 141–152.

Hardy, J. C. Techniques of measuring intraoral air pressure and rate of flow. *Journal of Speech and Hearing Research*, 10 (1967) 650–654.

Hardy, J. C. and Arkebauer, H. J. Development of a test for velopharyngeal competence during speech. *Cleft Palate Journal*, 3 (1966) 6–21.

Hardy, J. C., Netsell, R., Schweiger, J. W., and Morris, H. L. Management of velopharyngeal dysfunction in cerebral palsy. *Journal of Speech and Hearing Disorders*, 34 (1969) 123–137.

Harrington, R. A study of the mechanism of velopharyngeal closure. *Journal of Speech Disorders*, 9 (1944) 325–345.

Harrington, R. A note on a lingua-velar relationship. *Journal of Speech Disorders*, 11 (1946) 25.

Hattori, S., Yamamoto, K., and Fujimura, 0. Nasalization of vowels in relation to nasals. *Journal of the Acoustical Society of America*, 30 (1958) 267–274.

Hering, R., Hopppe, W., and Kraft, E. Uber elektromyographische Untersuchungen von Patienten mit Gaumenspalten. *Stoma*, 18 (1965) 24–36.

Hess, D. A. A new experimental approach to assessment of velopharyngeal adequacy: Nasal monometric bleed testing. *Journal of Speech and Hearing Disorders*, 41 (1976) 427–443.

Hess, D. A. and McDonald, E. T. Consonantal nasal pressure in cleft palate speakers. *Journal of Speech and Hearing Research*, 3 (1960) 201–211.

Hirano, M., Takeuchi, Y. and Hiroto, I. Intranasal sound pressure during utterance of speech sounds. *Folia Phoniatrica*, 18 (1966) 369–381.

Hixon, T. J. Turbulent noise sources for speech. *Folia Phoniatrica*, 18 (1966) 168–182.

Hixon, T. J., Bless, D. M., and Netsell, R. A new technique for measuring velopharyngeal orifice area during sustained phonation: An application of aerodynamic forced oscillation principles. *Journal of Speech and Hearing Research*, 19 (1976) 601–607.

Hixon, T. J., Saxman, J. H. and McQueen, H. D. A respirometric technique for evaluating velopharyngeal competence during speech. *Folia Phoniatrica*, 19 (1967) 203–219.

Hogan, V. M. A clarification of the surgical goals in cleft palate speech and the introduction of the lateral port control (L.P.C.) pharyngeal flap. *Cleft Palate Journal*, 10 (1973) 331–345.

Horii, Y. An accelerometric approach to nasality measurement: A preliminary report. *Cleft Palate Journal*, 17 (1980) 254–261.

Horii, Y. An accelerometric measure as a physical correlate of perceived hypernasality in speech. *Journal of Speech and Hearing Research*, 26 (1983) 476–480.

Horii, Y. and Monroe, N. Auditory and visual feedback of nasalization using a modified accelerometric method. *Journal of Speech and Hearing Research*, 26 (1983) 472–475.

House, A. S. and Stevens, K. N. Analog studies of the nasalization of vowels. *Journal of Speech and Hearing Disorders*, 21 (1956) 218–232.

Hultzen, L. S. Apparatus for demonstrating nasality. *Journal of Speech Disorders*, 7 (1942) 5–6.

Hutchinson, J. M., Robinson, K. L., and Nerbonne, M. A. Patterns of nasalance in a sample of normal gerontologic subjects. *Journal of Communication Disorders*, 11 (1978) 469–481.

Hyde, S. R. Nose trumpet: Apparatus for separating the oral and nasal outputs in speech. *Nature*, 219 (1968) 763–765.

Isshiki, N., Honjow, I., and Morimoto, M. Effects of velopharyngeal incompetence upon speech. *Cleft Palate Journal*, 5 (1968) 297–310.

Itoh, M., Sasanuma, S., and Ushijima, T. Velar movements during speech in a patient with apraxia of speech. *Brain and Language*, 7 (1979) 227–239.

Kantner, C. E. The rationale of blowing exercises for patients with repaired cleft palates. *Journal of Speech Disorders*, 12 (1947) 281–286.

Kelleher, R. E., Webster, R. C., Coffey, R. J., and Quigley, L. F. jr. Nasal and oral air flow in normal and cleft palate speech; velocity and volume studies using warm-wire flow meter and two-channel recorder. *Cleft Palate Bulletin*, 10 (1960) 66.

Kline, L. S. and Hutchinson, J. M. Acoustic and perceptual evaluation of hypernasality of mentally retarded persons. *American Journal of Mental Deficiency*, 85 (1980) 153–160.

Künzel, H. J. Photoelektrische Untersuchungen zur Velumhöhe bei Vokalen: Erste Anwendung des Velographen. *Phonetica*, 34 (1977) 352–370.

Künzel, H. J. Reproducibility of electromyographic and velographic measurements of the velopharyngeal closure mechanism. *Journal of Phonetics*, 6 (1978) 345–351.

Künzel, H. J. Röngenvideographische Evaluierung eines photoelecktrischen Verfahrens zur Registrierung der Velumhöhe beim sprechen. *Folia Phoniatrica*, 31 (1979a) 153–166.

Künzel, H. J. Some observations on velar movement in plosives. *Phonetica*, 36 (1979b) 384–404.

Künzel, H. J. First applications of a biofeedback device for the therapy of velopharyngeal incompetence. Folia Phoniatrica, 34 (1982) 92100.

Li, C. H. and Lundervold, A. Electromyographic study of cleft palate. Plastic and Reconstructive Surgery, 21 (1958) 427–432.

Lintz, L. B. and Sherman, D. Phonetic elements and perception of nasality. Journal of Speech and Hearing Research, 4 (1961) 381–396.

Lippman, R. P. Detecting nasalization using a low-cost miniature accelerometer. Journal of Speech and Hearing Research, 24 (1981) 314–317.

Lotz, W. K., Shaughnessy, A. L., and Netsell, R. Velopharyngeal and nasal cavity resistance during speech production. Paper presented at the Convention of the ASHA, 1981.

Lubker, J. F. An electromyographic-cinefluorographic investigation of velar function during normal speech production. Cleft Palate Journal, 5 (1968) 1–18.

Lubker, J. F. Velopharyngeal orifice area: A replication of analog experimentation. Journal of Speech and Hearing Research, 12 (1969) 218–222.

Lubker, J. F. and Curtis, J. F. Electromyographic-cinefluorographic investigation of velar function during speech. Journal of the Acoustical Society of America, 40 (1966) 1272(A).

Lubker, J. F. and Moll, K. L. Simultaneous oral-nasal air flow measurements and cinefluorographic observations during speech production. Cleft Palate Journal, 2 (1965) 257–272.

Lubker, J. F., Schweiger, J. W., and Morris, H. L. Nasal airflow characteristics during speech in prosthetically managed cleft palate speakers. Journal of Speech and Hearing Research, 13 (1970) 326–338.

Massengill, R., jr. Hypernasality. Springfield, IL: Thomas, 1972.

Massengill, R., jr. Early diagnosis of abnormal palatal mobility by the use of cinefluorography. Folia Phoniatrica, 18 (1966) 256–260.

Massengill, R., jr. and Brooks, R. A study of the velopharyngeal mechanism in 143 repaired cleft palate patients during production of the vowel /i/, the plosive /p/, and a /s/ sentence. Folia Phoniatrica, 25 (1973) 312–322.

Massengill, R., jr. and Bryson, M. A study of velopharyngeal function as related to perceived nasality of vowels, utilizing a cinefluorographic television monitor. Folia Phoniatrica, 19 (1967) 45–52.

Massengill, R., jr., Quinn, G., Barry, W. F., jr., and Pickrell, K. The development of rotational cinefluorography and its application to speech research. Journal of Speech and Hearing Research, 9 (1966) 256–265.

McDonald, E. T. and Koepp-Baker, H. Cleft palate speech: An integration of reserch and clinical observation. Journal of Speech and Hearing Disorders, 16 (1951) 9–20.

McWilliams, B. J. Some factors in the intelligibility of cleft-palate speech. Journal of Speech and Hearing Disorders, (1954) 524–527.

McWilliams, B. J. and Bradley, D. P. Rating of velopharyngeal closure during blowing and speech. Cleft Palate Journal, 2 (1965) 46–55.

Moll, K. L. Cinefluorographic techniques in speech research. Journal of Speech and Hearing Research, 3 (1960) 227–241.

Moll, K. L. Velopharyngeal closure on vowels. Journal of Speech and Hearing Research, 5 (1962) 30–37.

Moll, K. L. 'Objective' measures of nasality. Cleft Palate Journal, 1 (1964) 371–374.

Moll, K. L. Photographic and radiographic procedures in speech research. ASHA Reports, 1 (1965a) 129–139.

Moll, K. L. A cinefluorographic study of velopharyngeal function in normals during various activities. Cleft Palate Journal, 2 (1965b) 112–122.

Moll, K. L. and Daniloff, R. G. Investigation of the timing of velar movements during speech. Journal of the Acoustical Society of America 50 (1971) 678–684.

Moller, K. T., Martin, R. R., and Christiansen, R. L. A technique for recording velar movement. Cleft Palate Journal, 8 (1971) 263–276.

Moller, K. T., Path, M., Werth, L. J., and Christiansen, R. L. The modification of velar movement. Journal of Speech and Hearing Disorders, 38 (1973) 323–334.

Morris, H. L. The oral manometer as a diagnostic tool in clinical speech pathology. Journal of Speech and Hearing Disorders, 31 (1966) 362–369.

Morris, H. L. Etiological bases for speech problems. In Spriestersbach, D. C. and Sherman, D. (Eds.). Cleft Palate and Communication. New York: Academic Press, 1968. Pp. 119–168.

Morris, H. L. and Smith, J. K. A multiple approach for evaluting velopharyngeal competency. Journal of Speech and Hearing Disorders, 27 (1962) 218–226.

Morris, H. L., Spriestersbach, D. C. and Darley, F. L. An articulation test for assessing competency of velopharyngeal closure. Journal of Speech and Hearing Research, 4 (1961) 48–55.

Moser, H. M. Diagnostic and clinical procedures in rhinolalia. Journal of Speech Disorders, 7 (1942) 1–4.

Müller, E. M. and Brown, W. S., jr. Variations in the supraglottal air pressure waveform and their articulatory interpretation. In Lass, N. J. (Ed.). Speech and Language: Advances in Basic Research and Practice vol. 4. New York: Academic Press, 1980. Pp. 317–389.

Netsell, R. Evaluation of velopharyngeal function in dysarthria. *Journal of Speech and Hearing Disorders*, 34 (1969) 113–122.

Netsell, R. and Daniel, B. Dysarthria in adults: Physiologic approach to rehabilitation. *Archives of Physical Medicine and Rehabilitation*, 60 (1979) 502–508.

Niimi, S., Bell-Berti, F., and Harris, K. S. Dynamic aspects of velopharyngeal closure. *Folia Phoniatrica*, 34 (1982) 246–257.

Ohala, J. J. Monitoring soft palate movements in speech. *Journal of the Acoustical Society of America*, 50 (1971) 140A.

Pigott, R. W. The nasendoscopic appearance of the normal palatopharyngeal valve. *Plastic and Reconstructive Surgery*, 43 (1969) 19–24.

Pigott, R. W., Bensen, J. F., and White, F. D. Nasendoscopy in the diagnosis of velopharyngeal incompetence. *Plastic and Reconstructive Surgery*, 43 (1969) 141–147.

Pitzner, J. C. and Morris, H. L. Articulation skills and adequacy of breath pressure ratios of children with cleft palate. *Journal of Speech and Hearing Disorders*, 31 (1966) 26–40.

Plattner, J., Weinberg, B., and Horii, Y. Performance of normal speakers on an index of velopharyngeal function. *Cleft Palate Journal*, 17 (1980) 205–215.

Powers, G. R. Cinefluorographic investigation of articulatory movements of selected individuals with cleft palates. *Journal of Speech and Hearing Research*, 5 (1962) 59–69.

Quigley, L. F., jr., Shiere, F. R., Webster, R. C. and Cobb, C. M., Measuring palatopharyngeal competence with the nasal anemometer. *Cleft Palate Journal*, 1 (1964) 304–314.

Quigley, L. F., jr., Webster, R. C., Coffey, R. J., Kelleher, R. E., and Grant, H. P. Velocity and volume measurements of nasal and oral airflow in normal and cleft palate speech, utilizing a warm-wire flowmeter and two-channel recorder. *Journal of Dental Research*, 42 (1963) 1520–1527.

Redenbaugh, M. A. and Reich, A. R. Correspondence between an accelerometric nasal/voice amplitude ratio and listeners' direct magnitude estimation of hypernasality. *Journal of Speech and Hearing Research*, 28 (1985) 273–281.

Sawashima, M. and Ushijima, T. Use of the fiberscope in speech research. *Annual Bulletin of the Research Institute of Logopedics and Phoniatrics* (University of Tokyo), 5 (1971) 25–34.

Sawashima, M. and Ushijima, T. The use of fiberscope in speech research. In Hirschberg, J., Szépe, Gy., Vass-Kovács, E (Eds.). *Papers in Interdisciplinary Speech Research*. Budapest: Adadémiai Kiadó, 1972. Pp. 229–231.

Schwartz, M. F. Relative intra-nasal sound intensities of vowels. *Speech Monographs*, 35 (1968a) 196–200.

Schwartz, M. F. The acoustics of normal and nasal vowel production. *Cleft Palate Journal*, 5 (1968b) 125–140.

Schwartz, M. F. Acoustic measures of nasalization and nasality. In Bzoch, K. R. (Ed.). *Communicative Disorders Related to Cleft Lip and Palate*. Boston: Little, Brown, 1972. Pp. 194–200.

Seaver, E. J., III, and Kuehn, D. P. A cineradiographic and electromyographic investigation of velar positioning in non-nasal speech. *Cleft Palate Journal*, 17 (1980) 216–226.

Shaw, N. and Gilbert, H. R. A respirometric technique for evaluating velopharyngeal closure in children. *Journal of Speech and Hearing Research*, 25 (1982) 476–480.

Shelton, R. L., jr. and Blank, J. L. Oronasal fistulas, intraoral air pressure and nasal air flow during speech. *Cleft Palate Journal*, 21 (1984) 91–99.

Shelton, R. L., jr., Brooks, A. R., and Youngstrom, K. A. Articulation and patterns of palatopharyngeal closure. *Journal of Speech and Hearing Disorders*, 29 (1964) 390–408.

Shelton, R. L., jr., Brooks, A. R., and Youngstrom, K. A. Clinical assessment of palatopharyngeal closure. *Journal of Speech and Hearing Disorders*, 30 (1965) 37–43.

Shelton, R. L., jr., Harris, K. S., Sholes, G. N., and Dooley, P. M. Study of nonspeech voluntary palate movements by scaling and electromyographic techniques. In Bosma, J. F. (Ed.). *Second Symposium on Oral Sensation and Perception*. Springfield, IL: Thomas, 1970. Pp. 432–441.

Shelton, R. L., jr., Knox, A. W., Arndt, W. B., jr., and Elbert, M. The relationship between nasality score values and oral and nasal sound pressure level. *Journal of Speech and Hearing Research*, 10 (1967) 549–557.

Shelton, R. L., jr., Paesani, A., McClelland, K. D., and Bradfield, S. S. Panendoscopic feedback in the study of voluntary velopharyngeal movements. *Journal of Speech and Hearing Disorders*, 40 (1975) 232-244.

Sherman, D. The merits of backward playing of connected speech in the scaling of voice quality disorders. *Journal of Speech and Hearing Disorders*, 19 (1954) 312–321.

Skolnick, M. L. Videofluoroscopic examination of the velopharyngeal portal during phonation in lateral and base projections—a new technique for studying the mechanics of closure. *Cleft Palate Journal*, 7 (1970) 803–816.

Smith, B. E. and Weinberg, B. Prediction of velopharyngeal orifice area: A re-examination of model experimentation. *Cleft Palate Journal*, 17 (1980) 277–282.

Smith, H. Z., Allen, G., Warren, D. W., and Hall, D. J. The consistency of the pressure-flow technique for assessing oral port size. *Journal of the Acoustical Society of America,* 64 (1978) 1203–1206.

Smith, S. The electro-aerometer. *Speech Pathology and Therapy,* 3 (1960) 27–33.

Spriestersbach, D. C. Assessing nasal quality in cleft palate speech of children. *Journal of Speech and Hearing Disorders,* 20 (1955) 266–270.

Spriestersbach, D. C. The effects of orofacial anomalies on the speech process. *ASHA Reports,* 1 (1965) 111–128.

Spriestersbach, D. C., Darley, F. L., and Rouse, V. Articulation of a group of children with cleft lips and palates. *Journal of Speech and Hearing Disorders,* 21 (1956) 436–445.

Spriestersbach, D. C. and Powers, G. R. Nasality in isolated vowels and connected speech of cleft palate speakers. *Journal of Speech and Hearing Research,* 2 (1959a) 40–45.

Spriesterrsbach, D. C. and Powers, G. R. Articulation skills, velopharyngeal closure, and oral breath pressure of children with cleft palates. *Journal of Speech and Hearing Research,* 2 (1959b) 318–325.

Stevens, K. N., Kalikow, D. N., and Willemain, T. R. A miniature accelerometer for detecting glottal waveforms and nasalization. *Journal of Speech and Hearing Research,* 18 (1975) 594–599.

Stevens, K. N., Nickerson, R. S., Boothroyd, A., and Rollins, A. M. Assessment of nasalization in the speech of deaf children. *Journal of Speech and Hearing Research,* 19 (1976) 393–416.

Subtelny, J., Kho, G., McCormack, R. M., and Subtelny, J. D. Multidimensional analysis of bilabial stop and nasal consonants—cineradiographic and pressure-flow analysis. *Cleft Palate Journal,* 6 (1969) 263–289.

Subtelny, J. D., Koepp-Baker, H., and Subtelny, D. Palatal function and cleft palate speech. *Journal of Speech and Hearing Disorders,* 26 (1961) 213–224.

Subtelny, J. D., McCormack, R. M., Subtelny, J. D., Worth, J. H., Cramer, L. M., Runyon, J. C., and Rosenblum, R. M. Synchronous recording of speech with associated physiologic pressure flow dynamics: Instrumentation and procedures. *Cleft Palate Journal,* 5 (1968) 93–116.

Taub, S. The Taub oral panendoscope: A new technique. *Cleft Palate Journal,* 3 (1966a) 328–346.

Taub, S. Oral panendoscope for direct observation and audiovisual recording of velopharyngeal areas during phonation. *Transactions of the American Academy of Ophthalmology and Otolaryngology,* Sept-Oct 1966b, 855–857.

Thompson, A. E. and Hixon, T. J. Nasal air flow during normal speech production. *Cleft Pal-*

ate Journal, 16 (1979) 412–420.

Ushijima, T., Sawashima, M., Hirose, H., Abe, M. and Harada, T. A kinesiological aspect of myasthenia gravis: An electromyographic study of velar movements during speech. *Annual Bulletin of the Research Institute of Logopedics and Phoniatrics,* 10 (1976) 225–232.

van Demark, D. R. Predictability of velopharyngeal competency. *Cleft Palate Journal,* 16 (1979) 429–435.

van Demark, D. R. and Morris, H. L. A preliminary study of the predictive value of the IPAT. *Cleft Palate Journal,* 14 (1977) 124–130.

van Demark, D. R. and Swickard, S. L. A preschool articulation test to assess velopharyngeal competency: Normative data. *Cleft Palate Journal,* 17 (1980) 175–179.

van den Berg, J. Modern research in experimental phoniatrics. *Folia Phoniatrica,* 14 (1962) 81–149.

van Hattum, R. J. Articulation and nasality in cleft palate speakers. *Journal of Speech and Hearing Research,* 1 (1958) 383–387.

Vealey, J., Bailey, C., II, and Belknap, L., II. Rheadeik: To detect the escape of nasal air during speech. *Journal of Speech and Hearing Disorders,* 30 (1965) 82–84.

Warren, D. W. Velopharyngeal orifice size and upper pharyngeal pressure-flow patterns in normal speech. *Plastic and Reconstructive Surgery,* 33 (1964a) 148–161.

Warren, D. W. Velopharyngeal orifice size and upper pharyngeal pressure-flow patterns in cleft palate speech: A preliminary study. *Plastic and Reconstructive Surgery,* 34 (1964b) 15–26.

Warren, D. W. Nasal emission of air and velopharyngeal function. *Cleft Palate Journal,* 4 (1967) 148–156.

Warren, D. W. Perci: A method for rating palatal efficiency. *Cleft Palate Journal,* 16 (1979) 279–285.

Warren, D. W. and Devereux, J. L. An analog study of cleft palate speech. *Cleft Palate Journal,* 3 (1966) 103–114.

Warren, D. W., Duany, L. F., and Fischer, N. D. Nasal pathway resistance in normal and cleft lip and palate subjects. *Cleft Palate Journal,* 6 (1969) 134–140.

Warren, D. W. and DuBois, A. B. A pressure-flow technique for measuring velopharyngeal orifice area during continuous speech flow. *Cleft Palate Journal,* 1 (1964) 52–71.

Warren, D. W. and Mackler, S. B. Duration of oral port constriction in normal and cleft palate speech. *Journal of Speech and Hearing Research,* 11 (1968) 391–401.

Warren, D. W. and Ryon, W. E. Oral port constriction, nasal resistance, and respiratory aspects of cleft palate speech: An analog study. *Cleft Palate Journal,* 4 (1967) 38–46.

Warren, D. W., Wood, M. T., and Bradley, D. P. Respiratory volumes in normal and cleft palate speech. *Cleft Palate Journal,* 6 (1969) 449–460.

Watterson, T. and Emanuel, F. Effects of oral-nasal coupling on whispered vowel spectra. *Cleft Palate Journal* 18 (1981) 24–38.

Williams, W. N. Applications of radiologic measures. In Bzoch, K. R. (Ed.). *(Communicative Disorders Related to Cleft Lip and Palate.* Boston: Little, Brown, 1972. Pp. 163–171.

Williams, W. N. and Eisenbach, C. R. II. Assessing VP function: The lateral still techinque vs. cinefluorography. *Cleft Palate Journal,* 18 (1981) 45–50.

Willis, C. R. and Stutz, M. L. The clinical use of the Taub oral panendoscope in the observation of velopharyngeal function. *Journal of Speech and Hearing Disorders,* 37 (1972) 495–502.

Worth, J. H., Runyon, J. C., and Subtelny, J. D. Integrating flowmeter for measuring unimpaired oral and nasal flow. *IEEE Transactions on Bio-medical Engineering,* 15 (1968) 196–200.

Yules, R. B., Josephson, J. B., and Chase, R. A. A dehypernasality trainer. *Behavior Research Methods and Instrumentation,* 1 (1969) 160.

Zemlin, W. R. and Fant, G. The effect of a velopharyngeal shunt upon vocal tract damping times: An analog study. *Speech Transmission Laboratory Quarterly Progress and Status Report,* 4 (1972) 6–10.

Zwitman, D. H., Gyepes, M. T., and Sample, F. The submentovertical projection in the radiographic analysis of velopharyngeal dynamics. *Journal of Speech and Hearing Disorders* 38 (1973) 473–477.

Zwitman, D. H., Gyepes, M. T., and Ward, P. H. Assessment of velar and lateral wall movement by oral telescope and radiographic examination in patients with velopharyngeal inadequacy and in normal subjects. *Journal of Speech and Hearing Disorders,* 41 (1976) 381–389.

Zwitman, D. H., Sonderman, J. C., and Ward, P. H. Variations in velopharyngeal closure assessed by endoscopy. *Journal of Speech and Hearing Disorders,* 39 (1974) 366–372.

CHAPTER 11

Speech Movements

Speech sounds are produced by speech movements. Abnormal sounds are made by abnormal movements—of the chest wall, larynx, pharynx, palate, tongue, or facial structures. The diagnosis of speech disorders is, at base, the process of determining which movements are inadequate, in what ways, under what circumstances. Often that determination is based on correlates of motor behavior—air pressure, sound intensity, air flow rates, and the like. But it is frequently useful, and sometimes necessary, to monitor the movements themselves. Given that much of the speech system is not readily accessible and that important movements can be very small and extremely fast, the problems involved in observing important movements are often not simple. Other chapters have considered special aspects of speech motor behavior, such as vocal fold displacement or velopharyngeal closure. This chapter is concerned primarily with articulatory and chest wall movements in a more general sense. Of the many possible ways of moni-

toring the position of speech structures, only a few will be discussed here. The focus will be on those that are relatively innocuous, practicable in the clinical setting, and likely to be cost effective. A short discussion of electromyography is included because it figures very prominently in the research literature and because it can be used, by appropriate medical personnel, if necessary, to obtain information of great value to the speech clinician. In fact, speech pathologists in medical settings might often need to interpret electromyographic data that are part of the records of patients referred for rehabilitation.

Obtaining valid and reliable information about the movements of the organs of speech and using that information to design a course of therapy demands a firm understanding of the mechanisms of motor behavior in general and of speech motor control in particular. The literature in this area is extensive, but good overviews, at various levels of sophistication, have been prepared by Abbs and Kennedy (1982),

Kennedy and Abbs (1982), Abbs and Eilenber (1976), and Daniloff, Schuckers, and Feth (1980).

ELECTROMYOGRAPHY

Biological Principles

The structural unit of muscular activity is the muscle fiber, which contracts when appropriately excited. If it is not held at a fixed length it becomes shorter, but its overall tension (the force with which it pulls on the structures to which it is attached) remains relatively constant. Hence muscle contraction that results in length change is called *isotonic*. On the other hand, if muscle shortening is prevented (for example, by simultaneous contraction of opposing muscles) an *isometric* contraction occurs, and muscle tension rises significantly. Many muscle actions are a combination of isometric and isotonic contraction. Muscle fibers are capable of contraction only: Elongation to precontractile length must be effected by an external force, such as an opposing muscle.

Contraction is controlled by *motoneurones*, each of which synapses on many individual muscle fibers. If a motoneurone is activated it stimulates *all* of the muscle fibers that it innervates, making them *all* contract. This minimal unit of muscle action—a motoneurone and all of its associated muscle fibers—was named a *motor unit* by Liddell and Sherrington (1925). The number of muscle fibers in a motor unit varies widely. Muscles that are capable of only gross control have many muscle fibers per motoneurone (large motor units). The average motor unit in gastrocnemius, for instance, has more than 1700 muscle fibers (Buchthal and Schmalbruch, 1980). On the other hand, muscles that can be controlled very precisely have very small motor units. The cricothyroid motor unit size has been calculated to be between about 30 and 165 (Faaborg-Andersen, 1957; English and Blevins, 1969). Anatomically, the motor unit is not an isolated entity. Its muscle fibers are dispersed throughout a large region of the gross muscle mass. Muscle fibers lying next to each other are very likely to be members of quite different motor units. The effect of this dispersion is that a single motoneurone does not stimulate a localized contraction somewhere in a muscle, but rather it causes some small amount of contraction throughout the muscle.

Synaptic transmission from a motoneurone causes a wave of electrical activity to sweep along each of the muscle fibers in its motor unit. The electrical wave is associated with the chemical actions of contraction (Huxley, 1965; Porter and Franzini-Armstong, 1965; Hoyle, 1970). If it shows electrical activity, a muscle fiber must be contracting. Similarly, if a muscle fiber is contracting, there must be electrical activity. The magnitude of the electrical wave (called a *muscle action potential* or *MAP*) is several tens of millivolts at the muscle itself. It is strong enough to cause an electrical disruption in the muscle fiber's environment up to a distance of several centimeters with rapidly-diminishing strength. The force of a muscle's contraction is increased by more frequent synaptic stimulation of each motor unit and by activating a greater number of motor units (Akazawa and Fujii, 1981; Sussman, MacNeilage, and Powers, 1977).

The detection and recording of MAPs is called *electromyography (EMG)*. It was developed by neurophysiologists (e.g., Adrian and Bronk, 1929; Smith, 1934; Denny-Brown, 1949) and was quickly applied to the study and evaluation of muscle and nerve pathology (Weddell, Feinstein, and Pattle, 1944; Basmajian, 1974). By the 1950s electromyographic investigation of speech activity was well under way (Draper, Ladefoged, and Whitteridge, 1959, 1960; Faaborg-Andersen, 1957; Sawashima, Sato, Funasaka and Totsuka, 1958). Brief reviews of EMG in various areas of speech research have been published by Fromkin and Ladefoged (1966), Cooper (1965), Gay and Harris (1971), and Harris (1981).

While electromyography reveals a great deal about muscle activity, it provides very little information about structural movement. A muscle contracts in a context of many other opposing or augmenting forces. The precontractile status of the muscle, the activity of its antagonists, and the loading upon it are all significant. So are the biomechanical properties of the larger tissue matrix in which muscle activation occurs. In short, the electromyogram shows the magnitude of a single force vector among the great many that might be acting simultaneously. It is only rarely possible to conclude that a given movement is causally related to particular MAPs. It is to clarify causal relationships that researchers frequently monitor both motion and EMG simultaneously (for example, Gay, Ushijima, Hirose, and Cooper, 1974; Abbs, 1973a,b; Sussman, MacNeilage, and Hanson, 1973).

Instrumentation

Electrodes

Muscle action potentials are detected by conductors, called *electrodes*, placed in the region of the electrical disturbance. Although such electrodes might seem to be simple devices, subject only to straightforward and obvious design principles, this is far from the case. A great many criteria must be satisfied for precision work. The models of electrical behavior at the electrode to tissue junction are quite complex (Geddes, 1972; Cobbold, 1974) and well beyond the scope of this discussion. For the present purposes electrodes can be divided into two comprehensive classes: intramuscular and surface. Aside from pragmatic considerations, the choice between the two types (and among the subcategories within each) depends on the kind of information needed.

Electrodes are used in pairs with a differential amplifier (see Chap. 2). The EMG signal is the difference in the voltages seen by the two electrodes. All of the tissue between them contributes to this difference. The smaller the electrodes and the closer they are to each other, the smaller the vol-

ume of muscle tissue contributing to the net electrical input. Moving the electrodes as close as possible to the muscle fibers to be observed also limits the sampled tissue volume. If the electrodes can be made small enough and if they can be kept very close together, it is possible to observe the electrical response of a single muscle fiber. This information is needed by the research physiologist and the physician who must diagnose neuromuscular disorders. Intramuscular electrodes allow them to limit the volume of muscle being observed to a sufficiently small size. Speech clinicians, however, are almost never interested in the response of a single muscle fiber. What matters to them is the behavior of the muscle as an integral structure. For their purposes fairly large electrodes that are not in intimate contact with the muscle mass can often be very useful if certain limitations are understood.

No matter what kind of electrode system is decided on, at least three important criteria must be met. The electrodes

1. must not interfere with or alter normal motor function;
2. must be able to move with the muscle without generating spurious signals (movement artifacts); and
3. must be usable in confined areas, such as the oral cavity.

INTRAMUSCULAR ELECTRODES. Intramuscular electrodes are used when it is important that the volume of muscle being sampled is kept small or when the activity of only one of several muscles in an overlapping arrangement is to be examined.

Needle electrodes. Originally, intramuscular electrodes were of the needle type. *Monopolar needle electrodes* (Figure 11-1A) simply use the bare tip of a needle as an electrode. Two monopolar needles are inserted into the muscle for recording of the electrical activity in the zone between them. Inserting an insulated wire into the needle so that only its end is exposed creates a *concentric electrode* (Figure 11-1B).

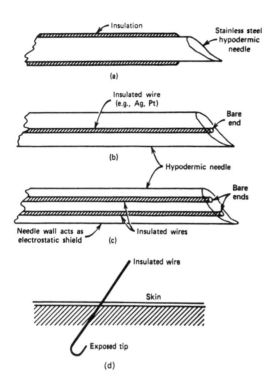

FIGURE 11-1. Electromyography electrodes. (A) Monopolar needle; (B) concentric monopolar; (C) bipolar; (D) hooked wire. (From Cobbold, R. S. C. *Transducers for Biomedical Measurements: Principles and Applications.* Figure 10.14, p. 438. © 1974 by John Wiley and Sons, Inc. Reprinted by permission of John Wiley and Sons, Inc.)

The needle and the wire serve as electrodes in this arrangement, and the sampled region is the zone between their exposed tips. If two insulated wires are carried in the needle, the resulting *bipolar electrode* (Figure 11.1C) samples the region between their bare ends while the shaft of the needle serves as a shield to screen out electrical interference.

Although needle electrodes have been used successfully to investigate behavior of the larynx (Rea, Templer, and Davis, 1978; Hiroto, Hirano, Toyozumi, and Shin, 1967; Zenker and Zenker, 1960; Fink, Basek, and Epanchin, 1956; Buchthal and Faaborg-Andersen, 1964; Faaborg-Andersen, 1965) pharynx and velopharyngeal port (Basmajian and Dutta, 1961), and facial muscles

(Leanderson, Persson, and Öhman, 1971) among others, they are not ideally suited to examination of speech behavior. Their rigidity and large size may restrict muscle activity. Shear forces acting on them, when muscles move beneath the skin, cause needle displacement that produces electrical artifacts and significant patient discomfort.

Hooked-wire electrodes were developed by Basmajian and Stecko (1962) to circumvent these problems. They are made (Figure 11-1D) by passing a loop of extremely fine insulated wire through a hypodermic needle. The insulation is removed from the loop, the bare wire is cut, and the two free ends are folded back over the needle tip. After sterilization, the needle is inserted into the muscle and then withdrawn, leaving the wire ends hooked on the muscle fibers. The needle is slipped off the trailing wires, which remain the only thing penetrating the skin. Their presence produces very little discomfort, and they are much less prone to displacement by muscle activity. After testing, a fairly gentle tug removes the wire electrodes from the muscle. Hooked wires have become the electrodes of choice for examining the speech musculature. Techniques have been developed for inserting them into almost all of the muscles of the vocal tract (Hirose, 1971, 1977; Hirano and Ohala, 1969; Bole and Lessler, 1966; Gay, Strome, Hirose, and Sawashima, 1972; Hirose, Gay, Strome, and Sawashima, 1971; Shipp, Fishman, Morrissey, and McGlone, 1970; Shipp, Deatsch, and Robertson, 1968; Dedo and Hall, 1969; Minifie, Abbs, Tarlow, and Kwaterski, 1974).

Because the tip of an intramuscular electrode cannot be seen, special verification procedures must be followed to prove that it is where it is supposed to be and that it is not picking up signals from surrounding muscles. In general, placement verification is done by observing the electromyographic output during maneuvers that are known to require contraction of the target muscle in relative isolation from those around it.

Unfortunately articulatory actions are very complex, and there is a serious paucity of information upon which to make unequivocal placement verifications for many muscles. Therefore, the tester will often need to fall back on a somewhat subjective, but accurately informed, judgment of placement made against a firm background knowledge of vocal tract structure and function. Some suggested tests of electrode placement are provided by Hirose (1971), Shipp, Fishman, Morrissey, and McGlone (1970), Shipp, Deatsch, and Robertson (1968) Kennedy and Abbs (1979) and 0'Dwyer, Quinn, Guitar, Andrews, and Neilson (1981).

SURFACE ELECTRODES Surface electrodes, which are completely noninvasive, are a viable alternative for some purposes. Attached to the skin, they detect electrical activity in a fairly large volume under them. This makes them too nonspecific for most research purposes. They can provide signals very similar to those of intramuscular electrodes, however, if the muscle being sampled is close to the surface* and clearly separate from nearby muscles (Abbs and Watkin, 1976; Netsell, Daniel, and Celesia, 1975). The vigorous speech movements of many vocal tract structures makes firm attachment of the electrodes to the skin or mucous membrane imperative. Any movement of the electrode relative to the skin surface will produce artifacts in the output signal. Electrodes have been specially designed to facilitate cementing them to the skin (Cole, Konopacki, and Abbs, 1983). But beyond using chemical adhesives, there are two relatively simple and harmless ways of achieving firm electrode placement:

1. Workers at Haskins Laboratories (Cooper, 1965; Harris, Rosov, Cooper, and Lysaught, 1964) made surface electrodes out of hollow silver jewelry beads. A bead is cut in half and fitted with a side tube that is connected by plastic tubing to a vacuum manifold. A stranded wire connected to the electrode passes through the vacuum tube to the vacuum chamber, where it is connected to the input leads from the amplifier. The vacuum inside the hemispheric electrode keeps it firmly in place. Electrodes of this type can be made sufficiently small and unobtrusive to be used successfully even on the surface of the tongue (MacNeilage and Sholes, 1964; Huntington, Harris, and Sholes, 1968).

2. Surface electrodes can also be painted on the skin. An acceptable conductive paint can be made by suspending 10 g of silver powder in 10 g of Duco cement thinned with a few milliliters of acetone. A drop of this mixture is applied at the chosen site and allowed to dry. The bared end of a very thin wire is laid on the spot of silver, and another drop of conductive liquid applied. This is allowed to harden into a silver and wire "sandwich." The wire is connected to the EMG amplifier (Allen, Lubker, and Harrison, 1972).* Complete specifications for this method are provided by Hollis and Harrison (1970). Allen, Lubker, and Turner (1973) have suggested that a very simple surface electrode can be made by simply attaching a loop of bare copper wire to the skin with a quick-setting cyanoacrylate cement, but the method has not yet been thoroughly evaluated.

The Electromyogram and Signal Processing

EMG signals are very small—ranging from 200 μV or less up to about 1 mV. Very high amplifier gain (on the order of 10,000) is often needed to get an output of suffi-

---

*Some specialized "surface" electrodes have been designed to record from muscles deep within body cavities. Hixon, Siebens, and Minifie (1969), for instance, designed such an electrode for the diaphragm, and Lastovka, Sram, and Sedlacek (1984) have described a bipolar electrode that can be placed within the larynx.

---

*Conductive paint intended for electromyography is available from Micro Circuits, Inc., New Buffalo, MI.

cient amplitude for recording. Furthermore, the input impedance of the amplifier must be as high as possible (well into the megohm range) to avoid electrical loading of the electrodes (see Chap. 2). The combination of a very small signal and very high input impedance makes the system susceptible to noise. The electrode wires that go to the amplifier act as antennas, picking up stray electromagnetic radiation. Because the wires must be kept as short as possible, it is common practice to put a preamplifier very close to the subject and to use its output as the signal to the EMG amplifier itself. Noise reduction is also facilitated by using differential amplifiers with high (100 dB or better) common mode rejection ratios (see Chap. 3). (A small EMG system, incorporating special surface electrodes with built-in ultrahigh-impedance preamplifiers is available from Ampel Systems Canada, London, Ontario. It has proven to be very effective and easy to use in several studies of motor control.)

The appearance of the electromyogram will depend on the volume of muscle "seen" by the electrodes and the nature of the motor task being examined. If the active region between the electrodes is very small (as with intramuscular bipolar electrodes), individual muscle action potentials may be recorded, especially if the muscle is not very active (Figure 11-2A). The frequency of the "spikes" of electrical activity can range up to more than 40 per second, making the "raw" electromyogram during a speech event look like the one shown in Figure 11-2B. Note that the frequency of the spikes changes from a relatively quiescent resting rate to a much higher rate. The number of spikes per second is a direct measure of the degree of muscle activation.

Normal muscle contraction is actually the result of excitation of many motor units. Because the fibers belonging to a given motor unit are widely dispersed, the several muscle fibers lying between the electrodes are very likely to be members of different motor units, and their firing will, therefore, be asynchronous. Most often the

EMG signal is the sum of the electrical actions occurring at quasi-random times with respect to each other. This kind of summation results in an *interference pattern* (colloquially often referred to as *hash*), as shown in Figure 11-2C. Surface electrodes always yield such a pattern because they are influenced by many motor units in the comparatively enormous muscle volume they sample.

Most often, EMG signals are rectified and integrated for analysis. This is the best way of demonstrating the "amount" of electrical activity, and it has been found (Lippold, 1952; Bigland and Lippold, 1954) that the amplitude of the integrated signal is directly proportional to the force of an isometric contraction. A simple rectifier with an RC filter (see Chap. 2) is adequate for this processing. The optimal RC time constant (averaging time) will vary with the muscle being observed and the task being evaluated. Fromkin and Ladefoged (1966) point out that it should be long compared to the interval between electrical spikes, but short compared to the rate of change of activity in the muscle. The longer the averaging time the more individual MAPs are leveled to create a smooth curve showing electrical activity over time. However the smoothing also levels the peaks and troughs that indicate muscle activity and quiescence: Fine details of EMG changes over time are lost in this averaging. Figure 11-3 clearly shows the loss of temporal resolution as the averaging time is increased. If a pen writer is used as the output device (as opposed to, say, an oscilloscope), the poor frequency response of the pen system represents a large increase in the averaging time of the entire emg instrumentation system. Peaks of EMG activity may be very poorly demonstrated in the resulting record. In cases in which the magnitude of EMG bursts is important, a relatively simple circuit devised by Doyle and Allon (1980) might prove useful. It holds the peak value of a transient burst of activity for a preset amount of time, stretching it out long enough for good display on a chart record.

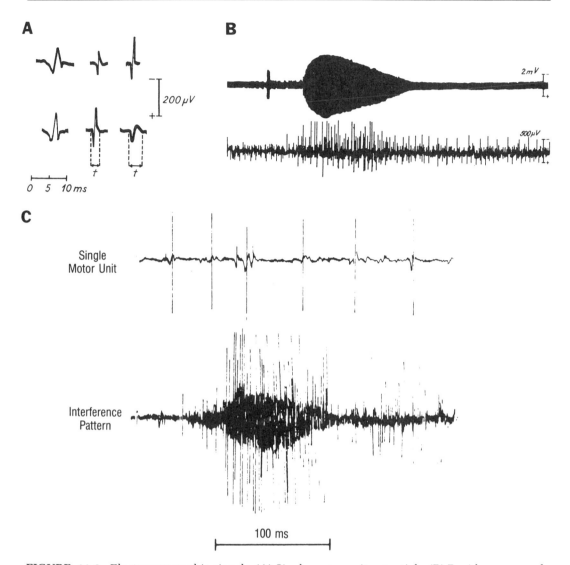

FIGURE 11-2. Electromyographic signals. (A) Single motor unit potentials; (B) Rapid sequence of "spikes." Note the change in impulse frequency, indicating a change in the level of muscle excitation; (C) EMG interference pattern, resulting from the superposition of many random spikes. (From Abbs, J. H., and Watkin, K. L. Instrumentation for the study of speech physiology. In Lass, N. J. (Ed.) *Contemporary Issues in Experimental Phonetics.* New York: Academic Press, 1976. Pp. 41-75. Figure 2.4, p. 45. Reprinted by permission.)

There is a certain "capriciousness" in the very complex muscle activity of speech. Minor differences in muscle activation occur from one repetition of an utterance to the next. These variations may interfere with an accurate assessment of what a given muscle actually does during a speech task. To mitigate this problem some laboratories have developed computer averaging techniques. These are discussed in detail in Cooper (1965), Fromkin and Ladefoged (1966), Port (1971), Gay and Harris (1971) and Kewley-Port (1977). Basically the technique involves sampling many repetitions of the same utterance. The EMG data are stored in a computer and are temporally aligned at some reference point chosen by the system user. The values for each

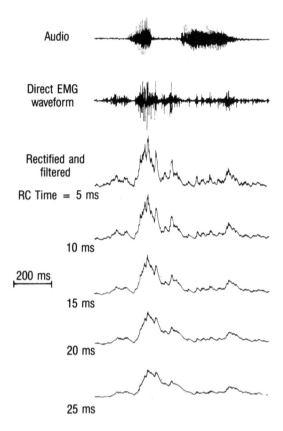

Audio

Direct EMG
waveform

Rectified and
filtered

RC Time = 5 ms

10 ms

200 ms

15 ms

20 ms

25 ms

FIGURE 11-3. Rectified and averaged EMG records of the utterance /æpæ/, with averaging time increasing from top to bottom. (From Abbs, J. H. and Watkin, K. L. Instrumentation for the study of speech physiology. In Lass, N. J. (Ed.) *Contemporary Issues in Experimental Phonetics.* New York, Academic Press, 1976. Pp. 41-75. Figure 2.7, p. 53. Reprinted by permission.)

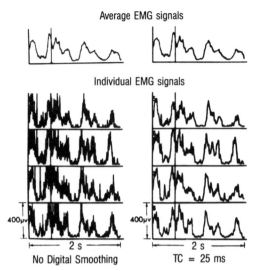

Average EMG signals

Individual EMG signals

400µv

400µv

2 s

2 s

No Digital Smoothing

TC = 25 ms

FIGURE 11-4. EMG averaging. The top trace represents the average of a total of 10 EMG recordings made during repetitions of a single utterance. (Only 4 of the 10 EMGs are shown.) The "line-up point" is shown by the vertical line. It corresponds to the offset of voicing during the utterance. Averaging of both "raw" (left) and smoothed (right side, time constant = 25 ms) are shown. (From Kewley-Port, D. EMG signal processing for speech research. *Haskins Laboratories Status Report on Speech Research,* SR-50 (1977) 123-146. Figure 4, p. 140. Reprinted by permission.)

of the samples at each point in time are averaged to produce a final output in which events that are present in every one of the samples are emphasized, but those that are unique are de-emphasized. Figure 11-4 illustrates the results achieved by this kind of averaging process.

Biofeedback

A very promising clinical use of surface electrom biofeedback of speech motor performance. Typically the patient is provided with an auditory signal whose frequency varies with the amplitude of the EMG volt-

age. The tone can be generated by using the amplified and averaged electromyographic potentials as the input to a voltage-to-frequency converter, which is available as an inexpensive integrated circuit. More complex circuits can combine signals from two or more muscles (with a different tone representing each) and inhibit the tone when muscle activity drops below a predetermined minimal value (Helmer, 1975). The patient, of course, is instructed to control the audible tone (in ways specified by the therapist) by means of muscle control. Biofeedback has been successfully used to reduce facial hypertonicity (Netsell and Cleeland, 1973), increase labial muscle activity after neural anastomosis (Daniel and Guitar, 1978), normalize perilaryngeal muscle tension in hyperfunctional voice disorders (Stemple, Weiler, Whitehead, and Komray, 1980), and reduce the frequency of stuttering moments (Guitar, 1975).

PALATOGRAPHY

Palatography provides information on the exact location of articulatory tongue-palate contact. Various forms of the technique date from the latter part of the 19th century, and were used in many of the important early studies of normal and disordered speech (Rousselot, 1897 1901; Scripture, 1902; Stetson, 1928; Gumpertz, 1931; Moses, 1939)* Palatography has been somewhat ignored during much of this century, but interest in it seems to be reviving. It is a moderately simple procedure that can provide with certain limitations a great deal of information about the precise location and timing of articuatory contacts that can be of inestimable value to the speech clinician (see Hardcastle and Morgan, 1982).

Palatographic methods may be classed as direct or indirect, according to whether an artifical palate is used. In both cases the contact surface is coated with a powder (such as talc, flour, or a mixture of powdered charcoal and cocoa) that is wiped away by lingual contact. The need for the powder can be obviated by the recently developed electronic devices that sense tongue contact with metallic points on the surface of an artificial palate.

Indirect Palatography

For *indirect palatography* an artificial palate generally made of acrylic is formed on a plaster cast of the patient's mouth. (Specific instructions for forming a metal-foil palate are given by Judson and Weaver, 1965, p. 160.) Just before use, it is coated with a powder that contrasts with the base material. It is carefully fitted over the patient's palate, the test utterance is produced,

and the plate is removed and examined. The powder will have been removed wherever there was tongue contact. A permanent record of the contact areas can be made by sketching them on an outline of the palate or (better) by photographing the plate. The artificial palate can be cleaned and reused as often as necessary.

Indirect palatography has a number of obvious drawbacks. The presence of the artificial palate might change articulatory patterns in unknown ways. Then too, it is not usually possible to extend the prosthesis very far over the velum without eliciting gagging. Therefore, linguavelar contacts cannot usually be detected with the technique. Most important from a practical point of view, however, is the fact that construction of the plate is an expensive and time-consuming process. On the other hand, the method has two significant advantages. First, the vertical dimension of tongue contact is accurately shown. Second, the ability to remove the pattern from the mouth makes undistorted photography easy.

Direct Palatography

For *direct palatography* the powder is dusted directly onto the patient's hard palate and velum. The test utterance is then produced, and the wipe-off pattern assessed. Because no artificial palate is involved, this method is simple, fast, and inexpensive. Also, there is nothing to interfere with articulation, and contact anywhere on the palate or velum is demonstrable.

Permanently recording the results, however, is more complicated than for indirect palatography. The easiest way is to insert a moderately large mirror into the mouth and photograph its reflection of the palate. However, the angle at which the photograph is taken (which can vary significantly from one trial to another) can cause distortion of the image. To minimize this problem, Ladefoged (1957) proposed a simple arrangement of mirrors (Figure 11-5)

---

*The history of palatography is sketched in Moses, (1940, 1964) and in Abercrombie (1957).

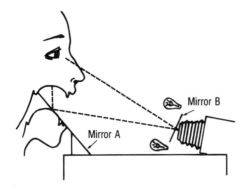

FIGURE 11-5. Camera and mirror arrangement for accurate photographs of direct palatograms. (From Ladefoged, P. use of palatography. *Journal of Speech and Hearing Disorders,* 22 (1957) 764-774. Figure 1, p. 765. © American Speech-Language-Hearing Association, Rockville, MD. Reprinted by permission.

that assures a relatively constant camera angle. The patient positions his mouth around mirror A until he sees his entire palate in mirror B. A photograph taken when this condition is met will be at approximately a right angle to the plane of the patient's teeth. The photograph, of course, does not depict depth, but for cases in which the vertical dimension is important, Ladefoged 1957 and Bloomer (1943) have suggested methods of generating contour lines of the palate. In addition, Witting (1953) has proposed a method for numerically describing the contact pattern.

Electropalatography

Electropalatography uses a special artificial palate with an array of exposed electrodes that can sense tongue contact. Associated circuitry turns on lamps on a display panel to show which electrodes have been touched. Electrical detection offers significant advantages, quite beyond the convenience of not having to bother with powder coatings. The electrodes are always ready—they need not be prepared after each contact. This means that continuous palatography is possible: A whole series of different contact patterns during

running speech can be observed on the display or recorded for later analysis. This in turn permits determination of the exact temporal duration and sequencing of many articulatory events. Electropalatography is, therefore, commonly called *dynamic palatography*.

Instrumentation

Although several different electropalatographs have been described (Kuzmin, 1962; Kozhnevnikov, Granstrem, Kuzmin, et al., 1968; Kydd and Belt, 1964; Hardcastle, 1970, 1972; Rome, 1964; Fujimura, Shibata, Kiritani, et al., 1968; Kiritani, Kakita, and Shibata, 1977), they all depend on the same basic principle: The tongue serves as a conductor that connects an electrical signal from a "sending" to a "receiving" electrode. In the early electropalatographs, the electrodes were arranged in sending and receiving pairs; tongue contact connected the members of each pair. More recent instruments use a modification of this system devised by Kydd and Belt (1964) that achieves improved reliability and greater spacial resolution. The *Edinburgh electropalatograph* (Hardcastle, 1970, 1972) and the somewhat more advanced Rion Model DP-01 electropalatograph are representative of the better available instruments.

Figure 11.6 schematizes the Edinburgh device (Hardcastle, 1970). The detector system is carried on a thin acrylic palate, custom made to fit the patient's mouth. Forty silver electrodes are exposed on its oral surface. Each is soldered to its own very thin wire, which is laminated into the plastic. The forty wires emerge at the plate's posterior corners. In use, the wire bundles pass behind the last molars and exit at the corners of the mouth.

Each of the forty electrodes is a receiver. The sending "electrode" is the tongue itself. This is arranged by connecting the patient to a 20 kHz oscillator by means of an electrode attached somewhere outside of the oral cavity. The entire oral region thus conducts the signal, which is coupled to an

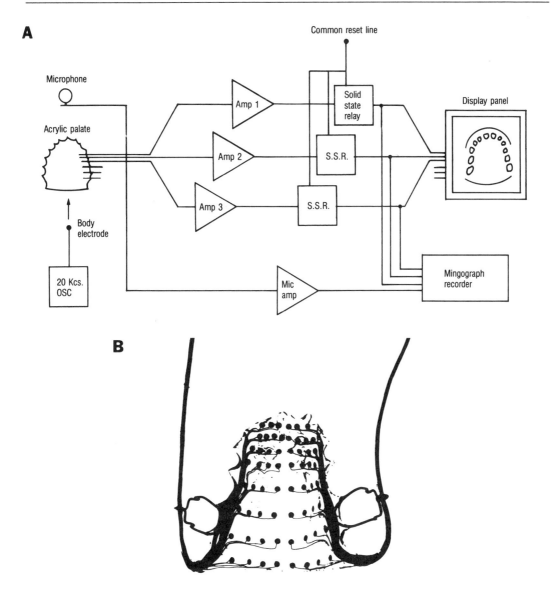

FIGURE 11-6. The "Edinburgh" electropalatograph. (A) Block diagram. (From Hardcastle, W. J. The use of electropalatography in phonetic research. *Phonetica*, 25 (1972) 197-215. Figure 1, p. 203. Reprinted by permission.) (B) Electrodes and wiring on the artificial palate. (From Hardcastle, W. J. Electropalatography in speech research. *University of Essex Language Centre Occasional Papers*, 9 (1970) 54-64. Figure 1, p. 56. Reprinted by permission.)

electrode when it is touched by the tongue. A high-input-impedance amplifier, tuned to pass only 20 kHz signals, is provided for each electrode. When tongue contact is made with a given electrode, its amplifier's output activates a circuit that lights a lamp on the display panel. (Hardcastle [1972] provides construction details of the acrylic plate and schematic diagrams of the associated circuits.)

The output display consists of 40 lamps arranged on a panel according to the position of the electrode each represents on the artificial palate. Normally the lights turn off as soon as tongue contact is terminated, but a system of relays is included in the display system to "freeze" it until it is manually reset. A static palatogram can thereby be generated when necessary. An electrical output is provided from each lamp circuit for connection to an external recording device.

The Rion model DP-01 electropalatograph is specifically designed for clinical use (Figure 11-7). It has 63 active gold electrodes embedded in its acrylic palate (whose wiring is done by printed-circuit methods). Each is a sending electrode. The common receiver is also on the palatal structure, in contact with the roof of the mouth. The electrodes are scanned 64 times per second by a multiplexer in the system's circuitry. The display is similar to that of the Edinburgh instrument: an array of lamps, each representing a palate electrode, that are turned on to indicate tongue contact. For therapy a plastic overlay is provided on which the contact pattern that the patient is to achieve is drawn. A digital memory can store the pattern of electrode activation for each of 64 consecutive scans of the array. The stored information can be displayed later in slow motion for careful analysis.

The major problem with any· electropalatograph is that of obtaining a permanent record. It is possible to feed the output signals to a chart recorder, but only a few palatal points can be accommodated, since each requires a separate pen. A simpler method is to photograph the display panel, using motion pictures for dynamic palatograms. Rion sells a special printer that produces printouts of the patterns stored in their intrument's memory.

The on-or-off nature of each of the individual data (i.e., contact) points immediately suggests the possibility of computer processing of palatograms. There has been some work done to achieve just this (Fujii, Fujimura, and Kagaya, 1971; Fujimura, Tatsumi, and Kagaya, 1973; Tatsumi, 1972; Fletcher, McCutcheon, and Wolf, 1975; McCutcheon, Fletcher, and Wolf, 1975), and the increasing availability and versatility of microcomputer systems may encourage further effort in this direction. Electropalatography has proven very useful to researchers and has stimulated modern work in the tradition of the early phoneticians (Palmer, 1973; Harley, 1972; Fujii, 1970; Butcher and Weiher, 1976; Miyawaki, 1972; Miyawaki, Kiritani, Tatsumi, and Fujimura, 1974). But it shares the problems of any form of indirect palatography: possible interference with articulation, limited ability to detect posterior contact, and the expense of artificial palates. Beyond this, the electrodes represent discrete points on the palate. The spatial resolution of the contact pattern is inversely proportional to the distance between the electrodes: The more densely packed they are, the better the accuracy of the output.

A word of caution

There is no doubt that palatograms, like those shown in Figure 11-8, can be of use to the clinician.They can, for example, show a patient how close his productions are to a standard model. Electropalatography could well play a role in computer-assisted articulation therapy. But there are important cautions that the therapist must keep in mind.

1. Stimuli must be carefully selected to provide the information needed. *Never* should an isolated consonant be used.
2. An acoustically acceptable speech sound can result from many different tongue placements.
3. Early users of palatography (Moses, 1939; Shohara and Hanson, 1941) realized that there is great variability among speakers in contact pattern for a given phone. Furthermore, the contact pattern of a consonant will be altered as the vowel environment changes. Indeed, the contact pattern is subject to significant *random* variation.
4. Hamlet, Bunnell, and Struntz (1986) have recently pointed out a important bias that may enter the interpretation of palatograms. "The lateral, midsaggital

A

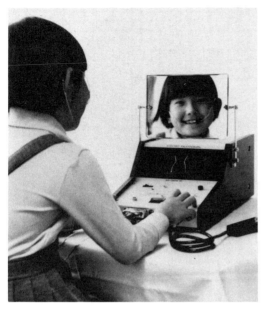

B

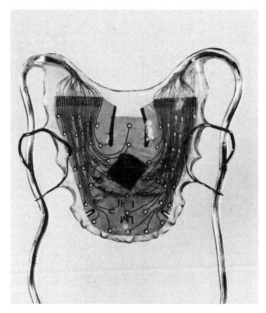

FIGURE 11-7. (A) The Rion electropalatograph. The patient can watch his or her own oral movements in the mirror above the instrument's display panel. (B) Wires emerging from the corners of the mouth connect to the 64 electrodes on the artificial palate. (Courtesy of Rion Trading Co., Tokyo, Japan.)

view of the vocal tract," they remind us, "has become a standard format for illustrating tongue activity in speech." Because of this, we tend to be poorly informed about contact patterns near the lateral margins of the palate. We also tend to assume that contact patterns are symmetrical about the midline. Their recent studies demonstrate quite clearly that there is likely to be considerable asymmetry of contact in normal speakers. Furthermore, there is also likely to be temporal asymmetry: contact on one side may be established before contact on the other. Neither asymmetry necessarily signals abnormality.

Considering these cautions, we must conclude that requiring a patient to match a therapist's palatogram precisely, or seeking an invariant tongue contact for a phoneme in all contexts, constitutes misuse of the technique. Palatography is of maximal a value for assessment of grossly abnormal

articulation and for tracking patient progress in approximating a more normal articulatory constriction.

DIADOCHOKINESIS

The evaluation of diadochokinesis—the ability to perform rapid repetitions of relatively simple patterns of oppositional contractions—has long been a part of the standard speech evaluation. The rationale for such testing rests on the assumption that it provides insight into the adequacy of the patient's neuromotor maturation and integration. Tests of diadochokinesis are viewed as screens for neurologic disability.

There has always been considerable controversy about the value of diadochokinetic tests as diagnostic or prognostic indicators. Early studies of individuals frequently included such non-oral diadochokinetic tasks as finger tapping (e.g., Heltman and

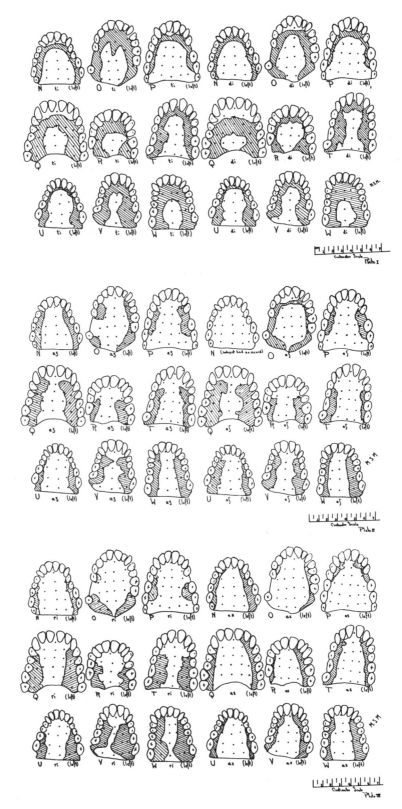

FIGURE 11-8. Specimen palatograms. (From Moses, E. R., Jr. Palatography and speech improvement. *Journal of Speech Disorders*, 4 (1939) 103-114. Plates I, II, and III, pp. 107, 109, 111. © American Speech-Language-Hearing Association, Rockville, MD. Reprinted by permission.)

Peacher, 1943; Strother and Kriegman, 1943). While there may be a common timing mechanism underlying such tasks and speech (Tingley and Allen, 1975; Albright, 1948), both research and professional experience showed them to be of little value to speech clinicians. They have largely been abandoned. Diadochokinetic rates for nonspeech movements of the articulators were also commonly determined, on the assumption that they represented a simpler motor substrate upon which speech movements were built (Fairbanks and Spriestersbach, 1950; Evans, 1952; Westlake, 1951, 1952). However, a number of studies (Heltman and Peacher, 1943; Irwin, 1957; Hixon and Hardy, 1964) have established that the relationship is at best very weak and that diadochokinetic rates for spoken syllables are generally significantly greater than for analogous nonspeech movements. Current practice limits diadochokinetic tests to spoken material.

Test Procedure

Although it is a fairly simple test, there is no single standardized procedure for eliciting the diadochokinetic performance or, for that matter, for measuring the repetition rate. Generally, the patient is simply instructed that, when told to begin, he is to repeat the test utterance as rapidly as possible and for as long as possible at comfortable pitch and loudness. It is common for the tester to demonstrate the task and to elicit at least one practice trial to be sure the patient correctly understands the instructions.

Rate measurement

Although appealing, the temptation to simply listen with a stopwatch, counting the patient's syllables "live,"is best resisted. It is very difficult to count accurately at the speed that is usually required. Special electronic counter circuits (e.g., Irwin and Becklund, 1953) can be used. But they may represent more sophistication than is

needed. One easy way to get accurate results is to play a recording of the task into a graphic level recorder (see Chap. 4) set for a fast writing speed. (An ordinary pen recorder can also be used if the speech signal is first rectified.) It is usually a simple matter to count the number of peaks per unit time on the paper record. In the absence of a pen recorder, a tape-recorded test can be played back with as much speed reduction as possible, slowing the repetitions to an easily counted rate. (When played back at half speed, 1 s of recording equals 0.5 s of real time.)

A decision must be made about what is to be counted. (The notes to Table 11-1 give just some of the alternatives.) Some prefer to count all syllables for the first 5 s. Others begin counting from the second second, thereby allowing for an onset adjustment period. Still others take a two-second sample from the middle of the syllable train. Whatever the sample, rate is usually expressed as the mean number of utterances per second. (An alternative, the time required to produce a predetermined number of repetitions, is discussed later.) Obviously, in addition to assessing the adequacy of the rate, it is important for the clinician to evaluate articulatory precision and rate variability during the task.

Expected Results

Testing is most often done for the syllables /pʌ/, /tʌ/, and /kʌ/, and for /pʌtʌkə/. Table 11-1A summarizes some of the data available for these four utterances. The limited information available for other syllables are similarly summarized in Table 11-1B. Details of sample elicitation and measurement techniques are tabulated in the accompanying notes.

Time-by-count method

Fletcher (1972) and Allen (1974) recommend that diadochokinetic rate be assessed by determining the amount of time required to produce a given number of repetitions

TABLE 11-1A. Diadochokinetic Rates for /p/, /t/, and /k/ in Normal Speakers

Age Range	Sex	N	Diado Rate Mean	S.D.	Range	Source
			/p/			
5	M/F	12	4.22			a
6	M/F	10	4.48			a
6	M	30	3.49	.383	2.51–4.47*	b
6	F	30	3.67	.419	2.60–4.74*	b
7	M	20	4.34	.589	2.72–5.92*	b
7	F	20	4.38	.501	3.00–5.76*	b
7– 9	M/F	8	4.70			a
9	M	20	4.56	.407	3.44–5.68*	b
9	F	20	4.40	.499	3.03–5.77*	b
9	M	10	4.8	.49		c
9	F	10	4.4	.47		c
10	M	10	4.9	.64		c
10	F	10	4.7	.76		c
11	M	20	4.80	.476	3.49–6.11*	b
11	F	20	4.88	.239	4.22–5.54*	b
11	M	10	5.5	.64		c
11	F	10	5.2	.52		c
13	M	20	5.17	.643	3.40–6.94*	b
13	F	20	5.44	.417	4.29–6.59*	b
15	M	20	5.86	.611	4.18–7.54*	b
15	F	20	5.44	.477	4.13–6.75*	b
18–39	M	28	7.0	1.0	5.4 –9.4 *	d
18–38	F	31	6.9	0.6	5.8 –7.8 *	d
19–28	M	20	6.0	0.66		f
18–26	F	25	5.9	0.35		f
25.7(= X̄)	M/F	20/20	7.0			h
65–76	M	10	6.0	0.82		f
65–76	F	12	6.7	0.93		f
68–89	M	27	5.4	1.2	2.8 –8.2 *	d
66–93	F	30	5.0	1.2	1.3 –7.0 *	d
			/t/			
5	M/F	12	4.17			a
6	M/F	10	4.49			a
6	M	30	3.33	.365	2.40–4.26*	b
6	F	30	3.51	.423	2.41–4.61*	b
7	M	20	4.14	.422	2.98–5.30*	b
7	F	20	4.33	.518	2.90–5.76*	b
7– 9	M/F	8	4.66			a
7–12	M/F	21/24	5.8	.75		i
9	M	20	4.49	.484	3.16–5.82*	b
9	F	20	4.32	.503	2.93–5.71*	b
9	M	10	4.6	.50		c
9	F	10	4.5	.65		c
10	M	10	5.0	.98		c
10	F	10	4.9	.82		c

11	M	20	4.75	.537	3.27−6.23*	b
11	F	20	4.84	.49	3.49−6.19*	b
11	M	10	5.5	.99		c
11	F	10	4.9	.47		c
13	M	20	5.09	.660	3.27−6.91*	b
13	F	20	5.22	.581	3.62−6.82*	b
15	M	20	5.77	.604	4.11−7.43*	b
15	F	20	5.38	.541	3.89−6.87*	b
18−39	M	28	6.9	1.1	4.2 −9.4	d
18−38	F	31	6.8	1.0	4.8 −8.4	d
19−28	M	20	6.0	0.96		f
18−26	F	25	5.8	0.37		f
25.7(=X̄)	M/F	20/20	7.1			h
65−76	M	10	5.8	0.69		f
65−76	F	12	6.5	0.44		f
68−69	M	27	5.3	1.0	3.0 −6.8	d
66−93	F	30	4.8	1.1	2.2 −6.8 *	d

/k/

5	M	12	3.85			a
6	M	10	4.26			a
6	M	30	3.18	.319	2.37−3.99*	b
6	F	30	3.28	.392	2.28−4.28*	b
7	M	20	4.02	.402	2.91−5.13*	b
7	F	20	3.88	.408	2.76−5.00*	b
7− 9	M/F	8	4.16			a
7−12	M/F	21/25	5.3	.72		i
9	M	20	4.19	.519	2.76−5.62*	b
9	F	20	3.94	.450	2.70−5.18*	b
9	M	10	4.2	.51		c
9	F	10	4.1	.53		c
10	M	10	4.6	.92		c
10	F	10	4.4	.53		c
11	M	20	4.52	.578	2.93−6.11*	b
11	F	20	4.46	.446	3.23−5.69*	b
11	M	10	4.9	.44		c
11	F	10	4.6	.55		c
13	M	20	4.84	.639	3.08−6.60*	b
13	F	20	4.76	.498	3.39−6.13*	b
15	M	20	5.27	.733	3.25−7.29*	b
15	F	20	5.00	.517	3.58−6.42*	b
18−39	M	28	6.2	.8	5.0 −8.2	d
18−38	F	31	6.2	.8	4.6 −8.2	d
19−28	M	20	5.4	.54		f
18−26	F	25	5.2	.60		f
25.7(=X̄)	M/F	20/20	6.2			h
65−76	M	10	5.8	.62		f
65−76	F	12	5.9	.83		f
68−89	M	27	4.9	1.0	2.6 −6.8	d
66−93	F	30	4.4	1.1	2.2 −6.4	d

TABLE 11-1B. Diadochokinetic Rates for /pʌtʌkʌ/ and Other Phones

Age Range	Sex	N	Diado Rate Mean	S.D.	Range	Source
			/pʌtʌkʌ/			
5	M/F	12	3.43			a
6	M/F	10	3.80			a
7– 9	M/F	8	3.85			a
9	M	10	4.3	.68		c
9	F	10	4.8	.72		c
10	M	10	5.0	.80		c
10	F	10	5.0	.47		c
11	M	10	5.0	.54		c
11	F	10	5.3	.58		c
18–39	M	28	5.8	1.0	4.0–8.2	d
18–38	F	31	6.3	0.9	3.8–7.8	d
68–89	M	26	4.4	1.3	2.4–7.0	d
66–93	F	30	3.6	1.3	1.4–6.2	d
			/ʌ/			
18–39	M	28	5.1	1.0	2.6–7.0	d
18–38	F	31	5.3	0.8	3.0–6.8	d
68–89	M	27	4.1	0.9	2.6–6.0	d
66–93	F	29	3.9	1.3	1.8–6.6	d
			/h/			
20–39	F	40	5.46	0.57		g
40–59			5.72			g
60–80			5.54	0.75		g
57 (median)	M	17	5.6 +		4.1–7.6	e
			/i/			
19–28	M	20	4.7	0.67		f
18–26	F	25	4.9	0.57		f
65–76	M	10	4.8	0.63		f
65–76	F	12	5.1	0.86		f

Sources:

a. Yoss and Darley, 1974. Specific testing procedure not given. Compared to dyspraxic children.

b. Irwin and Becklund, 1953. Special counter system ("Sylrater"). "Three trials of about 5 s each were . . . given for each test. The peak or maximum rate for each subject for each test item was recorded."

c. Blomquist, 1950. Subjects were schoolchildren. Told to repeat test syllable "as rapidly and as regularly as possible, then to do it again, then a third time." Spectrogram used to calculate mean number of repetitions in the 2.35 s displayed for each sample. Three of the four repetitions were analyzed for each child.

d. Ptacek, Sander, Maloney, and Jackson, 1966. Subjects asked "to take a deep breath and produce the sounds as rapidly as possible until stopped by the examiner" after demonstration. Seven-second samples, first and last seconds excluded from count, resulting in data based on mean repetition rate in 5 s.

e. Canter, 1965. Measurement of graphic readout. Comparison to Parkinsons patients. Vowels were schwa and /ɑ/.

f. Kreul, 1972. "Each diadochokinetic movement was demonstrated with standard instructions, and the subjects were instructed to produce the sounds 'just as rapidly as you can, keeping the sounds clear and distinct'." Single trial for each subject. Data are the number of sounds, to the nearest half, produced in a 2 s sample.

g. Shanks, 1970. Subjects instructed to repeat syllable /hʌ/ as rapidly as possible at comfortable pitch and loudness. Three practice trials, 5 s each, followed by three 5 s trials that were tape recorded. First 3 s of each sample were written by a graphic vocal recorder. The "number of peaks present on 9 [3 s, 3 trials] one-second intervals of the tracings was counted to establish the rate of syllable repetition per second."

h. Lundeen, 1950. Two 3 s practice sessions. Data are based on mid 5 s of a 7 s sample.

i. Dworkin, 1978. Mean number of repetitions on 3 3 s trials. Data are rates per 3 s. Compared with lispers.

*95% confidence limits.

†Median.

of the test utterance. Some clinicians may find that the counting task is simplified by this method, although half-speed playback of a recording of the task helps greatly. "Time-by-count" diadochokinetic rates of normal speakers are summarized in Table 11-2.

Speech disorders

Speech diadochokinetic rates have been found to be slower than normal in a wide range of speech disorders. The effect has been verified not only in cases of upper motoneurone pathology, but in cases of "functional" dyslalia as well. Table 11-3 provides a sample of the available data.

ARTICULATOR MOVEMENT

Instrumental measurement of the motion of the organs of speech is not difficult in theory. In principle, any of a fairly large selection of transduction and recording techniques could be used and, in fact, have been. No matter what transduction system (the combination of transducer, signal-processing elements, display and perhaps storage device) is assembled, it must meet certain criteria. The validity of the information gathered will depend on the system's physical characteristics and on the subject's response to the instrumentation.

From the mechanical and electrical point of view, the measurement apparatus must have a response to motion that is, if not linear, then at least governed by some invariant mathematical function. It should be adequately sensitive to motion, without being too sensitive. Many speech movements are small, and there must be adequate gain to detect them unambiguously. At the same time the very slight physiological tremor that is a normal aspect of muscle contraction should be ignored: It consititutes noise in the output record. Also, the gain must not be so great as to

TABLE 11-2. Diadochokinetic Rates for Normal Speakers (Time by Count Method)*

Age	Mean or S.D.	/pʌ/ (20)	/tʌ/ (20)	/kʌ/ (20)	/fʌ/ (20)	/lʌ/ (20)	/pʌtʌ/ (15)	/pʌkʌ/ (15)	/tʌkʌ/ (15)	/pʌtʌkʌ/ (10)
6	M	4.8	4.9	5.5	5.5	5.2	7.3	7.9	7.8	10.3
	SD	0.8	1.0	0.9	1.0	0.9	2.0	2.1	1.8	3.1
7	M	4.8	4.9	5.3	5.4	5.3	7.6	8.0	8.0	10.0
	SD	1.0	0.9	1.0	1.0	0.8	2.6	1.9	1.8	2.6
8	M	4.2	4.4	4.8	4.9	4.6	6.2	7.1	7.2	8.3
	SD	0.7	0.7	0.7	1.0	0.6	1.8	1.5	1.4	2.1
9	M	4.0	4.1	4.6	4.6	4.5	5.9	6.6	6.6	7.7
	SD	0.6	0.6	0.7	0.7	0.5	1.6	1.5	1.7	1.9
10	M	3.7	3.8	4.3	4.2	4.2	5.5	6.4	6.4	7.1
	SD	0.4	0.4	0.5	0.5	0.5	1.5	1.4	1.2	1.5
11	M	3.6	3.6	4.0	4.0	3.8	4.8	5.8	5.8	6.5
	SD	0.6	0.7	0.6	0.6	0.6	1.1	1.2	1.3	1.4
12	M	3.4	3.5	3.9	3.7	3.7	4.7	5.7	5.5	6.4
	SD	0.4	0.5	0.6	0.4	0.5	1.2	1.5	1.1	1.6
13	M	3.3	3.3	3.7	3.6	3.5	4.2	5.1	5.1	5.7
	SD	0.6	0.5	0.6	0.5	0.5	0.8	1.5	1.3	1.4

From Fletcher, S. G. Time-by-count measurement of diadochokinetic syllable rate. *Journal of Speech and Hearing Research*, 15 (1972) 763-770. Table 1, p. 765. 1978 C. C. Publications, Inc., Tigard, OR. Reprinted by permission.

*Tabled data are the times in seconds required to achieve the number of repetitions indicated below the syllable description. Measured by stopwatch after 2 practice trials of about 3 s each. 24 males and 24 females in each group. Total = 384 subjects.

TABLE 11-3A. Diadochokinetic Rates in Various Disorders: *Syllables per Second*

Diagnosis	Age	Sex	N	Phoneme	Mean (S.D.)	Reference
Functional artic	5 yr	M/F	12	/p/	3.94 .	a
				/t/	3.76 .	a
				/k/	3.50 .	a
	6 yr	M/F	10	/p/	4.34	a
				/t/	4.02*	a
				/k/	3.64*	a
	7–9 yr	M/F	8	/p/	3.86*	a
				/t/	3.81*	a
				/k/	3.48	a
"Lispers"	7.5–12 yr	M/F	21 + 24	/t/	5.3* (0.75)	b
				/d/	5.2* (0.79)	b
				/k/	4.6* (0.69)	b
				/g/	4.5* (0.62)	b
Cerebral palsy	4 yr 4 mo– 16 yr 2 mo (mean = 10 yr 6 mo)			/d/	2.33 (0.96)	c
Parkinsonism	56 yr 8 mo†	M	17	/b/	5.4 + (range: 0–7.4)	d
				/d/	4.8 + (range: 0–7.8)	d
				/g/	3.6 + (range: 0–7.6)	d
				/ha/	3.4 + (range: 0–5.6)	d
	55.8 yr (36–71 yr)	M/F	23	/p/	6.2 (1.01)	e
				/t/	6.1 (0.82)	e
				/k/	5.4 (0.88)	e

overdrive the system when a fairly large movement occurs.

Frequency response is another critical variable. Speech structures can move at velocities of several tens of centimeters per second, and acceleration can exceed 500 cm/s/s. The measurement system's bandwidth must extend high enough to track such movements without distortion. At the other end of the scale, the frequency response obviously must extend down to 0 Hz (DC). (The deleterious effects of an inadequate frequency response are illustrated for detection of air pressure changes in Figure 7-13 of Chap. 7. The same considerations discussed there apply in the present

TABLE 11-3B. Time required for a Given Number of Syllables (Time by Count): Means and Standard Deviations

/p/ (20)	/t/ (20)	/k/ (20)	/pʌtʌ/ (15)	/pʌtʌkʌ/ (10)	Source
Moderately severely hearing impaired (M/F, N = 7, mean age = 16.9 years (S.D. = 1.46)					
4.41 (0.85)	4.67 (1.03)	4.78 (0.87)	8.34 (1.91)	9.92 (2.59)	f
Severely hearing impaired (M/F, N = 13, mean age = 17.82 years (S.D. = 0.66)					
4.67 (0.98)	5.11 (1.26)	5.71 (1.45)	9.19 (2.04)	10.45 (4.29)	f
Profoundly hearing impaired (M/F, N = 10, mean age = 17.54 years (S.D. = 0.97)					
6.61 (2.30)	7.24 (2.41)	7.97 (2.73)	11.53 (3.52)	11.96 (3.80)	f

a. Yoss and Darley, 1974. Subjects had normal hearing, IQ > 90, language development no more than 6 months below CA, no apparent organic etiology.

b. Dworkin, 1978. Scores reported in article are number of repetitions per 3 s, converted for this table to repetitions per second.

c. Hixon and Hardy, 1964. Includes 25 spastic quadriplegics and 25 athetoid paraplegics, range of involvement from mild to severe. Data converted from reported number of repetitions per 10 s. Score is mean of three trials of each task.

d. Canter, 1965. No surgery or drugs within 48 hours of testing. "Measures of articulatory diadochokineses were correlated with clarity of articulation" (p. 223).

e. Kreul, 1972. Surgical patients. Three trials per task, 2 s sample.

f. Robb, Hughes, and Frese, 1985. Prelingual high-school students at a state school for the deaf.

*Significantly lower than normals tested in same study.

†Median.

case.) The system must also be appropriately damped. This means that it must be able to follow rapid changes in signal level with minimal overshoot (in terms of voltage in the electronic elements, or pen position on a chart recorder). As shown in Figure 11-9, overdamped systems are sluggish in their response to sudden change; underdamped systems oscillate or "ring." More complete consideration of mechanical and electrical criteria for measurement of physical events is provided by Abbs and Watkin (1976), Geddes and Baker (1968), and Cobbold (1974).

It should be obvious that the measurement system should not expose the patient to significant risk, nor should it cause any change in speech function. It should also be acceptable to the patient in a psychological sense.

In general, tracking movements of the tongue is more difficult than measuring lip or jaw motion. It is here that the theoretical ease of obtaining an adequate record meets the structural realities of the human body. The bases of the difficulty are apparent. First, the complex muscular arrangement of the tongue allows an almost infinite variety of movements. Second, tongue displacements can be very rapid. Stetson (1951) claimed to have observed tongue-tip trills at a rate of over 30 per second. Finally, the tongue acts in a very confined space, almost totally enclosed. Except for its most anterior portion, it is not directly observable, by eye or by instrument, from outside. Monitoring its behavior by inserting transducers into the vocal tract entails the very real possibility that articulatory behavior will be changed.

A

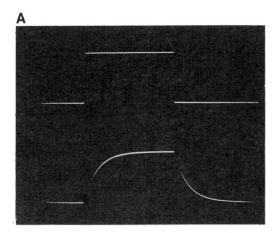

B

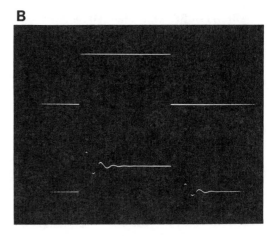

FIGURE 11-9. Effects of damping. (A) Response of an overdamped system to a square wave. The output (bottom) changes only slowly after a sudden change in the input (top). (B) Response of an underdamped system to the same square-wave input. The system response (bottom) is very fast, but unstable. There is considerable overshoot, and oscillation (called "ringing") occurs as the output settles down to a final value.

A great deal of ingenuity has gone into the search for better ways of observing the movements of the articulatory structures. Real progress has been made in the last 15 to 20 years. Only some of the instruments developed, however, have achieved widespread use among researchers, and almost none finds routine use in the clinic. It is the purpose of the brief review that follows to survey a few of the more practical approaches, those that hold promise for the rehabilitation specialist of tomorrow. Given this intent, radiographic techniques will be ignored, although they have been invaluable to researchers and to speech pathologists in special settings. Even though ways have been found to reduce radiation exposure dramatically (Kiritani, 1977; Umegaki, Tateno, and Iinuma, 1977; Fujimura, Kiritani, and Ishida, 1973; Kiritani, Tateno, Iinuma, and Sawashima, 1977; Kiritani, Itoh, and Fujimura, 1975), x-ray procedures are not likely to be routine in speech pathology.*

*It is not unlikely that new technology that can visualize internal structures without x-rays will provide much safer ways of obtaining the same information in the relatively near future. Nuclear magnetic resonance in particular seems to hold the best promise. It is clearly explained in Pykett (1982).

Macmillan and Kelemen (1952), Shelton, Brooks, Youngstrom, Diedrich, and Brooks (1963), Fletcher, Shelton, Smith, and Bosma (1960), Moll (1960, 1965), Kent (1972), and Perkell (1969) provide good summaries of various x-ray methods and their applicability to the evaluation of vocal tract movements.

Strain Gauge Systems

Strain gauges are an obvious choice for transducing structural movement. Several investigators have described strain-gauge systems for measuring lip and jaw motion. Almost all use a single basic configuration. Strain gauges are mounted on a flexible metal strip that is anchored at one end to a stable support (Figure 11-10A) to form a cantilever. Movement of the free end of the cantilever bends the metal strip, causing tension in the strain gauge mounted on the convex surface and compression of the one on the concave face (Figure 11-10B). Wiring the strain gauges together with two other resistors to form a Wheatstone bridge (see Chap. 2), as shown in Figure 11-10C, creates a very sensitive displacement detec-

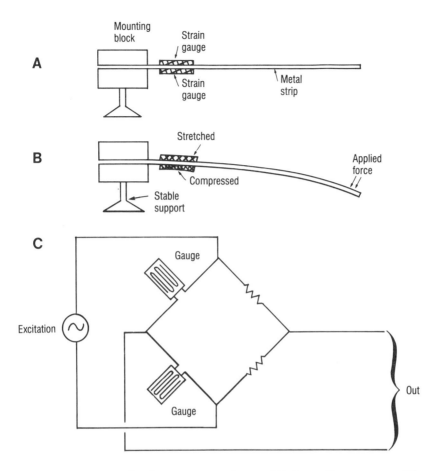

FIGURE 11-10. Strain gauge displacement transducers. (A) A cantilever system. (The gauges are shown proportionally much thicker than they would really be.) (B) Deformation of the upper and lower gauges by a force applied to the end of the cantilever. (C) Arrangement of the gauges in a Wheatstone bridge.

tor.* To track the movement of the lips or mandible, the free end of the cantilever is attached in some way to an appropriate place on the subject's face.

A number of factors must be taken into account in designing such a transducer. Most important among them is the *loading factor*, the force required to bend the metal strip, which acts as a spring. If too much force is needed the spring will cause the soft tissue to be deformed. The point at

which the transducer is attached will then not move in the same way as the rest of the surrounding structures, and an inaccurate measure will result. In extreme cases articulatory gestures may be distorted. Minimizing the loading factor is achieved by reducing the stiffness of the cantilever. The dynamic response of the transducer is also important. Accurate transduction requires that the cantilever's mechanical characteristics give it a resonant frequency well above the highest frequency components of the movement being measured. This objective is accomplished by minimizing the mass of the transducer system. Fortunately, strain gauges are inherently sensitive de-

*With different cantilever characteristics and a modified design strain gauges can also be used to evaluate the force of articulatory displacement. Such an evaluation may be useful in the assessment of motor impairments. See Barlow and Abbs (1983).

vices, and so obtaining adequate sensitivity requires no special design precautions. Also, using two gauges as shown assures a high degree of temperature stability.

Even with carefully designed transducers, some tissue deformation due to loading is bound to occur. The question is whether the problem is likely to be a serious one for the clinician. Kuehn, Reich, and Jordan (1980) found that strain-gauge measures of jaw displacement differed from X-ray determinations of mandibular movement by anywhere from 0.67 to 2.31 mm in the superior-inferior direction and from 0.52 to 1.28 mm in the anterior-posterior plane. Furthermore, the timing of the transducer signal was often slightly out of phase with mandibular movement. The error was not systematically related to the nature of the speech task and was apparently due to soft-tissue loading. The minimum discrepancies found by Kuehn et al. are probably acceptable in the clinical setting; the maximal errors may not be. The final judgment must be made in the context of the information required. It is probably wise, however, to pay close attention to relevant design factors when assembling a strain-gauge system. Abbs and Gilbert (1973) and Müller and Abbs (1979) provide excellent guidance in this regard.

Simple phosphor-bronze cantilevers can serve quite adequately, and have been used successfully by researchers (Sussman and Smith, 1970a,b, 1971; Sussman, MacNeilage, and Hanson, 1973). An engineering analysis by Müller and Abbs (1979) has resulted in an improved transducer that is no doubt the best available at this time. It is shown schematically in Figure 11-11. The basic cantilever (Figure 11-11A) is made of a thin (.005 inch thick) tapered piece of stainless steel on which the strain gauges are mounted. A relatively rigid stainless steel wire extends from its distal end and attaches to the subject, as discussed later in this section. The ridigity of the wire forces most of the bending to occur in the area where the gauges are placed. This arrangement creates an effective increase in length without adding significant mass and, at the same time, preserves sensitivity.

A single cantilever can only transduce motion in one plane—either vertical or horizontal. But lip and jaw movements are complex and certainly not restricted to a single direction. An ingenious modification of their transducer system allowed Abbs and his coworkers to track movements in two directions simultaneously. As shown in Figure 11-11B and C, they mounted the first flexible sheet to the end of another sheet at a 90° angle . Each cantilever can bend in only one direction (across its thickness), therefore each responds only in a single sensitive plane. The rod, however, is free to move in both planes. A pair of strain gauges on each of the segments monitors each of the directions separately.

The transducer system can be attached to the subject by adhesive-taping a small plate soldered to the end of the wire to the subject's face. But any side-to-side movement of the face can distort the output. An alternative attachment scheme (Müller and Abbs, 1979) minimizes this problem (Figure 11-11D). A small jewelry bead is cemented to a flexible plastic disc, which can be attached to the skin with double-surfaced adhesive tape. The wire is held in a hole drilled through the bead. The hole is somewhat larger than the wire's diameter so the wire can slide back and forth in case of side-to-side motion.

The Abbs strain gauge system has proven itself quite reliable in numerous studies (Abbs, 1973a,b; Abbs and Netsell, 1973; Folkins and Abbs, 1975, 1976; Hughes and Abbs, 1976; Abbs, Folkins, and Sivarajan, 1976; McClean, 1977). It is reasonably simple to assemble at very modest cost.

Obviously, any externally anchored measurement system imposes the requirement that the position of the transducer remain absolutely constant with respect to the head. Abbs and Stivers (1978) devised a special cephalostat (head holder) that fixes the head in one position, while the transducers are mounted on a separate stable support near the subject's face. A very sim-

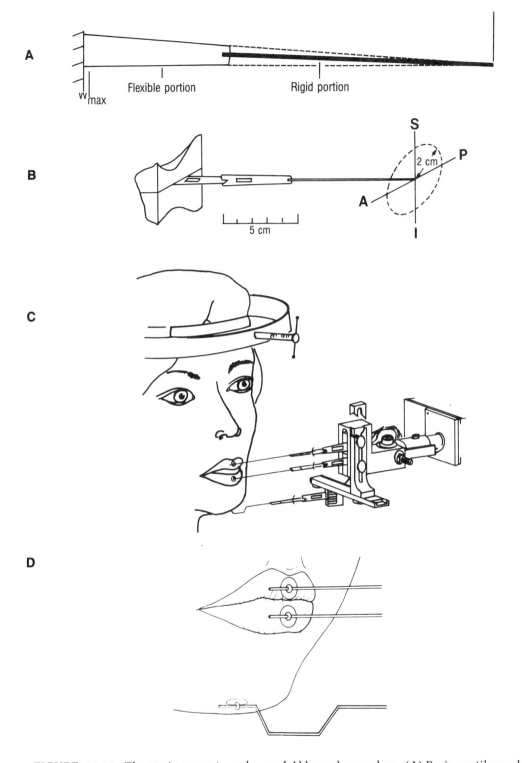

FIGURE 11-11. The strain gauge transducer of Abbs and coworkers. (A) Basic cantilever design. (B) Two dimensional transducer. (C) Mounting of the transducers for measurement. (D) Mylar disk/glass bead attachment technique. (From Müller, E. M. and Abbs, J. H. Strain gauge transduction of lip and jaw motion in the midsagittal plane: Refinement of a prototype system. *Journal of the Acoustical Society of America*, 65 (1979) 481-486. Figures 2 and 3, p. 483; Figures 5 and 6, p. 484. Reprinted by permission.)

ple system that is better suited to clinical purposes (especially with younger children) is the one described by Sussman and Smith (1970a,b) and by Hixon (1972) that is shown in Figure 11-12. A somewhat more elaborate head-mount that permits several transducers to be used on different facial regions has been designed of lightweight tubular aluminum (Barlow, Cole, and Abbs, 1983) and is available commercially. The transducers are clamped to a vertical rod that is suspended from an adjustable head band. In this way the relative position of the transducer is kept constant with respect to the face, while the patient is afforded some degree of mobility.

Capacitative transduction

The capacitance, C, of a pair of electrodes is $C = K(A/d)$, where A is the area of the electrodes facing each other, d is the distance between them, and K is the dielectric constant (a measure of insulating ability) of the medium separating them (see Chap. 2). In a given situation the area of the electrodes (assuming they do not slide past each other) and the dielectric constant are both unchanging. This being the case, $C \propto 1/d$—capacitance is inversely proportional to the distance separating the capacitor plates. If the plates are attached to body structures, it should be possible to transduce the distance between them by applying high.frequency signals and determining the inter-plate capacitance with appropriate circuitry.

In fact this principle has been applied to measurement of speech-organ movement. Mansell and Allen (1970), for instance, attached a small plate to one lip and mounted the other on a separate support a fixed-distance away. Intraoral capacitative techniques have been developed by Cole (1972) and by Hillix, Fry, and Hershman (1965). The latter's system employs a silicone-coated plate fixed to the palate. On the plate are two active elements of copper foil, one for the anterior, and the other for the posterior half of the palate. The capacitance between either of the palatal

plates and the tongue varies inversely with the distance between them. In theory it is, therefore, possible to achieve simultaneous measures of front and back tongue position. In practice, however, the output is very nonlinear, changing only slightly until the tongue-palate distance is less than 1/4 inch, after which the output change is very rapid.

The chief advantage of capacitative transduction is that the plates can be made very thin and loading of the structures being observed can be minimized. But this advantage is overridden by very serious limitations—the nonlinearity of the output, the inconvenience of being able to monitor only very small areas, and the near-impossibility of achieving a calibration in terms of absolute distances. For reasons involving fundamental electronic theory, several of the problems will likely prove very refractory. The availability of alternate transduction methods makes it unlikely that capacitative transduction will be intensively developed.

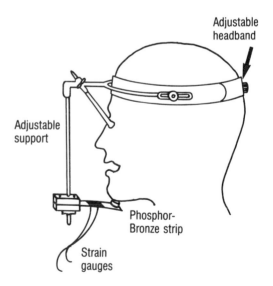

FIGURE 11-12. Head-band support for lip and jaw motion. (From Hixon, T. J. Some new techniques for measuring the biomechanical events of speech production: One laboratory's experiences. In *Orofacial Function: Clinical Research in Dentistry and Speech Pathology* (ASHA Reports, no. 7). Washington, D.C.: American Speech and Hearing Association, 1972. Pp. 68-103. Figure 7, p. 83. Reprinted by permission.)

Ultrasound

The term *ultrasound* refers to any sound signal above the frequency range of human hearing. Technically, ultrasound waves can range from 20 thousand to 20 million hertz (20 kHz - 20 MHz), but clinical ultrasound generally has a frequency above 1 MHz. An ultrasound signal can be passed into the body from a special transducer in contact with the body surface. The sound waves travel in a straight line, penetrating the structural layers as they go. For instance, the beam of ultrasound from a transducer applied to the neck just over the thyroid ala would pass through the skin, underlying fat, fascia, muscle, thyroid cartilage, and vocal folds, finally reaching the air space of the glottis. Each of the tissues has different acoustic transmissive properties: Some pass the ultrasound with relative ease, while others are comparatively poor ultrasound conductors. It is a general principle of the physics of sound that part of a sound beam will be reflected at the interface between two substances of differing transmissive properties. Every time the beam crosses the border between different tissues, part of the sound energy is reflected back toward the source while the remainder of the beam continues on until the next interface, when another portion is reflected and the remainder continues. Air is an extremely poor conductor of ultrasound, so that when an airspace is encountered, almost all of the ultrasound energy is reflected, and the transmission of the beam is effectively ended. The ultrasound reflections are a series of echos that can be detected by the transducer on the body surface. The longer it takes for an echo to be received, the further from the transducer a reflecting interface between tissues must be. It is a simple matter, then, to determine how deep under the surface the various tissue layers are: We need only time the returning echoes. Since the anatomy of a body region is generally well known, it is a fairly simple matter to associate given echoes with the boundaries between specific structures. At the intensities used in clinical

work, ultrasound has no apparent injurious effects.

There are two major forms of ultrasound data display. In the *A-mode* a beam begins sweeping across an oscilloscope screen when the ultrasound is pulsed into the tissue. Echoes show as spikes along the scope's horizontal axis. The position of a spike along the horizontal line, therefore, corresponds to the distance of the reflecting interface from the body surface, while the height of the spike indicates the strength of the echo and the amount of acoustic-transmissive difference between the tissues being traversed. The A-mode display is one-dimensional, provides limited information, and is difficult to interpret. It is not, therefore, the preferred display format.

B- (or *brightness*) *mode* displays cause the line being drawn on the scope screen to vary in brightness according to the strength of the echoes. If the transducer rotates slightly as rapidly-repeated pulses are sent into the tissue, the echoes from an entire sector can be detected. When the many B-mode lines are drawn next to each other on the oscilloscope screen in a sequence that corresponds to the transducer position at the time each on was generated, a two-dimensional black and white "picture" of the tissues is built up. Since the entire scanning process can be repeated very rapidly, it is possible to produce many complete sector scans every second, and thereby produce a "motion picture" of activity within the body. Such images are becoming increasingly familiar to everyone, thanks to their widespread application in cardiology and especially in obstetrics, where they are used to evaluate the status of the fetus *in utero*.

Minifie, Kelsey, Zagzebski, and King (1971) used echo ultrasound to visualize the longitudinal contour of the dorsal surface of the tongue. An ultrasound transducer was moved along the anterior midline of the neck and underside of the jaw, from the level of the layrnx to the mental symphysis. Transverse contours were generated by moving the transducer under the jaw along the coronal axis. A complete scan required about 3 s, during which the patient had to maintain a stable articulatory position. While the results were clear and impressive only static positions could be visualized, and there was some discrepancy between the ultasound and simultaneous X-ray measures.

A different system has been devised by Schuette, Shawker, and Whitehouse (1978) and applied to observation of tongue structure and movement by Sonies and her coworkers (Morrish, Stone, Sonies, Kurtz, and Shawker, 1984; Shawker and Sonies, 1984; Shawker, Sonies, and Stone, 1984; Shawker, Sonies, Stone, and Baum, 1983; Sonies, 1982; Sonies, Baum, and Shawker, 1984; Sonies, Shawker, Hall, Gerber, and Leighton, 1981; Sonies, Stone, and Shawker, in press). The transducing crystal is scanned across the structures being observed by rotating it, rather than sliding it along the surface. The rotation is done by a motor, covers a moderately wide angle, and is repeated at least 30 times per second. The transducer scans are synchronized with a TV monitor on which the ultrasound echos are displayed after digital processing. Soft-tissue structures are delineated quite clearly (Figure 11.13). Mathematical methods for describing the configuration of the tongue are being developed (Stone, Sonies, Shawker, Weiss, and Nadel, 1983; Morrish, Stone, Sonies, Kurtz, and Shawker, 1984).

Beyond probing the larynx (discussed in Chap. 6), echo ultrasound has been used with moderate success to track position changes of the pharyngeal wall (Kelsey, Hixon, and Minifie, 1969; Hawkins and Swisher, 1978; Kelsey, Woodhouse, and Minifie 1969), in one case by using a 20-transducer array to visualize a significant length of the structure (Skolnick, Zagzebski, and Watkin, 1975).

Transmission ultrasound measures distance by determination of the time required for an ultrasound pulse to travel through a structure from a transmitter to a receiver. The technique, therefore, observes only the small area under the probe. This can be an advantage if the distance between two well-defined points is wanted. Watkin and Zagzebski (1973) used transmission ultrasound to determine the displacement of a point on the tongue using the instrument setup diagrammed in Figure 11-14. The transmitter was placed under the jaw, and a very small receiver was cemented to the tongue. The pulse-transit time in this arrangement is a direct correlate of the height of the receiver above the transmitter. However, there is a problem with this method. The ultrasound transmission path must not have any air spaces in it, or the pulse will be almost completely reflected. This means, of course, that the tongue-tip tracking is not likely to be feasible.

Ultrasound techniques are relatively new

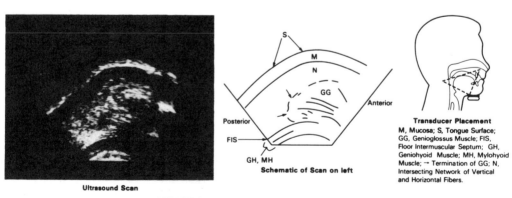

Ultrasound Scan

Schematic of Scan on left

GH, MH

Transducer Placement
M, Mucosa; S, Tongue Surface; GG, Genioglossus Muscle; FIS, Floor Intermuscular Septum; GH, Geniohyoid Muscle; MH, Mylohyoid Muscle; → Termination of GG; N, Intersecting Network of Vertical and Horizontal Fibers.

MIDLINE SAGITTAL SCAN OF MID-TONGUE.

FIGURE 11-13. Ultrasound visualization of the tongue in the sagittal plane. (Courtesy of Dr. B. Sonies.)

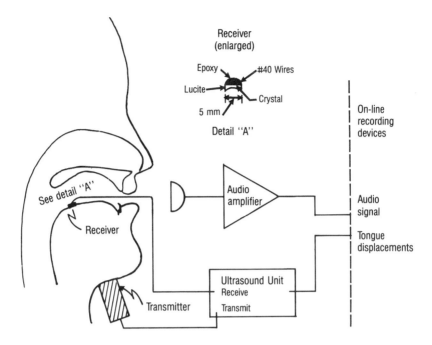

FIGURE 11-14. Transmission ultrasound monitoring of tongue motion. The ultrasound transmitter is in contact with the body surface just below the tongue mass, while the receiver is attached to the tongue's surface. (From Watkin, K. L. and Zagzebski, J. A. Cn-line ultrasonic technique for monitoring tongue displacements. *Journal of the Acoustical Society of America,* 54 (1973) 544-547. Figure 1, p. 544. Reprinted by permission.)

and are not fully developed by any means. A system optimized for vocal tract examination is not yet commercially available. But diagnostic ultrasound instruments are common in most hospitals. Speech pathologists may want to begin to take advantage of them.

Optical Transduction

Researchers in fields concerned with limb movement and locomotion have often attached small bright lamps to various body parts and tracked their trajectories using television or motion pictures. (Cavanagh, 1978; Grieve, Miller, Mitchelson, Paul, and Smith, 1975). The same basic principle, with sophisticated refinements that generate outputs showing the position of each light source, has been used by Sonoda and Wanishi (1982). Their instrument allows simultaneous tracking in real time of eight different points on the lips and jaw. The light sources are very small *light-emitting diodes* (LEDs) that serve as point sources of infrared illumination. The heart of the instrument is a special rectangular optoelectronic detector that produces small currents at its electrodes in response to a spot of light shining on it. The detector's characteristics inherently provide the means (with relatively simple electronics) for determining exactly where, in two dimensions, the spot shone on it.

For use, the LEDs are attached to the points of interest on the speaker's face, and the detector (with a lens system) is set up facing him, about 50 cm away. The outputs are analog voltages of the position of each of the LEDs that can be monitored on an oscilloscope or written by a pen recorder. Temporal resolution is 4 ms; spatial resolution is on the order of 0.05 to .01 mm.

Television is an obvious choice for monitoring the movement of any light source. When coupled to a video processor, it is possible to do an on-line analysis that determines the position of the light source in the camera's field. This method has been applied by McCutcheon, Fletcher, and Hasegawa (1977). Instead of an LED, they attached a small reflector (a 0.5 mm. glass bead) to the point on the lips or jaw to be tracked. When the face was brightly lit, the reflector acted as an effective light source. Digital circuits associated with the television system were able to detect the reflector with a spatial resolution of up to 0.3 mm and to track it at speeds up to 45 cm/s. The proliferation of computer technology and the associated reduction in the cost of digital equipment would tend to indicate that with further development, a system such as this one could be very prac-

tical and an attractive addition to the average speech clinic in the relatively near future.

Tongue motion has been transduced optically by a reflected-light detector devised by Chuang and Wang (1978). It takes advantage of the fact that the intensity of a reflected beam of light diminishes inversely with the length of the light's path. Small LED light sources and photosensitive detectors were arranged from front to back along the midline of an artificial palate, as shown in Figure 11-15. The light reaching each detector from its associated source is inversely proportional to the distance of the reflecting surface of the tongue from the artificial palate. Because of several characteristics in the physics of the situation (discussed in detail by the authors) the intensity to distance relationship is not linear, but the volt-

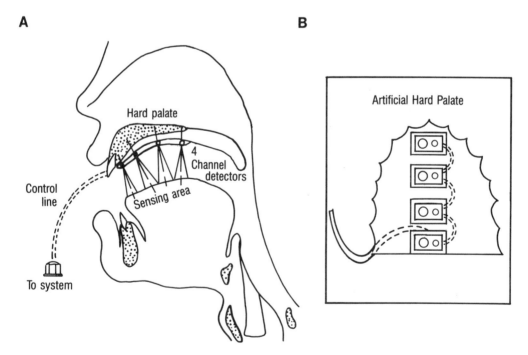

FIGURE 11-15. Optical scanning system for tongue motion. (A) Arrangement of the light sources and photodetectors on an artificial palate. (B) System in place. (From Chuang, C.-K. and Wang, S.-Y. Use of optical distance sensing to track tongue motion. *Journal of Speech and Hearing Research,* 21 (1978) 482-496. Figures 2 and 6, pp. 486 and 490. © American Speech-Language-Hearing Association, Rockville, MD. Reprinted by permission.)

age outputs can be linearized by means that are not very elaborate, assuming that extreme precision is not necessary.

Electromagnetic Transduction

The magnetometer system originally developed for monitoring chest wall activity (see the section on "Chest Wall Movement" in this chapter) can be used to track jaw and tongue movement as well. Hixon (1971a,b; 1972) used a single generator coil, driven at 1530 Hz, and two sensor coils, positioned as shown in Figure 11-16. The voltage induced in either of the sensors is inversely proportional to the cube of its distance from the generator. Therefore, as the mandible moves, the distance of the generator coil from one or both of the sensors changes, and the sensors' outputs var accordingly. The arrangement shown tracks mandibular movement in two directions—vertical and horizontal. Hixon (1972) also suggested that tongue motion might be tracked by placing a sensor coil on the surface of the tongue to transduce its distance from a generator under the jaw. A system very similar to this was, in fact, tried by Perkell and Oka (1980). They obtained useful data, but reported that several technical problems remained to be worked out.

The cubic nature of the magnetometer's voltage transfer function means that the voltage analog produced is a nonlinear function of distance. The nonlinearity grows less significant as the change in distance becomes a smaller proportion of the total separation of the coils. The system is convenient in that it is easily set up and requires no head restraint. It is also innocuous, entailing no meaningful risk. Despite the nonlinearity of its output, it provides an excellent display of relative motion.

An interesting variation of the magnetometer method has been devised by van der Giet (1977). It requires two pairs of generator coils, each pair driven at a different frequency. The two coils in each pair are wired to produce magnetic fields of equal intensity but opposite polarity. The coils are not located on the speaker's head, but on supports nearby. Their arrangement in space produces two sets of graded electromagnetic fields. Because of the polarity opposition of the members of each pair, the overlapping fields they generate sum to a

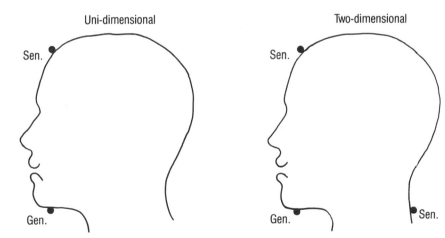

FIGURE 11-16. Placement of magnetometers to track vertical (left) and vertical and horizontal (right) motions of the mandible. (From Hixon, T. J. Some new techniques for measuring the biomechanical events of speech production: One laboratory's experiences. In *Orofacial Function: Clinical Research in Dentistry and Speech Pathology* (ASHA Reports, no. 7). Washington, D.C.: American Speech and Hearing Association, 1972. Pp. 68-103. Figure 10, p. 87. Reprinted by permission.)

single field that has maximal strength near one coil, diminishes to zero strength midway between the two coils, and then has maximal strength with opposite polarity near the other coil. If the speaker is placed within the two sets of electromagnetic fields, a sensing coil placed anywhere on the head will have a voltage induced whose amplitude, frequency, and phase characteristics indicate exactly where in the active field it lies. Clearly, significant computation is required to ascertain a sensing coil's absolute location in space, but this is handled by a computer. The increased complexity of this system is the price paid for a very important benefit: Almost any number of sensing coils can be used simultaneously, making it possible to track many separate points moving in different planes during single speech act. While not yet ready for everyday clinical application, further developmentof this technique may produce a convenient tool for the speech pathologist.

CHEST-WALL MOVEMENT

The *chest-wall* is defined by the physiologist to include the rib cage, diaphragm, abdominal contents, and anterior abdominal wall. Its movements store a volume of air for speech and pressurize it to an appropriate level. All of the acoustic energy radiated in the speech signal derives from that pressurization. The ventilatory system is the power generator for speech, and the chest wall is the motor which drives that generator.

A general review of the structure and function of the chest wall will not be attempted here. Good basic summaries have been prepared by Minifie, Hixon, and Williams (1973); Daniloff, Schuckers, and Feth (1980), and Zemlin (1981). More advanced consideration of breathing for speech is available in Bouhuys, (1968) and Wyke (1974). A number of points do need to be emphasized, however, because failure to keep them in mind has often led to signifi-

cant confusion and erroneous impressions of the quality of chest-wall function during speech production.

Most important, perhaps, is the fact that the chest wall is a two-part system, with (in the physiologist's phrase) two *degrees of freedom* of movement (Konno and Mead, 1967). One part is the rib cage, which is the primary wall of the thorax itself. The other part includes the diaphragm, which forms the floor of the thorax and the roof of the abdomen. Each part is independently movable. The muscles of the rib cage act to enlarge or diminish the size of the thorax by increasing the anteroposterior and, to a lesser extent, the transverse diameter of the enclosed space (Agostoni, Mognoni, Torri, and Saracino, 1965; Konno and Mead, 1967). The diaphragm is dome-shaped. Its flattening on contraction results in an increase in the height of the thoracic space as well as elevation and spreading of the ribs. At the same time, flattening of the diaphgram also displaces the visceral structures that lie just under it. (Hence, the abdomen's contents are considered part of the chest wall.) The displaced visceral volume appears as a bulge of the anterior abdominal wall, the only resilient region of the abdominal enclosure. The bulge has the same volume as that added to the thorax by diaphragmatic movement. The diaphragm, like any other muscle, cannot return to its precontraction position by its own power; something else must push it back into its original shape. The restorative force is provided by the anterior abdominal muscles that have been protruded. Their contraction forces the viscera back against the diaphragm, thereby returning it to its original dome-shaped condition. This, of course, reduces the volume of the thorax again. Enlargement of the thorax results in a decrease of the pressure of the gas within it. If the airway is patent, outside air at the relatively higher atmospheric pressure will flow along the pressure gradient into the lungs. (Note that the lungs fill because the thorax enlarges. The thorax does not enlarge to accommodate the increasing size of the lungs.) Any action that enlarges the thoracic space can be said to be inspiratory, while any action that decreases thoracic size can be called expiratory. Thoracic volume can be increased by movement of the rib cage or by movement of the diaphragm (which shows as abdominal motion). Since the rib cage muscles and the diaphragm-abdominal muscles can function independently, it is clear that one set could be acting to enlarge the rib cage, while the other operates to diminish its size. The net change in the lung volume is the sum of the actions of the two chest wall components. If the rib cage is enlarging while the diaphragm contracts, then both parts are contributing to inspiration. But if the rib cage muscles cause a decrease in its size while the diaphragm is contracting, the net flow of air will be inspiratory if the diaphragmatic displacement causes a greater volume change than the rib cage muscles do, or expiratory if the rib cage contraction makes a greater contribution to the thoracic volume change than the diaphragm does. The point here is that *there is no way of knowing whether inspiration or expiration is in progress by watching only the rib cage or the abdomen*. Both parts must be observed, and their relative contribution to thoracic volume change must be known before any observation of ventilatory movement can inform the observer about which ventilatory phase is in progress.

Movements of the chest-wall system are frequently very small, but even small changes can have a meaningful effect on the lung volume or the lung pressure. Furthermore, these small changes occur in a very massive structure, one which is very difficult to see all at once in its entirety. Worse, the movements can be very rapid, on the order of 100 ms or so (Baken, Cavallo, and Weissman, 1979; Baken and Cavallo, 1981), making assessment by simple visual observation still more difficult, and less reliable. Hence, there is a need for monitoring instrumentation that can accurately show what the system is doing in a way that can be easily followed by the observer.

Bellows Pneumograph

For many years the prime means of monitoring chest wall motion was a pneumatic device called the bellows pneumograph (Figure 11-17). Essentially an accordion-pleated tube, it is strapped around the rib cage and abdomen. As chest wall enlargement occurs, the bellows becomes longer, and hence the volume of the air space within it increases. This causes the pressure in the bellows to drop. A rubber hose attached to the pneumograph couples the change in its air pressure to a pressure transducer (see, for example, Isshiki and Snidecor, 1965 or Snidecor and Isshiki, 1965) or to a pneumatic linkage system that drives a pen producing a chart record of ventilatory motion.

This system is still used in *polygraphs* (*lie detectors*). While it may be adequate for that purpose, it does not meet the transduction needs of the speech pathologist. Often, no electrical output is provided, hence recording the breathing data or displaying them along with other variables is difficult. More important is the very poor frequency response of this kind of system and the significant loading of the chest wall that it might represent. While electronic secondary transducers have been incorporated into bellows pneumographs (thus solving some display and data-storage problems), the other limitations are inherent in the physics of the system and are largely irreducible. The bellows pneumograph, then, is not the transducer of choice.

Magnetometers

The coupling between the two coils of a transformer is inversely proportional to the cube of the distance separating them if the axes of the coils are parallel. Therefore, if an AC signal is applied to one coil the voltage induced in the other (see Chap. 2) will vary as a function of the distance between them. The electromagnetic field created by current flow in a coil easily penetrates nonmetallic materials. Therefore, if a signal-carrying coil is attached to the body wall,

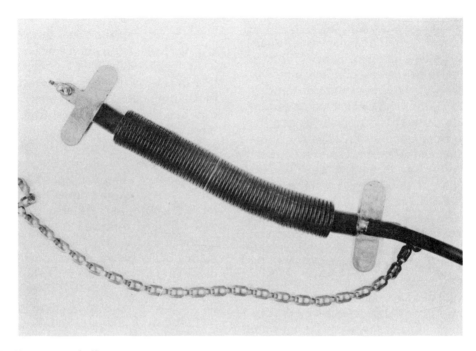

FIGURE 11-17. A bellows pneumograph. As the device is stretched its volume increases and the pressure of the air within it drops. The pressure change can be sensed by a transducer or can be used to drive a pen directly.

a voltage will be induced in another coil on the other side of the body. The magnitude of the induced voltage will be inversely related to the distance straight through the body that separates them.

This principle was exploited by Mead, Peterson, Grimby, and Mead (1967), whose measurement system is schematized in Figure 11-18. For each part of the chest wall a pair of identical coils is used. One coil of each pair (the generator) is driven by an oscillator and produces an alternating electromagnetic field. The body offers negligible resistance to the passage of the electromagnetic radiation, which induces an alternating voltage in the other coil (the sensor). That voltage diminishes proportional to the cube of the body diameter, but, if the change in distance between the coils is small compared to the total distance (which is indeed generally the case with breathing motions), the voltage change closely approximates linearity. The distance measurement can, therefore, be quite accurate

(Bancroft, 1978). Two pairs of coils can be used, one for each chest-wall component, if the two generators are driven at different, and nonharmonic, frequencies. While each sensor will pick up both generator signals, filtering in the detection circuit (see Chap. 2) will pass only one frequency for each sensor. This system has been used extensively in research on the ventilatory mechanics of speech by Hixon (1972), Hixon, Goldman, and Mead (1973), Hixon, Mead, and Goldman (1976), and Forner and Hixon (1977). The magnetometer system is very simple to use and can provide a clean stable output if the coils are firmly attached to the body wall. The electromagnetic radiation is harmless and poses no significant risk to most patients (Rolfe [1971] describes its successful application as an apnea monitor for premature infants). However, one should probably avoid using it with those having cardiac pacemakers or other electronic implants. Magnetometers and their associated circuitry are com-

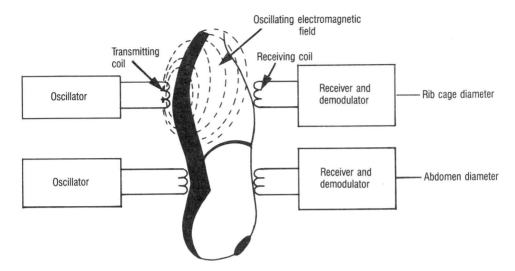

FIGURE 11-18. Magnetometry for detecting chest wall movements. Two pairs of coils are used. One pair for the rib cage and the other for the abdomen. One coil in each pair is a "transmitter" that generates an oscillating electromagnetic field that passes through the body. The other coil serves as a "receiver" that transduces the magnetic energy to an electrical signal. The strength of the magnetic field diminishes in a regular way with distance, so changes in the distance between the two coils results in changes in the strength of the detected signal.

mercially available from Lexington Instruments, Waltham, MA.

Impedance Plethysmography

Body parts offer resistance to the flow of electrical current. The magnitude of that resistance depends on the geometry of the structure and its tissue composition. It is easy to see that, as it expands and contracts, the resistance of the thorax is likely to alter significantly. The changes reflect not only a change in rib cage shape, but variation in composition caused by the addition and loss of intrathoracic air. When an electrical current is passed through the thorax, its resistance (which can be measured by any of a number of standard techniques) does indeed change across the breathing cycle. (The theoretical bases of this phenomenon are considered in some detail by Pacela, 1966 and Allison, 1970.) Researchers have used this method primarily in an attempt to find a way of monitoring lung volume without invasion or incumbrance of the airway (Goldensohn and Zablow, 1959; Geddes, Hoff, Hickman Hinds, and Baker, 1962; Geddes, Hoff, Hickman, and Moore, 1962; Allison, Holmes, and Nyboer, 1964; Kubicek, Kinnen, and Edin, 1964; Geddes and Baker, 1968; Khalafalla, 1970).

There are a great many problems with impedance plethysmography. The relationship between the resistance and actual dimensional change is unknown, for instance. Even more important, from a practical point of view, is the fact that the subject must be part of a live electrical circuit. The risks, with properly designed equipment, are not major. But they are unnecessary: better means of monitoring are available.

Mercury Strain Gauges

Whitney 1949 constructed an elastic strain gauge by filling the narrow bore of a rubber tube with mercury. As the tube is stretched, the increase in the length of the mercury column and the decrease in its cross-sectional area cause a moderately large change in its electrcial resistance. At relatively low AC frequencies, it behaves as an essentially pure resistance, without significant reactance. Therefore, its resistance is easily determined by making it one arm of a Wheatstone bridge (see Chap. 2). The gauge (shown in Figure 11-19A) is thin, lightweight, very flexible, non-loading, and inexpensive.

Movements of the chest wall can be recorded by taping mercury strain gauges across the anterior hemicircumference of the rib cage and abdomen (Baken, 1977), as shown in Figure 11-19B. The gauges can be used with very simple circuitry. Normally all that is required is an oscillator of some sort and a resistance bridge with an amplifier at its output (Baken and Matz, 1973). If, for any reason, extreme sensitivity is required, a special impedance-matching bridge can be used (Elsner, Eagan, and Andersen, 1959). Frequency response is more than adequate for tracking the move-

ments of speech and resolution of a fraction of a millimeter is easily achieved. This means of measuring chest-wall behavior is attractive because it is unencumbering and essentially free of risk. It is easy to use: The strain gauges can be attached with ordinary adhesive tape. A mercury strain gauge system can be inexpensively built by almost any technician using gauges available from Parks Electronics Laboratories, Beaverton, OR.

Variable Inductance Plethysmography

The *respiratory inductive plethysmograph* (available commercially as the "Respitrace" from Ambulatory Monitoring, Inc., Ardsley, NY) uses a rather unusual transduction principle. The inductance of a coil of wire depends on a number of factors, one of which is its diameter. If a wire is

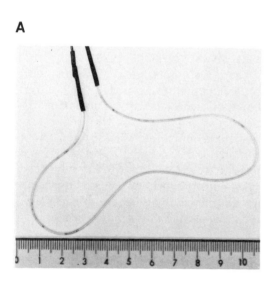

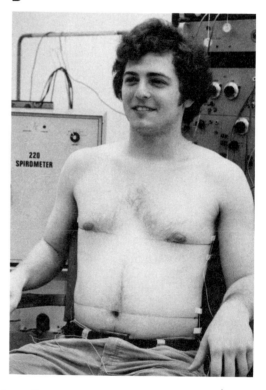

FIGURE 11-19. Whitney gauge transduction of body wall motion. (A) A Whitney gauge is a thin elastic tube filled with mercury. (B) Transducers in place for evaluating rib cage and abdominal movement.

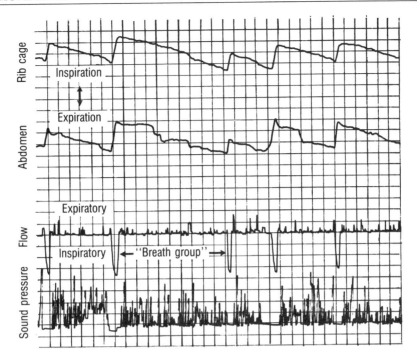

FIGURE 11-20. Record of normal ventilatory movements during reading. From top to bottom the traces are: rib cage hemicircumference, abdominal hemicircumference, airflow, and sound pressure.

wrapped around the torso, the inductance of the single-turn coil it forms will change according to the circumference of the loop. If this single coil can be made stretchable, so that it can change size with body movement, then its inductance will always be an analog of instantaneous torso size.

It is easy to put this inductance change to practical use. There are many oscillator circuits in which the frequency of oscillation is determined by the value of an inductor. If the inductor is the loop around the chest wall, then the frequency of oscillation will be an analog of chest-wall circumference. Put another way, the size of that part of the chest wall within the wire loop is automatically encoded in a frequency-modulated signal. Standard frequency demodulation techniques can be used to retrieve a DC voltage that represents chest-wall size (Sackner, Nixon, Davis, Atkins, and Sackner, 1980; Cohn, Watson, Weisshaut, Stott, and Sackner, 1975; Watson, 1979; Sackner, 1980).

In the Respitrace the inductive transducer is a zig-zag of wire attached to an elastic

band. This is fitted around the rib cage or abdomen, forming the wire into an expandable loop. (The transducers can be stabilized on the subject by an overfitting elastic-mesh vest.) The loop is connected to a minature oscillator that is also carried on the subject. The output of the oscillator is connected by a cable to the demodulating circuitry that produces a voltage output representing the size (cross-sectional area) of the body enclosed by the transducing loop. In practice, of course, two transducers are used, one for the rib cage and the other for the abdomen.

Expected Results

Figure 11-20 illustrates a record of chest-wall behavior during reading by a normal male. Mercury strain gauge transducers were positioned as shown in Figure 11-19. The speech signal was transduced by a probe microphone on the upper lip. In addition, airflow was recorded by a face mask and pneumotachograph system (see Chap. 8). The airflow data are helpful in interpreting the chest-wall movement record.

The specific details of normal chest-wall movement patterns will naturally vary according to the nature of the speech task. Figure 11-20, however, is typical in its essential characteristics. Inspirations are rapid and are accomplished by cooperative inspiratory motions of both the rib cage and abdomen. While the rib cage and abdomen also contribute together to the expirations of speech, note that they do not move in the same way. Abdominal motions are less "smooth" than rib cage movements, because the abdominal system is used to adjust pressure and meet the requirements of word stress and the like. Careful inspection of the chest-wall traces will show that the rib cage and abdomen do not begin expiratory movements simultaneously. This so-called *asynchrony* is normal and may be related to the way in which the chest wall is adjusted for speech (Baken, Cavallo, and Weissman, 1979; Baken and Cavallo, 1981). Typically, the abdomen begins contraction about 100 ms before the rib cage does, and the pattern is seen in very young children and singers, as well as in untrained adult speakers (Wilder and Baken, 1974; Gould and Okamura, 1974). ∎

SELECT BIBLIOGRAPHY

Abbs, J. H. The influence of the gamma motor system on jaw movement during speech. *Journal of Speech and Hearing Research*, 16 (1973a) 175-200.

Abbs, J. H. Some mechanical properties of lower lip movement during speech. *Phonetica*, 28 (1973b) 65-75.

Abbs, J. H. and Eilenberg, G. R. Peripheral mechanisms of speech motor control. In Lass, N. J. (Ed.), *Contemporary Issues in Experimental Phonetics*. New York: Academic Press, 1976. Pp. 139-168.

Abbs, J. H., Folkins, J. W., and Sivarajan, M. Motor impairment following blockage of the infraorbital nerve. *Journal of Speech and Hearing Research*, 19 (1976) 19-35.

Abbs, J. H. and Gilbert, B. N. A strain gage transduction system for lip and jaw motion in two dimensions: Design criteria and calibration data. *Journal of Speech and Hearing Research*, 16 (1973) 248-256.

Abbs, J. H. and Kennedy, J. G. III. Neurophysiological processes of speech movement control. In Lass, N. J., McReynolds, L. V., Northern, J. L., and Yoder, D. E. (Eds.), *Speech, Language, and Hearing, Vol. I: Normal Processes*. Philadelphia: Saunders, 1982. Pp. 84-108.

Abbs, J. H. and Netsell, R. W. An interpretation of jaw acceleration during speech. *Journal of Speech and Hearing Research*, 16 (1973) 421-425.

Abbs, J. H. and Stivers, D. A new cephalostat for speech physiology research. *Journal of the Acoustical Society of America*, 64 (1978) 1174-1175.

Abbs, J. H. and Watkin, K. L. Instrumentation for the study of speech physiology. In Lass, N. J. (Ed.), *Contemporary Issues in Experimental Phonetics*. New York: Academic Press, 1976. Pp. 41-75.

Abercrombie, D. Direct palatography. *Zeitschrift für Phonetik*, 10 (1957) 21-25.

Adrian, E. D. and Bronk, D. W. The discharge of the impulses in motor nerve fibers. II. The frequency of discharge in reflex and voluntary contractions. *Journal of Physiology*, 67 (1929) 119-151.

Agostoni, E., Mognoni, R., Torri, G., and Saracino, F. Relation between changes of rib cage circumference and lung volume. *Journal of Applied Physiology*, 20 (1965) 1179-1186.

Akazawa, K. and Fujii, K. Physical properties of muscular tissue: Determination of firing rate, number, and size of motor units. In Stevens, K. N. and Hirano, M. (Eds.), *Vocal Fold Physiology*. Tokyo: University of Tokyo Press, 1981. Pp. 61. 81.

Albright, R. W. The motor abilities of speakers with good and poor articulation. *Speech Monographs*, 15 (1948) 164-172.

Allen, G. D. On counting to twenty: An aid to measuring diadochokinetic syllable rate. *Journal of Speech and Hearing Disorders*, 39 (1974) 110-111.

Allen, G. D., Lubker, J. F., and Harrison, E., Jr. New paint-on electrodes for surface electromyography. *Journal of the Acoustical Society of America*, 52 (1972) 124.

Allen, G. D., Lubker, J. F., and Turner, D. T. Adhesion to mucous membrane for electromyography. *Journal of Dental Research*, 52 (1973), 391.

Allison, R. D. Bioelectric impedance measurements—introduction to basic factors in impedance plethysmography. In Allison, R. D. (Ed.), *Basic Factors in Bioelectric Impedance Measurements*. Pittsburgh: Instrument Society of America, 1970. Pp. 1-70.

Allison, R. D., Holmes, E. L., and Nyboer, J. Volumetric dynamics of respiration as measured by electrical impedance plethysmography.

Journal of Applied Physiology, 19 (1964) 166-172.

Baken, R. J. Estimation of lung volume change from torso hemicircumferences. *Journal of Speech and Hearing Research*, 20 (1977) 808-812.

Baken, R. J. and Cavallo, S. A. Prephonatory chest wall posturing. *Folia Phoniatrica*, 33 (1981) 193-203.

Baken, R. J., Cavallo, S. A., and Weissman, K. L. Chest wall movements prior to phonation. *Journal of Speech and Hearing Research*, 22 (1979) 862-872.

Baken, R. J. and Matz, B. J. A portable impedance pneumograph. *Human Communication*, 2 (1973) 28-35.

Bancroft, J. C. A quantitative evaluation of magnetometers with lung volume estimates. Paper presented at the annual convention of the American Speech and Hearing Association, 1978.

Barlow, S. M. and Abbs, J. H. Force transducers for the evaluation of labial, lingual, and mandibular motor impairments. *Journal of Speech and Hearing Research*, 26 (1983) 616-621.

Barlow, S. M., Cole, K. J., and Abbs, J. H. A new head-mounted lip-jaw movement transduction system for the study of motor speech disorders. *Journal of Speech and Hearing Research*, (1983) 283-288.

Basmajian, J. V. *Muscles Alive*. Baltimore: Williams and Wilkins, 1974.

Basmajian, J. V. and Dutta, C. R. Electromyography of the pharyngeal constrictors and levator palati in man. *Anatomical Record*, 139 (1961) 561-563.

Basmajian, J. V. and Stecko, G. A new bipolar electrode for electromyography. *Journal of Applied Physiology*, 17 (1962) 849.

Bigland, B. and Lippold, 0. C. J. The relation between force velocity and integrated electrical activity in human muscles. *Journal of Physiology*, 123 (1954) 214-224

Blomquist, B. L. Diadochokinetic movements of nine-, ten-, and eleven-year-old children. *Journal of Speech and hearing Disorders*, 15 (1950) 159-164.

Bloomer, H. A palatograph for contour mapping of the palate. *Journal of the American Dental Association*, 30 (1943) 1053-1057.

Bole, C. T. II and Lessler, M. A. Electromyography of the genioglossus muscles in man. *Journal of Applied Physiology*, 21 (1966) 1695-1698.

Bouhuys, A. (Ed.) *Sound Production in Man (Annals of the New York Academy of Sciences*, vol. 155) New York: New York Academy of Sciences, 1968.

Buchthal, F. and Faaborg-Andersen, K. Electromyography of laryngeal and respiratory muscles: Correlation with phonation and respiration. *Annals of Otology, Rhinology, and Laryngology*, 73 (1964) 118-123.

Buchthal, F. and Schmalbruch, H. Motor units of mammalian muscles. *Physiological Review* 60 (1980) 90-142.

Butcher, A. and Weiher, E. An electropalatographic investigation of coarticulation in VCV sequences. *Journal of Phonetics*, 4 (1976) 59-74.

Canter, G. J. Speech characteristics of patients with Parkinson's disease: III. Articulation, diadochokinesis, and overall speech adequacy. *Journal of Speech and Hearing Disorders*, 30 (1965) 217-224.

Cavanagh, P. R. Instrumentation and methodology of applied and pure research in biomechanics. In Landry, F. and Orbin, W. A. R. (Eds.) *Biomechanics of Sports and Kinanthropology*. Miami: Symposia Specialists, 1978.

Chuang, C..K. and Wang, W. S.-Y. Use of optical distance sensing to track tongue motion. *Journal of Speech and Hearing Research*, 21 (1978) 482-496.

Cobbo1d, R. S. C. *Transducers for Biomedical measurements: Principles and Applications*. New York: Wiley, 1974.

Cohn, M. A., Watson, H Weisshaut R., Stott, F. and Sackner, M. A. A transducer for non-invasive monitoring of respiration. In Stott, F. D., Rafferty, E. B., Sleigh, P., and Gouldring, L. (Eds.) *Proceedings of the Second International Symposium on Ambulatory Monitoring*. New York: Academic Press, 1975. Pp. 119-128.

Cole, K. J., Konopacki, R. A., and Abbs, J. H. A miniature electrode for surface electromyography during speech. *Journal of the Acoustical Society of America*, 74 (1983) 1362-1366.

Cole, R. M. Electrical capacitance measures of oropharyngeal functions. In Bzoch, K. R. (Ed.), *Communicative Disorders Related to Cleft Lip and Palate*. Boston: Little, Brown, 1972. Pp. 172-177.

Cooper, F. S. Research techniques and instrumentation. *ASHA Reports* 1 (1965) 153-168.

Daniel, B. and Guitar, B. EMG feedback and recovery of facial and speech gestures following neural anastomosis. *Journal of Speech and Hearing Disorders*, 43 (1978) 9-20.

Daniloff, R., Schuckers, G., nd Feth, L. *The Physiology of Speech and Hearing*. Englewood Cliffs, N. J.: Prentice-Hall, 1980.

Dedo, H. H. and Hall, W. N. Electrodes in laryngeal electromyography: Reliability comparison. *Annals of Otorhinolaryngology*, 78 (1969) 172-179.

Denny-Brown, D. Interpretation of the electromyogram. *Archives of Neurology and Psychiatry*, 61 (1949) 99-128.

Doyle, F. J. and Allon, R. The preservation of amplitude information in burst phenomena in physiological recordings. *Behavior Research Methods and Instrumentation*, 12 (1980) 51-54.

Draper, M. H., Ladefoged, P., and Whitteridge, D. Respiratory muscles in speech. *Journal of Speech and Hearing Research*, 2 (1959) 16-27.

Draper, M. H., Ladefoged, P., and Whitteridge, D. Expiratory pressures and air flow during speech. *British Medical Journal*, 18 (1960) 1837-1843.

Dworkin, J. P. Protrusive lingual force and lingual diadochokinetic rates: A comparative analysis between normal and lisping speakers. *Language, Speech. and Hearing Services in Schools*, 9 (1978) 8-16.

Elsner, R. W., Eagan, C. J., and Andersen, S. Impedance matching circuit for the mercury strain gauge. *Journal of Applied Physiology*, 14 (1959) 871-872.

English, D. T. and Blevins, C. E. Motor units of laryngeal muscles. *Archives of Otolaryngology*, 89 (1969) 778-784.

Evans, M. Efficiency is the goal in cerebral palsied speech. *Crippled Child*, 29 (1952) 19-21.

Faaborg-Andersen, K. Electromyographic investigation of intrinsic laryngeal muscles in humans. *Acta Physiologica Scandinavica*, 41 Suppl. 140 (1957) 1-147.

Faaborg-Andersen, K. Electromyography of laryngeal muscles in human: Technics and results. *Current Problems in Phoniatrics and Logopedics*, 3 (1965) 1-72.

Fairbanks, G. and Spriestersbach, D. C. A study of minor organic deviations in "functional" disorders of articulation: 1. Rate of movement of oral structures. *Journal of Speech and Hearing Disorders*, 15 (1950) 60-69.

Fink, B. R., Basek, M., and Epanchin, V. The mechanism of opening of the human larynx. *Laryngoscope*, 66 (1956) 410-425.

Fletcher, S. G. Time-by-count measurement of diadochokinetic syllable rate. *Journal of Speech and Hearing Research*, 15 (1972) 763-770.

Fletcher, S. G. and Hasegawa, A. Speech modification by a deaf child through dynamic orometric modeling and feedback. *Journal of Speech and Hearing Disorders*, 48 (1983) 178-185.

Fletcher, S. G., McCutcheon, M. J., and Wolf, M. B. Dynamic palatometry. *Journal of Speech and Hearing Research*, 18 (1975) 812-819.

Fletcher, S. G., Shelton, R. L. Jr., Smith, C. C., and Bosma, J. F. Radiography in speech pathology. *Journal of Speech and Hearing Disorders*, 25 (1960) 135-144.

Folkins, J. W. and Abbs, J. H. Lip and jaw motor control during speech: Responses to resistive loading of the jaw. *Journal of Speech and Hearing Research*, 18 (1975) 207-2.

Folkins, J. W. and Abbs, J. H. Additional observations on responses to resistive loading of the jaw. *Journal of Speech and Hearing Research*, 19 (1976) 820-821.

Forner, L. L. and Hixon, T. J. Respiratory kinematics in profoundly hearing-impaired speakers. *Journal of Speech and Hearing Research*, 20 (1977) 373-408.

Fromkin, V. and Ladefoged, P. Electromyography in speech research. *Phonetica*, 15 (1966) 219-242.

Fujii, I. Phoneme identification with dynamic palatography. *Annual Bulletin of the Research Institute of Logopedics and Phoniatrics*, 3 (1970) 67-68.

Fujii, I., Fujimura, 0., and Kagaya, R. Dynamic palatography by use of a computer and an oscilloscope. *Proceedings of the Seventh International Congress on Acoustics*, 1971, 113-116.

Fujimura 0. Kiritani, S., and Ishida, H. Computer controlled radiography for observation of movements of articulatory and other human organs. *Computers in Biology and Medicine*, 3 (1973) 371-384.

Fujimura, O., Shibata, S., Kiritani, S., Simada, Z., and Satta, C. A study of dynamic palatography. *Proceedings of the Sixth International Congress on Acoustics*, 1968, 21-24.

Fujimura, 0., Tatsumi, I. F., and Kagaya, R. Computational processing of palatographic patterns. *Journal of Phonetics*, 1 (1973) 47-54.

Gay, T. and Harris, K. Some recent developments in the use of electromyography in speech research. *Journal of Speech and Hearing Research*, 14 (1971) 241-246.

Gay, T., Strome, M., Hirose, H., and Sawashima, M. Electromyography of the intrinsic laryngeal muscles during phonation. *Annals of Otology, Rhinology, and Laryngology*, 81 (1972) 401-409.

Gay, T., Ushijima, T., Hirose, H., and Cooper, F. S. Effect of speaking rate on labial consonant-vowel articulation. *Journal of Phonetics*, 2 (1974) 47-63.

Geddes, L. A. *Electrodes and the Measurement of Bioelectric Events*. New York: Wiley, 1972.

Geddes, L. A. and Baker, L. E. *Principles of Applied Biomedical Instrumentation*. New York: Wiley, 1968.

Geddes, L. A., Hoff, H. E., Hickman, D. M., Hinds, M., and Baker, L. Recording respiration and the electrocardiogram with common electrodes. *Aerospace Medicine*, 33 (1962) 891.

Geddes, L. A., Hoff, H. E., Hickman, D. M., and Moore, A. G. The impedance pneumograph. *Aerospace Medicine*, 33 (1962) 28-33.

Goldensohn, E. S. and Zablow, L. An electrical impedance spirometer. *Journal of Applied Physiology*, 14 (1959) 463-464.

Gould, W. J. and Okamura, H. Respiratory training of the singer. *Folia Phoniatrica*, 26 (1974) 275-286.

Grieve, D. W., Miller, D. I., Mitchelson, D., Paul, J. P., and Smith, A. J. *Techniques for the Analysis of Human Movement*. Princeton, NJ: Princeton Book Co., 1975.

Guitar, B. Reduction of stuttering frequency using analog electromyographic feedback. *Journal of Speech and Hearing Research*, 18 (1975) 672-685.

Gumpertz, F. Palatographische Untersuchungen an Stammlern mit Hilfe eines neuen künstlichen Gaumens. *Monatschriften Ohrenheilkeit*, 1931, 1095-1116.

Hamlet, S. L., Bunnell, H. T., and Struntz, B. Articulatory asymmetries. *Journal of the Acoustical Society of America*, 79 (1986) 1164-1169.

Hardcastle, W. Electropalatography in speech research. *University of Essex Language Centre Occasional papers*, 9 (1970) 54-64.

Hardcastle, W. J. The use of electropalatography in phonetic research. *Phonetica*, 25 (1972) 197-215.

Hardcastle, W. J. Instrumental investigations of lingual activity during speech: A survey. *Phonetica*, 29 (1974) 129-157.

Hardcastle, W. J. and Morgan, R. A. An instrumental investigation of articulation disorders in children. *British Journal of Disorders of Commuication*, 17 (1982) 47-65.

Harley, W. T. Dynamic palatography: A study of linguapalatal contacts during the production of selected consonant sounds. *Journal of Prosthetic Dentistry*, 27 (1972) 364-376.

Harris, K. S. Electromyography as a technique for laryngeal investigation. In Ludlow, C. L. and Hart, M. O. (Eds.). *Proceedings of the Conference on the Assessment of Vocal Pathology (ASHA Reports no. 11)*. Rockville, MD: American Speech-Language-Hearing Assn., 1981. Pp. 70-87.

Harris, K. S., Rosov, R., Cooper, F. S., and Lysaught, G. F. A multiple suction electrode system. *Electroencephalography and Clinical Neurophysiology*, 17 (1964) 698-700.

Hawkins, C. F. and Swisher, W. E. Evaluation of a real-time ultrasound scanner in assessing lateral pharyngeal wall motion during speech. *Cleft Palate Journal*, 15 (1978) 161-166.

Helmer, R. J. Modulator and filter circuits for EEG feedback. *Behavior Research Methods and Insrumentation*, 7 (1975) 15-18.

Heltman, H. J. and Peacher, G. M. Misarticulation and diadokokinesis in the spastic paralytic. *Journal of Speech and Hearing Disorders*, 8 (1943) 137-145.

Hillix, W. A., Fry, M. N., and Hershman, R. L. Computer recognition of spoken digits based on six nonacoustic measures. *Journal of the Acoustical Society of America*, 38 (1965) 790-796.

Hirano, M. and Ohala, J. Use of hooked-wire electrodes for electromyography of the intrinsic laryngeal muscles. *Journal of Speech and Hearing Research*, 12 (1969) 362-373.

Hirose, H. Electromyography of the articulatory muscles: Current instrumentation and technique. *Haskins Laboratories Status Report on Speech Research*, SR25/26 (1971) 73-86.

Hirose, H. Electromyography of the larynx and other speech organs. In Sawashima, M. and Cooper, F. S. (Eds.). *Dynamic Aspects of Speech Production*. Tokyo: University of Tokyo Press, 1977. Pp. 49-67.

Hirose, H., Gay, T., Strome, M., and Sawashima, M. Electrode insertion technique for laryngeal electromyography. *Journal of the Acoustical Society of America*, 50 (1971) 1449-1450.

Hiroto, I., Hirano, M., Toyozumi, Y., and Shin, T. Electromyographic investigation of the intrinsic laryngeal muscles related to speech sounds. *Annals of Otology, Rhinology, and Laryngology*, 76 (1967) 861-872.

Hixon, T. J. Magnetometer recording of jaw movements during speech. *Journal of the Acoustical Society of America* 49 (1971a) 104.

Hixon, T. J. An electromagnetic method for transducing jaw movements during speech. *Journal of the Acoustical Society of America*, 49 (1971b) 603-606.

Hixon, T. J. Some new techniques for measuring the biomechanical events of speech production: One laboratory's experiences. In *Orofacial Function: Clinical Research in Dentistry and Speech Pathology (ASHA Reports no. 7)*. Washington, DC: American Speech and Hearing Association, 1972. Pp. 68-103.

Hixon, T. J., Goldman, M. D., and Mead, J. Kinematics of the chest wall during speech production: Volume displacement of the rib cage, abdomen, and lung. *Journal of Speech and Hearing Research*, 16 (1973) 78-115.

Hixon, T. J. and Hardy, J. C. Restricted mobility of the speech articulators in cerebral palsy. *Journal of Speech and Hearing Disorders*, 29 (1964) 293-306.

Hixon, T. J., Mead, J., and Goldman, M. D. Dynamics of the chest wall during speech production: Function of the thorax, rib cage, diaphragm, and abdomen. *Journal of Speech and Hearing Research*, 19 (1976) 297-356.

Hixon, T. J., Siebens, A. A., and Minifie, F. D. An EMG electrode for the diaphragm. *Journal of the Acoustical Society of America* 46 (1969) 1588-1590.

Hollis, L. I. and Harrison, E. An improved surface electrode for monitoring myopotentials. *American Journal of Occupational Therapy,* 24 (1970) 28-30.

Hoyle, G. How is muscle turned on and off? *Scientific American,* April 1970, 84.

Hughes, 0. M. and Abbs, J. H. Labial mandibular coordination in the production of speech: Implications for the operation of motor equivalence. *Phonetica,* 33 (1976) 199-221.

Huntington, D. A., Harris, K. S., and Sholes, G. N. An electromyographic study of consonant articulation in hearing-impaired and normal speakers. *Journal of Speech and Hearing Research,* 11 (1968) 147-158.

Huxley, H. E. The mechanism of muscular contraction. *Scientific American,* January 1965, 18.

Irwin, J. V. and Becklund, 0. Norms for maximum repetitive rates for certain sounds established with the Sylrater. *Journal of Speech and Hearing Disorders,* 18 (1953) 149-160.

Irwin, 0. Correct status of a third set of consonants in the speech of cerebral palsied children. *Cerebral Palsy Review,* 18 (1957) 17-20.

Isshiki, N. and Snidecor, J. C. Air intake and usage in esophageal speech. *Acta Oto-laryngologica,* 59 (1965) 559-573.

Judson, L. S. and Weaver, A. T. *Voice Science* (2nd ed.). New York: Appleton-Century-Crofts, 1965.

Kelsey, C. A., Hixon, T. J. and Minifie, F. D. Ultrasonic measurement of lateral wall displacement. *IEEE Transactions on Bio-Medical Engineering,* BME-16 (1969) 143-147.

Kelsey C. A. Minifie F. D., and Hixon, T. J. Applications of ultrasound in speech research. *Journal of Speech and Hearing Research,* 12 (1969) 546-575.

Kelsey, C. A., Woodhouse, R. J., and Minifie, F. D. Ultrasonic observations of coarticulation in the pharynx. *Journal of the Acoustical Society of America* 46 (1969) 1016-1018.

Kennedy, J. G., III and Abbs. J. H. Anatomic studies of the perioral motor system: Foundations for studies in speech physiology. In Lass, N. J. (Ed.) *Speech and Language: Advances in Basic Research and Practice,* vol. 1. New York: Academic Press, 1979. Pp. 211-270.

Kennedy, J. G. III, and Abbs, J. H. Basic neurophysiological mechanisms underlying oral communication. In Lass, N. J., McReynolds, L. V., Northern, J. L., and Yoder, D. E. (Eds.). *Speech, Language, and hearing,* vol. I: *Normal Processes.* Philadelphia: Saunders, 1982. Pp. 53-83.

Kent, R. D. Some considerations in the cinefluorographic analysis of tongue movement during speech. *Phonetica,* 26 (1972) 16-32.

Kewley-Port, D. EMG signal processing for speech research. *Haskins Laboratories Status Report on Speech Research,* (1977) 123-146.

Khalafalla, A. S. Thoracic impedance measurement of respiration. In Allison, R. D. (Ed.). *Basic Factors in Bioelectric Impedance Measurements of Cardiac Output, Lung Volumes, and the Cerebral Circulation.* Pittsburgh: Instrument Society of America, 1970. Pp. 52-77.

Kiritani, S. Articulatory studies by the X-ray microbeam system. In Sawashima, M. and Cooper, F. S. (Eds.). *Dynamic Aspects of Speech production.* Tokyo: University of Tokyo Press, 1977. Pp. 171-190.

Kiritani, S., Itoh, K., and Fujimura, 0. Tongue-pellet tracking by a computer-controlled x-ray microbeam system. *Journal of the Acoustical Society of America,* 57 (1975) 1516-1520.

Kiritani, S., Kakita, K., and Shibata, S. Dynamic palatography. In Sawashima, M. and Cooper, F. S. (Eds.). *Dynamic Aspects of Speech Production.* Tokyo: University of Tokyo Press, 1977. Pp. 159-168.

Kiritani, S., Tateno, Y., Iinuma, T., and Sawashima, M. Computer tomography of the vocal tract. In Sawashima, M. and Cooper, F. S. (Eds.). *Dynamic Aspects of Speech Production.* Tokyo: University of Tokyo Press, 1977. Pp. 201-206.

Konno, K. and Mead, J. Measurement of the separate volume changes of rib cage and abdomen during breathing. *Journal of Applied Physiology,* 22 (1967) 407-422.

Kozhevnikov, V. A., Granstrem, M. P., Kuzmin, Y. I., Shupliakov, V. S., Vencov, A. V., Borozdin, A. N., Gerasimov, A. A., and Zhukov, S. J. System of devices for articulatory and acoustic study of continuous speech. *Zeitschrift für Phonetik,* 21 (1968) 123-128.

Kreul, E. J. Neuromuscular control examination (NMC) for Parkinsonism: Vowel prolongations and diadochokinetic and reading rates. *Journal of Speech and Hearing Research,* 15 (1972) 72-83.

Kubicek, W. G., Kinnen, E., and Edin, A. Calibration of an impedance pneumograph. *Journal of Applied Physiology,* (1964) 557-560.

Kuehn, D. P., Reich, A. R., and Jordan, J. E. A cineradiographic study of chin marker positioning: Implications for the strain gauge transduction of jaw movement. *Journal of the Acoustical Society of America* 67 (1980) 1825-1827.

Kuzmin, Y. I. Mobile palatography as a tool for acoustic study of speech sounds. *Proceedings of the Fourth International Congress of Acousticas,* 1962. P. G35.

Kydd, W. L. and Belt, D. A. Continuous palatography. *Journal of Speech and Hearing Disorders,* 29 (1964) 489-492.

Ladefoged, P. Use of palatography. *Journal of Speech nd Hearing Disorders*, 22 (1957) 764-774.

Lastovka, M., Sram, F. and Sedlacek, K. Elektromyographie bei funktionelle Dysphonien mit Hilfe der Oberflächenelektrode. *Folia Phoniatrica*, 36 (1984) 284-288.

Leanderson, R., Persson, A., and Öhman, S. Electromyographic studies of facial muscle activity in speech. *Acta Otolaryngologica*, 72 (1971) 361-369.

Lidell, E. G. T. and Sherrington, C. S. Recruitment and some other features of reflex inhibition. *Proceedings of the Royal Society*, 97B (1925) 488-503.

Lippold, 0. C. J. The relation between integrated action potentials in a human muscle and its isometric tension. *Journal of Physiology*, 117 (1952) 492-499.

Lundeen, D. J. The relationship of diadochokinesis to various speech sounds. *Journal of Speech and Hearing Disorders*, 15 (1950) 54-59.

Macmillan, A. S. and Kelemen, G. Radiography of the supraglottic speech organs. *Archives of Otolaryngology*, 55 (1952) 671-685.

MacNeilage, P. F. and Sholes, G. N. An electromyographic study ofthe tongue during vowel production. *Journal of Speech and Hearing Research* 7 (1964) 209-232.

Mansell, R. and Allen, R. A first report on the development of a capacitance transducer for the measurement of lip-excursion. *University of Essex Language Centre Occasional Papers* , 9 (1970) 88-115.

McClean, M. Effects of auditory masking on lip movements for speech. *Journal of Speech and Hearing Research*, 20 (1977) 731-741.

McCutcheon, M. J. Fletcher, S. G., and Hasegawa, A. Video-scanning system for measurement of lip and jaw motion. *Journal of the Acoustical Society of America* 61 (1977) 1051-1055.

McCutcheon, M., Fletcher, S., and Wolf, M. Palatometry and gnathometry in speech (PAGIS). Paper presented at the Annual Convention of the American Speech and Hearing Association, 1975.

Mead, J., Peterson, N., Grimby, G., and Mead, J. Pulmonary ventilation measured from body surface movements. *Science*, 156 (1967) 1383-1384.

Minifie, F. D., Abbs, J. H., Tarlow, A. and Kwaterski, M. EMG activity within the pharynx during speech production. *Journal of Speech and Hearing Research*, 17 (1974) 497-504.

Minifie, F. D., Hixon, T. J. and Williams, F. (Eds.). *Normal Aspects of Speech, Hearing, and Language.* Englewood Cliffs, NJ: Prentice-Hall, 1973.

Minifie, F. D., Kelsey, C. A., Zagzebski, J. A., and King, T. W. Ultrasonic scans of the dorsal surface of the tongue. *Journal of the Acoustical Society of America* 49 (1971) 1857-1860.

Miyawaki, K. A preliminary study of American English /r/ by use of dynamic palatography. *Annual Bulletin of the Research Institute of Logopedics and Phoniatrics*, 6 (1972) 19-24.

Miyawaki, K., Kiritani, S., Tatsumi, I., and Fujimura, O. Palatographic observation of VCV articulations in Japanese. *Annual Bulletin of the Research Institute of Logopedics and Phoniatrics*, 8 (974) 51-58

Moll, K. L. Cinefluorographic techniques in speech research. *Journal of Speech and Hearing Research*, 3 (1960) 227-241.

Moll, K. L. Photographic and radiographic procedures in speech research. *Proceedings of the Conference: Communicative Problems in Cleft Palate (ASHA Reports, no. 1).* Washington, DC: ASHA, 1965. Pp. 129-139.

Morrish, K. A., Stone, M., Sonies, B. C., Kurtz, D., and Shawker, T. Characterization of tongue shape. *Ultrasonic Imaging*, 6 (1984) 37-47.

Moses, E. R. jr. Palatography and speech improvement. *Journal of Speech Disorders*, 4 (1939) 103-114.

Moses, E. R. Jr. A brief history of palatography. *Quarterly Journal of Speech*, 26 (1940)

Moses, E. R. Jr. *Phonetics: History and Interpretation.* Englewood Cliffs, NJ: Prentice-Hall, 1964.

Muller, E. M. and Abbs, J. H. Strain gauge transduction of lip and jaw motion in the midsagittal plane: Refinement of a prototype system. *Journal of the Acoustical Society of America* 65 (1979) 481-486.

Netsell, R. and Cleeland, C. S. Modification of lip hypertonia in dysarthria using EMG feedback. *Journal of Speech and Hearing Disorders* 38 (1973) 131-140.

Netsell, R., Daniel, B., and Celesia, G. G. Acceleration and weakness in parkinsonian dysarthria. *Journal of Speech and Hearing Disorders*, 40 (1975) 170-178.

O'Dwyer, N. J., Neilson, P. D., Guitar, B. E., Quinn, P. T., and Andrews, G. Control of upper airway structures during nonspeech tasks in normal and cerebral-palsied subjects: EMG findings. *Journal of Speech and Hearing Research*, 26 (1983) 162-170.

O'Dwyer, N. J., Quinn, P. T., Guitar, B. E., Andrews, G. and Neilson, P. D. Procedures for verification of electrode placement in EMG studies of orofacial and mandibular muscles. *Journal of Speech and Hearing Research*, 24 (1981) 273-288.

Pacela, A. F. Impedance pneumography—A survey of instrumental techniques. *Medical and*

Biological Engineering 4 (1966) 1-15.

Palmer, J. M. Dynamic palatography—General implications of locus and sequencing patterns. Phonetica, 28 (1973) 76-85.

Perkell, J. S. Physiology of Speech Production: Results and Implications of a Quantitative Cineradiographic Study. Cambridge, MA: MIT Press, 1969.

Perkell, J. S. and Oka, D. Use of an alternating magnetic field device to track midsagittal plane movements of multiple points inside the vocal tract. Journal of the Acoustical Society of America, 67 (1980) S92.

Port, D. K. The EMG data system. Haskins Laboratories Status Report on Speech Research, SR 25/26 (1971) 67-72.

Porter, K. R. and Franzini-Armstrong, C. The sarcoplasmic reticulum. Scientific American, January 1965, 72.

Ptacek, P. H., Sander, E. K., Maloney, W. H., and Jackson, C. C. R. Phonatory and related changes with advanced age. Journal of Speech and Hearing Research, 9 (1966) 353-360.

Pykett, I. L. N[uclear] m[agnetic] r[esonance] imaging in medicine. Scientific American, May 1982, 78.

Rea, J. L., Templer, J. W., and Davis. W. E. Design and testing of a new electrode for laryngeal electromyography. Archives of Otolaryngology, 104 (1978) 685-686.

Robb, M. P., Hughes, M. C., and Frese, D. J. Oral diadochokinesis in hearing-impaired adolescents. Journal of Communication Disorders, 18 (1985) 79-89.

Rolfe, P. A magnetometer respiration monitor for use with premature babies. Bio-Medical Engineering, 6 (1971) 402-404.

Rome, J. A. An artificial palate for continuous analysis of speech. Quarterly Progress Report, Research Laboratory of Electronics (MIT), 74 (1964), 190-191.

Rousselot, P. J. Principes de phonétique expérimentale, vol. 1. Paris: Welter, 1897-1901.

Sackner, M. A. Monitoring of ventilation without a physical connection to the airway. In Sackner, M. A. (Ed.). Diagnostic Techniques in Pulmonary Disease, Part I. New York: Marcel Dekker, 1980. Pp. 503-537.

Sackner, J. D., Nixon, A. J., Davis, B., Atkins, N., and Sackner, M. A. Non-invasive measurement of ventilation during exercise using a respiratory inductive plethysmograph. American Review of Respiratory Disease, 122 (1980) 867-871.

Sawashima, M., Sato, M., Funasaka, S., and Totsuka, G. Electromyographic study of the human larynx and its clinical application. Japanese Journal of Otology, 61 (1958) 1357-1364.

Schuette, W. H., Shawker, T. H., and Whitehouse, W. C. An integrated television and real-time ultrasonic imaging system. Journal of

Clinical Ultrasound, 6 (1978) 271-272.

Scripture, E. W. The Elements of Experimental Phonetics. New York: Scribner's, 1902.

Shanks, S. J. Effect of aging upon rapid syllable repetition. Perceptual and Motor Skills, 30 (1970) 687-690.

Shawker, T. H., and Sonies, B. C. Tongue movement during speech: A real-time ultrasound evaluation. Journal of Clinical Ultrasound, 12 (1984) 125-133.

Shawker, T. H., Sonies, B., Hall, T. E., and Baum, B. F. Ultrasound analysis of tongue, hyoid, and larynx activity during swallowing. Investigative Radiology, 19 (1984) 82-86.

Shawker, T. H., Sonies, B. C., and Stone, M. Soft-tissue anatomy of the tongue and floor of the mouth: An ultrasound demonstration. Brain and Language, 21 (1984) 355-350.

Shawker, T. H., Sonies, B. C., Stone, M., and Baum, B. Real-time ultrasound visualization of tongue movement during swallowing. Journal of Clinical Ultrasound 11 (1983) 485-490.

Shelton, R. L. Jr., Brooks, A. R., Youngstrom, K. A., Diedrich, W. M., and Brooks, R. S. Filming speed in cinefluorographic speech study. Journal of Speech and Hearing Research, (1963) 19-26.

Shipp, T., Deatsch, W. W., and Robertson, K. A technique for electromyographic assessment of deep neck muscle activity. Laryngoscope, 78 (1968) 418-432.

Shipp, T., Fishman, B. V., Morrissey, P., and McGlone, R. E. Method and control of laryngeal emg electrode placement in man. Journal of the Acoustical Society of America, 48 (1970) 429-430.

Shohara, H. H. and Hanson, C. Palatography as an aid to the improvement of articulatory movements. Journal of Speech Disorders, 6 (1941) 115-124.

Skolnick, M. L., Zagzebski, J. A., and Watkin, K. L. Two dimensional ultrasonic demonstration of lateral pharyngeal wall movement in real time—a preliminary report. Cleft Palate Journal, 12 (1975) 299-303.

Smith, C. Action potentials from single motor units in voluntary contraction. American Journal of Physiology, 108 (1934) 629-638.

Snidecor, J. C. and Isshiki, N. Air volume and air flow relationships of six male esophageal speakers. Journal of Speech and Hearing Disorders, 30 (1965) 205-216.

Sonies, B. C. Oral imaging systems: A review and clinical applications. Journal of the National Student Speech Language Hearing Association, 10 (1982) 30-43.

Sonies, B. C., Baum, B. J., and Shawker, T. H. Tongue motion in the elderly: Initial in situ observations. Journal of Gerontology, 39 (1984) 279-283.

Sonies, B. C., Shawker, T. H., Hall, T. E., Gerber,

L. H., and Leighton, S. B. Ultrasonic visualization of tongue motion during speech. *Journal of the Acoustical Society of America,* 70 (1981) 683-686.

Sonies, B. C., Stone, M., and Shawker, T. Speech and swallowing in the elderly. *Journal of Gerontology,* in press.

Sonoda, Y. and Wanishi, S. New optical method for recording lip and jaw movements. *Journal of the Acoustical Society of America* 72 (1982) 700-704.

Stemple, J. C., Weiler, E., Whitehead, W. and Komray, R. Electromyographic biofeedback training with patients exhibiting a hyperfunctional voice disorder. *Laryngoscope,* 90 (1980) 471-476.

Stetson, R. H. Motor phonetics. *Archive Néerlandaise de Phonétique Expérimentale,* 3 (1928) 1-216.

Stetson, R. H. *Motor Phonetics.* Amsterdam: North-Holland, 1951.

Stone, M., Sonies, B. C., Shawker, T. H., Weiss, G., and Nadel, L. Analysis of real-time ultrasound images of tongue configuration using a grid-digitizing system. *Journal of Phonetics,* 11 (1983) 207.218.

Strother, C. R. and Kriegman, L. S. Diadochokinesis in stutterers and non-stutterers. *Journal of Speech Disorders,* 8 (1943) 323-335.

Sussman, H. M., MacNeilage, P. F., and Hanson, R. J. Labial and mandibular dynamics during the production of labial consonants: Preliminary observations. *Journal of Speech and Hearing Research,* 16 (1973) 397-420.

Sussman, H. M., MacNeilage, P. F., and Powers, R. K. Recruitment and discharge patterns of single motor units during speech production. *Journal of Speech and Hearing Research,* 20 (1977) 616-630.

Sussman, H. M. and Smith, K. U. Transducer for measuring mandibular movements. *Journal of the Acoustical Society of America,* 48 (1970a) 857-858.

Sussman, H. M. and Smith, K. U. Transducer for measuring lip movements during speech. *Journal of the Acoustical Society of America* 48 (1970b) 858-860.

Sussman, H. M. and Smith, K. U. Jaw movements under delayed auditory feedback. *Journal of the Acoustical Society of America,* 50 (1971) 685-691.

Tatsumi, I. F. Some computer techniques for dynamic palatography. *Annual Bulletin of the Research Institute of Logopedics and Phoniatrics,* 6 (1972) 15-18.

Tingley, B. M. and Allen, G. D. Development of speech timing control in children. *Child Development,* 46 (1975) 186-194.

Umegaki, Y., Tateno, Y., and Iinuma, T Low dose noninvasive X-ray techniques. In Sawashima, M. and Cooper, F. S. (Eds.). *Dynamic Aspects of Speech Production.* Tokyo: University of Tokyo Press 1977. Pp. 195-200.

van der Giet, G. Computer.controlled method for measuring articulatory activities. *Journal of the Acoustical Society of America,* 61 (1977) 1072-1076.

Watkin, K. L. and Zagzebski, J. A. On-line ultrasonic technique for monitoring tongue displacements. *Journal of the Acoustical Society of America,* 54 (1973) 544-547.

Watson, H. The technology of respiratory inductive plethysmography. *Proceedings of the Third International Symposium on Ambulatory Monitoring,* 1979.

Weddell, G., Feinstein, B., and Pattle, R. E. The electrical activity of voluntary muscle in man under normal and pathological conditions. *Brain,* 67 (1944) 178-257.

Westlake, H. Muscle training for cerebral palsied speech cases. *Journal of Speech and Hearing Disorders,* 16 (1951) 103-109.

Westlake, H. *A System for Developing Speech with Cerebral Palsied Children.* Chicago: National Society for Crippled Children and Adults, 1952.

Whitney, R. J. The measurement of changes in human limb-volume by means of a mercury-in-rubber strain gage. *Journal of Physiology,* 109 (1949) 5P-6P.

Wilder, C. N. and Baken, R. J. Respiratory patterns in infant cry. *Human Communication,* 3 (1974) 18-34.

Witting, C. New techniques of palatography. *Studia Linguistica,* 7 (1953) 54-68.

Wyke, B. (Ed.). *Ventilatory and Phonatory Control Systems.* York: Oxford, 1974.

Yoss, K. A. and Darley, F. L. Developmental apraxia of speech in children with defective articulation. *Journal of Speech and Hearing Research,* 17 (1974) 399-416.

Yoss, K. A. and Darley, F. L. Developmental apraxia of speech in children with defective articulation. *Journal of Speech and Hearing Research,* 17 (1974) 399-416.

Zemlin, W. R. *Speech and Hearing Science: Anatomy and Physiology.* Englewood Cliffs, NJ: Prentice-Hall, 1981.

Zenker, W. and Zenker, A. Über die Regelung der Stimmlippenspannung durch von aussen eingreifende Mechanismen. *Folia Phoniatrica,* 12 (1960) 1-36.

Appendices

APPENDIX A: CONVERSION TABLES

Using the Table: Multiply units given in the left column by the factor shown in the center to obtain the equivalent value in units given in the right column.

Multiply:	PRESSURE by:	To get:
microbars (μb) or dynes per square centimeter (d/cm^2)	1.0197×10^{-2}	millimeter of water (mm H$_2$O)
	7.5006×10^{-4}	millimeters of mercury (mm Hg)
	9.8692×10^{-7}	atmospheres (atm)
	4.0147×10^{-4}	inches of water (in H$_2$O)
	3.3456×10^{-5}	feet of water (ft H$_2$O)
	2.9530×10^{-5}	inches of mercury (in Hg)
millimeters of water (mm H$_2$O)	98.0637	microbars (μb)
	7.3554×10^{-2}	millimeters of mercury (mm Hg)
	9.6781×10^{-5}	atmospheres (atm)
	3.9370×10^{-2}	inches of water (in H$_2$O)
	3.2808×10^{-3}	feet of water (ft H$_2$O)
	2.8958×10^{-3}	inches of mercury (in Hg)
millimeters of mercury (mm Hg)	1.3332×10^{-3}	microbars (μb)
	13.5955	millimeters of water (mm H$_2$O)
	1.3158	atmospheres (atm)
	0.5352	inches of water (in H$_2$O)
	4.4605×10^{-2}	feet of water (ft H$_2$O)
	3.9369×10^{-2}	inches of mercury (in Hg)
atmospheres (atm)	1.0132×10^{6}	microbars (μb)
	1.0333×10^{4}	millimeters of water (mm H$_2$O)
	760.	millimeters of mercury (mm Hg)
	4.0679×10^{2}	inches of water (in H$_2$O)
	33.8995	feet of water (ft H$_2$O)
	29.9212	inches of mercury (in Hg)
inches of water (in H$_2$O)	2.4908×10^{3}	millimeters of water (mm H$_2$O)
	1.8683	millimeters of mercury (mm Hg)
	2.4582×10^{-3}	atmospheres (atm)
	8.3333×10^{-2}	feet of water (ft H$_2$O)
	7.3554×10^{-2}	inches of mercury (in Hg)
feet of water (ft H$_2$O)	2.9889×10^{4}	microbars (μb)
	3.0480×10^{2}	millimeters of water (mm H$_2$O)
	22.4192	millimeters of mercury (mm Hg)
	2.9499×10^{-2}	atmospheres (atm)
	.8826	inches of mercury (in Hg)
inches of mercury (in Hg)	3.3864×10^{4}	microbars (μb)
	3.4533×10^{2}	millimeters of water (mm H$_2$O)
	25.4000	millimeters of mercury (mm Hg)
	3.3421×10^{-2}	atmospheres (atm)
	13.5955	inches of water (in H$_2$O)
	1.1329	feet of water (ft H$_2$O)

MASS or WEIGHT

Multiply:	by:	To get:
grams (g)	3.5274×10^{-2}	ounces (oz)
	2.2046×10^{-3}	pounds (lb)
kilograms (kg)	2.2046	pounds (lb)
	35.2739	ounces (oz)
ounces (oz)	38.3495	grams (g)
	2.8349×10^{-2}	kilograms (kg)
	6.25×10^{-2}	pounds (lb)
pounds (lb)	4.5359×10^{2}	grams (g)
	0.4535	kilograms (kg)

LENGTH

Multiply:	by:	To get:
meters (m)	1×10^{3}	millimeters (mm)
	1×10^{2}	centimeters (cm)
	39.3700	inches (in)
	3.2808	feet (ft)
	1.0936	yards (yd)
millimeters (mm)	1×10^{-3}	meters (m)
	1×10^{-1}	centimeters (cm)
	3.937×10^{-2}	inches (in)
	3.2808×10^{-3}	feet (ft)
	1.0936×10^{-3}	yards (yd)
inches (in)	25.4000	millimeters (mm)
	2.5400	centimeters (cm)
	2.5400×10^{-2}	meters (m)
	8.3333×10^{-2}	feet (ft)
	2.7777×10^{-2}	yards (yd)
yards (yd)	9.1440×10^{2}	millimeters (mm)
	91.440	centimeters (cm)
	0.9144	meters (m)

AREA

Multiply:	by:	To get:
square inches (in^2)	6.4516×10^{2}	square millimeters (mm^2)
	6.4516	square centimeters (cm^2)
	6.4516×10^{-4}	square meters (m^2)
square millimeters (mm^2)	1.5499×10^{-3}	square inches (in^2)
	1×10^{-2}	square centimeters (cm^2)
	1×10^{-6}	square meters (m^2)
square centimeters (cm^2)	0.1549	square inches (in^2)
	1×10^{2}	square millimeters (mm^2)
	1×10^{-4}	square meters (m^2)
square meters (m^2)	1.5499×10^{3}	square inches (in^2)
	1×10^{6}	square millimeters (mm^2)
	1×10^{4}	square centimeters (cm^2)

VOLUME

Multiply:	by:	To get:
millimeters (mL)	6.1025×10^{-2}	cubic inches (in^3)
	1.0567×10^{-3}	U.S. quarts (qt)
liters (L)	61.0251	cubic inches (in^3)
	1.0567	U.S. quarts (qt)
U.S. quarts (qt)	0.9463	liters (L)
	946.231	milliliters (mL)
	57.75	cubic inches (in^3)
cubic inches (in^3)	1.6387×10^{-2}	liters (L)
	16.387	milliliters (mL)
	1.7316×10^{-2}	U.S. quarts (qt)

ANGLES

radians (rad)	5.7296	degrees (°)
degrees (°)	1.7453×10^{-2}	radians (rad)

TEMPERATURES

°Kelvin (absolute) (°K)
$= °C + 273.15$
$= 0.5555 (°F) + 255.3722$

°Fahrenheit (°F)
$= 1.8 (°K) - 459.67$
$= 1.8 (°C) + 32$

°Centigrade (°C)
$= °K - 273.15$
$= 0.5555 (°F) - 17.7777$

APPENDIX B: NORMAL ARTICULATORY MATURATION

Earliest Age (years-months) at which 75% of Children Correctly Produced Each Sound in Initial, Medial, and Final Positions

Sound	Boys	Girls	Combined
all plosives	3-0	3-0	3-0
m	3-0	3-0	3-0
n	3-0	3-0	3-0
g	3-0	3-0	3-0
h	3-0	3-0	3-0
f	3-0	3-0	3-0
v	3-0	3-6	3-6
θ	*	*	5-0
d	*	5-0	5-0
s	4-0	3-0	4-0
z	*	3-0	4-0
(sh)	3-6	4-0	4-6
(zh)	4-0	4-0	4-0
(ch)	3-6	4-0	4-0
(dj)	3-6	4-0	4-0
l	4-6	4-0	4-0
r	5-0	5-0	5-0
w	3-0	3-0	3-0

From Arlt, P. B. and Goodban, M. T. A comparative study of articulation acquisition as based on a study of 240 normals, aged three to six. *Language, Speech, and Hearing Services in Schools*, 7 (1976) 173-180. Table 1, p. 177. © American Speech-Language-Hearing Association, Rockville, MD. Reprinted by permission.

*Not produced correctly by 75% at oldest age tested.

All vowels were correctly produced by age 3-0.

Children of normal IQ and varied SES. Half-year age levels from 3-0 to 5-6, 20 boys and 20 girls per group (total = 240 Ss.).

APPENDIX C: THE RAINBOW PASSAGE*

	Cumulative Word Count
When the sunlight strikes raindrops in the air, they act	10
like a prism and form a rainbow. The rainbow is	20
a division of white light into many beautiful colors. These	30
take the shape of a long round arch, with its	40
path high above, and its two ends apparently beyond the	50
horizon. There is, according to legend, a boiling pot of	60
gold at one end. People look, but no one ever	70
finds it. When a man looks for something beyond his	80
reach, his friends say he is looking for the pot	90
of gold at the end of the rainbow.	98
Throughout the centuries men have explained the rainbow in various	108
ways. Some have accepted it as a miracle without physical	118
explanation. To the Hebrews it was a token that there	128
would be no more universal floods. The Greeks used to	138
imagine that it was a sign from the gods to	148
foretell war or heavy rain. The Norsemen considered the rainbow	158
as a bridge over which the gods passed from earth	168
to their home in the sky. Other men have tried	178
to explain the phenomenon physically. Aristotle thought that the rainbow	188
was caused by reflection of the sun's rays by the	198
rain. Since then physicists have found that it is not	208
reflection, but refraction by the raindrops which causes the rainbow.	218
Many complicated ideas about the rainbow have been formed. The	228
difference in the rainbow depends considerably upon the size of	238
the water drops, and the width of the colored band	248
increases as the size of the drops increases. The actual	258
primary rainbow observed is said to be the effect of	268
superposition of a number of bows. If the red of	278
the second bow falls upon the green of the first,	288
the result is to give a bow with an abnormally	298
wide yellow band, since red and green lights when mixed	308
form yellow. This is a very common type of bow,	318
one showing mainly red and yellow, with little or no	328
green or blue.	331

*From Fairbanks, G. *Voice and Articulation Drillbook* (second ed.). New York: Harper and Bros., 1960. P. 127.

Phonemic Analysis of the First Three Sentences
(as spoken by a "General American" speaker)

	Number	Percent
Total words		51
Total syllables		66
Total phonemes		177
Front vowels	21	11.8
Back vowels	7	3.9
Central vowels	24	13.6
Diphthongs	16	9.0
Total words and diphthongs	68	38.3
Voiced consonants and combinations	71	40.1
Voiceless consonants and combinations	38	21.4
Total consonants and combinations	109	61.5
Total voiced elements:		
Vowels		29.3
Diphthongs		9.0
Consonants		40.1
		78.4
Total voiceless elements		21.4

From Curry, E. T., Snidecor, J. C., and Isshiki, N. Fundamental frequency characteristics of Japanese Asai speakers. *Laryngoscope*, 38 (1973) 1759-1763. Table I, p. 1761. Reprinted by permission.

APPENDIX D:
FUNDAMENTAL FREQUENCIES OF THE MUSICAL (12-interval chromatic) SCALE (A = 440 Hz)

NOTE			OCTAVE							
			c^{-3}	c^{-2}	c^{-1}	c^{0}	c^{1}	c^{2}	c^{3}	c^{4}
	C		16.35	32.70	65.41	130.81	261.63	523.25	1046.50	2093.00
C#		D_b	17.32	34.65	69.30	138.59	277.18	554.37	1108.73	2217.46
	D		18.35	36.71	73.42	146.83	293.66	587.33	1174.66	2349.32
D#		E_b	19.45	38.89	77.78	155.56	311.13	622.25	1244.51	2489.02
	E		20.60	41.20	82.41	164.81	329.63	659.26	1318.51	2637.02
	F		21.83	43.65	87.31	174.61	349.23	689.46	1396.91	2793.83
F#		G_b	23.12	46.25	92.50	185.00	369.99	739.99	1479.98	2959.96
G#		A_b	25.96	51.91	103.83	207.65	415.30	830.61	1661.22	3322.44
	A		27.50	55.00	110.00	220.00	440.00	880.00	1760.00	3520.00
A#		B_b	29.14	58.27	116.54	233.08	466.16	932.33	1864.66	3729.31
	B		30.87	61.74	123.47	246.96	493.88	987.77	1975.53	3951.07

Multiple		Power of 10	Prefix	Symbol
1,000,000,000,000	trillion	10^{12}	tera	T
1,000,000,000	billion	10^{9}	giga	G
1,000,000	million	10^{6}	mega	M
1,000	thousand	10^{6}	kilo	K
100	hundred	10^{2}	hecto	h
10	ten	10^{1}	deka	dk*
0.1	tenth	10^{-1}	deci	d
0.01	hundreth	10^{-2}	centi	c
0.001	thousandth	10^{-3}	milli	m
0.000001	millionth	10^{-6}	micro	μ
0.000000001	billionth	10^{-9}	nano	n
0.000000000001	trillionth	10^{-12}	pico	p

EXAMPLES

20/1000 of a liter (L) = 20 milliliters (mL),
2 centiliters (cL) or .2 deciliters (dL)
6000 grams (g) = 6 kilograms (Kg), 60 hectograms (hg), or 600 dekagrams (dkg)

*da is also used.

APPENDIX F:
PLAYING TIME OF RECORDING TAPE*

Tape Length (ft)	Tape Speed (inches/sec)			
	15	7.5	3.25	1.875
4800	1h 4m	2h 8m	4h 16m	8h 32m
3600	0h 48m	1h 36m	3h 12m	6h 24m
2400	0h 32m	1h 4m	2h 8m	4h 16m
1800	0h 24m	0h 48m	1h 36m	3h 12m
1200	0h 16m	0h 32m	1h 4m	2h 8m
600	0h 8m	0h 16m	0h 32m	1h 4m
300	0h 4m	0h 8m	0h 16m	0h 32m

Note: Time shown is for a single direction. If tape is recorded on both sides, time available is double the tabled value.

*In hours and minutes.

APPENDIX G:
DECIBEL EQUIVALENTS OF PRESSURE AND POWER RATIOS

Pressure ratio	Power ratio	dB*	Pressure ratio	Power ratio	dB*
0.10000	0.0100	− 20.0	0.1178	0.0316	− 15.0
0.1023	0.0105	− 19.8	0.1820	0.0331	− 14.8
0.1047	0.0110	− 19.6	0.1862	0.0347	− 14.6
0.1072	0.0115	− 19.4	0.1905	0.0363	− 14.4
0.1096	0.0120	− 19.2	0.1950	0.0380	− 14.0
0.1122	0.0126	− 19.0	0.1995	0.0398	− 14.0
0.1148	0.0132	− 18.8	0.2042	0.0417	− 13.8
0.1175	0.0138	− 18.6	0.2089	0.0437	− 13.6
0.1202	0.0145	− 18.4	0.2138	0.0457	− 13.4
0.1234	0.0151	− 18.2	0.2188	0.0479	− 13.2
0.1259	0.0158	− 18.0	0.2239	0.0501	− 13.0
0.1288	0.0166	− 17.8	0.2291	0.0525	− 12.8
0.1318	0.0174	− 17.6	0.2344	0.0550	− 12.6
0.1349	0.0182	− 17.4	0.2399	0.0575	− 12.4
0.1380	0.0191	− 17.2	0.2455	0.0603	− 12.2
0.1416	0.0200	− 17.0	0.2512	0.0631	− 12.0
0.1445	0.0209	− 16.8	0.2570	0.0661	− 11.8
0.1479	0.0219	− 16.6	0.2630	0.0692	− 11.6
0.1514	0.0229	− 16.4	0.2692	0.0724	− 11.4
0.1549	0.0240	− 16.2	0.2754	0.0759	− 11.2
0.1585	0.0251	− 16.0	0.2818	0.0794	− 11.0
0.1622	0.0263	− 15.8	0.2884	0.0832	− 10.8
0.1660	0.0275	− 15.6	0.2951	0.0871	− 10.6
0.1698	0.0288	− 15.4	0.3020	0.0912	− 10.4
0.1738	0.0302	− 15.2	0.3090	0.0955	− 10.2
0.3162	0.1000	− 10.0	0.5623	0.3162	− 5.0
0.3236	0.1047	− 9.8	0.5754	0.3311	− 4.8
0.3311	0.1096	− 9.6	0.5888	0.3467	− 4.6
0.3388	0.1147	− 9.4	0.6026	0.3631	− 4.4
0.3467	0.1202	− 9.2	0.6166	0.3802	− 4.2
0.3548	0.1259	− 9.0	0.6310	0.3981	− 4.0
0.3631	0.1318	− 8.0	0.6457	0.4169	− 3.8
0.3715	0.1380	− 8.6	0.6607	0.4365	− 3.6
0.3802	0.1445	− 8.4	0.6761	0.4571	− 3.4
0.3890	0.1514	− 8.2	0.6918	0.4786	− 3.2
0.3981	0.1585	− 8.0	0.7079	0.5012	− 3.0
0.4074	0.1660	− 7.8	0.7244	0.5248	− 2.8
0.4169	0.1738	− 7.6	0.7413	0.5495	− 2.6
0.4266	0.1820	− 7.4	0.7586	0.5754	− 2.4
0.4365	0.1905	− 7.2	0.7762	0.6026	− 2.2
0.4467	0.1995	− 7.0	0.7943	0.6310	− 2.0
0.4571	0.2089	− 6.8	0.8128	0.6607	− 1.8
0.4677	0.2188	− 6.6	0.8318	0.6918	− 1.6
0.4786	0.2291	− 6.4	0.8511	0.7244	− 1.4
0.4898	0.2399	− 6.2	0.8710	0.7586	− 1.2
0.5012	0.2512	− 6.0	0.8913	0.7943	− 1.0
0.5129	0.2630	− 5.8	0.9120	0.8318	− 0.8

Pressure ratio	Power ratio	dB*	Pressure ratio	Power ratio	dB*
0.5248	0.2754	− 5.6	0.9333	0.8710	− 0.6
0.5370	0.2884	− 5.4	0.9550	0.9120	− 0.4
0.5495	0.3020	− 5.2	0.9772	0.9550	− 0.2
			1.000	1.000	0.0
1.000	1.000	0.0	1.7783	3.1623	5.0
1.0233	1.0471	0.2	1.8197	3.3113	5.2
1.0471	1.0965	0.4	1.8621	3.4674	5.4
1.0715	1.1483	0.6	1.9055	3.6308	5.6
1.0965	1.2023	0.8	1.9498	3.8019	5.8
1.1220	1.2589	1.0	1.9953	3.9811	6.0
1.1482	1.3183	1.2	2.0417	4.1687	6.2
1.1749	1.3804	1.4	2.0893	4.3652	6.4
1.2023	1.4454	1.6	2.1380	4.5709	6.6
1.2303	1.5136	1.8	2.1878	4.7863	6.8
1.2589	1.5849	2.0	2.2387	5.0119	7.0
1.2883	1.6596	2.2	2.2909	5.2481	7.2
1.3183	1.7378	2.4	2.3442	5.5954	7.4
1.3490	1.8197	2.6	2.3988	5.7544	7.6
1.3804	1.9055	2.8	2.4547	6.0256	7.8
1.4125	1.9953	3.0	2.5119	6.3096	8.0
1.4454	2.0893	3.2	2.5704	6.6070	8.2
1.4792	2.1878	3.4	2.6303	6.9183	8.4
1.5136	2.2909	3.6	2.6915	6.2444	8.6
1.5488	2.3988	3.8	2.7542	7.5858	8.8
1.5849	2.5119	4.0	2.8184	7.9433	9.0
1.6218	2.6303	4.2	2.8840	8.3177	9.2
1.6596	2.7542	4.4	2.9512	8.7097	9.4
1.6982	2.8840	4.6	3.0200	9.1202	9.6
1.7378	3.0200	4.8	3.0903	9.5500	9.8
3.1623	10.0000	10.0	5.6234	31.6230	15.0
3.3259	10.4713	10.2	5.7544	33.1134	15.2
3.3113	10.9648	10.4	5.8885	34.6740	15.4
3.3885	11.4816	10.6	6.0256	36.3081	15.6
3.4674	12.0227	10.8	6.1660	38.0192	15.8
3.5481	12.5893	11.0	6.3096	39.8110	16.0
3.6308	13.1826	11.2	6.4566	41.6873	16.2
3.7154	13.8039	11.4	6.6070	43.6519	16.4
3.8019	14.4545	11.6	6.7609	45.7092	16.6
3.8905	15.1357	11.8	6.9183	47.8634	16.8
3.9811	15.8490	12.0	7.0795	50.1192	17.0
4.0738	16.5960	12.2	7.2444	52.4812	17.2
4.1687	17.3781	12.4	7.4131	54.9546	17.4
4.2658	18.1971	12.6	7.5858	57.5445	17.6
4.3652	19.0547	12.8	7.7625	60.2565	17.8
4.4669	19.9528	13.0	7.9433	63.0963	18.0

APPENDIX G (continued)

Pressure ratio	Power ratio	dB*	Pressure ratio	Power ratio	dB*
4.5709	20.8731	13.2	8.1283	66.0700	18.2
4.6774	21.8778	13.4	8.3177	69.1837	18.4
4.7863	22.9988	13.6	8.5114	72.4443	18.6
4.8978	23.9833	13.8	8.7097	75.8585	18.8
5.0119	25.1190	14.0	8.9126	79.4336	19.0
5.1286	26.3029	14.2	9.1202	83.1772	19.2
5.2481	27.5425	14.4	9.3326	87.0972	19.4
5.3703	28.8405	14.6	9.5500	91.2020	19.6
5.4954	30.1997	14.8	9.7724	95.5002	19.8
			10.0000	100.0000	20.0

APPENDIX H:
COMMON ELECTRONIC SYMBOLS

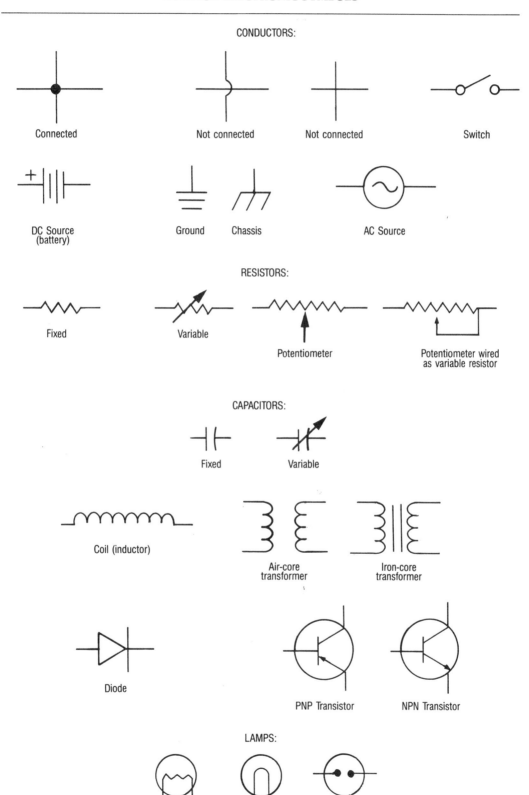

CONDUCTORS:

Connected

Not connected

Not connected

Switch

DC Source
(battery)

Ground

Chassis

AC Source

RESISTORS:

Fixed

Variable

Potentiometer

Potentiometer wired
as variable resistor

CAPACITORS:

Fixed

Variable

Coil (inductor)

Air-core
transformer

Iron-core
transformer

Diode

PNP Transistor

NPN Transistor

LAMPS:

(neon)

Author Index

Subject Index